Nutrition, Food, and Fitness

The Science of Wellness

Dorothy F. West, Ph.D.

*Chairperson, Department
of Social Sciences
Lithuania Christian College
Klaipeda, Lithuania*

Publisher
The Goodheart-Willcox Company, Inc.
Tinley Park, Illinois

Acknowledgments

The author and publisher are grateful to the following professionals who provided valuable input:

Contributing Author

Martha Dunn-Strohecker, Ph. D., CFCS
Author of Family and Consumer Sciences
    Textbooks and Management Consultant
Boston, Massachusetts

Reviewers

Carol Byrd-Bredbenner, Ph.D., R.D., F.A.D.A.
Extension Specialist and Professor of Nutrition
Rutgers, the State University of New Jersey
New Brunswick, New Jersey

Molly Kiefer, M.S.
Family and Consumer Sciences Teacher
Cary Grove High School
Cary, Illinois

LuAnn Soliah, Ph.D., R.D.
Associate Professor and Director of Dietetics
Baylor University
Waco, Texas

Introduction

Nutrition, Food, and Fitness: The Science of Wellness is a text that stresses the crucial role eating a nutritious diet plays in overall health. It also highlights the importance of making physical activity part of your daily routine. As you read this text, you will learn how your decisions affect your state of wellness. You will realize the need to adopt healthful eating and activity patterns as permanent lifestyle habits. You will also study how caring for your mental and social health is part of total wellness.

You will learn about nutrition science as you study the sources and functions of nutrients. You will read about weight management, eating disorders, food safety, and global hunger. You will study physical fitness, stress management, and substance abuse. You will also learn about consumer issues, trends, and careers. This information should help you make lifestyle choices for wellness.

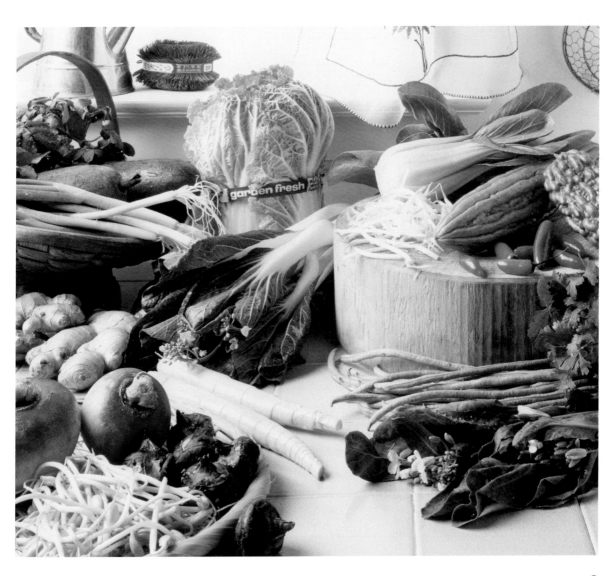

Contents

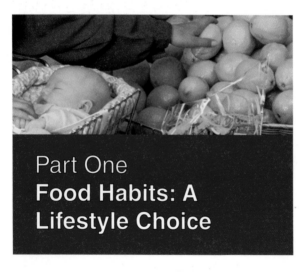

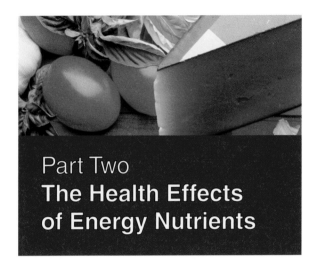

Part Two
The Health Effects of Energy Nutrients

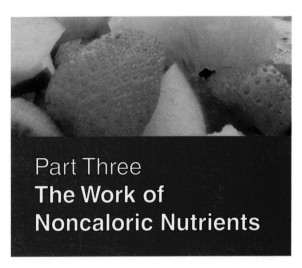

Part Three
The Work of Noncaloric Nutrients

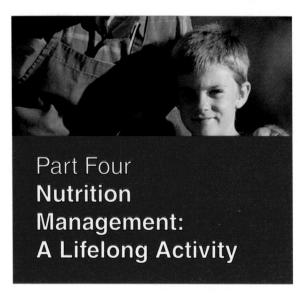

Part Four
Nutrition Management: A Lifelong Activity

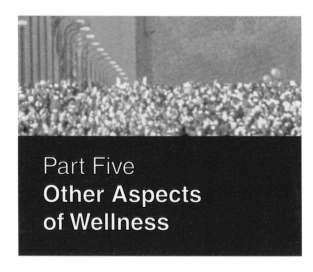

Part Five
Other Aspects of Wellness

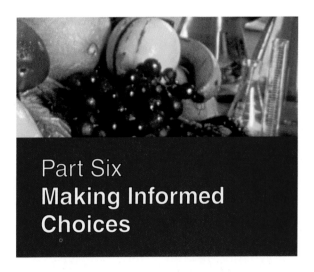

Part Six
Making Informed Choices

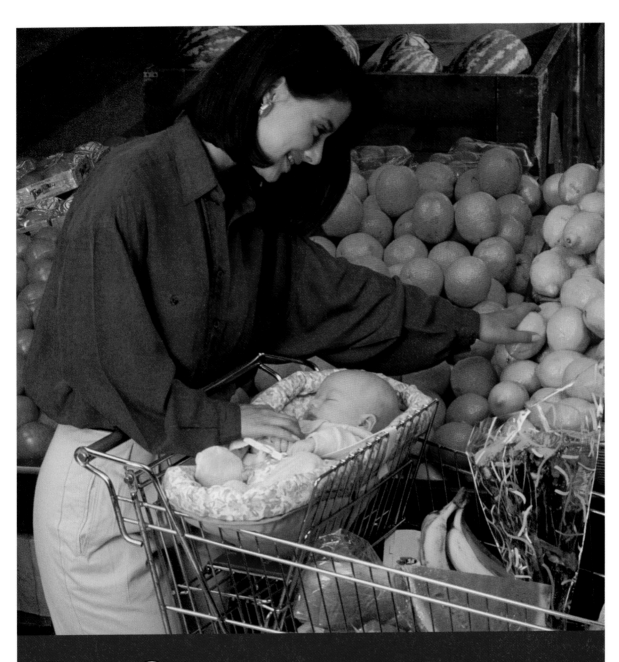

Part One
Food Habits:
A Lifestyle Choice

Chapter 1

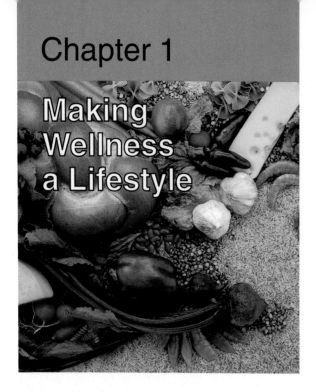

Making Wellness a Lifestyle

● Learn the Language

wellness
quality of life
premature death
optimum health
physical health
mental health
social health
holistic medicine
risk factor
environmental
  quality

diagnosis
diet
peer pressure
nutrition
nutrient
scientific method
hypothesis
theory
life expectancy

● Objectives

After studying this chapter, you will be able to
* explain the physical, mental, and social aspects of wellness.
* list factors that contribute to disease.
* predict how lifestyle choices you make will affect your health.
* describe the relationship between nutrition and health.

You make choices every day that affect how you feel, think, and act. You decide what you will eat and when you will sleep. You choose how physically active you will be, too. Your actions affect who you are now and the person you will become. It is your responsibility to make decisions that will benefit your health.

How healthy will you be 10 years from now? You could be healthier and in better physical shape than you are now! Choosing behaviors that promote health can have lifelong benefits. You can take steps to feel just as fit at age 50 as you do at age 15. See 1-1.

● What Is Wellness?

Wellness is the state of being in good health. Wellness is often associated with quality of life. *Quality of life* refers to a person's satisfaction with his or her looks, lifestyle, and responses to daily events. When people are in good health, they have a desire to stay fit and live a healthful lifestyle. They are energetic and have an enthusiastic outlook. They are able to successfully meet the challenges of each day. When people are not in good health, life's events can become harder to manage. This causes a decrease in quality of life.

Most people want to continually improve their quality of life as they grow and mature. Trying to achieve a high level of wellness is one way to improve quality of life.

● The Wellness Continuum

You can use a continuum to define your personal state of wellness. Premature death is at one end of the continuum and optimum health is at the other. *Premature death* is death that occurs due to lifestyle behaviors that lead to a fatal accident or the formation of an avoidable disease. *Optimum health* is a state of wellness characterized by peak physical, mental, and social well-being. See 1-2.

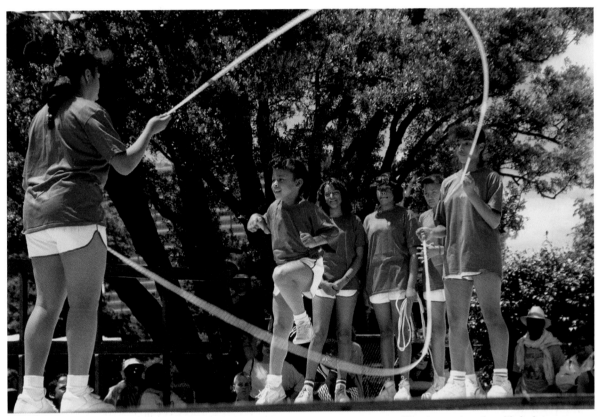

1-1 Making physical activity a lifestyle choice early in life can have a positive impact on health in later years.

Your health status determines your place along the wellness continuum. Being free from illness and having much energy indicate that you have a high level of physical wellness. If you are able to cope with life's challenges and maintain stable relationships, you exhibit mental and social wellness, too. This means you probably fall near the optimum health end of the continuum. A short-term decline in any of these areas may

Wellness Continuum		
Premature Death ⟵	⟶	**Optimum Health**
low energy level	moderate energy level	high energy level
frequent illness	some illness	infrequent illness and quick recovery from illness
inferior stress management skills	average stress management skills	superior stress management skills
poor social relationships	fair social relationships	excellent social relationships

1-2 Evaluate your physical, mental, and social health to determine where you fall along the wellness continuum.

temporarily move you toward the other end of the continuum. However, the key is your overall state of health *most* of the time. This is your wellness point.

If you are already at optimum health, you will want to find out how to maintain this state of wellness. If you are not at optimum health, you can learn how to change your lifestyle to move toward that goal. The key to achieving wellness rests with you. No one can force you to change. Moving toward optimum health happens because you want change to happen.

Once you begin taking steps to improve your health, you will start to notice the benefits. You might feel stronger and more alert. You may begin to feel better about yourself. Maybe you will find it easier to cope with the daily stresses of life. Perhaps you will feel more satisfied with your performance at home, school, work, and play. You may begin to experience better relationships with family members and friends. You may notice additional benefits of wellness in the future. Having optimum health will help you face the challenges of parenthood, career changes, and other aspects of active adult living.

● Aspects of Wellness

Wellness means much more than not being sick. It also means more than eating healthful foods and being physically fit. There are three major components of wellness. These are physical health, mental health, and social health. Each contributes to your total sense of wellness in special ways. Together they affect how you look, feel, and act.

● Physical Health

Physical health refers to the fitness of your body. It requires numerous body parts to work in harmony.

A number of factors can harm your physical health. For instance, getting too little rest will reduce your energy for exercising and doing chores. Eating too much or too fast may upset your stomach. Lack of physical activity, excess stress, poor sanitation, and reckless actions can also keep your body below peak performance level. Tobacco and alcohol and other drugs can harm physical health, too. Choosing lifestyle behaviors that avoid these factors will help you stay in good physical health. See 1-3.

Health care professionals use medicine, physical therapy, diet, and surgery to care for the physical health of their patients. They keep up on research about alternative treatments, such as use of herbs and nutrient supplements. As the costs of health care services rise, people are becoming more interested in learning how to prevent disease. Doctors often suggest that patients combine medical care with lifestyle changes. You will read more about making lifestyle changes later in this chapter.

● Mental Health

Mental health is related to the way you feel about yourself, your life, and the world around you. People with good mental health generally like themselves for who they are. They express positive attitudes and tend to act according to a set of socially acceptable values. They may also hold beliefs that help them see their relationship to a larger universe.

Irrational fears, stress, and depression may be signs of a mental health problem. If you are concerned about your mental health, you should talk to a trusted adult. Share concerns and problems with parents, teachers, counselors, or clergy persons. These people may be able to help you better understand who you are and what you want to become. Building effective communication and problem-solving skills can go a long way toward helping you improve your mental health.

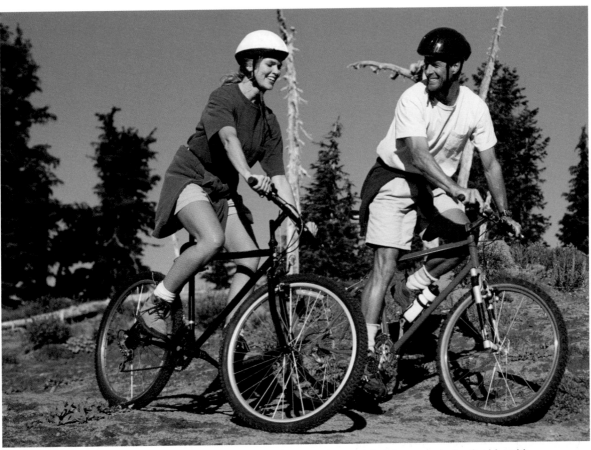

1-3 Getting regular exercise is an important requirement for maintaining good physical health.

● Social Health

Social health describes the way you get along with other people. Friends and family members help enrich your life. Social health can be negatively affected when disagreements occur and problems arise. Learning to resolve conflicts with others is an important skill that can help you achieve and maintain good social health. See 1-4.

Social health is related to an understanding and acceptance of roles. People have different role expectations for sons, daughters, husbands, wives, mothers, fathers, girlfriends, boyfriends, teachers, students, employers, and employees. You may want to analyze your roles for possible conflicts. For instance, you may be expected to be a follower in your role as an employee. However, you may be expected to be a leader in your

role as team captain. Learning appropriate ways to act in each role can contribute to your social wellness.

Social health affects a person's outlook on life and his or her personal state of wellness. For example, a teen on a first date might become so nervous that he gets an upset stomach. A student who worries about being accepted among friends may find it hard to fall asleep at night.

Building social skills allows you to improve your social health. One such skill is learning how to use good communication to resolve conflicts with others. Seeking and lending support to people who need your help is another important social skill. Building a positive self-image will also help you improve your relationships. Developing these skills will help you reach optimum social

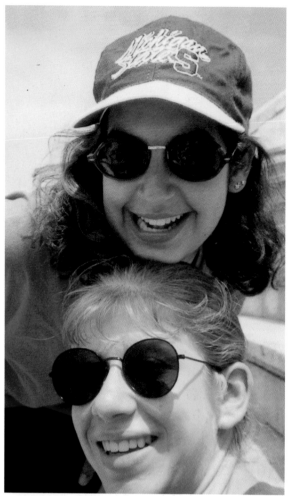

1-4 Positive interactions with friends contribute to a sense of social health.

health. Reaching this optimum level means you can work, play, and interact with others cooperatively. Optimum social health will contribute to your state of physical and mental health, too.

Learning about how people develop physically, mentally, and socially can positively affect your sense of wellness. You may feel reassured in knowing you are normal in your growth patterns.

● Holistic Approach to Wellness

Holistic medicine is an approach to health care that focuses on all aspects of patient care—physical, mental, and social. It

evolved because many medical doctors saw links among physical, mental, and social health. Treatment programs and medicine may not be enough to cure a physical illness. The effect of physical treatment can depend on mental and social health. Low self-esteem or loneliness can reduce a person's desire to get better. These factors can also delay the healing process by impairing the function of the body's immune system.

A holistic approach to wellness is well-rounded. You need to be aware of your physical, mental, and social health needs. You must manage time, money, and other resources to address your needs in all these areas. If you spend all your time working out, you may end up neglecting relationships. This would cause your social health to suffer at the expense of your physical health. If you spend all your money going out with friends, you may not be able to pay for school supplies. You would be neglecting your mental health in favor of your social health. Taking a holistic approach to wellness means making choices that fit together to promote all facets of health. See 1-5.

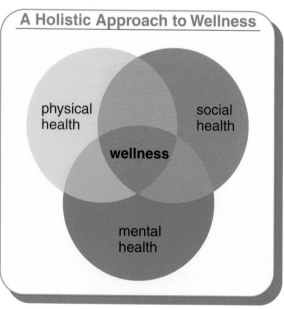

A Holistic Approach to Wellness

physical health

social health

wellness

mental health

1-5 Physical health, mental health, and social health all contribute to a total sense of wellness.

Factors That Affect Wellness

Why is it important to recognize the impact of health-related decisions in the teen years? The reason is your present actions and attitudes are shaping the person you will be in the future. It is hard to change a habit once you have established it. This is true for good habits as well as bad habits. Once you take on an unhealthful behavior, you are more likely to repeat it. Likewise, once you choose a healthful behavior, you can easily make it a regular part of your life.

Because you are responsible for making many decisions, you have much control over your personal state of wellness. You can engage in activities that will lead to the decline of your health. You can also follow practices that will help ensure good health.

Learning to improve your odds for a long and healthy life requires an understanding of the consequences of poor choices. It also involves recognizing wise choices. Studying information about nutrition, exercise, and health care will help you gain the knowledge you need.

Factors That Contribute to Disease

A *risk factor* is a characteristic or behavior that influences a person's chance of being injured or getting a disease. Researchers identify risk factors by studying the traits and actions of large groups of people. Then the researchers determine what effects these traits and behaviors have on the people's health.

Certain lifestyle habits, environmental conditions, and health care limitations are known to be risk factors you can control. Hereditary factors affect your risk of disease, too. Genetic research has not yet been able to find ways to prevent people from getting inherited diseases.

Unhealthful Lifestyle Choices

Heart disease, cancer, and stroke are three major causes of death among adults in the United States. The Centers for Disease Control and Prevention estimate lifestyle choices account for about half the factors contributing to these diseases. One example of a lifestyle choice is a decision about smoking. Smoking is a risk factor for cancer and heart disease. If you choose to smoke, you are at increased risk of getting these diseases. On the other hand, choosing not to smoke will lessen your chances of getting these diseases.

Other lifestyle choices include decisions about nutrition, stress management, and exercise. You will want to avoid choices in each of these areas that increase your risk of disease. Eating large amounts of fats and oils and few fruits, vegetables, and grain products is a poor nutritional practice. Failing to manage your time can increase your stress level, which can negatively affect your health. Spending little time being physically active can contribute to weight problems and other health risks.

Poor Environmental Quality

About one-fifth of the risk factors that contribute to leading causes of death are related to poor environmental quality. *Environmental quality* refers to the state of the physical world around you. It relates to the safety of the water you drink, the air you breathe, and the food you eat. It also pertains to your exposure to the elements. Pollutants in water and air and contaminants in food decrease the quality of your environment. Failing to obtain proper shelter puts you in a poor-quality environment, too. See 1-6.

Some jobs require people to assume greater environmental health risks than others. You may want to think about the safety of the work environment as you evaluate career choices. Compare the job of an urban construction worker with that of a sales representative. What environmental risk factors can you identify in each job?

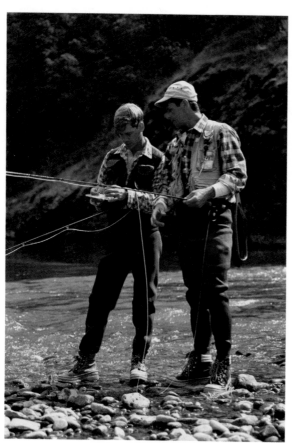

1-6 A high-quality environment that provides fresh air and clean water poses few health risks.

Jobs that require the use of heavy equipment and exposure to dangerous conditions add risk to health and safety.

Inadequate Health Care

Inadequate health care accounts for about 10 percent of the risk factors that contribute to leading causes of death. Medicine is not an exact science. Doctors cannot always assess symptoms and test results to easily reach a correct diagnosis. A **diagnosis** is the identification of a disease. Failing to *diagnose,* or recognize, a disease early enough can interfere with effective treatment. Some health care facilities lack the specialists or equipment needed to treat certain diseases. Sometimes facilities are not managed well or treatments are not given properly.

Inadequate health care is not always the fault of medical professionals. Patients sometimes interfere with the quality of their health care. Some patients fail to get regular checkups, which are needed to help physicians evaluate and maintain patients' health. Other patients do not seek medical care soon enough when they are experiencing symptoms. Some patients may delay going to see a doctor because they lack health insurance and cannot afford treatment. Others may hesitate out of fear.

Even when patients go to a physician, they can lessen the effectiveness of their care. They might not share important information with the physician. They might fail to follow the physician's advice. When you are a patient, you have a responsibility to play an active role in your medical care.

Heredity

Twenty-five percent of the factors that contribute to leading causes of death are hereditary. These factors are beyond your control. Genes you received from your parents determine your body structure and other physical traits. Genes can also affect your likelihood of developing certain diseases. For instance, if someone in your family has had cancer, you are at increased risk of developing cancer, too.

You cannot change who your biological parents are. Likewise, you cannot change the genes you inherit from them. However, you can keep yourself in good physical condition. This will help you avert the influence of genetic risk factors. It will also improve your body's ability to handle diseases if they do develop. For example, someone with a family history of Type II diabetes mellitus has an increased risk of developing this disease. However, this person can exert control over this risk factor by watching his or her diet. He or she can also get plenty of exercise and maintain a healthy body weight. Taking these steps can help this person avoid developing Type II diabetes. See 1-7.

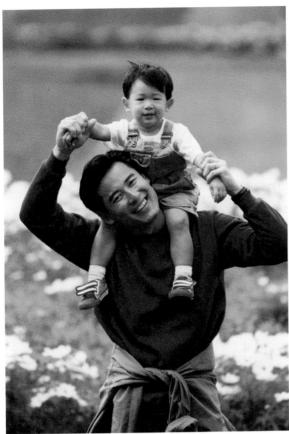

1-7 Some factors that affect health are inherited from parents.

example, you can choose to eat a diet rich in fruits, vegetables, and grain products. This will help reduce your risk of some cancers. The earlier you begin making healthful lifestyle choices, the more you will decrease your risk of early disease.

Health experts recommend adopting the following practices into your lifestyle:

- Provide your body with fuel throughout the day by eating three or more regularly spaced meals, including breakfast, 1-8.
- Supply your body with needed nutrients to support health, growth, and development.
- Sleep eight to nine hours each night.
- Maintain a healthy weight.
- Stay active. Accumulate at least 60 minutes of physical activity most days of the week.
- Do not smoke.
- Avoid drinking alcoholic beverages.
- Do not use street drugs. Carefully follow your physician's instructions when using prescription drugs.

Health-Promoting Choices

Studies show you have much control over the factors that influence your health. Health care experts have identified certain behaviors that make a difference in people's quality of life and wellness level. By choosing these behaviors regularly, you can promote good health and perhaps lengthen your life.

Choose a Healthful Lifestyle

Because you can control your lifestyle choices, you can also control some of your risks for disease. Your diet is one main lifestyle factor that has a strong correlation with many diseases. *Diet* refers to all the foods and beverages you consume. You have a large amount of control over your diet. For

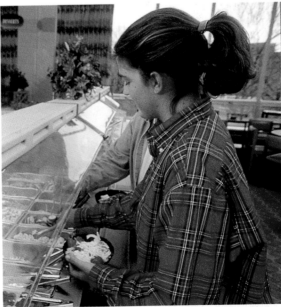

Photo courtesy of University Relations, MSU, Bruce A. Fox, photographer

1-8 Choosing balanced meals helps young adults reduce their risks of early disease.

Throughout this book, you will read about the impact of each of these practices on health. Although these behaviors may sound simple, many people fail to follow them. Instead they develop poor health habits. This may occur for a number of reasons. Some people take good health for granted. Perhaps they feel they are strong enough to withstand the strain of poor health habits. Others do not notice the slow toll such habits take on their health. For instance, frequently eating desserts and snack foods in place of fruits and vegetables deprives your body of needed nutrients. However, you may not notice the gradual decrease in energy level and other health effects caused by this eating habit.

Another reason people form poor health habits is they fail to realize how addictive some behaviors can be. Perhaps you have heard someone say, "I can quit drinking alcohol whenever I want." This person may not realize how physically and emotionally dependent on alcohol he or she has become. Most people need professional services to overcome addictions.

● Resist Negative Peer Pressure

Peer pressure can play a role in the development of health habits. **Peer pressure** is the influence people in your age and social group have on your behavior. The desire to be accepted leads many teens to try activities their peers encourage. This can often be good, such as when friends invite one another to become involved with a sport. However, peer pressure is negative when it encourages people to pursue activities that can endanger their health. Teens who urge their friends to smoke cigarettes, drink alcohol, or drive recklessly are using negative peer pressure. Negative peer pressure may play a role in making accidents and suicide leading causes of death among teens.

You can stand up against negative peer pressure and still come out a winner. Combating negative peer pressure requires self-confidence. You need to believe in your ability to evaluate the effect a choice will have on your health. You also need to be strong enough to say no to what you consider to be a poor choice. Be aware that people who have trouble resisting negative peer pressure may admire you for doing so.

● Improve Your Environment

You can do your share to make your environment a healthful one. Carpool or take public transportation to avoid polluting the air with car exhaust. Use cleaning products that will not pollute water supplies with harmful chemical wastes. Handle food carefully to avoid contamination that can cause illness. These are just a few of the many steps you can take to improve the quality of your environment.

Besides these personal efforts, you can work with others to improve the environmental quality of your area. Contact local industries about the efforts they are making to reduce their impact on the environment. Write to government officials if you have concerns about the quality of the air or water in your community. Talk with your employer about the benefits of creating a work environment that surpasses federal health and safety standards. These steps can help promote the health of many people.

● Choose Quality Health Care

Choosing quality health care will help you reduce health risks. The first step is to select a physician who has a reputation for providing quality care services. Also, choose facilities that can meet your needs and are approved by your health care provider. See your doctor for regular checkups. Seek your doctor's advice when you first notice a health problem. Research has shown that early detection of health problems is the best way to prevent serious illness. When you visit your doctor, describe your symptoms completely and accurately. Ask questions to be sure you understand your symptoms and treatment. See 1-9.

help you interact more positively with others, too (social health). Knowing these added benefits may be just the incentive you need to start eating breakfast.

Although you may be motivated to improve your health, you may not know how to start. Look at the questions in Chart 1-10. They can help you pinpoint areas where you might improve.

Once you have identified an area, set a goal for improvement. Then make a behavior change contract to help you achieve your goal. Write your goal at the top of a sheet of paper. Then set up a chart. In the first column of the chart, list specific steps you will take to reach the goal. For instance, suppose your goal is to improve your diet. You might list steps such as "Eat breakfast daily" and "Drink

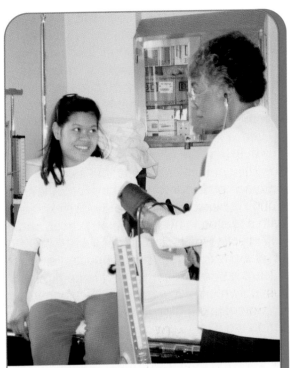

Questions Your Doctor Can Answer

What is causing these symptoms?

How long will the symptoms last?

Are these symptoms normal for someone in my age range?

What are my options for treatment?

What are the possible risks and side effects associated with prescribed medications or treatments?

1-9 Patients should feel free to ask their doctors questions.

● Making a Change

Changing one behavior can affect all aspects of your health. Knowing this can increase your motivation to make positive changes. For instance, you may have heard eating breakfast can help you concentrate better in school (mental health). However, this may not be enough to encourage you to eat breakfast. Eating breakfast can also help you maintain a healthy weight (physical health). It can moderate mood swings and

Lifestyle Choices That Promote Wellness

Do you
- avoid the use of tobacco?
- avoid the use of alcohol and street drugs?
- regularly eat a nutritious diet, including breakfast?
- manage your weight?
- get daily physical activity to maintain fitness?
- manage stress effectively?
- get enough sleep?
- carefully follow the instructions on medicine labels?
- wear protective clothing when participating in sports and fitness activities?
- avoid taking unnecessary risks?
- avoid unsafe sexual practices?
- take appropriate safety precautions when using equipment and machinery?
- enthusiastically participate in school and community activities?

1-10 If you can answer yes to most of these questions, you are making lifestyle choices that promote good health.

no more than one soft drink daily." List the days of the week across the top of the chart. Each day you complete a listed step, give yourself a check. This allows you to see the progress you are making toward your goal.

It will take time for you to notice most physical, mental, and social health benefits of a lifestyle change. Follow the listed steps and keep your chart for at least three weeks. After that time, evaluate the results of your efforts. Ask yourself what factors helped you complete steps that you marked with a check. Also ask yourself what kept you from completing steps left unchecked. For instance, you might notice that eating breakfast on weekends is easier because you have more time in the morning. You might find that limiting your soft drink consumption on weekends is hard when you are socializing with friends.

Your evaluation will help you set new goals and plan steps for achieving them. Try to consistently reach your goal for a period of six weeks. After this time, you will have formed a new habit that will be an ongoing part of your wellness lifestyle. Achieving optimum health is a lifelong process of consciously evaluating daily lifestyle choices.

Seeing positive results in one lifestyle area can affect your desire to change other areas. For instance, if you improve your eating habits, you are likely to have more energy. This may increase your willingness to begin an exercise program or join a sports team.

Your confidence that good health practices will improve your state of wellness will help you follow such practices. However, not all of your daily choices will be in the best interest of your health. Everyone skips a meal or overeats snack foods once in a while. Little harm is done unless you start making such choices on a regular basis.

● Nutrition and Wellness

One factor that has been shown to have a big impact on wellness is nutrition. **Nutrition** is the sum of the processes by which a person takes in and uses food

substances. There has been widespread growth in the study of nutrition in recent years. Scientists once thought foods contained just a few basic nutrients. **Nutrients** are the basic components of food that nourish the body. Today, scientists know of over 45 nutrients needed in the diet. See 1-11.

Growth in nutrition science is linked to growth in the field of epidemiology. *Epidemiology* is a branch of science that studies the incidence of disease in a population. After World War II, epidemiologists began exploring factors related to heart disease, cancer, and viral infections. One factor that really interested them was diet. They conducted studies to learn how eating patterns of large groups of people related to certain disease patterns.

Sometimes nutrition studies involve comparing the effects of various food choices. For instance, researchers might want to compare the health of people who eat meat with those who do not. They might compare

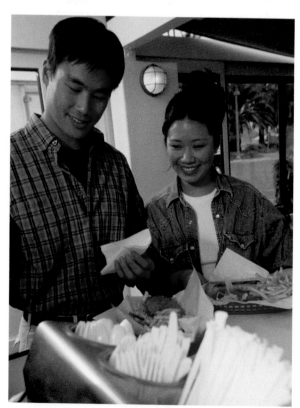

1-11 Eating food provides the body with needed nutrients.

the health effects of high-fiber diets with low-fiber diets. Researchers can also compare diet and lifestyle patterns among cultures.

What have researchers learned from all their nutrition studies? They have learned that eating specific foods cannot cause or prevent certain diseases. However, they have found that following certain eating patterns tends to increase or decrease a person's chances of illness. For instance, studies have shown that eating sugar does not cause diabetes. Nevertheless, eating a diet high in simple sugars can increase a person's risk of becoming overweight. This, in turn, can increase his or her risk of developing Type II diabetes.

Nutrition scientists continue to research the roles food components play in the human body. They use research methods to discover answers to questions about the links between diet and health. As a student of nutrition, you will use tools similar to those used by scientists. Correct use of these tools will help you understand and apply information covered in this text.

● Using the Scientific Method to Study Nutrition and Wellness

One tool scientists and dietitians use is the scientific method. The **scientific method** is the process researchers use to find answers to their questions. The process involves three key steps.

1. Make observations.
2. State a hypothesis. A **hypothesis** is a suggested answer to a scientific question. It can be tested and verified.
3. Devise experiments to test the hypothesis to determine if it is true. View the diagram in 1-12 to follow the steps of the scientific method.

The following example illustrates the use of the scientific method. A researcher becomes aware of statistics showing men do not tend to live as long as women. This prompts her to raise the question: Why do males have a shorter life expectancy than females? The researcher begins observing males and females. Through these observations, she

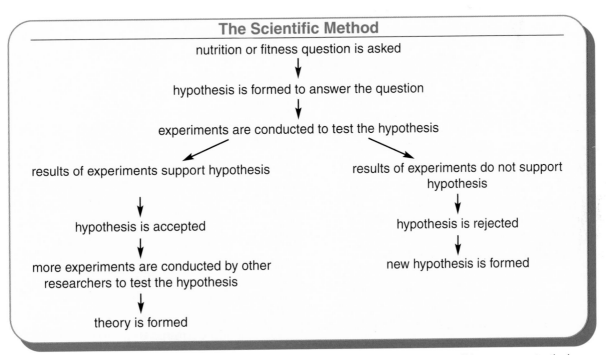

The Scientific Method

nutrition or fitness question is asked
↓
hypothesis is formed to answer the question
↓
experiments are conducted to test the hypothesis

results of experiments support hypothesis
↓
hypothesis is accepted
↓
more experiments are conducted by other researchers to test the hypothesis
↓
theory is formed

results of experiments do not support hypothesis
↓
hypothesis is rejected
↓
new hypothesis is formed

1-12 Through the scientific method, researchers are able to test and verify possible answers to their questions.

notes that men seem to exercise less than women. This causes her to form a hypothesis. The researcher's hypothesis states: Men do not live as long as women because men do not exercise as much as women. The researcher then compares the life spans of men and women who do the same amount of exercise. Suppose this test revealed that men who exercise as much as women have the same life expectancy as women. This would indicate the hypothesis is true. Conversely, suppose the testing revealed that men who exercise as much as women still have a shorter life expectancy. This would indicate the hypothesis is false.

If other researchers have conducted many experiments and reached the same conclusion, a theory forms. A **theory** is a principle that tries to explain something that happens in nature. Although it is based on evidence, a theory is not a fact. It still requires further testing.

There are many unanswered questions about diet, disease, and health that still need answers. Addressing the following questions helps researchers choose which food science, nutrition, and physical fitness topics to study:

- How is current technology affecting these areas?
- What gaps of knowledge currently exist related to the problems identified?
- How many people will be affected by learning about the information?
- Are resources available (money, time, staff, other resources) to do the research?
- How can current technology be used to advance research?
- Where will the study take place and who will participate?
- Are the rights of people protected, and is the physical environment left unharmed?

Evaluating Research Reports

You can learn about some of the latest findings and recommendations for improving your wellness level. Television and radio newscasts often include brief reports about the results of health and nutrition studies. Information is covered in greater detail in newspaper and magazine articles. Professional journals will present more technical information. Hundreds of health and nutrition Web sites on the Internet provide a wealth of data.

As you evaluate information, keep a number of points in mind. Identify the audience to which the report is directed. Is the information intended to update professionals or pique consumer interest? Be aware of who is relaying the information. Is it a media reporter or a health or nutrition professional? Take note of the size and length of the study. Did it involve 8 people observed for three weeks or 8,000 people observed for three years? Also keep in mind that many experiments are conducted to prove or disprove a theory. Not all experiments will yield the same results. A single study is not a sufficient basis for recommending changes in behavior.

Healthful Living in the United States

Studies show many people in the United States are not following the most healthful eating and physical activity patterns. Studies also show nutritional problems tend to increase as income levels decrease. A number of health and fitness problems are affecting the nation's state of wellness.

- About one-third of the people in the United States eat an inadequate diet.
- One out of three adults is overweight; one out of four is more than 20 percent overweight.
- Popular lifestyles include less and less physical activity, 1-13.
- Important nutrients are missing from the diets of some groups of people, such as teens and older adults.

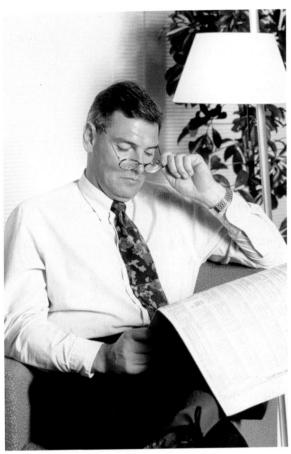

1-13 Many people fail to balance sedentary work and leisure activities with physical activity.

- Fat, cholesterol, sodium, and sugar intake are higher than recommended.

These problems arise for several reasons. Some people do not have enough money to acquire adequate nutrition. Others lack the information and skills needed to select a nutritious diet. Some people may not know they need to make changes. Still others simply choose to ignore current nutrition recommendations.

One reason some people give for disregarding nutrition recommendations is some nutrition messages are unclear or contradictory. Findings from one study seem to dispute the findings from another study. One source says to eat more fiber. Another

reference focuses on the importance of protein. Sports books say one thing; diet books say another; advertisements say something else. Even government nutrition guidelines change periodically. What is a health-conscious person supposed to believe as he or she tries to make wise lifestyle choices?

Education can help you sort out conflicting messages. Learning the scientific method and studying about functions and food sources of nutrients will help you assess media reports. Asking questions will also help you evaluate nutrition information. Finding out who conducted a study and how it was conducted can help you decide whether the results are valid.

Some nutrition studies have uncovered information so convincing it has changed the way people eat. For instance, researchers have found that people who eat high-fat diets are more likely to have heart disease. Identifying this link helped researchers discover that eating a lowfat diet can reduce the risk of heart disease. As people became aware of these findings, they began to change their eating habits. Consumers are now buying and eating more reduced-fat products than ever before. However, on the average, consumers are now eating more total calories and they are more likely to be overweight. These factors have kept the overall risk of heart disease from decreasing.

One result of improved eating habits over the last 100 years has been an increase in life expectancy. **Life expectancy** is the average length of life of people living in the same environment. Life expectancy in the United States is over 70 years. With improved health, life expectancy tends to increase.

Together, healthy people make a healthy nation. Following nutrition and physical activity guidelines will help you and your family maintain good health and contribute to the health of the nation.

Chapter 1 Review

Summary

Wellness involves being in good physical, mental, and social health. People can define their personal states of wellness as points on a continuum between premature death and optimum health.

A number of factors can negatively affect wellness by contributing to disease. Most of these factors are unhealthful lifestyle choices, over which you have control. Poor environmental quality, inadequate health care, and heredity can contribute to disease, too. You can counteract these factors by making health-promoting choices. Choose a healthful lifestyle and resist peer pressure to engage in unhealthful behaviors. Also, work to improve the quality of your environment and seek health care when you need it. You can set and work toward goals for improving behaviors that affect your health.

Nutrition and physical activity are two factors that have been shown to have a big impact on health. Experts use the scientific method to find answers to their questions about these factors. Their findings have led many people to change their lifestyle habits. However, a number of nutrition and fitness concerns still exist in the United States. With education, skills, and motivation, people can eat better to maintain better health.

Check Your Knowledge

1. What points lie at each end of the wellness continuum?
2. What are three resources health care professionals use to care for the physical health of their patients?
3. What are three signs of a mental health problem?
4. What are two social skills that can help teens improve their social health?
5. Why is it important to recognize the impact of health-related decisions in the teen years?
6. Name three factors that contribute to disease.
7. What are three of the major causes of death among adults in the United States?
8. List five lifestyle practices that health experts recommend people adopt.
9. Explain how to set up a behavior change contract for achieving a goal for personal improvement.
10. How many nutrients have scientists found to be needed in the diet?
11. What are the three key steps in the scientific method?
12. What are two factors that have contributed to health and wellness problems in the United States?

Put Learning into Action

1. Label one end of the room "Premature Death" and the other end of the room "Optimum Health." Stand between the two points to indicate where you place yourself on the wellness continuum. Explain to the class why you chose to stand where you did.
2. Interview a health care professional about the effects mental and social health can have on physical health. Summarize your findings in a written report.
3. Write a two-page opinion paper in response to the statement: If it's fun, it can't be a healthful lifestyle choice.
4. Contact the Department of Public Health or a community hospital for a health and wellness lifestyle questionnaire. Take the test and analyze the results. Identify your

major health risk areas and suggest methods for changing risk behaviors into health-promoting behaviors.

5. Contact local community health agencies to gather quantities of health information brochures. Use these to develop a "Wellness Information Corner" in your classroom. Make posters inviting students throughout your school to take advantage of this resource area.

Explore Further

1. Develop interview questions about diet, physical activity, and other lifestyle choices; environmental conditions; use of medical services; and heredity. Use your questions to interview an adult over age 70. Try to determine factors that contributed to his or her long life. Report conclusions to the class.

2. Investigate a health club, health care agency, or other community facility concerned with the health of clients. Write a description stating who may use this resource and how much it costs. Also, specify what the agency provides and the expected benefits of participation. Place your description in a notebook to create a community wellness resource directory.

3. Conduct research to create a list of Internet Web sites that offer information on wellness. Rate each site for accuracy and usability of information and credibility of source. Make a printout of your list and add it to the wellness resource directory created in Explore Further 2.

Chapter 2

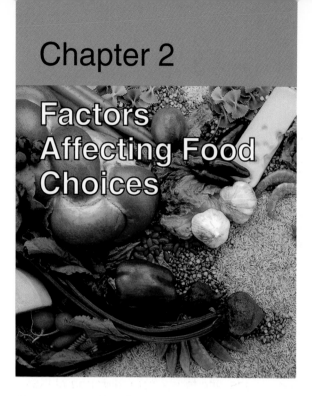

Factors Affecting Food Choices

What people eat says a lot about them. Food tells a story about where people live, what they do, and what they hold to be important. Food reflects people's history, and it will affect their future. In fact, one way to find out about a group of people is to study their daily food habits.

What factors affect people's food choices? When choosing food you probably think about what tastes good. However, you may not realize all the other factors that affect your daily food choices. Where you live and the people around you affect the foods you choose to eat. The resources available to you and your experiences with food are likely to shape your food choices, too. See 2-1.

● Learn the Language

culture	value
ethnic food	status food
soul food	staple food
food norm	technology
food taboo	aseptic packaging
kosher food	

● Objectives

After studying this chapter, you will be able to

- explain how culture influences people's food choices.
- describe how family and friends influence food choices.
- analyze the effect of emotions on the way people eat.
- relate how agricultural resources, technology, economic factors, and politics affect the availability of food.

● Food Is a Reflection of Culture

You may have had the experience of guessing where someone comes from by the way he or she speaks. Similarly, you might be able to guess where people come from

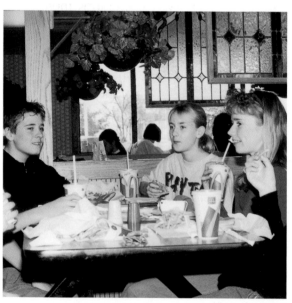

Nancy Konopasek

2-1 Friends are just one of many factors that affect people's food choices.

by some of the foods they eat. Like speech patterns, food habits are a reflection of culture. *Culture* refers to the beliefs and social customs of a group of people. It affects all aspects of your life, from where you live to how you dress.

What foods people serve for a meal is an example of cultural influence. Insects are a sweet delicacy in some cultures. However, people seldom serve them for meals in the United States. Families in the United States are far more likely to serve barbecued chicken, lasagna, or even moo shu pork than insects. Clearly, food practices vary from culture to culture.

While changes in culture appear minor from one year to the next, culture is never static. Culture changes over time as new ideas are introduced. For instance, in recent years, much information about health and fitness has been introduced. This information has caused people in the United States to become more health conscious. Many aspects of culture have reflected this change. Today, people are more likely to spend their time in health clubs than people in the past. They are more likely to spend their money on exercise equipment. They are also more likely to eat special lowfat foods. Ask your grandparents how often they ate lowfat yogurt and fat-free cookies when they were children. The difference between their response and that of children today reflects a change in culture.

What factors have helped shape your culture? Family members, friends, and other people who are close to you help pass along culture. Schools, religious organizations, and the media are also key influences.

● Historical Influences

Have you ever researched your family tree? Many people in the United States have roots based in other cultures. Maybe your ancestors came from Europe, Africa, Asia, or Latin America. When people came to the United States from these lands, they brought many foods and food customs with them.

When early settlers came to America, they found a vast amount of land. The climate was moderate and the soil was fertile. The settlers brought with them wheat, barley, oats, and rye. They found these grains grew well in this new land. They also brought fruits, vegetables, and herbs from their homelands. Figs, dates, broccoli, carrots, mint, and parsley are among the many foods these immigrants brought to America.

Many foods were being grown in America before the first settlers arrived. Native Americans grew corn, beans, potatoes, sweet potatoes, tomatoes, squash, chili peppers, and pumpkins. The settlers combined these foods with foods from their homelands to create a variety of dishes. These dishes are now part of America's diverse cuisine. See 2-2.

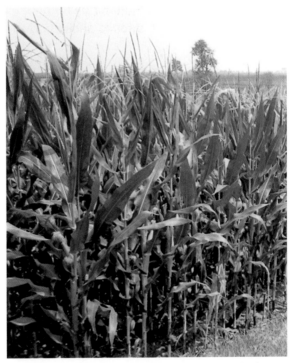

2-2 Native Americans were growing corn before the first settlers arrived. Today, the United States is the leading corn-producing nation.

● Ethnic Influences

Some of the foods you choose to eat may be based on your ethnic group. Groups of people who share common blood ties, land ties, or racial and religious similarities are called *ethnic groups.* What pulls group members together is their shared beliefs and group norms. Members of ethnic groups also share food traditions. **Ethnic foods** are foods that are typical of a given racial, national, or religious culture. For instance, **soul food** is traditional food of the African American ethnic group. Soul food includes such dishes as chitterlings, collard greens, and ham hocks. Sharing common foods helps build a sense of ethnic pride.

Ethnic groups have **food norms**, or typical standards and patterns related to food and eating behaviors. For example, most meals among the Pennsylvania Dutch include something sweet and something sour. The Pennsylvania Dutch often serve pickles or pepper cabbage as the sour element of a meal. Then they serve a sweet dessert at the end of the meal.

Some ethnic groups have special ways of selecting, buying, cooking, serving, eating, and storing foods. Group members take pride in these unique food habits. Many Italian cooks shop for food every day to get the freshest ingredients. Some Indian cooks prepare foods in a special oven called a *tandoor.* The British serve tea with cookies or sandwiches as a light meal in the late afternoon. These customs are ways of expressing deep-rooted ties to a common heritage.

Ethnic food traditions help build bonds of togetherness. Many ethnic groups serve special foods on certain days of the year to build positive emotions. The Japanese traditionally eat black beans on New Year's Day for good health and fortune for the new year. Jewish people eat apples and honey as part of their New Year celebration so the coming year will be sweet. What foods are part of your family's ethnic tradition?

You can recognize many ethnic foods by their ingredients, seasonings, and preparation methods. Ethnic ingredients are usually plentiful in the region from which the foods come. For instance, corn and beans grow well in Mexico. Therefore, many Mexican dishes feature corn and beans. Many ethnic cuisines get their characteristic flavors from a few typical seasonings. Spanish dishes are often flavored with onions, garlic, and olive oil. Middle Eastern foods are often seasoned with saffron, cumin, and ginger. Certain cooking methods also typify some ethnic cuisines. Chinese dishes are often stir-fried or steamed. Frying is typical of African cuisine.

Today in the United States, people seem to have a growing interest in and taste for ethnic foods. Specialty stores, farmers' markets, and supermarkets are beginning to carry more of the foods used in ethnic menus. Chinese, Mexican, Greek, and Thai are just a few of the many types of ethnic restaurants listed in the Yellow Pages. Many communities hold ethnic festivals, which allow visitors to try national specialties. See 2-3.

Throughout this century, many more international visitors, immigrants, and refugees are likely to come to the United States. A

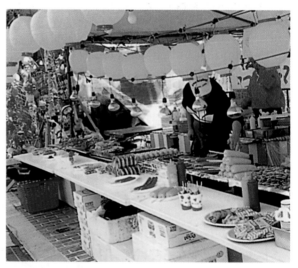

2-3 Ethnic festivals give people a chance to sample the flavors of another culture.

growing number of people from the United States will travel internationally for business, study, and recreation. This is likely to expand the range of ethnic foods available to you as you make food choices. Being willing to experience new tastes by trying different ethnic dishes will add variety to your diet.

Food Taboos

In most ethnic groups, social customs prohibit the use of certain edible resources as food. Such customs are called **food taboos**. Many people in the United States enjoy eating beef. Hindus living in India and other parts of the world, however, have a food taboo against eating beef. Their culture considers cows to be sacred. People in some Asian countries cannot understand why people in the United States do not savor dog stew. In the United States, there is a food taboo against eating dog meat.

No single diet pattern is acceptable to all people. People learn feelings about food through cultural experiences. What tastes good depends largely on what you were taught to believe tastes good.

Regional Influences

You may choose to eat some foods because they are popular in your region. Each region of the United States features some distinctive types of foods. This is because each region reflects different ethnic heritages and each heritage is typified by different foods. For instance, the Southwest has a large Mexican-American population. The tortillas, tacos, and tamales that are popular in the Southwest reflect this heritage. Many Asian people helped settle the Pacific Coast. They contributed rice dishes and the stir-fry cooking method to the cuisine of this region. See 2-4.

Religious Influences

Religious beliefs have influenced people's food choices for centuries. Certain religious groups have rules regarding what members

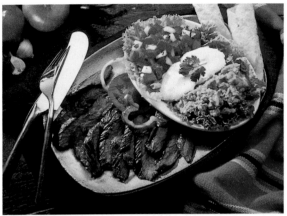

National Cattleman's Beef Association

2-4 Fajitas are a popular Southwestern dish that reflects Mexican influences.

may or may not eat. For example, many Orthodox Jews follow dietary laws based on their interpretation of the Old Testament. These laws forbid the eating of pork and shellfish. They also specify that meat and dairy foods may not be stored, prepared, or eaten together. Foods prepared according to these laws are called **kosher foods**.

Many other religions also have restrictions regarding food and drink. For instance, Muslims fast during the days of the ninth month of their calendar year. Seventh-Day Adventists eat a vegetarian diet. They also abstain from drinking alcohol, tea, and coffee because of their drug effects on the body.

Some members of religious groups view food customs as strict commandments. Others observe the customs to help keep traditions alive for future generations.

Social Influences on Food Choices

Have you noticed that food seems to taste better when you share it with people you know and like? Food often plays a role in social relationships with family members and friends. These people may influence the foods you choose to eat.

● Family

The family is a major influence on the diets of young eaters. You no doubt formed many of your beliefs about food when you were much younger. By watching your family members, you learned about table manners and how to eat certain foods. You learned about food traditions for holidays, birthdays, and other special occasions. You probably also adopted some of the food likes and dislikes of your family members. See 2-5.

Like culture, families change over time. Years ago, most households had two parents—a father who went off to work and a mother who stayed home. The mother was usually responsible for preparing food. Dinner was often served as soon as the father came home from work. Families have changed in many ways during the last century. The following changes have led to new trends in what, how, and when families eat:

- *More households are headed by working single parents.* A working single parent is likely to have only a limited amount of time for meal preparation. Families today often rely on preprepared foods to help save time. Meal preparation tasks may be shared among family members. The evening meal may be eaten later because preparation cannot begin until one or more family members arrive home.

- *Many dual-worker families have more income at their disposal.* Dual-worker families may be able to afford to buy more timesaving kitchen appliances and ready-made food products. They might have enough money to eat out more often. They might have sufficient means to hire someone to help with food preparation tasks, too.

- *The average family is smaller.* Manufacturers are offering many food products in smaller portion sizes to better suit smaller households.

- *Family members are increasingly mobile.* Working family members may commute to their jobs. Children and teens are frequently involved in a variety of activities. Busy schedules often keep family members from eating meals together. Many family members are in the habit of serving themselves whenever they are hungry.

Values make a difference in the kinds of changes seen in family food behaviors. **Values** are beliefs and attitudes that are important to people. Traditions, such as making special foods and eating together, are important values in many families. Such traditions can bring family members closer emotionally and socially. This is probably why about half the families in the United States still eat together at least once a day.

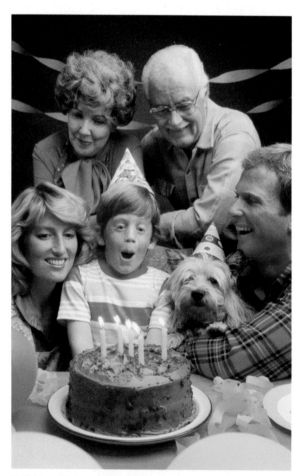

2-5 Families teach children about traditional foods for special occasions.

● Friends

Your friends and peers play a major role in determining what, where, and when you eat. Have you noticed that your friends like many of the same foods you like? Popular foods for teens include pizza, tacos, hamburgers, French fries, milk shakes, and soft drinks. Specific favorites may vary from one region of the country to another. However, some foods seem to be popular among teens everywhere.

Anywhere people gather you are likely to see food. Students eat lunch together in the school cafeteria. Fans eat hot dogs, popcorn, and nachos at sporting events. Friends enjoy sharing snacks and meals together at one of the more than 300 fast-food chains. Movie theaters, parties, church gatherings, and shopping malls are all places where people meet with friends and enjoy food. See 2-6.

Just as friends eat together almost anywhere, they also eat together almost anytime. Jogging partners may share breakfast after an early morning run. Neighbors may meet for midmorning coffee and rolls. Business associates often gather for lunch to discuss company decisions. A group of classmates may search the cupboards for an after-school snack. Couples and families enjoy sharing dinner in the evening at home and in restaurants. Teenagers may raid the refrigerator for a late-night study break.

When serving food to friends at a social event, people often choose foods that will help create a festive mood. Certain foods add special meaning to social events. Thanksgiving turkey and wedding cake are popular examples.

When people serve food to friends, they want to serve foods their friends will like. Sometimes foods that people perceive as being popular are not the most healthful. For instance, adults may serve cake and cookies at a card party. Teens may serve chips and soda to a group of friends. These foods are high in calories, fat, and sugar and low in other nutrients.

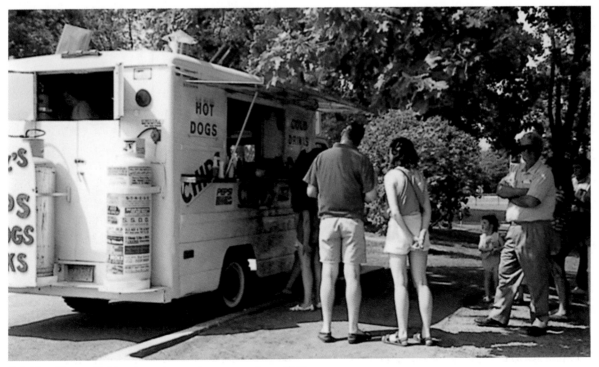

2-6 Food is available almost anywhere people gather.

You do not have to stop serving snack foods that are low in nutrients. However, you might want to offer your friends some healthful snacks, too. Fresh fruits or vegetables with a lowfat dip make tasty, healthful alternatives to high-fat, high-calorie snacks.

Peers affect eating behaviors as well as food choices. Teens commonly worry about body weight, complexion problems, and the impressions they make on others. Some teens try new eating behaviors that are reported to address these problems. Fad dieting is one such behavior that is popular among teens.

When choosing eating behaviors, just as when choosing foods, you need to keep health in mind. For instance, choosing to follow a fad diet to lose weight can be harmful. Fad diets often severely limit calories. Someone who restricts calorie intake during the teen years can inhibit his or her growth.

Are your choices based on nutrition knowledge or the influence of your peers? Examine how much your friends influence your eating behaviors and food choices. Think about the extent to which they affect when, where, and what you eat. Ask yourself if you tend to eat after school or in the evenings because you are with your friends. Evaluate whether you order popcorn at the movies or hot dogs at a basketball game because your friends are doing so. Do you find yourself ordering a cheese and sausage pizza because that is what your friends like? Becoming aware of how others affect the quality of your diet can help you improve your overall health.

● The Status of Foods

Sometimes people choose foods to tell a story about their social status. *Social status* is identified by a person's position in the community. Power and wealth influence social status.

Some foods are called *status foods*. **Status foods** are foods that have a social impact on others. Status foods are often served at special occasions to influence or impress important people. Caviar is a traditional status food served at social events of the rich and famous. See 2-7.

The status of a food often affects its cost but has little to do with its nutritional quality. For instance, filet mignon is a high-status food; hamburger is not. Filet mignon has no more nutritional value than hamburger, yet it costs about six times more.

Over time, the status level of foods can change. A low-status food can become a high-status food. For example, *quinoa* is a grain that might be considered a low-status food in Peru, where it is widely used. However, in the United States, quinoa is being marketed as an exotic, new grain. It is often available only in specialty stores and might, therefore, be viewed as a high-status food.

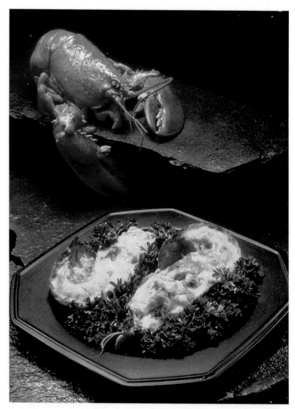

2-7 Due to its high price, lobster is a status food.

● Media

The media is a strong social influence on food choices. People may choose to prepare foods in a way shown in a newspaper or magazine or on a television program. They may choose to buy foods reported to have certain health benefits.

The media carry food advertisements. Television commercials have an especially strong impact on people's food choices. Commercials are designed to acquaint you with products. After you hear or see an ad over and over, you are more likely to buy the product.

Research shows that children in the United States view an average of 22,000 commercials a year. Children become socialized to want the foods they see advertised. More than half of the commercials are for foods high in calories, sugar, fat, and salt. Eating such foods instead of fresh fruits, vegetables, and whole grain cereals can harm children's health.

The effects of commercials on people's eating behaviors are hard to escape. The media portray young, thin people as the ideal of beauty. This entices some people to go on weight-loss diets to achieve the ideal. Without first consulting a dietitian or doctor, however, going on such diets can be dangerous.

● Emotions Affect Food Choices

People use food to do more than satisfy physical hunger. Many people choose to eat or avoid certain foods for emotional reasons. For example, suppose you ate a hot dog for lunch and later in the day you felt terribly sick. This may lead you to form a mental connection between hot dogs and illness. You may think, "Hot dogs make me sick, and I never want to eat one again!" Such an emotional response can outweigh hunger pangs and nutrition knowledge in its effect on your food choices. See 2-8.

Mental Connections with Foods and Eating Patterns

Food/Eating Pattern	Mental Connection
luncheon salads	femininity
meat and potatoes	masculinity
carving meats	strength, authority
expensive foods	status, elegance
sharing food	trust, friendship, hospitality
giving food as a gift	custom, affection
snacking	amusement, camaraderie
family dining	security
formal dining	tradition, ritual
eating alone	independence, loneliness, punishment
refusal to eat	sacrifice, retaliation
overeating	anxiety, greed, lack of self-control
fad dieting	insecurity, vanity

2-8 Emotional factors cause some people to form mental connections with certain foods and eating patterns. What foods create emotional responses for you?

● Emotional Responses to Food

Food evokes many emotional responses. People develop most of their emotional reactions toward foods in early life. For some people, food creates feelings of good luck and happiness. For others, food produces feelings of frustration or disgust. Play a word association game with a friend to learn more about your emotional response to food. What feelings come to mind when you hear the words *chocolate, liver, spinach,* and *ice cream?*

You learn some emotional responses to food in the context of family, school, community, religion, and the media. In other words, your culture affects how you will react to the food presented to you.

Some emotional responses to food may be associated with gender. Research has shown that some people connect maleness with hardy foods, such as steak and potatoes. Similarly, some people link femaleness with dainty foods, such as parfaits and quiches.

● Using Food to Deal with Emotions

Food not only evokes emotions, it can also be used to express emotions. Many people offer food as a symbol of love and caring. People show concern by taking food to neighbors and friends who have an illness or death in the family.

People often choose to eat certain foods to help meet emotional needs. For instance, a chocolate bar may cheer you up when you are depressed. Your grandmother's recipe for macaroni and cheese may comfort you when you are feeling lonely. A double scoop of ice cream might be just what you need to celebrate a good report card. Chicken noodle soup may nourish your emotions as well as your body when you have a cold.

Frustration can lead some people to eat more or less food than their bodies need.

Other people use food to help them deal with fears. Both types of people use the pleasure of eating to avoid thoughts that are annoying or scary. Have you ever found yourself wanting to snack heavily before a big event in your life? If so, you may have been associating food with emotional comfort.

Some feelings related to food can be harmful. Some teens and young adults, mainly girls, starve themselves to be very thin. This pattern of eating is grounded in emotions and requires the help of professional counselors. People must examine the way they use food to help put eating behaviors into a healthy perspective.

● Food Used for Rewards or Punishment

Foods can be used to manipulate behaviors. For instance, parents may use food to change a child's behavior. If parents want to encourage a child to do something, they may give a special treat. Cookies, ice cream, and candy are popular rewards for good behavior. See 2-9.

People who have been rewarded with food as children may continue to reward themselves with food as adults. They may select food rewards even when they are not hungry. Following this learned pattern of behavior can lead to weight management problems.

Sometimes parents take foods away from children as a punishment. For instance, a parent may withhold dessert when a child misbehaves at the dinner table. This can cause some children to develop negative emotions toward food and eating. Some children carry such negative associations into their adult years.

● Individual Preferences Affect Food Choices

You choose to eat many foods simply because you like them. What causes you to like some foods more than others? Your helps explain why members of the same family who have the same background often prefer different foods.

Although genes play an important role in determining taste preferences, your experiences with food affect your preferences, too. Suppose someone offers you a choice between fried grasshoppers and a hamburger. If you have eaten hamburgers but have never tried grasshoppers, you are more likely to choose the hamburger. Someone from China, where fried grasshoppers are a delicacy, might be more likely to choose the grasshoppers. People simply prefer what is familiar to them. See 2-10.

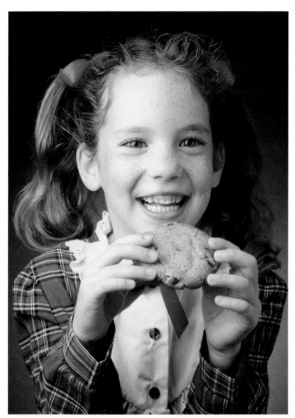

2-9 Some parents use cookies and other well-liked foods to reward their children.

emotions are one factor. You are likely to prefer foods that you associate with positive emotions, such as comfort and caring. However, you are apt to dislike foods that you associate with negative feelings, such as guilt and fear.

Your genes are partly responsible for your food preferences. You were born with personal preferences for certain tastes and smells. Everyone has taste buds that sense the tastes of sweet, salty, sour, and bitter. Just how you perceive each of these tastes, however, is part of your unique makeup. For instance, one person might wince in pain from the heat he or she feels when eating a jalapeño pepper. However, another person might hardly seem to notice the heat when eating one of these peppers. This difference in taste perception is due to genetics. It

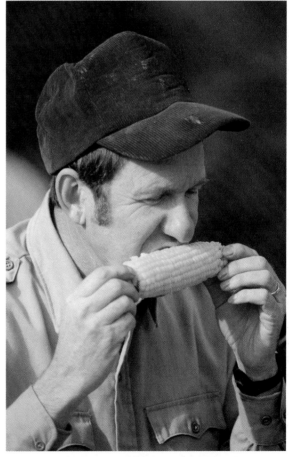

2-10 Most people prefer to eat foods that are familiar to them.

● The Influences of Agriculture, Technology, Economics, and Politics

Sometimes you have control over what is available to eat and sometimes you do not. When you buy food, you have control over what is in your cupboards. However, you have little control over what foods are available in the grocery store. Factors that can affect what foods are sold in stores include agriculture, technology, economics, and politics.

Most people in the United States have many foods available to them. This is not the case for many people throughout the world. In poor countries, agriculture, technology, economics, and politics affect more than the variety of foods available. These factors can affect whether there is food available at all.

● Agriculture and Land Use

Food production is plentiful when important resources are available to grow crops. These resources include

- fertile soil
- adequate water supply
- favorable climate
- technical knowledge
- human energy

The availability of these five resources differs greatly among regions throughout the world.

Crops need fertile soil in which their roots can take hold. Fertile soil supplies the nutrients plants need to grow. In some regions, the soil quality is too poor to support crop growth.

Quality of soil varies from area to area in the United States and throughout the world. The typical diet of a region usually is based on the foods that grow well there. For example, soil quality in the Andes Mountains of South America is too poor to support many types of crops. However, such hardy crops as potatoes grow well there, yielding large amounts in a small amount of acreage. Therefore, potatoes are a staple food in the countries through which the Andes extend, including Chile, Peru, and Bolivia. A ***staple food*** is a mainstay food in the diet. A staple food supplies a large portion of the calories people need to maintain health.

In Asia, rice grows well and is a staple food in the diet. Western Europe and the United States have conditions favorable for growing wheat. Bread made with wheat flour is a mainstay in the diets of these regions. Corn grows well in South American soil. Therefore, South American people eat many corn-based foods. Rye is a staple crop in Russia and northern Europe. This grain is used to make the hardy breads typical of this region. See 2-11.

Water availability affects food availability. Experts predict lack of freshwater will be one of the most serious concerns in this

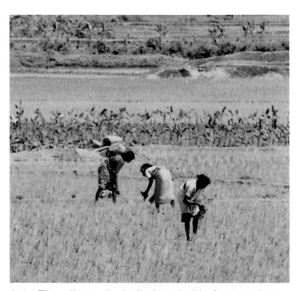

2-11 The climate in India is suitable for growing rice. Therefore, rice is a staple food in the diets of Indian people.

century. Rainfall is not always plentiful enough to fill the rivers and streams. Watering crops to increase yields creates a heavy draw on underground water supplies. Thus, water resources are at risk of being depleted.

Climate refers to the average temperatures and rainfall in a region. Different crops grow best in different climates. For instance, citrus fruits require warm temperatures for an extended time. Apples, on the other hand, cannot withstand long periods of warm weather. That is why most oranges come from warm regions like Florida, Israel, and Spain. Apples tend to grow well in cooler regions like Washington, Oregon, and Russia. Wherever the weather can sustain plant life, people can raise some type of food.

Technical knowledge is specialized information. It helps farmers get the most from their land. Through experience and scientific study, farmers have learned ways to increase crop production. They have discovered what nutrients crops need to grow. This helped them develop planting techniques and chemical fertilizers that replenish the soil with those nutrients. Farmers have determined how much water crops require, and they have installed elaborate watering systems to provide it. They have found what weeds and insects are damaging to plants. This has enabled them to take steps to control these pests.

Human energy is needed to plant seeds and harvest crops. In areas where the other four resources are available, a few people can produce an abundant food supply. When the other resources are scarce, however, many people may be needed to grow only small amounts of food. In the Midwestern United States, the soil is fertile and an ample amount of rain falls each year. The climate is suitable for growing crops such as corn, wheat, and soybeans. Farmers in this area are able to take advantage of the latest information about the most productive farming methods. These factors allow a Midwestern farmer to produce enough grain to feed thousands of people per year.

Consider the contrast presented by a farmer in a country such as Afghanistan. Much of the land is covered by mountains or desert, making it difficult to farm. Although some areas have fertile soil, rainfall is insufficient to support crop growth. Many farmers lack access to current technical knowledge. They are also unable to obtain high-quality seeds, modern machinery, and chemicals to help stimulate plant growth and control insects. In Afghanistan, many farmers barely produce enough food to feed their families.

Technology

Shoppers in the United States often find New Zealand kiwifruit and Mexican mangoes in the produce section of the supermarket. With the help of science and technology, foods from many lands are as close as the local grocery store.

In the last 75 to 100 years, many changes in technology and agriculture have influenced how food gets from farm to table. *Technology* is the application of a certain body of knowledge. Modern farming machinery, faster food processing systems, and rapid transportation are all examples of technological advances. The invention of new foods and food handling processes has increased the food supply. See 2-12.

Improved food packaging is another way in which technology has affected the food supply. Researchers try to design packaging materials that will keep food safe without adding much to the cost of products. Plastic is one such material that is commonly used in food packaging. Plastics keep food fresh and protect food from contaminants in the air and on unclean surfaces. Another factor researchers must keep in mind when designing packaging is its impact on the environment. One option being studied is biodegradable packaging that will break down in landfills.

A packaging technology that preserves quality and extends shelf life of food is called *aseptic packaging.* This process involves

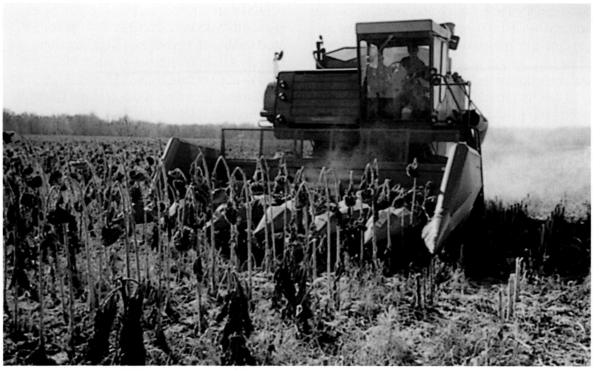

W. Funk

2-12 Technological advances in farm machinery have improved harvesting techniques and helped increase the food supply.

packing sterile food into sterile containers. It is done in a sterile atmosphere. Bacteria cannot grow in aseptic packages. Therefore, food does not need to be refrigerated to remain wholesome. This means perishable foods can be kept in places where there is no refrigeration.

Food products can now be safely and quickly transported all over the world. Staple foods can be stored for extended periods and then used during times of food shortages. These foods can be shipped to areas where food production is low and people want to buy them.

● The Economics of Food

Have you ever had to forego buying a candy bar because you were out of change? This is a minor example of the fact that it takes money to buy food. It also takes money to buy the seeds to grow food.

Economics has much to do with the availability of food. If a country cannot afford the agricultural supplies or other technological aids, such as tractors, food production is limited. If farmers cannot buy fertilizer, crop yields decrease. Poverty is a close relative of hunger.

Poor countries lack the resources to build food processing plants and store food safely. This can result in up to 40 percent of crops being lost to spoilage and contamination. Poor countries also lack the dollars to import food from other more productive countries. The nutritional status of the entire population can suffer when a country's economy cannot afford to produce adequate food.

● The Politics of Food

The degree to which a country's economic resources are used to address food problems depends largely on politics. The people with political power make most of the decisions in some countries. Those who have political power may decide what lands will be used for food production. They might determine what crops will be grown. Sometimes the decision is made to raise crops that can be sold to other countries. Money from these crops often goes to the people in power rather than the farmers who grew the crops. While the politicians get rich, the farmers remain too poor to buy food. Land that could be used to raise nutritious food for hungry people is being used for the exported crops instead. See 2-13.

Some political decision makers invest a large percentage of a country's economic resources in military power. Sometimes leaders make these decisions to increase their personal power. Sometimes they feel compelled to channel resources to the military to protect their country from hostile neighbors. In any case, money spent on the military is not available to help develop a country's agricultural production. It cannot be used to buy food from other countries, either.

Political leaders may even decide how food will be distributed. Food needed by hungry people may be given to the military. People with higher status may receive more

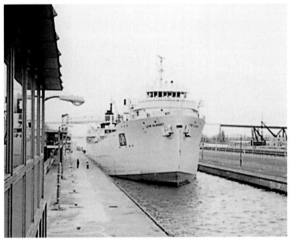

W. Funk

2-13 Many governments use land to raise crops for export rather than to produce food to feed people in their countries.

or better food than those who are poor. You will read more about how politics affect food availability in Chapter 24, "Nutrition and Health: A Global Concern."

Politics does not affect food only in other countries. The U.S. government sets many policies that relate to the food supply. Some policies concern food products that are imported from other countries. Some of these policies are intended to ensure the wholesomeness of foods. Other policies are designed to protect the market for products produced in the United States. Still other policies are made to keep trade relations friendly with other countries.

Many federal regulations mandate how food is to be produced and processed. The government requires that many foods, such as meat and poultry, be inspected to be sure they are wholesome. Guidelines state that manufacturers must pack foods in a sanitary setting. Laws require label information to be truthful. Federal acts designate what types of ingredients can be added to products, too. All these factors affect the foods that are available to you in the marketplace.

● Nutrition Knowledge Affects Food Choices

This chapter has addressed a number of factors that affect your food choices. As you have read, factors ranging from your culture to government policies have an impact on the foods you select. One other factor that influences your food choices is how much you know about nutrition.

To illustrate this point, answer the following question: Should you avoid vegetable oil because it is high in cholesterol? If you said yes, you would be agreeing with 68 percent of respondents to a nationwide survey. Unfortunately, you would be wrong. Vegetable oil, like all other foods from plant sources, contains no cholesterol. Therefore, you would be avoiding a food based on misinformation.

This example should help you see why correct information is so important. It can help you make knowledgeable food choices.

People have many beliefs about food and nutrition. The following are just a few examples reflecting a lack of knowledge that may lead people to make uninformed choices:

- *Certain foods have magical powers.* Eating fish will not make you a genius. Eating yogurt will not allow you to live to be over 100 years old. Eating an apple every day will not end your need for medical care. All nutritious foods have benefits for the body. However, you need to eat a variety of foods. No single food provides all the nutrients you need.

- *Taking vitamin and mineral pills eliminates the need to eat nutritious foods.* Some doctors suggest taking a multivitamin and mineral pill to help make up for lacks in the diet. However, no pill can replace the nutrients supplied by a nutritious diet. Depending on pills for good nutrition can interfere with a person's good dietary habits.

- *Foods grown without chemical pesticides have greater nutritional value than other foods.* Some people are concerned about the effects of chemicals used to control weeds and insects. They worry about the impact these chemicals may have on the environment and the food chain. However, farmers must use chemicals within safety guidelines set by government agencies. According to tests, foods grown with and without chemical pesticides have similar nutritional value.

- *Certain foods can cure diseases.* Some people have heard a story about British sailors years ago. The story reports how the sailors stopped dying of scurvy when they started eating citrus fruits. Many people want to believe eating certain foods can similarly cure such diseases as arthritis and cancer. What these people may not understand is that scurvy is a nutrient-deficiency disease. It is caused by a lack of vitamin C in the diet. It was not the citrus fruits themselves, but the vitamin C they contained, that cured the sailors. Some foods have been shown to be useful in preventing and treating certain diseases not caused by nutrient deficiencies. For instance, research has shown that regularly eating onions and garlic may help prevent some types of cancer. However, diet is only one of several factors that play a role in disease prevention and treatment.

Where do you look for information about nutrition? Friends and relatives may offer advice, but they may lack knowledge. You can find an abundance of nutrition information through books, magazines, television, and the Internet. However, be aware that details from these sources can be incomplete or inaccurate. For reliable information, look for materials reviewed by registered dietitians. These professionals have expert knowledge of nutrition. See 2-14.

Knowledge about your health is also important for making the best food choices. Certain illnesses like diabetes and hypertension require a modified diet. A qualified physician must correctly diagnose illnesses. Then a registered dietitian can help people with illnesses plan diets that will meet their special needs.

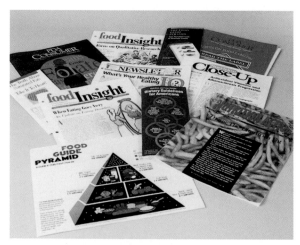

2-14 Choosing reliable reference materials will help you get accurate nutrition information.

Chapter 2 Review

Summary

Choosing foods goes beyond satisfying hunger. Many factors influence people's food choices. Food choices often reflect a person's culture. Studying history can reveal how some foods became associated with a particular culture. Many foods have importance to certain ethnic groups. When people from an ethnic group settle together, their foods may become associated with a certain region. Religious beliefs about food are also an aspect of cultural cuisine.

People often choose food for social reasons. Family members influence the food choices children make. Friends can also influence food choices, especially for teens. The way people perceive the status of certain foods can affect people's interest in eating them. The media impact people's desire and willingness to eat certain foods, too.

Emotions are another factor that affects food choices. Some foods produce emotional responses in people. In the same way, some emotions cause people to desire certain foods. Some people use food to reward or punish themselves or others. Of course, personal preferences may be one of the biggest factors governing which foods people choose.

Agriculture, technology, economics, and politics affect what foods are sold in the grocery store. Foods that grow well in a region are likely to be widely available in that region. However, technological advances have made it easier for foods from all over the world to reach local supermarkets. Even when people need locally grown foods, the foods may be shipped to other countries for economic reasons. People with political power make decisions that affect the availability of food products among people in a country.

A final factor that affects food choices is nutrition knowledge. People are more likely to choose foods that are good for them when they understand their nutritional needs.

Check Your Knowledge

1. What three factors can help identify ethnic foods?
2. Why are certain foods more common in some regions of the United States than others?
3. What are four trends that have influenced family eating habits?
4. True or false. High-status foods have more nutritional value than other foods.
5. What are two ways in which the media influence people's food choices and eating habits?
6. When do people develop most of their emotional reactions toward foods?
7. True or false. People who have been rewarded with food as children may continue to reward themselves with food as adults.
8. What are two factors that affect individual food preferences?
9. What five resources are needed to grow plentiful crops?
10. Name three technological advances that have improved the food supply in modern history.
11. How can lack of food processing plants and food storage facilities affect food availability in an economically disadvantaged country?
12. List three examples of lack of nutrition knowledge that may lead people to make misinformed food choices.

Put Learning into Action

1. Identify and/or prepare one of your favorite meals. Write an essay or tell the class what the meal says about you and your culture.
2. Make a list of all the food commercials aired within a one-hour time segment. Note the techniques used to promote each product. Indicate which products on the list you have tried or would like to try.

3. List several emotions you commonly experience, such as anger, love, and fear. Then list a food you associate with each emotion. Compare your list with other students to decide if certain emotions make you think of the same foods.

4. What aspect of technology do you think has had the greatest impact on food production in the last 50 years? Write a research report explaining your answer.

5. Plan to try one new food each week. Keep a diary of your personal reactions.

6. Choose a food product, such as a fresh vegetable, baked dessert, or dry cereal. Design a package for the product. Be prepared to discuss the cost, safety, and environmental impact of the packaging material you choose. Compare your choice of packaging material with the materials chosen by your classmates.

Explore Further

1. Research the dietary laws of an ethnic group. Find out where and why the laws originated. Summarize your findings in an oral presentation.

2. Examine the food section of a local newspaper. Identify articles and advertisements that might influence readers' food choices and eating habits.

3. Survey five of your friends. Ask them which, if any, foods are more masculine or feminine than others. Summarize your survey results in an article for the school newspaper.

4. Select one country from another continent. Research the country to find out about the characteristics of the land, water, and climate. Relate these factors to the food patterns of the people.

Chapter 3

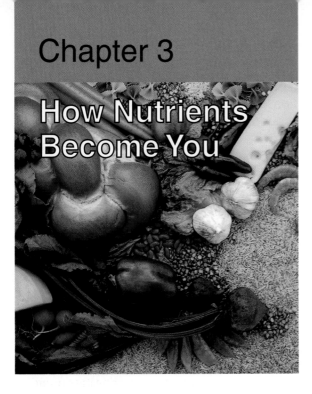

How Nutrients Become You

Learn the Language

kilocalorie
digestion
enzyme
gastrointestinal (GI)
 tract
mastication
peristalsis
gastric juices
chyme
bile
feces
absorption

villi
metabolism
ATP (adenosine
 triphosphate)
food allergy
diarrhea
constipation
indigestion
heartburn
ulcer
gallstones
diverticulosis

Objectives

After studying this chapter, you will be able to
- identify the six basic nutrient groups.
- distinguish the functions of the major parts of the digestive system.
- describe the processes of absorption and metabolism.
- explain factors affecting digestion and absorption.
- name common digestive disorders.

The phrase "You are what you eat" is a true statement. Food is your body's fuel. When you eat, your body breaks down food and the nutrients it contains into simpler elements. Energy is released and nutrients are used to help build, repair, and maintain body cells. Then your body discards the by-products of this process as waste. This chapter will help you picture the process of how your body uses food from beginning to end. See 3-1.

Food, Nutrients, and Energy

Food plays more roles than simply satisfying hunger. The food you eat becomes part of you. Nutrients from food are your body's source of fuel and building materials.

The Six Nutrient Groups

There are six groups of nutrients your body needs. They are carbohydrates, fats, proteins, vitamins, minerals, and water. You must obtain these substances from the foods you eat. Each nutrient has specific jobs to perform in the body. Each of these nutrients, in recommended quantities, is vital to good health. Without adequate amounts of these nutrients over time, your risk of various health problems will increase.

The Chemistry of Nutrition

Learning about health and nutrition requires some knowledge of chemistry. Your body and the foods you eat are composed of chemical elements. *Elements* are the simplest substances from which all matter is formed. *Matter* is anything that takes up space and has a measurable quantity. An *atom* is the smallest part of an element that can enter into a chemical reaction. A *molecule* is the smallest amount of a substance that has all the characteristics of the substance. Molecules are made up of two or more atoms that are bonded together. The

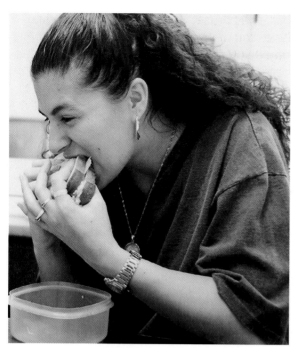

3-1 Eating is the beginning of a process your body uses to change food into materials for growth, repair, and maintenance.

atoms in a molecule may all be the same element, or they may be different elements. When atoms of different elements are bonded together, a *compound* is formed.

Hydrogen and oxygen are both elements. An atom of hydrogen can enter into a chemical reaction with another atom of hydrogen. These two atoms can be bonded together to form a hydrogen molecule. Two atoms of hydrogen can also bond to an atom of oxygen. The resulting substance would be a molecule of water. Because this molecule is made up of two different elements, water is a compound.

Five of the basic nutrient groups—carbohydrates, fats, proteins, vitamins, and water—are compounds. Minerals—the sixth basic nutrient group—are elements. There are at least 25 chemical elements involved in health and nutrition, including oxygen, hydrogen, carbon, nitrogen, sulfur, and cobalt.

It may be difficult to think of food as a list of chemicals. You do not need to carry out laboratory experiments to understand nutrition. However, having some chemistry background will help you grasp how nutrients interact in your body.

The Functions of Nutrients

Essential nutrients from food are used to
- build and repair body tissues
- regulate all body processes
- provide energy

When your body is performing all these functions in harmony, your potential for optimum wellness increases.

Build and Repair Body Tissues

Your body is made up of billions of cells. From before you are born until you die, cells divide. Each time a cell divides, it produces two new cells. These new cells account for your growth. New cells are also used to repair damaged body tissues and to replace old cells. All cells are formed with materials that come from food. Therefore, your body needs adequate amounts of nutrients to help make new cells. See 3-2.

Nutrient needs during periods of rapid growth are greater than at any other time. Such periods include the prenatal period, infancy, and adolescence. Lacking adequate nutrition during periods of growth may affect a person's physical size, strength, and health. His or her learning abilities and behavior patterns could be affected, too.

Every cell in your body contains genes. *Genes* carry hereditary information you received from your parents. Height, gender, skin color, and other details that are yours alone are on a genetic blueprint. However, good nutrition is necessary if you are to reach your full genetic potential. In other words, if your parents are tall, they may have passed along genes allowing you to become tall, too. However, your body needs nutrients to grow. If your diet does not provide these nutrients, you will not grow to your full height potential.

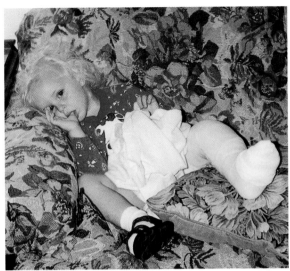

Frea Mars

3-2 A key function of nutrients is to help the body repair damaged tissues.

pump blood, move muscles, and provide heat. You need energy every minute of every day. If you go without food too long, your body will not have the energy needed to operate vital organs. The more active you are, the more energy you need to meet the physical demands placed on your body.

Chemical reactions that take place in your cells release energy from the nutrients you get from food. Carbohydrates and fats are the two main nutrients used for energy. Proteins may also be used, but the body prefers to save proteins for other vital functions. Vitamins, minerals, and water do not provide energy. However, the body needs these nutrients to help regulate the release of energy from carbohydrates, fats, and proteins. If just one nutrient is missing from the diet, energy release will be hampered.

● Regulate Body Processes

A second function of nutrients is to keep body processes running smoothly. For instance, the circulation of body fluids requires a balance of essential nutrients. Maintaining the correct acid-base level in the blood is a function of nutrients. Digestion, absorption, and metabolism are also processes that rely on proper amounts of nutrients.

The chemical reactions that control body processes are complex. However, these reactions normally work well. You will not usually need to think about which foods cause which chemical reactions. Instead, you need only to focus on eating a nutritious diet. This will ensure you are getting the nutrients you need to help your organs and tissues work properly. See 3-3.

● Provide Energy

A third key function of nutrients is to provide energy. Food is to your body what gasoline is to a car. It is a source of energy for performance. The quality of the food you eat affects how well your body will run.

Energy is necessary for all life processes to occur. Your body needs energy to breathe,

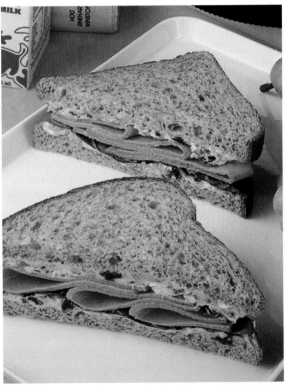

National Cattleman's Beef Association

3-3 A balanced diet includes a variety of foods, which provide the nutrients needed to keep your body running right.

The Energy Value of Food

The energy value of food is measured in units called **kilocalories**. A kilocalorie is the amount of heat needed to raise one kilogram of water one degree Celsius. Kilocalories may also be called *calories.* (The prefix *kilo* means 1,000. A kilocalorie is 1,000 times larger than the calorie unit used in your chemistry or physics classes.)

As mentioned earlier, only certain nutrients provide energy. Each gram of carbohydrate in a food product supplies the body with 4 kilocalories of energy. Fats provide 9 kilocalories per gram. Proteins yield 4 kilocalories per gram. Water, vitamins, and minerals do not yield energy. Therefore, they have no calorie content. The more calories in a food, the more energy it will provide. See 3-4.

Alcohol provides 7 calories per gram consumed. However, alcohol is not considered a nutrient because it does not promote growth, maintain cells, or repair tissues. Alcohol is a drug. If consumed in excess, its harmful effects outweigh any positive energy contributions it might make to the diet.

The Process of Digestion

What happens to a piece of food after you put it in your mouth? A detailed answer to this question would describe the complex process of digestion. **Digestion** is the process by which your body breaks down food, and the nutrients in food, into simpler substances. The blood can then carry these simple substances to cells for use in growth, repair, and maintenance.

Digestion occurs through mechanical and chemical means throughout the digestive system. *Mechanical digestion* happens as food is crushed and churned. Chewing food is an observable form of mechanical digestion.

In *chemical digestion,* food is mixed with powerful acids and enzymes. **Enzymes** are a type of protein produced by cells that cause specific chemical reactions. For example, digestive enzymes cause food particles to break apart into simpler substances.

As food is digested, it passes through a muscular tube leading from the mouth to the anus. This tube is called the **gastrointestinal (GI) tract**. The GI tract is about 25 to 30 feet in length. Each section performs important functions.

In the Mouth

Food enters the GI tract through the mouth. **Mastication,** or chewing, is the first step in the digestive process. The teeth and tongue work together to move food and crush it into smaller pieces. This process prepares food for swallowing. Chewing your

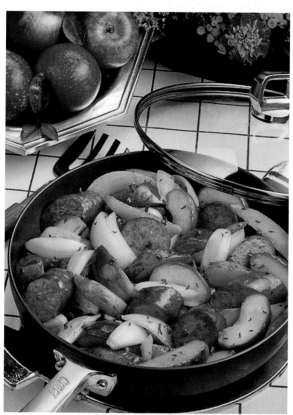

National Cattleman's Beef Association

3-4 The calories in this dish come from carbohydrates in the apples and potatoes and fat and protein in the sausage. The onions have a high water content and, therefore, provide few calories.

food well aids digestion because the body can break down small food particles faster than large particles.

There are about 9,000 taste buds that cover the surface of the tongue. These taste buds sense the flavors of food. This taste sensation, along with good food odors and the thought of food, trigger salivary glands in your mouth. These glands produce and secrete a solution called *saliva.* Saliva is a mixture of about 99 percent water plus a few chemicals. One of these chemicals is an enzyme called *salivary amylase.* This enzyme, found only in the mouth, helps chemically break down (digest) the starches in foods. See 3-5.

Saliva plays other important roles in the digestive process besides the breakdown of starches. Without saliva, your mouth is dry and food seems to have little taste. Saliva moistens, softens, and dissolves food. It also helps cleanse the teeth and neutralize mouth acids.

● In the Esophagus

As you chew, the muscles of your mouth and tongue form the food into a small ball. Your tongue moves this ball of food to the back of your mouth and you swallow it. As you swallow, food passes from the mouth to the stomach through the esophagus. The *esophagus* is a tube about 10 inches long. It connects the mouth to the stomach.

The esophagus is only one of two tubes in the throat. The other is the *trachea,* which is sometimes called the windpipe. When you swallow food, a flap of skin called the *epiglottis* closes to keep food from entering the trachea.

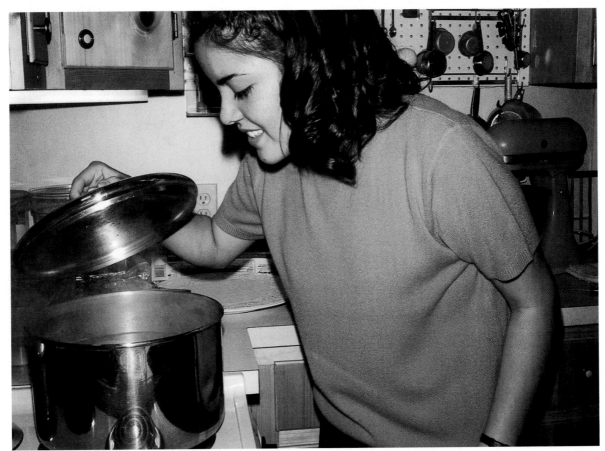

3-5 Appetizing smells, such as those from cooking food, trigger glands in the mouth to secrete saliva.

Breathing automatically stops when you swallow food to help prevent choking.

A series of squeezing actions by the muscles in the esophagus, known as **peristalsis**, helps move food through the tube. Peristalsis is involuntary. It happens automatically when food is present. You cannot feel or control the muscles as they move the food toward the stomach. Peristaltic action occurs throughout the esophagus and intestine to help mechanically move and churn food.

In the Stomach

When you eat, the stomach produces gastric juices to prepare for digesting the oncoming food. The term *gastric* means stomach. **Gastric juices** contain hydrochloric acid, digestive enzymes, and mucus. The mixture of gastric juices and chewed and swallowed food combine in the stomach. This mixture is called **chyme**.

The acid in the stomach is almost as strong as battery acid found in a car. The stomach wall has a thick lining, called the *mucosa*. The mucosa secretes mucus. *Mucus* is a thick fluid that helps soften and lubricate food. It also helps protect the stomach from its strong acidic juices.

Protein digestion begins in the stomach. The major gastric enzyme that begins to chemically break down protein is *pepsin*.

Most people can hold about one quart of food in their stomachs. Food generally remains in the stomach two to three hours, depending on the type of food. Liquids leave the stomach before solids. Carbohydrates and proteins digest faster than fats. Fatty foods stay in the stomach the longest. From the stomach, chyme moves to the small intestine. See 3-6.

In the Small Intestine

About 95 percent of digestion occurs in the small intestine. The small intestine is coiled in the abdomen in circular folds. It has three sections: the duodenum, the jejunum, and the ileum. The *duodenum* is the first section and is about 12 inches long. The *jejunum*

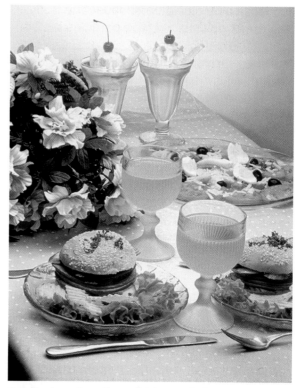

3-6 During digestion of this meal, liquids (apple juice) would leave the stomach first. They would be followed first by the carbohydrates (bun, fruit), then by the proteins (meat, eggs), and finally by the fats (potato chips, ice cream).

is the middle section and is about 4 feet long. The *ileum* is the last section and is 5 feet in length. When stretched, the small intestine measures about 20 feet in length and 1 inch in diameter.

It takes about 5 to 14 hours for food to travel from the mouth through the small intestine. During this time, strong muscular contractions constantly mix and churn food, aiding in mechanical digestion. Peristalsis moves food through the small intestine.

The small intestine needs a less acidic environment than the stomach to perform its work. The *pancreas,* an elongated gland behind the stomach, helps create the correct environment. The pancreas secretes *bicarbonate,* which neutralizes hydrochloric acid that has come from the stomach with the partially digested food.

The pancreas also produces digestive enzymes that aid in the chemical digestion that takes place in the small intestine. These enzymes break down proteins, fats, and carbohydrates into their most basic parts so your body can use them. *Amino acids* are the most basic parts of proteins. *Monosaccharides* are the most basic parts of carbohydrates. *Fatty acids, glycerol,* and *monoglycerides* are the most basic parts of fats. *Proteases* break down proteins into amino acids. *Lipases* are fat-digesting enzymes, which break down fats into fatty acids, glycerol, and monoglycerides. *Saccharidases* break carbohydrates into monosaccharides (simple sugars).

The liver is also involved in the chemical digestion that happens in the small intestine. The *liver* is a large gland that sits above the stomach. It produces a digestive juice called **bile**, which aids fat digestion. Bile helps disperse fat in the water-based digestive fluids. This gives enzymes in the fluids access to the fat so they can break it down. Bile is stored in a muscular sac called the *gallbladder* until it is needed for digestive purposes. It is secreted into the first part of the small intestine (duodenum). See 3-7.

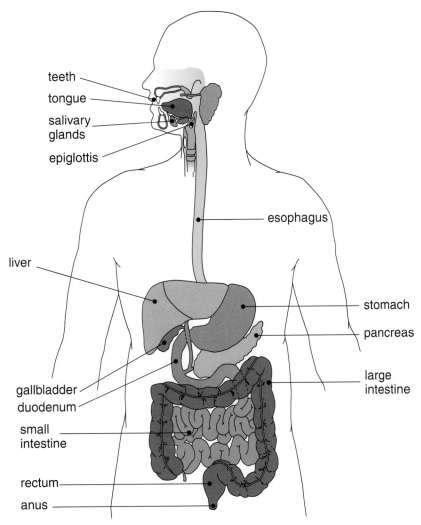

teeth
tongue
salivary glands
epiglottis
esophagus
liver
stomach
pancreas
gallbladder
duodenum
small intestine
large intestine
rectum
anus

3-7 Each part of the digestive system performs important functions in breaking down food for use in the body.

In the Large Intestine

The small intestine is connected to the large intestine, which is sometimes called the *colon*. The large intestine measures about 3½ feet in your body, or 5 to 6 feet when stretched. Very little digestion occurs in the large intestine. The main job of the large intestine is to reabsorb water. (Chyme is very liquid when it enters the large intestine.)

Chyme usually stays in the colon for about one to three days before elimination. During this time, water is absorbed through the walls of the colon. Useful bacteria in the colon work on fiber. They also help manufacture small amounts of some vitamins.

Solid wastes that result from digestion are called **feces**. These wastes include mucus, bile pigments, fiber, sloughed off cells from the lining of the large intestine, and water. The end of the large intestine is called the *rectum*. Feces collect here until they are ready to pass from the body through the *anus*.

Absorption of Nutrients

After being digested in the small intestine, the nutrients in food are ready for absorption. **Absorption** is the passage of nutrients from the digestive tract into the circulatory or lymphatic system. Most nutrients pass through the walls of the small intestine. However, alcohol and a few other drugs can be absorbed in the stomach. Alcohol can be absorbed in the mouth, too.

The inside surface area of the small intestine is about 600 times larger than that of a smooth tube. This is because the wall of the small intestine is pleated with thousands of folds. The folds are covered with villi. **Villi** are tiny, fingerlike projections that give the lining of the small intestine a velvetlike texture. Each cell of every villus is covered with *microvilli,* which are like microscopic hairs that help catch nutrient particles.

Some nutrients can dissolve in water. They are called *water-soluble nutrients.*

These nutrients include amino acids from proteins, monosaccharides from carbohydrates, minerals, most vitamins, and water. Tiny blood vessels in the villi, called *capillaries,* absorb water-soluble nutrients into the bloodstream. Then these nutrients are carried to the liver through the portal vein.

Some nutrients can dissolve in fat. They are called *fat-soluble nutrients.* These nutrients include a few vitamins as well as fatty acids, glycerol, and monoglycerides from fats. Lymph vessels in the villi, called *lacteals,* absorb fat-soluble nutrients into the lymphatic system. These nutrients then make their way to the bloodstream. See 3-8.

The large intestine finishes the job of absorption. Small amounts of water and some minerals are absorbed in the large intestine. Bacteria, plant fibers, and sloughed off cells from the lining of the large intestine make up the remaining waste material.

Metabolism

Once nutrients are digested and absorbed, the circulatory system takes over. The circulatory system carries nutrients and oxygen to individual cells. All the chemical changes that occur as cells produce energy and materials needed to sustain life are known as **metabolism**.

During metabolism, cells make some compounds. They use some of these compounds for energy and store others for later use. For example, cells can make new proteins to be used for growth. The body will slough off worn cells and replace them with new cells.

Through metabolism, cells break down some nutrients to release energy. The body stores this energy as **ATP (adenosine triphosphate)**. ATP is the source of immediate energy found in muscle tissue. When the body needs energy, chemical reactions break down ATP to release energy. Every cell makes ATP to help meet all your energy needs.

The body must discard waste products that result from cell metabolism. Waste

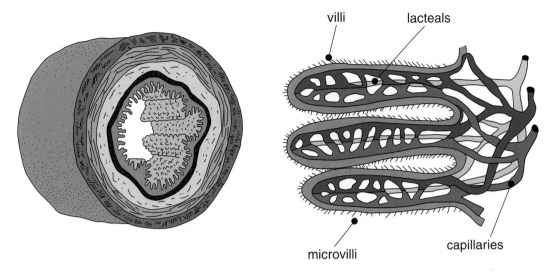

villi   lacteals

microvilli

capillaries

3-8 Villi lining the small intestine increase the surface area through which nutrients can be absorbed into the capillaries and lacteals.

products leave the body through the kidneys, lungs, and skin. The *kidneys* are part of the urinary system. They act like a filter to remove wastes and excess water from the blood and form *urine,* a liquid waste material. The urine collects in the *bladder* until it is excreted. Drinking six to eight glasses of water daily helps keep waste products flushed out of your system.

Breath from your lungs and perspiration through your skin also excrete waste products from cell metabolism. The harder and faster you breathe, as when exercising, the more moisture and carbon dioxide you lose.

Factors Affecting Digestion and Absorption

Have you ever been nervous or worried and felt food sitting in your stomach like a rock? The GI system usually works as it should. However, sometimes people have problems. Factors that affect this complex system include your eating habits and emotions. Food allergies and physical activity can affect

digestion, too. Healthy lifestyle choices can help you avoid many GI problems. See 3-9.

Eating Habits

The foods you choose and how you eat them can affect digestion. If you eat too little food or your diet lacks variety, you may be missing important nutrients. The lack of a single nutrient can affect how your body will digest and absorb other nutrients. To ensure normal digestion, choose a nutritious diet that includes a wide range of foods.

Be sure to include fresh fruits and vegetables and whole grain products in your varied diet. These plant foods are high in an indigestible material called *fiber.* Fiber helps strengthen intestinal muscles the way weight training helps strengthen arm and leg muscles. Fiber forms a mass in the digestive tract that creates resistance against which the muscles of the intestine can push.

Eating too much food too quickly places stress on the mechanical and chemical reactions needed for normal digestion. To avoid such stress, take time to enjoy your food instead of rushing through a meal. Also, be aware of the size of your portions.

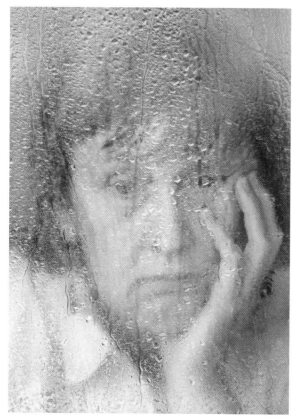

3-9 Emotions like anxiety and depression can interfere with normal digestion.

Eat moderate amounts of food rather than stuff yourself.

The makeup of a meal affects how long it will take your body to digest. Foods high in fat take longer to digest than foods high in carbohydrates or protein. In the stomach, fats separate from the watery part of the chyme and float to the top. They are the last food component to leave the stomach. A steak dinner, including baked potato with sour cream, oily salad dressing, and chocolate cream pie, is high in fat. This meal will take longer to digest than a high-carbohydrate meal, such as spaghetti, bread, and fruit salad. Because fats take longer to digest, you will feel full longer after eating the high-fat meal.

You should be aware of the wholesomeness of the foods you choose. Spoiled and contaminated foods are unsafe and can cause intestinal problems. Symptoms of these problems often include nausea, stomach cramps, and other intestinal disturbances. Illnesses caused by some contaminated foods can even lead to death. (You will find more information about foodborne illnesses in Chapter 20, "Keeping Food Safe.")

Emotions

Emotions like fear, anger, and tension can lead to digestive difficulties. You can avoid most of these problems by making a few lifestyle changes. Making a point of reducing stress and tension while eating will aid digestion. Try to enjoy food in a peaceful, quiet, cheerful atmosphere. Avoid family quarrels at mealtime. Also, chew foods slowly and thoroughly to ease swallowing. Taking these steps will help promote normal digestion. See 3-10.

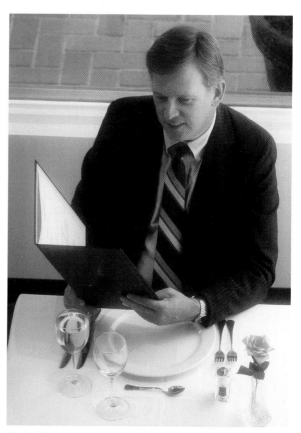

3-10 Dining in a relaxed atmosphere aids normal digestion.

● Food Allergies

The *immune system* is the body's defense system. It is made up of the tonsils, thyroid, lymph glands, spleen, and white blood cells. The immune system protects the body against disease and foreign materials. It produces proteins called *antibodies.* Antibodies combat foreign materials that get into your bloodstream.

A **food allergy** is a reaction of the immune system to certain proteins found in food. The protein that stimulates the immune system to produce antibodies is called an *allergen.* When an allergen enters the body, the release of antibodies leads to allergy symptoms. Vomiting, stomach pain, and intestinal distress are common symptoms of a food allergy. However, some people experience skin rashes, swelling, and breathing problems.

Which foods can cause allergies? Most people are allergic to only one or two foods. The foods most often identified with allergic reactions are nuts, eggs, milk, soybeans, and wheat. People who are allergic to such foods must eliminate or limit them. They must also carefully read labels to be sure prepared foods do not contain allergens.

Experts cannot predict who will develop allergies or how allergies will affect people. Heredity seems to play a role in the development of some allergies. Very small amounts of an allergen may be a problem for one person. Another person may be able to tolerate much more of the same substance. Allergic reactions can change over a life span. As some children get older, their allergies go away. However, other people develop new allergies as adults.

Food allergies should not be confused with *food sensitivities.* These are reactions to food that do not involve the production of antibodies by the immune system. For instance, some people are sensitive to milk because they lack the enzyme needed to digest the sugar in milk (lactose). Sometimes people react to food for psychological reasons rather than physical reasons. A person's worry about eating a food may be enough to cause a digestive upset. Separating food allergies from food sensitivities is not always easy. A medical exam is the best way to determine how a food is involved in the reactions that occur.

● Physical Activity

Physical activity can improve health in many ways. It can aid digestion and metabolism. Physical activity stimulates a healthy appetite and strengthens the muscles of internal organs. It helps move food through the GI tract. It also helps reduce stress, and it adds to your total sense of well-being. For a healthy digestive system, include some physical activities in your lifestyle. See 3-11.

● Digestive Disorders

Most people experience digestive disorders from time to time. Consumers spend many dollars on medications to relieve these problems. Most of these medications are not needed. The digestive system normally

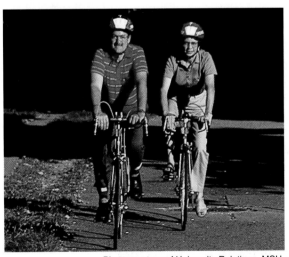

Photo courtesy of University Relations, MSU,
Bruce A. Fox, photographer

3-11 Physical activity stimulates a healthy appetite and helps the digestive system function properly.

functions better without drugs. To help avoid problems, focus on eating a nutritious diet. Be sure to include a variety of high-fiber fruits, vegetables, and whole grain products.

Long-term illnesses, including ulcer and gallstones, can have more serious effects on digestion. They can alter the kinds and amounts of nutrients that reach the cells. Such illnesses require medical supervision.

● Diarrhea

Diarrhea is frequent expulsion of watery feces. Food sensitivity, harmful bacteria, and stress are just a few of the factors that can cause diarrhea. Diarrhea causes food to move through the digestive system too quickly for nutrients to be fully absorbed. In addition, diarrhea can lead to a loss of body fluids. Drinking plenty of water will help restore fluid losses when diarrhea occurs. Prolonged diarrhea may be a sign of other health problems and indicates a need to see a doctor.

● Constipation

Constipation occurs when chyme moves very slowly through the large intestine. When this happens, too much water is reabsorbed from the chyme. This causes the feces to become hard, making bowel movements painful. Straining during elimination can lead to the added problem of hemorrhoids. *Hemorrhoids* are swollen veins in the rectum.

Constipation can result from erratic eating habits, low fiber intake, and lack of physical activity. Drinking too little water and failing to respond to a bowel movement urge can also add to this problem.

Many people use laxatives when they are constipated. However, the body can start to depend on the use of laxatives. Therefore, laxatives can worsen constipation. A better approach to treating and preventing constipation is to choose a diet high in fiber. Get regular physical activity and be sure to drink plenty of water, too. See 3-12.

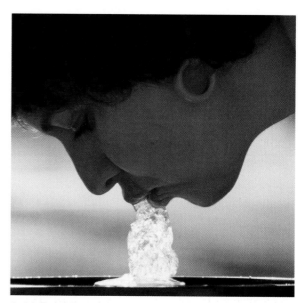

3-12 Drinking plenty of water can help prevent constipation.

● Indigestion

Indigestion is a difficulty in digesting food. Indigestion may be caused by stress, eating too much or too fast, or eating particular foods. Symptoms of indigestion may include gas, stomach cramps, and nausea.

People often take antacids for indigestion. *Antacids* are medications that neutralize stomach acids. However, taking too many antacids can alter the acidity levels of the stomach and interfere with nutrient absorption rates. Frequent use of antacids can also cause constipation. Instead of taking antacids, try to modify your diet. Avoid eating too much of one food or too many calories at one meal. Avoid eating foods that seem to upset your stomach. Also, eat in a relaxed atmosphere to help reduce stress.

● Heartburn

Heartburn is a burning pain in the middle of the chest, but it has nothing to do with the heart. It is caused by stomach acid flowing back into the esophagus. This is known as *reflux.*

Many people have heartburn after a meal now and then. Antacids can help relieve occasional discomfort. However, you should see a doctor if you have ongoing or recurrent heartburn. This may be a sign of a more serious condition called *gastroesophageal reflux disease (GERD).* This disease is common among older adults. If left untreated, it can cause damage to the esophagus and other complications.

Ulcer

An *ulcer* is an open sore in the lining of the stomach or small intestine. This disease is caused by a bacterium. The ulcerated area becomes inflamed, and the person who has the ulcer experiences a burning pain.

Some people get ulcers more quickly than others. People may have a hereditary tendency for the disease. Those who are under stress or use alcohol or aspirin excessively may also be at greater risk. You can avoid factors that contribute to ulcers by making healthful lifestyle choices.

Doctors generally prescribe antibiotic therapy for ulcer patients. Doctors also encourage ulcer patients to eat a nutritious diet. They recommend increasing physical activity and decreasing stress levels. They tell patients getting enough sleep and restricting the use of alcohol, tobacco, and caffeine are important, too. See 3-13.

Gallstones

Gallstones are small crystals that form from bile in the gallbladder. Bile, which is produced by the liver to help digest fat, is stored in the gallbladder. When food is present in the small intestine, the gallbladder contracts to release bile. When gallstones are blocking the duct between the gallbladder and the small intestine, this contraction causes severe pain. The presence of gallstones may slow fat digestion and cause fluids to pool and back up into the liver.

The treatment of gallstones often requires medical supervision. A physician may recommend a diet low in fats. In severe cases, the doctor may remove the gallbladder.

Diverticulosis

Diverticulosis is a disorder in which many abnormal pouches form in the intestinal wall. When these pouches become inflamed, the condition is called *diverticulitis.*

Diverticulosis can occur when intestinal muscles become weak, such as when the diet is too low in fiber. A high-fat diet and an inactive lifestyle can also increase the risk of getting this disease. The best prevention method is to eat a high-fiber diet, which will help keep intestinal muscles toned.

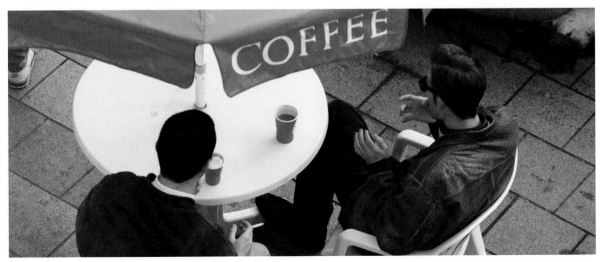

3-13 Ulcer patients who drink coffee would be wise to switch to decaf. They should also give up the use of tobacco.

Chapter 3 Review

Summary

Your body needs six types of nutrients—carbohydrates, fats, proteins, vitamins, minerals, and water. These nutrients, like your body, are made up of chemical elements. Your body uses them to build and repair tissues and control body processes. Carbohydrates, fats, and proteins are also used to provide energy. Energy is measured in units called calories or kilocalories.

Your body breaks down the food you eat through a process called digestion. Digestion occurs in the gastrointestinal (GI) tract. The GI tract includes the mouth, esophagus, stomach, small intestine, and large intestine. Throughout the GI tract, crushing and churning help digest food mechanically. Enzymes and other fluids help digest food chemically.

After digestion, your bloodstream is able to absorb nutrients and carry them to your cells. Most absorption takes place in the small intestine. Once nutrients reach your cells, they undergo changes to produce energy and materials needed to sustain life. Together, these changes are known as metabolism.

Several factors can affect digestion and absorption. These include eating habits, emotions, food allergies, and physical activity. Lifestyle behaviors that improve the digestive processes include eating a nutritious diet and reducing personal stress. Drinking six to eight glasses of water daily and getting regular physical activity can improve digestion, too.

The digestive system is complex. Normally all works well, but problems sometimes occur. Diarrhea, constipation, indigestion, ulcers, gallstones, and diverticulosis are among the digestive disorders that trouble some people. You can prevent most digestive problems by forming healthful lifestyle habits that aid digestion.

Check Your Knowledge

1. Name the six nutrient groups and give the three main functions of nutrients in your body.
2. How is the energy value of food measured?
3. What is the difference between mechanical digestion and chemical digestion?
4. Name four functions of saliva.
5. How does the epiglottis help prevent you from choking on food while eating?
6. What is the function of mucus secreted in the stomach?
7. Describe the function of three digestive enzymes that help break down foods in the small intestine.
8. What is the main job of the large intestine?
9. What are the water-soluble and fat-soluble nutrients and how are they absorbed?
10. How does metabolism provide for the body's energy needs?
11. List four factors that affect digestion and absorption.
12. Describe two digestive disorders and recommended treatment for each.

Put Learning into Action

1. Make a chart listing the six nutrient groups. Identify which groups are chemical compounds and which are elements. Also identify how much energy per gram each nutrient provides.
2. Make a poster illustrating the digestive system. Label and list key functions of each part.
3. Prepare a collage or bulletin board illustrating healthful lifestyle choices that can help people avoid problems with digestion and absorption.

4. Visit a store that sells medications for digestive disorders. List the various disorders and identify the names of drugs available to "treat" each one. Which disorder seems to offer the greatest variety of drug choices? Talk to the pharmacist to learn why so many choices are available. Report your findings in class.

Explore Further

1. Research how and where alcohol is digested, absorbed, and metabolized in the body. Report to the class the effects of alcohol on the liver, kidneys, and other organs.

2. Research one specific organ of the digestive system. Become an "expert" on the location and functions of the organ and its relationship to other organs. Write a report discussing how to maintain the health of the organ. Also discuss disorders and treatments of the organ.

3. Critique a research article reporting the latest findings on the causes, prevention, and treatment of a particular digestive disease. Diseases to investigate might include diverticulosis, irritable bowel syndrome (spastic colon), and stomach or colon cancer.

Chapter 4

Nutrition Guidelines

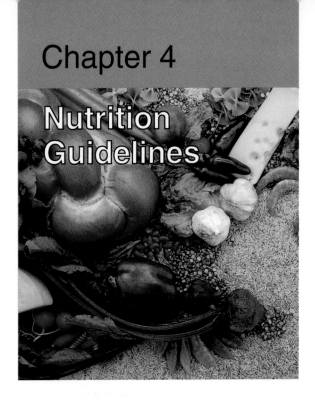

● **Learn the Language**

Dietary Reference Intakes (DRIs)
Recommended Dietary Allowance (RDA)
Estimated Average Requirement (EAR)
Adequate Intake (AI)

Upper Tolerable Intake Level (UL)
Food Guide Pyramid
serving size
Dietary Guidelines for Americans
Daily Values
nutrient density
food diary

● **Objectives**

After studying this chapter, you will be able to

- discuss how the Recommended Dietary Allowances (RDAs) and Dietary Reference Intakes (DRIs) are used.
- identify the recommended number of daily servings and serving sizes for each food group in the Food Guide Pyramid.
- summarize the advice offered in the Dietary Guidelines for Americans.
- use percent Daily Values on food labels to evaluate a food's contributions to daily nutrient needs.
- describe how to evaluate a food's nutrient density.
- collect and analyze data about your current eating habits and use the Food Guide Pyramid to plan nutritious menus.

People are often curious about how their bodies work. They also want to know what they can do to help keep their bodies healthy. You can find answers to many questions about these topics by studying food, exercise, and lifestyle choices. See 4-1.

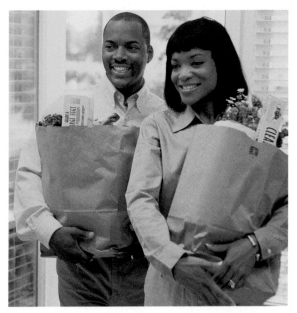

4-1 Many people want to know what foods they should choose to keep their bodies healthy.

This chapter will help you use the basic scientific tools common to the study of nutrition. You will read about guidelines for planning a healthful diet. You will then evaluate your eating pattern and practice applying the guidelines to your food choices.

● Tools for Planning a Healthful Diet

Health experts have been challenged to inform people about how to meet their nutritional needs. Many boards, councils, and committees have worked to develop tools to help people plan and evaluate their diets. These tools continue to be revised as new information is discovered.

● Dietary Reference Intakes

The Food and Nutrition Board of the Institute of Medicine, National Academy of Sciences is developing a new diet planning tool. This tool, the *Dietary Reference Intakes (DRIs)*, is a set of nutrient reference values. They can be used to plan and assess diets for healthy people. These values are based on the most recent findings on nutrients. The purpose of the DRIs is to prevent diseases caused by a lack of nutrients. They are also intended to prevent chronic diseases linked to nutrition, such as heart disease and diabetes.

The Food and Nutrition Board is releasing information about the DRIs in a series of reports. Until all DRI reports are released, health professionals must use a combination of DRIs and RDAs to evaluate people's diets. *RDAs,* or *Recommended Dietary Allowances*, are a planning tool that has been published since 1943. RDAs are suggested levels of nutrient intake to meet the needs of most healthy people. The RDAs include recommendations for energy needs and a number of nutrients. RDAs are not available for every known nutrient. This is because information about some nutrients is incomplete. The RDAs are revised from time to time to reflect new research findings.

The latest revisions involve a major shift from using the RDAs to using the DRIs. The DRIs include four types of nutrient reference standards. The first of these is the *Estimated Average Requirement (EAR).* This is a nutrient recommendation estimated to meet the need of half the healthy people in a group. If a group of people consumes a nutrient at this level, half would be fine and half would be deficient.

Newly revised RDAs are the second type of nutrient reference values grouped under the DRI umbrella. RDAs are based on EARs. The RDAs are roughly 20 percent higher than the EARs to cover the nutrient needs of most people.

Adequate Intake (AI) is another type of value set for nutrients. This value is determined for nutrients for which research is inconclusive. An EAR cannot be established for these nutrients. Therefore, no RDA can be determined. As more research becomes available, AIs for some nutrients may be replaced by EARs and RDAs. AIs are used for all nutrients for infants under the age of one year.

The *Upper Tolerable Intake Level (UL)* is the fourth reference standard. It represents the maximum level at which a nutrient is unlikely to cause harm to most people. Daily intake of a nutrient above the UL could cause a poisonous reaction. Not enough information is available to set ULs for all nutrients.

You can use DRIs for diet planning. You should aim to include the AI or RDA amount of each nutrient in your diet. Keep in mind that the DRIs are just one type of standard. To fully evaluate your diet, you must also look at your overall eating pattern and health condition. Such factors as medications and diseases can affect your nutrient needs, 4-2. A true nutrient lack or excess can be determined only through medical tests. You can find a chart listing the RDAs and DRIs in Appendix B.

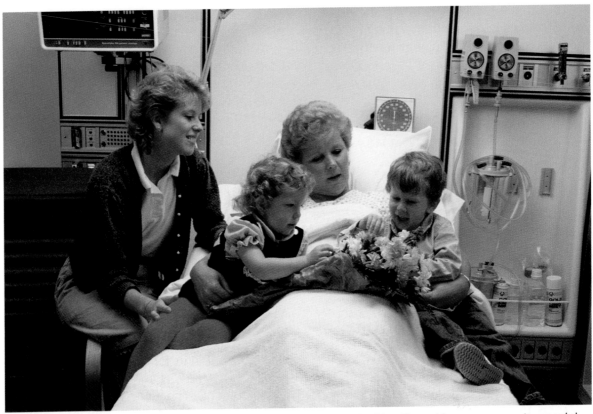

4-2 DRIs are useful in assessing only the diets of healthy people. Health problems can create special nutrient needs.

The Food Guide Pyramid

In 1992, the United States Departments of Agriculture (USDA) and Health and Human Services (HHS) devised the **Food Guide Pyramid** based on research. The Pyramid is a visual tool used to help people plan healthful diets. It divides foods into five main groups. It also recommends a range of daily servings people should eat from each group. For good health, you need some foods from all the food groups. Following the Pyramid can help you reduce risks of major chronic diseases common in the United States. See 4-3.

The Pyramid shows the *breads, cereals, rice, and pasta group* should form the base of a healthful diet. Most active teenage females should eat 9 servings from this group each day. Most teenage males should eat 11 daily servings. These foods are excellent sources of carbohydrates and fiber.

Foods from the *vegetable group* and the *fruit group* are also important sources of fiber. They form the second tier, or layer, of the Pyramid. Teenage females should eat four servings from the vegetable group and three servings from the fruit group each day. Teenage males need five daily servings from the vegetable group and four servings from the fruit group. Foods in these groups are good sources of vitamins and minerals, too.

Two groups that are high in protein form the third tier of the Pyramid. These are the *milk, yogurt, and cheese group* and the *meat, poultry, fish, dry beans, eggs, and nuts group*. All teens need three daily servings from the milk group and two to three servings from the meat and beans group.

Food Guide Pyramid
A Guide to Daily Food Choices

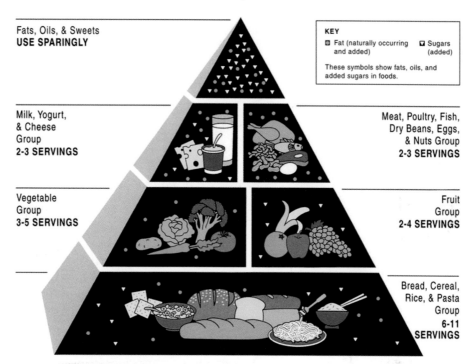

Fats, Oils, & Sweets
USE SPARINGLY

KEY
■ Fat (naturally occurring and added)   ▢ Sugars (added)

These symbols show fats, oils, and added sugars in foods.

Milk, Yogurt, & Cheese Group
2-3 SERVINGS

Meat, Poultry, Fish, Dry Beans, Eggs, & Nuts Group
2-3 SERVINGS

Vegetable Group
3-5 SERVINGS

Fruit Group
2-4 SERVINGS

Bread, Cereal, Rice, & Pasta Group
6-11 SERVINGS

4-3 Using the Food Guide Pyramid to plan daily food choices can help you get the balance of nutrients you need.

At the top of the Pyramid, you see fats, oils, and sweets. This section includes such foods as candy, butter, margarine, table syrups, cakes, cookies, and many snack foods. You should use these foods sparingly because they provide few nutrients.

The location of the groups in the Pyramid reflects a healthful eating pattern. This pattern promotes a diet higher in carbohydrates and fiber and lower in sugar, fats, cholesterol, and sodium. Foods in all groups of the Pyramid can contain fats and sugar. However, carefully choosing foods from the first three tiers of the Pyramid will help you get a nutritious diet.

Determining Daily Servings Needed

The Food Guide Pyramid recommends a range of daily servings for each food group. The number of servings you need depends on several factors. Your age, sex, body size, and activity level all affect your particular needs. Teens tend to need more servings than adults. Young adults usually need more servings than senior citizens. Females generally require fewer servings than males. Large people need more servings than smaller people. Active people usually need more servings than inactive people. People who are trying to reduce their weight may reduce the number of servings they eat. Those trying to gain weight need to add servings.

Serving Sizes

You need to know how much food equals a serving. *Serving size* is the amount of a food item normally eaten at one time. See 4-4. Serving sizes for two- to three-year-old children can be smaller. However, young children still need the minimum number of servings from each food group.

How Big Is a Serving?

Breads, Cereals, Rice, and Pasta

1 slice of bread

½ hamburger bun

1 small roll

3 or 4 small crackers

½ cup cooked cereal, rice, or pasta

1 ounce ready-to-eat cereal (about 1 cup)

Vegetables

½ cup chopped raw or cooked vegetables

1 cup leafy raw vegetables

¾ cup juice

Fruits

1 apple, banana, or orange

½ cup canned fruit

¼ cup dried fruit

¾ cup juice

Milk, Yogurt, and Cheese

1 cup milk

8 ounces yogurt

1½ ounces natural cheese

2 ounces process cheese

Meat, Poultry, Fish, Dry Beans, Eggs, and Nuts

2½ to 3 ounces cooked lean meat, poultry, or fish

1 egg, ½ cup cooked beans, 2 tablespoons peanut butter, or ½ cup tofu equals 1 ounce of lean meat

4-4 To use the Food Guide Pyramid effectively, you need to know how much food equals a serving.

Serving sizes can make a difference when figuring your needs for the day. Servings can add up quicker than you think. Eating portions that are larger than the recommended serving size will cause you to eat more calories than you need. For example, you may think of a cup of pasta as one serving, but it actually counts as two servings.

Sometimes visualizing a serving of ice cream, meat, or macaroni and cheese is difficult. You may want to measure a few foods to visualize a serving size. This will help you more accurately estimate how many servings you eat throughout the day.

Read the labels on food products to help you figure the serving size of packaged foods. Serving size is not up to the manufacturer. Food labeling laws require that serving sizes be uniform and reflect the amounts people usually eat. They must be expressed on the label in common household and metric measures.

● Dietary Guidelines for Americans

The United States Departments of Agriculture and Health and Human Services publish the ***Dietary Guidelines for Americans.*** These 10 recommendations were developed to help healthy people age two and over know what to eat to stay healthy. The Dietary Guidelines are general enough for people of all lifestyles and cultures to follow.

The Dietary Guidelines were developed because many people in the United States eat unhealthful diets. The average American diet is too high in fats, cholesterol, and sugar. It is too low in the nutrients found in whole grains, vegetables, and fruits. Such dietary patterns are linked with an increased risk of heart disease, stroke, cancer, and liver disease. These diseases are among the leading causes of death in the United States. Following the Dietary Guidelines can help people aim for fitness, build a healthy base, and choose sensibly for good health. See 4-5.

Aim for a healthy weight. Follow a lifestyle that combines sensible food choices with regular physical activity. These efforts will help you stay within a healthy weight range. Being overweight is linked with high blood pressure, heart disease, stroke, some forms of diabetes, and certain cancers. Underweight people are more likely to have trouble recovering from surgery and some diseases. Maintain a healthy weight to avoid developing weight-related health problems.

Dietary Guidelines for Americans

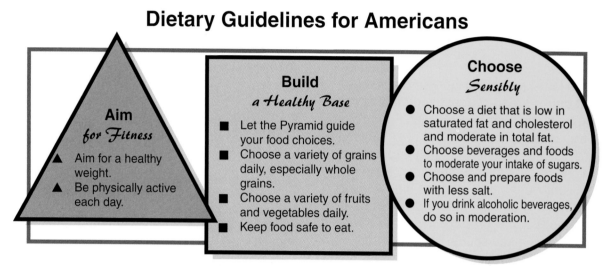

Aim
for Fitness

▲ Aim for a healthy weight.
▲ Be physically active each day.

Build
a Healthy Base

■ Let the Pyramid guide your food choices.
■ Choose a variety of grains daily, especially whole grains.
■ Choose a variety of fruits and vegetables daily.
■ Keep food safe to eat.

Choose
Sensibly

● Choose a diet that is low in saturated fat and cholesterol and moderate in total fat.
● Choose beverages and foods to moderate your intake of sugars.
● Choose and prepare foods with less salt.
● If you drink alcoholic beverages, do so in moderation.

4-5 The Dietary Guidelines for Americans help people answer the question, what should I eat to stay healthy?

Be physically active each day. Being physically active involves moving the body. Physical activity helps reduce the risk of heart disease and makes it easier to maintain or lose weight. During your teen years, you should try to spend at least 60 minutes a day in moderate physical activity. Throughout adulthood, you should try to accumulate at least 30 minutes of physical activity most, if not all, days of the week. Choose activities you enjoy, such as in-line skating or bicycling with friends. Even tasks like raking leaves and cutting the grass count as physical activity. You do not have to do all your activity at one time. You can gather minutes of physical activity all through the day.

Let the Pyramid guide your food choices. No one food can supply all the nutrients in the amounts you need. The Food Guide Pyramid can help you choose a variety of foods for a nutritious diet. If a food group is not a part of your diet, seek guidance to help ensure you get all the nutrients you need.

Choose a variety of grains daily, especially whole grains. Whole grains, such as wheat, rice, and oats, help form the base of a nutritious diet. Vitamins, minerals, and other substances in whole grain foods may help protect you against many chronic diseases. Grain products are naturally low in fats and high in fiber. Fiber promotes healthy bowel function. Active teens need 6 to 11 servings of grain foods per day.

Choose a variety of fruits and vegetables daily. Include plenty of different fruits and vegetables with your meals and snacks. Fruits and vegetables provide essential vitamins, minerals, fiber, and other substances that are important for health. Eat a variety of fruits and vegetables to get a diet rich in different nutrients.

Keep food safe to eat. Healthful foods are selected, prepared, and stored with safety in mind. Safe foods are free from harmful bacteria, viruses, parasites, and chemical contaminants. Ways to keep food safe to eat are discussed in Chapter 20.

Choose a diet that is low in saturated fat and cholesterol and moderate in total fat. A healthful diet must include some fat. However, diets high in fat, saturated fat, and cholesterol are linked to heart disease, stroke, and certain types of cancer. Excess fat in the diet also increases the risk of obesity because fat is a concentrated source of calories. No more than 30 percent of your total day's calories should come from fat. No more than 10 percent of your total calories should come from saturated fats.

Choose beverages and foods to moderate your intake of sugars. Sugars include white sugar, brown sugar, honey, molasses, and table syrups. Foods high in sugars include jams, jellies, candies, and desserts. Soft drinks are the largest source of added sugars in the average U.S. diet. Foods high in sugars supply calories but not many nutrients. Excess calories contribute to overweight. Sugars also contribute to tooth decay. Limit your intake of foods high in sugar and brush your teeth after eating. See 4-6.

Choose and prepare foods with less salt. Salt is a key source of dietary sodium, which is linked with high blood pressure. Restricting salt may help reduce your risk of developing high blood pressure. Much dietary sodium also comes from processed foods and beverages. Read labels to examine the sodium content of foods. Also, limit the amount of salt you add to foods during preparation and at the table.

If you drink alcoholic beverages, do so in moderation. Alcohol merely supplies calories to the diet. Drinking alcohol can be harmful to health. Alcohol can be a contributing factor in accidents, and drinking alcohol can lead to addiction. Excessive alcohol consumption may cause cirrhosis of the liver and inflammation of the pancreas. Damage to the heart and brain and an increased risk for many cancers are also associated with high alcohol consumption.

For teens and children, drinking alcoholic beverages is illegal as well as unhealthful. Children, teens, and pregnant women should completely avoid consuming alcohol. Nursing mothers, alcoholics, and anyone taking medication or planning to drive or operate machinery should also avoid alcohol.

● Using Variety, Moderation, and Balance

Variety, moderation, and *balance* are three words that sum up the spirit of healthful

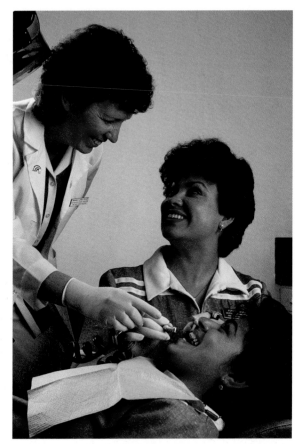

4-6 Choosing a diet moderate in sugars will help reduce the risk of tooth decay.

eating with the Dietary Guidelines. Variety means you should include many different types of foods in your diet. Moderation means you should avoid eating too much of any one type of food. Balance involves selecting some foods that are lower in salt, sugars, saturated fats, cholesterol, and calories. This will help offset food choices that are higher in those components. You also need to choose foods in amounts that are equal to your calorie needs.

The Dietary Guidelines for Americans help people look at eating behaviors with a lifestyle perspective. One day's meals are not nearly as important as the total picture. Work toward improving your eating patterns over the long haul to build a healthful lifestyle.

● The Daily Values on Food Labels

Food labels are another tool that can help you plan your diet. Nutrition Facts on food labels are presented in an easy-to-use form.

As you read the nutrition panel, you will see the term *Daily Value.* **Daily Values** are recommended nutrient intakes based on daily calorie needs. Daily Values for carbohydrate, fat, and protein used as references on food labels are based on a 2,000-calorie diet. The amounts of nutrients in a serving of a food product are expressed as a percentage of these Daily Values.

Most food labels do not have enough room to list all nutrients for each age range and sex. Therefore, labels highlight only the nutrients most important to the health of today's consumer. Percent Daily Values are listed for fat, saturated fat, cholesterol, sodium, carbohydrate, fiber, vitamin A, vitamin C, calcium, and iron.

Learn to use the percent Daily Values to see how foods contribute to your daily nutrient needs. Ask yourself what combination of foods you can eat throughout the day to get 100 percent of your Daily Values. You can also use the percent Daily Values to compare the nutrient content of different brands and products. For instance, you might compare the protein content of two brands of baked beans. Then you might compare the protein in baked beans with the protein in a canned chicken dinner. Such comparisons will help you get the most nutrition for your food dollar. (You will read more about how to use food labels in Chapter 22, "Making Wise Consumer Choices.") See 4-7.

● Nutrient Density

Is a baked potato better for you than a bag of potato chips? You can use nutrient density as a tool to help you answer this question. **Nutrient density** is a comparison

Nutrition Facts		
Serving Size 1 cup (228g)		
Servings Per Container 2		
Amount Per Serving		
Calories 260	Calories from Fat 120	
		% Daily Value*
Total Fat 13g		20%
Saturated Fat 10g		50%
Cholesterol 60mg		20%
Sodium 330mg		14%
Total Carbohydrate 31g		10%
Dietary Fiber 5g		20%
Sugars 10g		
Protein 5g		
Vitamin A 15%	•	Vitamin C 8%
Calcium 20%	•	Iron 2%

* Percent Daily Values are based on a 2,000 calorie diet. Your daily values may be higher or lower depending on your calorie needs:

		Calories:	2,000	2,500
Total Fat	Less than		65g	80g
Sat Fat	Less than		20g	25g
Cholesterol	Less than		300mg	300mg
Sodium	Less than		2,400mg	2,400mg
Total Carbohydrate			300g	375g
Dietary Fiber			25g	30g

Calories per gram:
Fat 9 • Carbohydrate 4 • Protein 4

4-7 Nutrition Facts on a food label list the percent Daily Value of various nutrients in each serving of the product.

of the nutrients provided by a food with the calories provided by the food. It is an evaluation of the nutritional quality of a food.

Calculating nutrient density involves looking at a person's daily nutrient and calorie needs. A food that provides a greater percentage of nutrient needs than calorie needs has a *high nutrient density.* A food that provides a lesser percentage of nutrient needs than calorie needs has a *low nutrient density.*

To understand how nutrient density is computed, look at Chart 4-8. Assume a teenage girl needs 2,200 total calories and

Potato Chips

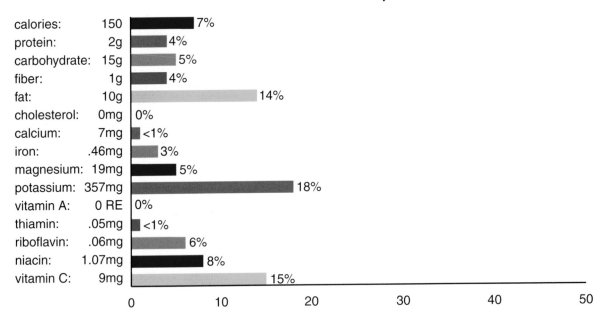

calories:	150	7%
protein:	2g	4%
carbohydrate:	15g	5%
fiber:	1g	4%
fat:	10g	14%
cholesterol:	0mg	0%
calcium:	7mg	<1%
iron:	.46mg	3%
magnesium:	19mg	5%
potassium:	357mg	18%
vitamin A:	0 RE	0%
thiamin:	.05mg	<1%
riboflavin:	.06mg	6%
niacin:	1.07mg	8%
vitamin C:	9mg	15%

Baked Potato

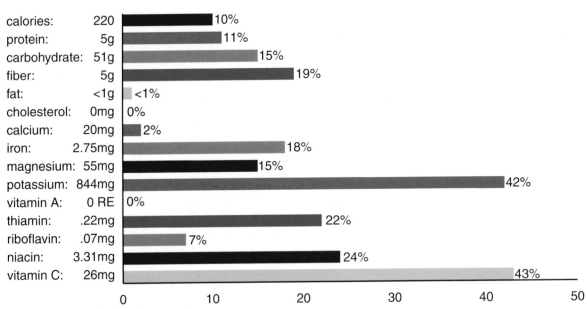

calories:	220	10%
protein:	5g	11%
carbohydrate:	51g	15%
fiber:	5g	19%
fat:	<1g	<1%
cholesterol:	0mg	0%
calcium:	20mg	2%
iron:	2.75mg	18%
magnesium:	55mg	15%
potassium:	844mg	42%
vitamin A:	0 RE	0%
thiamin:	.22mg	22%
riboflavin:	.07mg	7%
niacin:	3.31mg	24%
vitamin C:	26mg	43%

4-8 You can evaluate the nutrient density of a food by comparing the nutrients it provides with the calories it provides.

15 milligrams of iron for the day. As you can see, the potato chips provide 150 calories and 0.46 milligrams of iron per serving. This means the chips supply 7 percent of the young woman's daily calorie needs (150 ÷ 2,200 = .07). However, they supply only 3 percent of her iron needs (0.46 ÷ 15 = .03). This indicates that the chips have a low

nutrient density for iron. By comparison, the baked potato provides 220 calories and 2.75 milligrams of iron. This indicates the baked potato supplies 10 percent of the teen's calorie needs ($220 \div 2,200 = .10$). It also supplies 18 percent of her iron needs ($2.75 \div 15 = .18$). Therefore, the baked potato has a high nutrient density for iron.

You can analyze the ratio of a wide variety of nutrients to calories. A food can have a low density for one nutrient and a high density for another nutrient. Look again at the potato chips. They provide higher percentages of potassium and vitamin C than of iron or thiamin. Comparing serving for serving, however, the baked potato offers more nutrients than the potato chips overall.

You can use your knowledge about nutrient density to help you better the quality of your diet. If your diet does not provide the recommended amounts of nutrients, you can substitute foods to improve it. If you are currently eating foods that have a low nutrient density, substitute foods that have a higher nutrient density.

You may have heard people use terms like *junk food* or *health food* to describe a food's quality. As you begin to analyze foods, you will find there is no such thing as a perfect food. Likewise, there are few foods that supply absolutely no nutrients. Therefore, *junk food* and *health food* are less useful than the terms *low nutrient density* and *high nutrient density.* Every food has the potential to make a dietary contribution. For this to happen, you must make variety, moderation, and balance a part of your diet.

Using Food Recommendations and Guidelines

You now know about a variety of diet planning tools. The next step is to learn how to use them to improve your diet.

Keep a Food Diary

Before you can determine whether you are getting enough nutrients, you need to know what foods you are eating. One way to be aware of what you eat is to keep a food diary. A **food diary** is a record of the kinds and amounts of foods and beverages consumed for a given time. This includes snacks and foods eaten away from home. It also includes condiments, such as catsup, pickles, salad dressings, syrups, and jellies. See 4-9.

You need a complete diary if you want a true analysis of your diet. You will find it easy to forget what you ate if you wait too long to record information. Keeping a pad and pencil handy will help you remember to write down each food item you eat.

For your diet analysis to be valid, you need to accurately estimate your portion sizes. Look at measuring utensils to help you become familiar with the size of amounts like one tablespoon and one cup. Remember that a 3-ounce portion of meat or chicken is about the size of a deck of playing cards. Find out how many ounces your cups, bowls, and glasses hold. This will help you correctly list in your food diary the amounts of foods you consume.

You might want to record what you eat for several days. This will give you a more accurate picture of your eating habits than you will get from a one-day record. You will also get a better account if you record your diary on typical days. Avoid keeping a record on birthdays, holidays, and other days when you are likely to follow different eating patterns.

Analyze Your Diet

Use the information recorded in your food diary to see if you are meeting your daily nutrient needs. A number of software programs are available that can help you quickly analyze your diet with a computer. Most of these programs include a database of *food composition tables.* These tables are a reference guide listing the nutritive

Food Diary

Meal	Amount	Food
Breakfast	2 1.25-ounce packages	instant cinnamon oatmeal
	½ cup	sliced peaches
	1 cup	fat free milk
Snack	¼ cup	raisins
Lunch	1	toasted cheese sandwich
	½ cup	sautéed zucchini
	1	apple
	12 ounces	juice blend
Snack	15	toasted tortilla chips
	2 tablespoons	salsa
Dinner	3 ounces	grilled salmon steak
	½ cup	cooked broccoli
	1 cup	pasta salad with carrots, celery, onions, and olives
	2	whole wheat rolls
	1 cup	fat free milk
	½ cup	frozen lowfat vanilla yogurt
Snack	1	banana

4-9 Keeping a food diary can help you evaluate the nutritional quality of the foods you are eating.

values of many foods in common serving sizes. You can enter data into the computer about the foods you ate. The program can then tell you such information as the calorie and nutrient values of those foods. You can make a detailed printout showing how your daily nutrient values compare to the RDAs and DRIs. This comparison will show you which nutrient needs you have and have not met. See 4-10.

If your analysis indicates your diet is low in some nutrients, refer to Chapters 5 through 9. These chapters discuss sources and functions of many nutrients. They can help you find out what foods you might eat to improve your diet.

If you do not have access to diet analysis software, you can analyze your diet yourself. Make a chart with columns for the foods you ate, calories, and all the major nutrients.

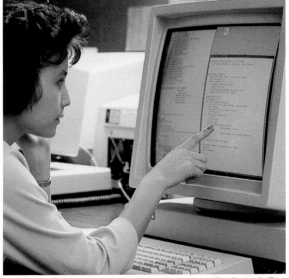

Photo courtesy of University Relations, MSU, Bruce A. Fox, photographer

4-10 Diet analysis software can help you identify nutrients that may be lacking in the foods you eat.

List the foods recorded in your food diary in the first column. Look up each food in the food composition tables found in Appendix C, "Nutritive Values of Foods." Write the amounts of nutrients supplied by each food in the appropriate columns of your chart. After you have filled in all the information for each food, total the amounts in all the nutrient columns. Compare these totals to the RDAs and DRIs.

As you complete your chart, remember to think about serving sizes. Compare the amount of each food you consumed to the serving size listed in the table. If your serving size differs, you will have to adjust the nutrient amounts you list in your chart. For instance, the serving size listed in the table for milk is 1 cup. If you drank 1½ cups, you will have to multiply the quantity of each nutrient listed for milk by 1.5.

You can also use the Food Guide Pyramid to help you analyze your diet. Does your food diary show you are getting the recommended number of daily servings from each food group? The different groups are good sources of different nutrients. Eating the recommended number of servings from each group every day will help you get all the nutrients you need. However, if you are missing a couple of servings, you may be missing some nutrients, too.

● Plan Menus Using the Food Guide Pyramid

Your diet analysis may show you are eating too much of some foods and not enough of others. Planning menus using the Food Guide Pyramid can help you correct such problems. The sample menus in 4-11 show how you might include the recommended number of servings throughout the day. Following this type of menu plan will help you get the balance of nutrients you need.

Eating right may be easier and tastier than you think. The Food Guide Pyramid is flexible enough for anyone to use. It can suit

Menu Planning with the Food Guide Pyramid

Poached Egg on Whole Wheat Toast
Cantaloupe
Fat Free Milk

Blueberry Bagel
Lowfat Strawberry Yogurt

Tomato Stuffed with Tuna Salad
Rye Crackers
Iced Tea
Grapes

Vegetables with Lowfat Dip

Broiled Chicken Breast
Wild Rice Pilaf
Glazed Carrots
Romaine Lettuce with Cilantro-Lime Dressing
Cloverleaf Rolls
Fat Free Milk
Ambrosia

Popcorn

4-11 Using the Food Guide Pyramid can help you plan nutritious meals that provide needed nutrients from a variety of foods. Plan meal and snack menus that include the number of daily servings recommended for most teens.

different family lifestyles, ethnic backgrounds, and religious beliefs. It can accommodate all your favorite foods.

Menu planning with the Pyramid involves a bit more than counting the number of servings from each food group. You also need to think about which foods you choose from each group. Keeping a few tips in mind will help you limit fat, cholesterol, added sugars, and sodium. See 4-12.

Tips for Using the Food Guide Pyramid

Bread, Cereal, Rice, and Pasta Group

Choose whole grain bread and cereal products often. They are rich in fiber.

Avoid adding salt or oil to cooking water when preparing rice or pasta.

Add only half the recommended amount of butter or margarine when preparing pasta and rice mixes.

Read labels to find cereal choices that are low in added sugars.

Choose regular and quick-cooking hot cereals instead of instant products, which tend to be high in sodium.

Choose high-fat cakes and doughnuts less often than bread, rice, and pasta, which tend to be low in fat.

Vegetable Group

Choose fresh vegetables over canned when possible. They are usually lower in sodium.

Use herbs rather than butter and salt to season cooked vegetables.

Choose baked and steamed vegetables over battered and fried varieties.

Fruit Group

Choose whole fruits for a fiber advantage over fruit juices.

Choose fruits canned in juice rather than syrup to limit added sugars.

Milk, Yogurt, and Cheese Group

Use fat free milk and lowfat yogurt over whole milk products.

Look for reduced-fat cheeses as an alternative to regular cheese products.

Use plain, nonfat yogurt as an alternative to sour cream.

Opt for frozen yogurt instead of ice cream.

Meat, Poultry, Fish, Dry Beans, Eggs, and Nuts Group

Choose lean cuts of meat with little visible fat or marbling.

Choose light meat poultry pieces. They are lower in fat than dark meat pieces.

Remove skin from poultry before eating to reduce fat.

Chill meat stocks and gravies and skim off fat before serving.

Limit your use of processed luncheon meats, which tend to be high in fat and sodium.

Choose canned fish packed in water over oil-packed varieties.

When choosing meat alternatives, opt for dried beans more often than nuts. Dried beans are high in fiber, and they lack the high fat content of nuts.

Fats, Oils, and Sweets

Keep portions moderate in size when serving your favorite sweet and high-fat foods.

4-12 These tips will help you make wise choices when selecting foods from each group in the Food Guide Pyramid.

Summary

Experts have developed a number of tools to help people evaluate their diets and make wise food choices. The Dietary Reference Intakes (DRIs) are nutrient recommendations healthy people can use to evaluate their diets. The Food Guide Pyramid gives a range of daily servings for five food groups to help people plan sound diets. The Dietary Guidelines for Americans are ten recommendations designed to help people know what to eat to maintain good health. Daily Values on food labels show how servings of food products contribute to daily nutrient needs. Nutrient density helps people compare the nutrients foods provide with the calories they provide.

You can learn how to use all these tools to improve your diet. Start by using a food diary to keep track of the kinds and amounts of foods and beverages you consume. Then use the information you collect and diet analysis software to see if you are meeting your daily nutrient needs. You should also note the number of servings from each group in the Food Guide Pyramid you eat each day. Use the recommendations of the Pyramid to plan balanced menus that will help you meet nutrient needs.

As you learn to use the tools for planning a healthful diet, you will hear a few messages repeated. Balance your diet by eating a variety of foods from all the food groups. Always use moderation when selecting foods. Eat plenty of grains, vegetables, and fruits. To avoid certain health risks, avoid alcohol and consume only limited amounts of foods high in saturated fat, cholesterol, sugar, and salt.

Check Your Knowledge

1. True or false. There is an RDA for every known nutrient.
2. How many servings from each group in the Food Guide Pyramid should you include in your daily menu plans?
3. True or false. Foods in all groups of the Food Guide Pyramid can contain fats and sugars.
4. Give one example of a serving size for each food group in the Food Guide Pyramid.
5. Why were the Dietary Guidelines for Americans developed?
6. What do the Dietary Guidelines recommend for teens in terms of physical activity?
7. What is the recommended limit for saturated fat in the diet?
8. Daily Values used as references on food labels are based on a _____ calorie diet.
9. What determines if a food has a high nutrient density?
10. Give two tips for keeping a food diary that will increase the validity of a diet analysis.
11. What are food composition tables?
12. Give one tip for making wise choices when selecting foods from each group in the Food Guide Pyramid.

Put Learning into Action

1. Choose three food products from each of two food groups of the Food Guide Pyramid. Study the Nutrition Facts panels on all six products. In a brief oral report, summarize your conclusions about the nutrients provided by each of the two food groups.
2. With your classmates, develop questions to use in surveying people about how well they follow the Dietary Guidelines for Americans. Also develop a rating scale respondents can use in answering the questions. Then survey two people from different demographic groups. Compile your findings with those of your classmates. Summarize your general conclusions in an article for the school newspaper.

3. Find one of your favorite foods listed in Appendix C, "Nutritive Values of Foods." Compare the nutrients the food provides with your daily nutrient needs as shown in Appendix B, "Recommended Nutrient Intakes." Prepare a bar graph similar to Figure 4-8 to illustrate the percentage of each nutrient need met by the food. Write a brief report describing the food's nutrient density.

● Explore Further

1. Investigate how the DRIs are being developed. Choose a specific nutrient for which DRIs have been determined. Write a report explaining how the DRIs compare to the previous edition of RDAs for this nutrient. Include reasons given in the DRI report for any changes in recommendations.

2. Keep a food diary for three days. List all foods and beverages consumed, including snack foods and condiments. Note the amount of each item you consumed in common serving sizes. Use your diary and nutrient analysis software to identify nutrients in which your intakes are low. Suggest ways to improve your diet.

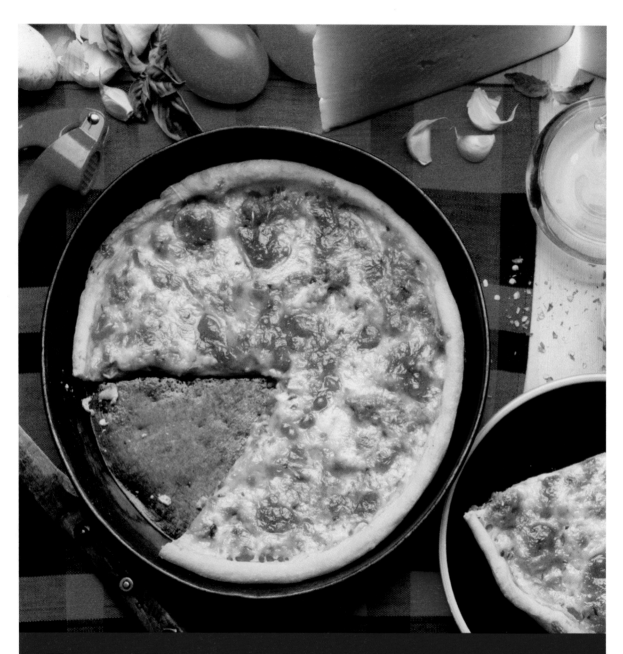

Part Two
The Health Effects of Energy Nutrients

Chapter 5

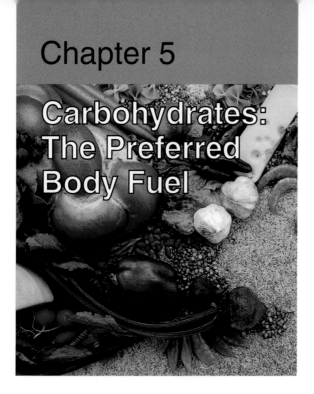

Carbohydrates: The Preferred Body Fuel

● Objectives

After studying this chapter, you will be able to
- describe the three types of carbohydrates.
- list the functions of carbohydrates.
- explain how the body uses carbohydrates.
- use food labels to meet your carbohydrate needs.
- evaluate the role of carbohydrates in a variety of health issues.

What comes to mind when you hear the word *carbohydrates?* If you are thinking potatoes, bread, rice, spaghetti, or fruits, you are correct. If your thoughts lead you to fattening foods, you might think differently after you read this chapter.

Carbohydrates are one of the six essential nutrients and are your body's main source of energy. They are the sugars, starches, and fibers in your diet. Except for the natural sugar in milk, nearly all carbohydrates come from plant sources.

Carbohydrates should form the bulk of your diet. Many nutrition experts recommend 55 to 60 percent of your daily calories should come from carbohydrates. The Food Guide Pyramid shows a variety of carbohydrate foods make up the foundation of a healthful diet.

● Types of Carbohydrates

Carbohydrates are made of three common chemical elements: carbon, hydrogen, and oxygen. These elements are bonded together to form *saccharides,* or sugar units. The elements can be combined in several ways. The arrangement of the elements determines the type of sugar unit. Sugar units may be linked in various arrangements to form different types of carbohydrates. See 5-1.

● Monosaccharides

Monosaccharides are carbohydrates composed of single sugar units. (The prefix *mono-* means one.) These are the smallest carbohydrate molecules. The three monosaccharides are glucose, fructose, and galactose. **Glucose** is sometimes called *blood sugar* because it circulates in the bloodstream. It is the body's source of energy. *Fructose* has the sweetest taste of all sugars. It occurs naturally in fruits and honey.

Carbohydrate Structures

Monosaccharides

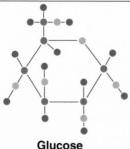

Glucose   **Fructose**

Both monosaccharide molecules contain 6 carbon atoms, 12 hydrogen atoms, and 6 oxygen atoms. However, the elements are arranged differently in each molecule.

Disaccharides

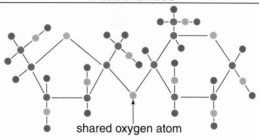

shared oxygen atom

Sucrose

A molecule of fructose bonded to a molecule of glucose forms the disaccharide sucrose. The two molecules share an oxygen atom. Notice that this disaccharide contains one fewer oxygen atom and two fewer hydrogen atoms than the two separate monosaccharide molecules. This is because a molecule of water (H_2O) was released when the bond was formed.

Polysaccharides

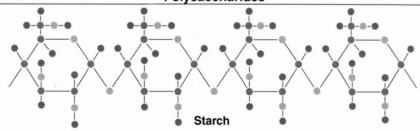

Starch

This is just a small part of a starch chain, which is made up of many glucose molecules bonded together.

Key
● carbon atom
● hydrogen atom
● oxygen atom

5-1 Carbohydrates are all made of different arrangements of carbon, hydrogen, and oxygen.

Galactose does not occur alone as a monosaccharide in foods. Instead, it is found bonded to glucose. Together, these two monosaccharides form the sugar in milk. See 5-2.

Disaccharides

The **disaccharides** are made up of two sugar units. (The prefix *di-* means two.) The body splits disaccharides into monosaccharides during digestion. The disaccharides are sucrose, maltose, and lactose. All the mono- and disaccharides are collectively referred to as **sugars**.

Sucrose is the sugar you use in recipes or add to foods at the table. It is made of one glucose molecule and one fructose molecule that are bonded together. Sucrose is found in many foods. Beet sugar, cane sugar, molasses, and maple syrup are concentrated sources of sucrose.

Lactose is found in milk. It is made of one glucose molecule and one galactose molecule that are bonded together. Lactose serves as a source of energy for breast-fed infants.

Maltose is made of two glucose molecules that are bonded together. It is formed during the digestion of starch. It may also be found in certain grains, such as malt.

Polysaccharides

Polysaccharides are carbohydrates that are made up of many sugar units. (The prefix *poly-* means many.) These units are linked in long, straight chains or branched chains. Like the disaccharides, the polysaccharides must be broken down during digestion. Starches and fibers are polysaccharides.

Starch is a polysaccharide that is the storage form of energy in plants. Starch is made of many glucose molecules that are bonded together. Grain products, such as breads and cereals, and starchy vegetables, such as corn, potatoes, and legumes, are high in starch. See 5-3.

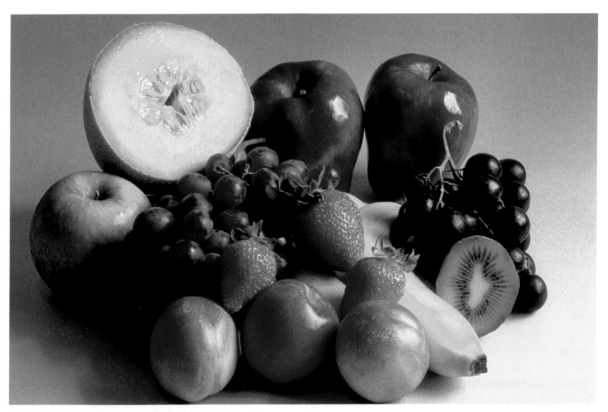

5-2 Fructose is the sugar found in fruit.

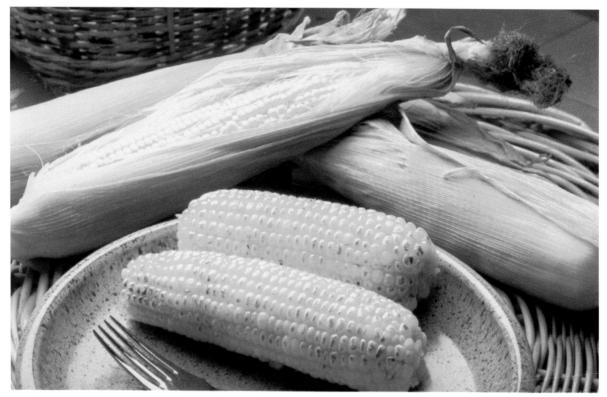

5-3 Corn plants store energy as starch in kernels of grain. When you eat these starchy kernels, they become a source of energy for you.

Fibers are polysaccharides that make up the tough, fibrous cell walls of plants. These carbohydrates are found only in plant foods. Human digestive enzymes cannot digest fibers, but bacteria in the digestive tract can break down some fibers. Because most fibers pass through the digestive system unchanged, these carbohydrates provide almost no energy (calories). *Cellulose, gums,* and *pectin* are some types of fibers.

Because of their simple molecular structures, monosaccharides and disaccharides are considered **simple carbohydrates**. When people talk about eating simple carbohydrates, they are generally referring to foods that are high in simple sugars. Such foods include table sugar, candy, syrups, and soft drinks. Polysaccharides have a larger, more intricate molecular structure. Therefore, they are considered **complex carbohydrates**. When people talk about eating

complex carbohydrates, they are referring to foods that are high in starch and fiber. Breads, cereals, rice, pasta, and vegetables are all sources of complex carbohydrates. See 5-4.

The distinction between simple and complex carbohydrates is important when making food choices. Choosing more food sources of complex carbohydrates and fewer sources of simple carbohydrates has health and nutrition benefits. You will read about these benefits later in the chapter.

● The Functions of Carbohydrates

Carbohydrates serve four key functions. They provide energy, spare proteins, assist in the breakdown of fats, and provide bulk in the diet.

Types and Classifications of Carbohydrates

Simple Carbohydrates	
Monosaccharides	**Disaccharides**
Glucose	Sucrose
Fructose	Lactose
Galactose	Maltose
Complex Carbohydrates	
Polysaccharides	
Starch	Fiber

5-4 The arrangement of atoms and sugar units that make up carbohydrates determines their type and classification.

Produce Energy

Meeting the energy needs of all your cells as they work to sustain life is your body's main goal. Carbohydrates provide 4 calories of energy per gram. Carbohydrates are the preferred source of energy because your body can use them so efficiently. However, if you do not consume enough carbohydrates, your body will draw mainly on proteins for fuel needs.

Spare Proteins

If necessary, your body can use proteins as an energy source. Your body is less efficient in using proteins for energy than it is in using carbohydrates. More importantly, if you eat too little carbohydrate, your body will not be able to use proteins to build and maintain cell structures. By eating adequate amounts of carbohydrates, you spare the proteins. That means you allow the proteins to be used for their more vital roles. See 5-5.

Break Down Fats

If the diet is too low in carbohydrates, the body cannot completely break down fats. Incompletely broken down fats form compounds called *ketone bodies.* These compounds then collect in the bloodstream, causing the blood to become more acidic than normal. This acidity can damage cells and organs. This condition is called *ketosis.* A person in ketosis

has a characteristic "nail polish remover" smell to his or her breath. He or she also feels nauseous and weak. If the ketosis continues, the person can go into a coma and die.

Provide Bulk in the Diet

One other important function of carbohydrates is to add bulk to the diet. Fiber is the carbohydrate responsible for this task. It helps promote normal digestion and elimination of body wastes.

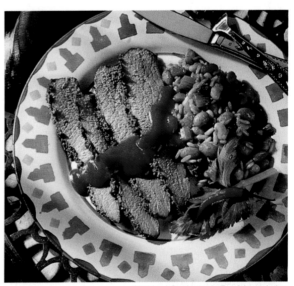

National Cattleman's Beef Association

5-5 In this meal, the carbohydrates in the beans and rice supply energy, allowing the proteins in the meat to be used for other functions.

Like the muscles in your arms and legs, the muscles in your digestive tract need a healthy workout. Fiber is the solid material that provides this workout, helping intestinal muscles retain their tone.

Fiber acts like a sponge. It absorbs water, which softens stools and helps prevent constipation. Softer stools are easier to pass, reducing the likelihood of *hemorrhoids,* which are swollen veins in the rectum. Some fibers form gels that add bulk to stools. This helps relieve diarrhea.

Bulk in the diet has added benefits for people who are trying to lose weight. As fiber swells, it helps you feel full. Fiber also slows the rate at which the stomach empties. Fibrous food sources are usually lower in calories than foods high in fat, too. See 5-6.

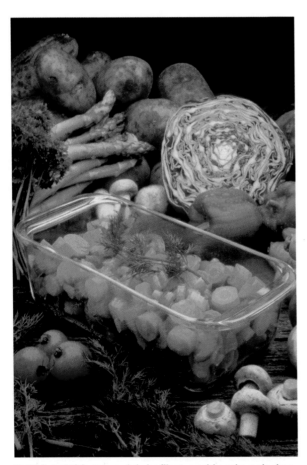

5-6 Vegetables are rich in fiber and low in calories.

● **Other Benefits of Fiber in the Diet**

Fiber has been shown to have many benefits besides providing bulk in the diet. Current interest in fiber stems from observations made by British scientists around 1923. They noted African populations had lower rates of certain GI tract diseases, such as colon cancer, than Western industrialized populations. This led the scientists to study eating pattern differences. They found people in Western countries had rather low fiber intakes. In contrast, people in the African nations tended to have high fiber intakes. The scientists hypothesized the difference in the disease rate could be related to the difference in fiber consumption.

A variety of studies have been carried out to find out more about the role fiber plays in promoting wellness. Research results indicate including plenty of fiber in a lowfat diet appears to have many health benefits. For example, dietary fiber can help prevent *appendicitis,* which is an inflammation of the appendix. It may lower the risks of heart and artery disease. Dietary fiber may reduce the risk of colon cancer. It also helps control diabetes mellitus.

● **Different Fibers Have Different Effects**

Fibers vary in their composition and the jobs they perform in the GI tract. **Soluble fibers** can dissolve in water and develop a gel-like consistency. These are the fibers that help lower blood cholesterol levels. Oat bran, legumes, and apple and citrus pectins are sources of soluble fiber. See 5-7.

Insoluble fibers do not dissolve in water. These fibers are associated with reducing cancer risks. Wheat bran and whole grains are high in insoluble fiber.

As you can see, both types of fiber have positive effects on health. Many plant foods contain a combination of fibers. Eating a variety of fruits, vegetables, and whole grains will give you the full range of benefits from dietary fiber. These foods also provide other nutrients, including starch, protein, vitamins, and minerals.

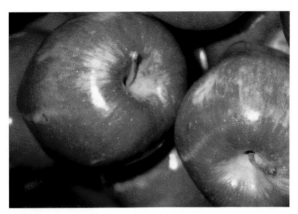

5-7 Apple pectin is a soluble fiber.

● How Your Body Uses Carbohydrates

Eating carbohydrates, regardless of their source, sets off a complex chain of events in your body. The way your body uses carbohydrates is explained here in simplified terms.

All carbohydrates must be in the form of glucose for your cells to use them as an energy source. To get them into this form, your digestive system first breaks down poly- and disaccharides from foods into monosaccharides. The monosaccharides are small enough to move across the intestinal wall into the blood. They travel via the blood to the liver. Any fructose and galactose in the blood is converted to glucose in the liver.

When the amount of glucose in the blood rises (this happens after you eat), a hormone called insulin is released from the pancreas. **Hormones** are chemicals produced in the body and released into the bloodstream to regulate specific body processes. **Insulin** helps the body lower blood glucose back to a normal level. It does this by triggering body cells to burn glucose for energy. It also causes muscles and the liver to store glucose.

If your cells do not have immediate energy needs, they store the glucose they took in from the bloodstream. They convert the glucose to glycogen. **Glycogen** is the body's storage form of glucose. Two-thirds of your body's glycogen is stored in your muscles for use as an energy source during muscular activity. Your liver stores the other one-third of the glycogen for use by the rest of your body. See 5-8.

Your liver can store only a limited amount of glycogen. You need to eat carbohydrates throughout the day to keep your glycogen stores replenished. However, suppose you eat more carbohydrates than your body can immediately use or store as glycogen. In this case, your liver will convert the excess carbohydrates into fat. An unlimited amount of fat can be stored in the fatty tissues of your body. Unlike glycogen stores, fat stores cannot be converted back into glucose.

If a candy bar and a sandwich both end up as glucose, you may wonder why it matters which you eat. The candy bar provides little more than simple sugars. The sandwich, on the other hand, supplies vitamins, minerals, and protein as well as complex carbohydrates.

In addition, complex carbohydrates take longer to digest than simple carbohydrates. This gives complex carbohydrates greater satiety value. **Satiety** is a term used to describe the feeling of fullness you have after eating food. The sandwich is higher in complex carbohydrates. Therefore, you are likely to feel full longer after eating the sandwich than after eating the candy bar.

● Meeting Your Carbohydrate Needs

Many popular foods, including breads, pasta, ice cream, and baked goods, are rich sources of carbohydrates. Even so, the typical diet in the United States falls short of the daily recommendation for carbohydrates. Most experts agree the average diet also has an excess of simple carbohydrates and too few complex carbohydrates.

How does your diet compare with this average? Do you often choose foods like milk shakes, candy, soft drinks, and pastries that

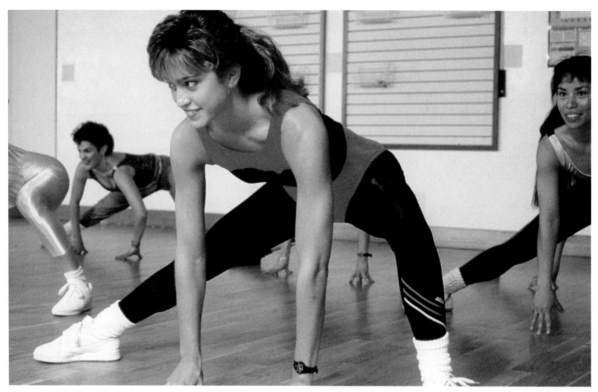

5-8 During physical activity, your body uses glycogen stored in the muscles for energy.

are high in simple sugars? Do you choose complex carbohydrates like rice, vegetables, and legumes less often? Just what are your carbohydrate needs, and how can you choose foods to meet them?

● Sugars

You can divide sugars in foods into two categories. The first category includes sugars that occur naturally in foods. These sugars include lactose in milk and fructose in fruits. Naturally occurring sugars are generally accompanied by other nutrients in foods. Therefore, they do not cause great concern among nutrition experts.

The second category of sugars includes sugars added to foods at the table or during processing. These sugars are sometimes called *refined sugars*. **Refined sugars** are carbohydrate sweeteners that are separated from their natural sources for use as food additives. They come from such sources as

sugar cane, sugar beets, and corn. Refined sugars function as more than sweetening agents. They may also be added to foods to increase bulk or aid in browning. See 5-9.

Soft drinks are the main source of sugar in teen diets. Many other foods that are high in sugar, such as candy, cakes, cookies, and donuts, are high in fat, too. Eating too many of these foods can mean too many calories and not enough nutrients. This can lead to overweight and malnutrition.

Many processed foods, such as catsup and cereals, are also high in added sugars. Although sugar is an excellent source of simple carbohydrates, it contributes no other nutrients to foods. In other words, sugars increase the calories a food provides without increasing the nutrients it provides. This means added sugars reduce the nutrient density of processed foods. (Review Chapter 4, "Nutrition Guidelines," for more information about nutrient density.)

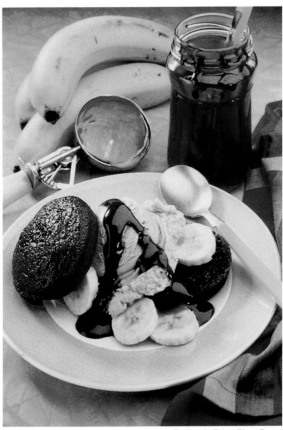

California Dried Plum Board

5-9 Most desserts get their sweet taste from refined sugars.

sources of refined sugars. Many experts recommend reducing this figure. They suggest limiting added sugar intake to no more than 25 percent of total calorie intake. That means someone who needs 2,000 calories a day should obtain no more than 500 calories from refined sugars. Sugars, as well as starches, provide 4 calories per gram. Therefore, this person's daily limit for refined sugars is about 125 grams. For reference, a teaspoon of sugar equals about 4 grams of carbohydrates. This means a person following a 2,000-calorie diet should limit intake to about 31 teaspoons of sugar a day. That is the number of teaspoons in three to four cans of most regular soft drinks.

You may be surprised how quickly sugars can add up in your diet. A bowl of sweetened cereal for breakfast might contain 3 teaspoons of refined sugar. A carton of fruit-flavored yogurt for lunch would provide 7 more teaspoons. A soft drink and a small package of chocolate candies for a snack furnish 16 to 20 teaspoons. A piece of cake with dinner would add another 9 teaspoons. This totals at least 35 teaspoons of refined sugars. This is more than the recommended daily limit for a 2,000-calorie diet.

● Starches

As mentioned, starches are the preferred source of fuel for your diet. Your body can burn them efficiently for energy, and they have greater satiety value than simple sugars. Many starchy foods are also excellent sources of vitamins, minerals, and fiber. See 5-10.

Nutrition experts recommend a minimum of 20 percent of your calories should come from complex carbohydrates. A person needing 2,000 calories a day should be consuming at least 400 calories a day from starches. This equals about 100 grams of starches per day.

Following the Food Guide Pyramid will help you achieve this goal. The breads, cereals, rice, and pasta group is an excellent

Another group of foods that often includes much added sugar is reduced fat and fat free products. Many consumers are aware that foods high in fat are also high in calories. To limit their calorie intake, consumers are buying products like reduced fat crackers and fat free cookies. However, these products often have as many calories as regular crackers and cookies. This is because manufacturers often add sugar to products when they remove fat. Some consumers mistakenly think they can eat more when they choose reduced fat snacks. These consumers may end up gaining weight rather than losing it.

People in the United States are eating more sweets than ever before. Soft drinks, candy, pastries, and other sweets are major source of foods high in starch. Foods in the vegetable group and legumes from the meat and beans group are high in starch, too.

● Fiber

The DRI for fiber is 38 grams per day for males ages 14 through 50. The DRI is 26 grams per day for 14- to 18-year old females. For women ages 19 through 50, the DRI decreases to 25 grams daily. These recommendations are based on intakes that have been shown to help protect against heart disease. For most people, meeting these recommendations means at least doubling their current intakes of fiber.

You can begin increasing your fiber intake by choosing whole grain products in place of refined grain products whenever possible. *Whole grain* products contain all three edible parts of the grain kernel: the bran, the germ, and the endosperm. The *bran* is the outer layer of the grain, which is a good source of fiber. The *germ* is the nutrient-rich part of the

kernel. The *endosperm* is the largest part of the kernel and contains mostly starch. *Refined* grain products have had the bran and germ, and consequently most of the fiber, removed during processing. White flour and white rice are examples of refined grain products. See 5-11.

Some people use fiber supplements to add fiber to their diets. A **supplement** is a concentrated source of a nutrient, usually in pill, liquid, or powder form. Supplements do not offer the range of nutritional benefits provided by food sources of nutrients.

For most people, fiber supplements are unnecessary. Meeting your fiber needs is fairly easy if you eat the recommended number of servings from the Food Guide Pyramid. An average serving of most whole grain breads and cereals, vegetables, and fruits provides two grams of fiber. Dry beans provide up to eight grams per serving.

As you change your eating habits, it is a good idea to increase your intake of dietary fiber slowly. This helps your body adjust. A

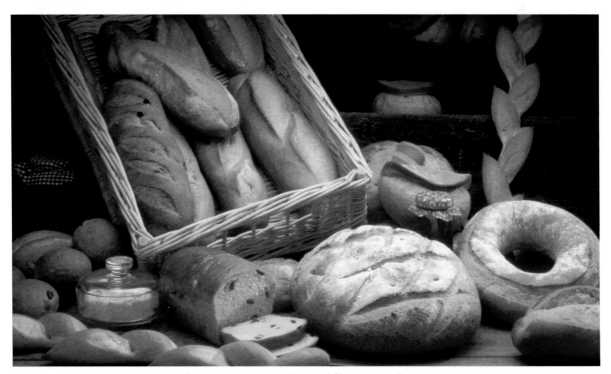

5-10 Whole grain breads supply vitamins, minerals, and fiber as well as starch.

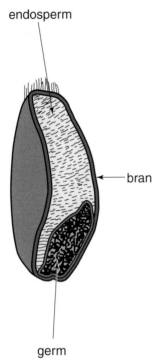

endosperm

bran

germ

5-11 The germ and the fiber-rich bran layer are removed when grains are refined. Choose whole grain bread and cereal products for the nutrients contained in all three parts of the kernel.

sudden large increase of dietary fiber may cause digestive discomfort. Also, be sure to drink plenty of water as you increase your fiber intake.

Using Food Labels to Meet Your Carbohydrate Needs

Reading food labels can help you meet your carbohydrate needs. Total carbohydrates provided by foods are listed on Nutrition Facts panels in grams. The number of grams includes both naturally occurring and added carbohydrates. Underneath this figure, you will see the number of grams of dietary fiber and sugars per serving.

Reading the ingredient lists on food labels can help you identify foods that contain added carbohydrates. Ingredient lists can also help you spot foods that are high in refined sugars. Ingredients are listed in order of weight, with the most predominant ingredient being listed first. Only added carbohydrates will be listed as ingredients. Check to see if sugar appears near the beginning of the list. Also, check to see if more than one type of sugar is listed. These are both indications a product is high in refined sugars. See 5-12.

Health Questions Related to Carbohydrates

As you read about the importance of carbohydrates in your diet, you may find yourself thinking of specific questions. Many teens and their parents want to know the answers to these frequently asked questions.

Are Starchy Foods Fattening?

Some people believe eating foods high in starch causes weight gain. Starchy foods are rich in carbohydrates. Gram per gram, carbohydrates have the same amount of calories (4) as protein. They have less than half the calories (9) of fat.

One reason some people think starchy foods are fattening may be related to the way these foods are served. Pasta is often served with cream sauce, rice with gravy, and baked potatoes with sour cream. Such high-fat toppings can send the total calories in carbohydrate dishes soaring. Consider the example of a slice of bread, which has about 12 grams of carbohydrate and 65 calories. Spreading the bread with a teaspoon of butter would add 4 grams of fat and 36 more calories. If you are trying to cut calories out of your diet, try limiting the fatty toppings, not the carbohydrates.

Carbohydrates Added to Foods

Type of Carbohydrate	Functions
Starches – arrowroot, cornstarch, potato starch, rice flour, tapioca, wheat flour	Provide bulk and structure, stabilize gels, thicken foods
Gums and pectins – algin, carageenan, gum agar, gum Arabic, gum tragacanth, karaya gum	Mimic the texture and viscosity of fat, thicken and stabilize mixtures
Simple sugars – brown sugar, corn sweetener, corn syrup, dextrose, fructose, glucose, high-fructose corn syrup, honey, invert sugar, lactose, maltose, molasses, sucrose	Add sweetness, enhance browning, form syrups, preserve foods

5-12 Food scientists have found many beneficial uses for carbohydrates as additives to food products. Become familiar with these names of carbohydrates, which are among those that appear on food labels.

Is Sugar a Hazard to Your Teeth?

There is a clear connection between sweets and *dental caries* (tooth decay). People who eat much sugar are likely to have a higher incidence of tooth decay than people who eat less sugar. However, sugar is not the only culprit. Starches can promote tooth decay, too.

Bacteria that live in the mouth feed on the carbohydrates in food particles. The bacteria form a sticky substance called *plaque* that clings to teeth. As the bacteria grow, they produce acid that eats away the protective tooth enamel, forming pits in the teeth. In time, these pits can deepen into cavities.

The risk of dental caries depends on two main factors: the type of food and when you eat it. Sticky, carbohydrate foods, like raisins, cookies, crackers, and caramels, tend to cling to teeth. They are more harmful than foods that are quickly swallowed and removed from contact with the teeth. Likewise, sugars and starches eaten between meals tend to be more harmful to tooth enamel than carbohydrates consumed at meals. This is because particles from between-meal snacks tend to remain in the mouth for longer periods. Carbohydrates eaten during meals are removed from the mouth by beverages and other foods eaten with them.

Avoiding sticky carbohydrate-rich foods between meals is good advice for keeping teeth healthy. If you do eat sticky foods, drink plenty of water to wash the teeth. If brushing and flossing your teeth are possible, this is even better. See 5-13.

People who care for young children should know tooth damage can begin in early infancy. Regularly allowing a baby to sleep with a bottle in his or her mouth can destroy the baby's teeth. The acids formed

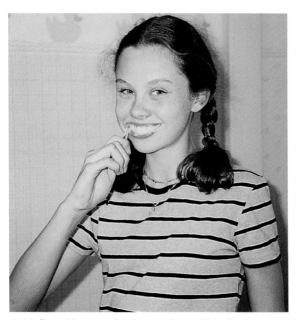

5-13 Brushing teeth after eating will help prevent a buildup of plaque that can lead to tooth decay.

by constant contact of bacteria with sugars in the milk will erode the baby's tooth enamel. After feeding, caregivers should gently clean babies' gums and teeth by wiping them with a soft, clean cloth.

● Does Sugar Cause Hyperactivity?

Hyperactivity is a condition in which a person seems to be in constant motion and is easily distracted. Children with this condition may disrupt their classmates and have trouble concentrating on their schoolwork. Many teachers and parents have observed children are more active after parties and other events at which sweets are served. This has led some people to believe sugar causes hyperactivity.

Although researchers have conducted many studies, they have found no proof that consuming sugars causes behavior changes in most people. It is true eating sugars gives children energy needed to fuel activity. However, children at a party may exhibit rowdy behavior simply because they are excited. After all, eating and playing with friends are fun, social activities. Caregivers may find leading children in less-active games at the end of a party helps reduce post-party excitement. See 5-14.

Caregivers should also keep in mind that children who eat large amounts of sweets may be missing some important nutrients. If you know a child who has trouble concentrating, look at his or her total diet. Eating a well-balanced diet that includes fewer sweets and more nutritious snacks can help improve performance.

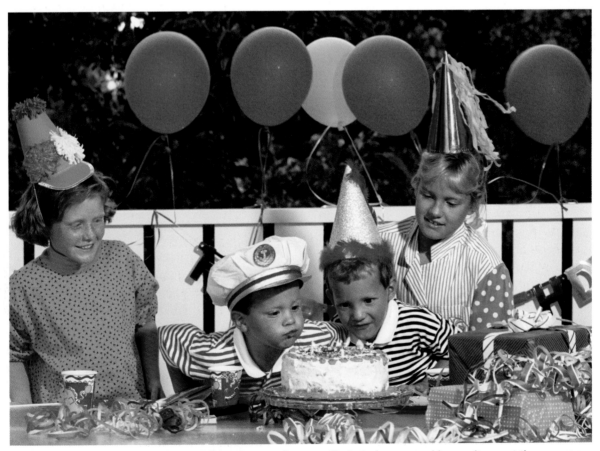

5-14 Unruly behavior following a children's party is more likely to be caused by excitement than sugar consumption.

● Is Sugar Addictive?

Some people seem to crave sweets all the time. There are those who believe this type of craving qualifies as an *addiction,* or a habitual need.

Experiments have shown that if animals do not have a nutritious diet, they will eat excessive amounts of sugar. When the animals are allowed to eat a variety of foods, they seem to be less dependent on sugar. This indicates the animals did not truly need the sugar. Therefore, *addiction* is not the best word to use to explain the animals' excessive use of sugar.

Research has shown people are born with a preference for sweet-tasting foods. However, people may not respond to sugar in the same way as test animals. Researchers now seem to think the need for sugar is more psychological than physiological. In other words, people seem to eat sweets because they enjoy them, not because they are addicted to them.

● Will Too Much Sugar Cause Diabetes?

Diabetes mellitus is a lack of or an inability to use the hormone insulin. Sugars and starches in the foods you eat are converted to glucose, which then enters the bloodstream. Insulin regulates the blood glucose level by stimulating cells to pull glucose from the bloodstream. When the body does not make enough insulin, or fails to use insulin correctly, glucose builds up in the bloodstream.

There are two main types of diabetes. In Type I, or *insulin-dependent* diabetes, the pancreas is not able to make insulin. This type of diabetes occurs most often in children and young adults. People with Type I diabetes must take daily injections of insulin to maintain normal blood glucose levels.

In Type II, or *noninsulin-dependent* diabetes, body cells do not respond well to the insulin the pancreas makes. This type of

diabetes is much more common, and it usually occurs in adults over age 40. People who are overweight and eat diets high in refined carbohydrates and low in fiber are at greater risk of developing this type of diabetes. People in the later stages of this disease may require insulin injections. In the earlier stages, however, Type II diabetes can often be controlled with diet and physical activity. See 5-15.

Both types of diabetes tend to run in families. Symptoms of both types include excessive hunger and thirst accompanied by weakness, irritability, and nausea. Changes in eyesight; slow healing of cuts; drowsiness; and numbness in legs, feet, or fingers are symptoms, too.

In both types of diabetes, the blood glucose level rises too high. Although eating sugar increases the blood glucose level, it does not cause diabetes to develop. However, diabetics need to regulate their sugar intake by following a diet plan prescribed by a physician or registered dietitian.

● What Is Hypoglycemia?

Hypoglycemia refers to a low blood glucose level. An overproduction of insulin causes blood sugar to drop sharply two to four hours after eating a meal. The central nervous system depends on a constant supply of glucose from the blood. Low blood sugar causes physical symptoms of sweating, shaking, headaches, hunger, and anxiety.

A medical test is required to diagnose true hypoglycemia. This condition is rare and may point to a more severe health problem. Many people who believe they have hypoglycemia may just be reacting to stress.

The dietary advice for hypoglycemics is sensible for all people. That is, avoid eating large amounts of sugar all at once. Also, eat nutritious meals at regular intervals.

● What Is Lactose Intolerance?

Lactose intolerance is an inability to digest lactose, the main carbohydrate in

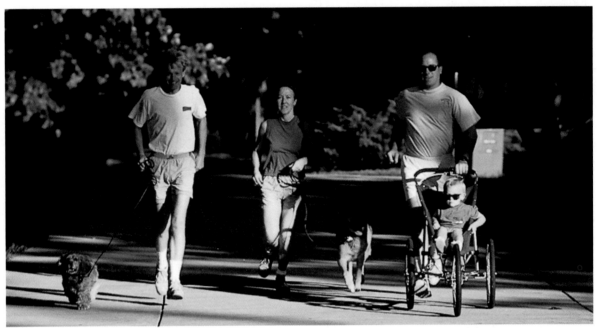

Photo courtesy of University Relations, MSU, Bruce A. Fox, photographer

5-15 Regular physical exercise plays an important role in controlling Type II diabetes.

milk. This condition is caused by a lack of the digestive enzyme *lactase,* which is needed to break down lactose. People who are lactose intolerant may experience gas, cramping, nausea, and diarrhea when they consume dairy products.

Lactose intolerance is common throughout the world. It occurs more often among nonwhite populations and tends to develop as people age.

Milk and milk products are the chief sources of calcium and vitamin D in the diet. These nutrients help build strong bones and teeth. They are especially important for children and pregnant women. People who do not consume dairy products must use care to eat and drink adequate sources of calcium and vitamin D.

People who are unable to drink milk must meet their calcium needs from other sources. Some people can tolerate small amounts of milk if they consume it with a meal. They may also be able to consume milk alternates like yogurt, cheese, and buttermilk. Lactose in these products is changed to lactic acid or broken down into glucose and galactose during the culturing process. Another option is to take lactase pills or add lactase drops to dairy foods. See 5-16.

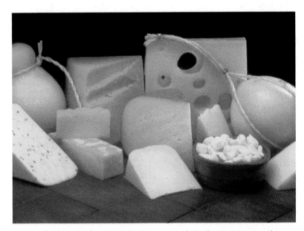

5-16 Someone who is lactose intolerant may be able to digest cheese more easily than milk.

Summary

Carbohydrates are sugars, starches, and fibers in the diet. Simple carbohydrates are called *sugars.* They include the mono- and disaccharides. Complex carbohydrates include starches and fibers. They are also called *polysaccharides.* Breads, pasta, rice, vegetables, fruits, milk, yogurt, legumes, and sweets are all sources of carbohydrates.

Carbohydrates supply four calories per gram and are the body's most important energy source. They spare proteins in the diet for other important functions. Carbohydrates also help with fat metabolism, and they provide bulk in the diet as fiber. In addition, fiber may help people manage weight and lower risks of heart disease, cancer, and intestinal disorders.

During digestion, carbohydrates are broken down and converted into glucose with the help of the liver. The bloodstream delivers glucose to cells where it is used for energy or converted to glycogen for storage. Insulin from the pancreas helps regulate this process. Excess carbohydrates are converted into fat.

Carbohydrates should make up a large portion of your diet. About half of your daily calories should come from complex carbohydrates. However, many experts recommend limiting your intake of refined sugars to no more than 10 percent of daily calories. They also suggest most people increase their intake of dietary fiber. Reading food labels can help you meet these dietary goals.

Some people have concerns about including carbohydrates in their diets. These people may be relieved to know carbohydrates are not fattening, although they are often served with high-calorie toppings. Sugars and starches that remain in contact with the teeth promote dental caries, but good dental hygiene can reduce problems. Also, sugar has not been proven to cause hyperactivity, nor has it been shown to be addictive.

A number of health questions are related to carbohydrates. Diabetes Type I and Type II affect how the body responds to carbohydrates, but sugar does not cause diabetes. Hypoglycemia, which is a low blood glucose level, can often be controlled by regularly consuming meals high in complex carbohydrates. Lactose intolerance, which is an inability to digest milk sugar, may be controlled through careful use of dairy products.

Check Your Knowledge

1. Name two monosaccharides and two disaccharides.
2. How do simple carbohydrates differ from complex carbohydrates?
3. If the diet does not provide enough carbohydrates, how will the body meet its needs for energy?
4. What are two benefits of fiber in the diet for people who are trying to lose weight?
5. True or false. A person is likely to feel full longer after eating a soft pretzel than after eating cotton candy.
6. Where is the body's glycogen stored and how is it used?
7. Why do refined sugars in the diet cause greater concern among nutrition experts than naturally occurring sugars?
8. If a person needs 3,000 calories per day, about how many of those calories should come from complex carbohydrates?
9. List three food sources of fiber.
10. What two factors affect the risk of dental caries?
11. What is the difference between Type I diabetes and Type II diabetes?
12. What causes lactose intolerance?

Put Learning into Action

1. Write an entertaining and informative public service announcement for television or radio that encourages people to increase their fiber intake.

2. Make a list of snacks that are high in refined sugars. Then make a list of snack alternatives that are high in naturally occurring sugars and/or complex carbohydrates.

3. Analyze five cereal product labels. Make a chart and record the amount of total carbohydrate, dietary fiber, and sugars in each product. Also list all the types of refined sugars included in each product.

4. Review the ingredient lists on three canned or frozen entrees to identify the carbohydrate additives. Try to find out the major function of each additive listed. You may use the Internet to learn more about the purpose of food additives. Share your findings in class.

5. Prepare a bulletin board or showcase showing how to use information about carbohydrates found on food labels.

6. Interview a dentist to find out more about the relationship between nutrition and dental health.

Explore Further

1. Keep a food intake diary listing all the foods and beverages you consume for three days. Be sure to include serving sizes. Put a star by each item that is a source of simple carbohydrates. Use diet analysis software to determine how many calories, grams of carbohydrates, and grams of fiber you consumed each day. Calculate what percentage of each day's calories came from carbohydrates. Also estimate what percentage of your calories come from simple carbohydrates.

2. Evaluate your school lunch program for the availability of whole grain products and other high-fiber foods. Meet with the foodservice director to discuss the nutritional quality of school meals. Inquire about the ratio of carbohydrates to fats and proteins.

3. Research how to adjust recipes to reduce refined sugars and increase fiber. Adjust one of your favorite recipes. Prepare the original version and the adjusted version of the recipe. Compare the appearance, taste, and texture of the two products in a written evaluation.

4. Research one of the health questions related to carbohydrates discussed in the chapter. Write a report identifying causes, symptoms, treatment, and recommended diet patterns.

Chapter 6

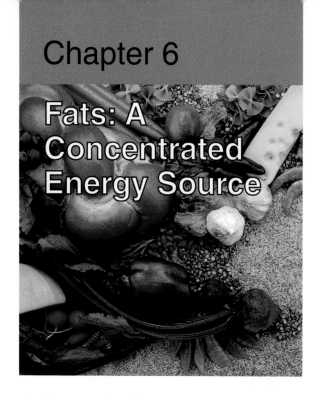

Fats: A Concentrated Energy Source

● Learn the Language

lipid	chylomicron
triglycerides	lipoprotein
fatty acid	very low-density
saturated fatty acid	lipoprotein (VLDL)
unsaturated fatty acid	low-density
monounsaturated	lipoprotein (LDL)
fatty acid	high-density
polyunsaturated fatty	lipoprotein (HDL)
acid	coronary heart
hydrogenation	disease (CHD)
rancid	plaque
trans-fatty acid	atherosclerosis
phospholipids	heart attack
lecithin	stroke
emulsifier	hypertension
sterols	blood lipid profile
cholesterol	omega-3 fatty acids
essential fatty acid	cancer
adipose tissue	fat replacer

● Objectives

After studying this chapter, you will be able to

- describe the characteristic differences between saturated and unsaturated fatty acids.
- list five functions of lipids in the body.
- summarize how the body digests, absorbs, and transports lipids.
- explain the role fats play in heart health.
- identify 10 heart-health risk factors.
- make food choices that follow recommended limits for dietary fats and cholesterol.

Fat seems to be a common topic on the health and nutrition front these days. "Americans are eating too much fat." "How many grams of fat are in that food?" "Have you tried the latest lowfat diet?" You might hear comments like these through the media, at the grocery store, and even in the halls at school. See 6-1.

There are some good reasons to be concerned about fat. Too much fat in the diet is linked to a variety of health problems. However, fats are not all bad. In fact, fats perform many important functions in the body. You need to eat foods containing some fat every day. The goal is to choose foods with the right amount of fat for a healthful diet.

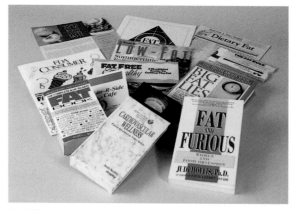

6-1 Studying nutrition can help you sort fact from fiction when reviewing the abundance of popular materials that focus on fat.

What Are Lipids?

You are familiar with the word *fat,* but the word *lipid* may be new to you. **Lipid** is a broader term for a group of compounds that includes fats, oils, lecithin, and cholesterol. Lipids can be grouped into three main classes: triglycerides, phospholipids, and sterols.

What Are Triglycerides?

Triglycerides are the major type of fat found in foods and in the body. Triglycerides consist of three fatty acids attached to a *glycerol* molecule. **Fatty acids** are organic compounds made up of a chain of carbon atoms to which hydrogen atoms are attached. The last carbon atom at one end of the chain forms an *acid group* with two oxygen atoms and a hydrogen atom. Fatty acid chains vary in length. The most common fatty acids in food have 16 to 18 carbon atoms.

Saturated and Unsaturated Fatty Acids

Fatty acids can be saturated or unsaturated. **Saturated fatty acids** have no double bonds in their chemical structure. They have a full load of hydrogen atoms. An **unsaturated fatty acid** has at least one double bond between two carbon atoms in each molecule. If a double bond is broken, two hydrogen atoms can be added to the molecule. The number of double bonds and hydrogen atoms in the fatty acid chain determine the degree of saturation. A **monounsaturated fatty acid** has only one double bond between carbon atoms. A **polyunsaturated fatty acid** has two or more double bonds. See 6-2.

Nearly all fats and oils contain a mixture of the three types of fatty acids. For instance, corn oil is 13 percent saturated, 25 percent monounsaturated, and 62 percent polyunsaturated. The fats in meat and dairy products, including beef fat, lard, and butterfat, tend to be high in saturated fatty acids. Fats from plants are usually higher in unsaturated fatty acids. Olive and peanut oils are high in monounsaturated fatty acids. Corn, safflower, and soybean oils are high in polyunsaturated fatty acids. The tropical oils, such as coconut and palm oils, are an exception to the rule about fats from plants. These oils are high in saturated fatty acids.

The prevalent type of fatty acid determines whether a lipid is liquid or solid at room temperature. Lipids that are high in saturated fatty acids tend to be solid at room temperature. Lipids that are high in unsaturated fatty acids tend to be liquid at room temperature. This is because unsaturated fats have a lower melting point than more highly saturated fats. This is why chicken fat will melt at a lower temperature than butterfat, which is more highly saturated.

Unsaturated fatty acids can be hydrogenated. **Hydrogenation** is the process of breaking the double carbon bonds in unsaturated fatty acids and adding hydrogen. This process converts liquid oils into solid fats. For instance, hydrogen is added to some of the double bonds in unsaturated liquid vegetable oil to make solid margarine.

Besides changing the texture, the main reason for hydrogenating oils is to improve their keeping quality. Oils turn rancid if they are exposed to air or stored for a long time. **Rancid** describes a food oil in which the fatty acid molecules have combined with oxygen. This causes them to break down, and the oil spoils. Rancid oils have an unpleasant smell and taste. Food manufacturers often prefer to use hydrogenated fats over unsaturated oils. The longer shelf life of the hydrogenated fats saves the manufacturers money and improves consumer satisfaction.

When oils are partially hydrogenated, some of the unsaturated fatty acids in the oils change their molecular shapes. These fatty acids are known as **trans-fatty acids.** Research shows trans-fatty acids act much like saturated fats in the body. Trans-fatty acids, like saturated fats, are linked to a risk of heart disease. Staying within recommended

Types of Fatty Acids

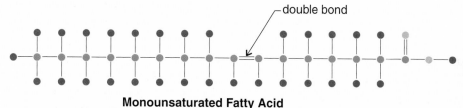

Saturated Fatty Acid

The carbon atoms in the chain are all linked with single bonds. The chain is saturated with as many hydrogen atoms as the carbon atoms can hold.

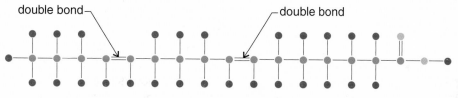

Monounsaturated Fatty Acid

The chain of carbon atoms contains one double bond. The two carbon atoms linked by the double bond could each hold another hydrogen atom.

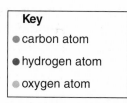

Polyunsaturated Fatty Acid

The chain of carbon atoms contains more than one double bond. Each of the carbon atoms linked by double bonds could hold another hydrogen atom.

Key
- carbon atom
- hydrogen atom
- oxygen atom

6-2 The number of double bonds and hydrogen atoms determine whether a fatty acid is saturated, monounsaturated, or polyunsaturated.

limits for total fat and saturated fat in your diet will help you avoid health risks.

● Other Lipids

So far, you have learned about three types of fatty acids that form the triglycerides found in food. There are two other classes of lipids. They are phospholipids and sterols.

● Phospholipids

Phospholipids are lipids that have a phosphorus-containing compound in their chemical structure. *Lecithin* is a phospholipid.

Lecithin is made by the liver, so it is not essential to the diet. However, lecithin is found in many foods, including egg yolks. You will see *lecithin* on the ingredient lists of some food products. Soya lecithin is added to chocolate candy and commercially baked products.

Lecithin, like other phospholipids, is an **emulsifier.** It is a substance that can mix with water and fat. This is why adding egg yolk to oil and vinegar will form a mixture that will not separate—mayonnaise. The lecithin in the egg yolk keeps the oil particles suspended in the watery vinegar. See 6-3.

In the body, lecithin is part of cell membranes. Some health food stores claim lecithin is a magical nutrient, but it is not. Lecithin supplements have no known benefits to your health. This is because lecithin is broken down when it is digested. Therefore, your body no longer recognizes it as lecithin when it is absorbed.

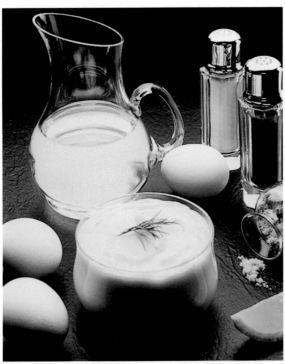

American Egg Board

6-3 Egg yolk contains lecithin, which acts as an emulsifier in mayonnaise by keeping oil droplets suspended in watery vinegar.

● **Sterols**

The third class of lipids are called **sterols.** Sterols have a complex molecular structure. They include some hormones, vitamin D, and cholesterol.

Cholesterol is a white, waxy lipid made by the body that is part of every cell. Your body uses cholesterol to make sex hormones and bile acids. Cholesterol is found only in animal tissues. It is never present in plants. Therefore, plant foods, such as peanut butter and corn oil margarine, contain no cholesterol.

All animal foods, including milk, cheese, hamburgers, eggs, and butter, contain cholesterol. It is abundant in egg yolks, organ meats (liver and kidney), crab, and lobster. Cholesterol is not essential in the diet because the body manufactures it.

● Functions of Lipids

Lipids serve many important functions in the body. You need a number of fatty acids for normal growth and development. Your body can make most of these. However, two polyunsaturated fatty acids, *linoleic acid* and *linolenic acid,* are called **essential fatty acids.** Your body cannot make them. You must get them from your diet. If your diet is missing these nutrients, the skin, reproductive system, liver, and kidneys may all be affected. Most people include plenty of fats and oils in their diets, so lacks of the essential fatty acids are rare.

Lipids provide a concentrated source of energy. All lipids, whether butter, margarine, corn oil, or some other type of fat or oil, provide 9 calories per gram. In comparison, proteins and carbohydrates provide only 4 calories per gram. Your body can conveniently store fat calories for future energy needs.

The body stores a large share of lipids in **adipose tissue**. About half of this tissue is just under your skin. It serves as an internal blanket that holds in body heat. The fat cells in adipose tissue can expand to hold an almost unlimited amount of fat. See 6-4.

Body fat surrounds organs, such as the heart, and liver. This fat acts like a shock absorber. It helps protect the organs from the bumps and bruises of body movement.

Vitamins A, D, E, and K dissolve in fat. They are carried into your body along with the fat in foods. Lipids also help move these vitamins around inside your body.

Lipids are part of the structure of every cell. You need lipids for the formation of healthy cell membranes. They are also used to make some hormones, vitamins, and other secretions.

Fats play roles in foods as well as in your body. Both naturally occurring and added fats affect the tastes, textures, and aromas of foods. Fats make meat moist and flavorful. They make biscuits tender and pie crusts flaky. Fats help fried foods become brown and crisp. They disperse the compounds that allow you to smell bacon cooking, too.

● Lipids in the Body

You probably include sources of fat in your diet throughout the day. You may have an egg for breakfast, a cheese sandwich for lunch, and a pork chop for dinner. How does your body use the fats in foods to perform vital functions?

● Lipid Digestion and Absorption

Remember that most of the fats in foods are triglycerides. After chewing and swallowing, fat reaches the stomach along with carbohydrates, proteins, and other food elements. The fat separates from the watery contents of the stomach and floats in a layer on top.

When fats reach the small intestine, they are mixed with bile, which acts as an emulsifier. Bile helps break fats into tiny droplets and keeps them suspended in watery digestive

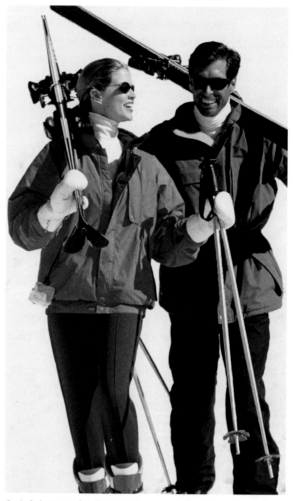

6-4 A layer of adipose tissue under the skin helps insulate the body in cold weather.

fluid. Breaking fat into tiny droplets increases its surface area. This makes it easier for pancreatic enzymes to break triglycerides down into glycerol, fatty acids, and monoglycerides. (A *monoglyceride* is one fatty acid attached to a glycerol molecule.) Bile's emulsifying effect improves the absorption of the fat by the cells lining the intestine.

● Lipid Transport in the Body

Lipids travel in the bloodstream to tissues throughout the body. Glycerol and short-chain fatty acids resulting from fat digestion pass through the intestinal lining directly into the bloodstream. Monoglycerides and long-chain fatty acids are converted back into triglycerides. Balls of these triglycerides are thinly coated with cholesterol, phospholipids, and proteins, forming **chylomicrons.** Chylomicrons carry absorbed dietary fat to body cells. They are absorbed into the lymphatic system. Then they move into the bloodstream.

Keep in mind that blood is made up mostly of water, which does not mix well with fats. The protein and phospholipid coat on chylomicrons allows fats to remain dispersed in water-based blood. This helps fats from your diet move efficiently through your blood vessels to the tissues where they are needed.

Chylomicrons are one type of lipoprotein. **Lipoproteins** are a combination of fats and proteins that helps transport fats in the body. **Very low-density lipoproteins (VLDL)** are a second type. They carry triglycerides and cholesterol made by the liver to body cells. Once in the bloodstream, some of the triglycerides in VLDL are broken down into glycerol and fatty acids and released. Losing triglycerides causes VLDL to become more dense and contain a larger percentage of cholesterol. At this point, VLDL become **low-density lipoproteins (LDL)**. LDL carry cholesterol through the bloodstream to body cells. A fourth type of lipoproteins is the **high-density lipoproteins (HDL)**. HDL pick up cholesterol from around the body and transfer it to other lipoproteins for transport back to the liver. The liver processes this returned cholesterol as a waste product for removal from the body. You will read more about LDL and HDL later in this chapter.

Lipid Use for Energy

Enzymes on the lining of blood vessels break down the triglycerides in chylomicrons and VLDL into glycerol and fatty acids. Body cells can take up fatty acids from the bloodstream. Cells can break fatty acids down further to release energy for immediate

needs. If the cells do not have immediate energy needs, they can rebuild the fatty acids into triglycerides. The cells store these triglycerides for future energy needs.

Most cells can store only limited amounts of triglycerides. However, fat cells can hold an almost limitless supply. When needed, fat cells can break down stored triglycerides. They send fatty acids through the bloodstream to other body cells that use lipids for fuel.

Fats and Heart Health

Fats in the diet and in the body play a major role in the health of your heart. **Coronary heart disease (CHD)** refers to disease of the heart and blood vessels. It is the leading cause of death in the United States.

Arteries are the blood vessels that carry oxygen and nutrients to body tissues. Fatty compounds made up largely of cholesterol can attach to the inside walls of arteries, forming a buildup called **plaque**. Plaque begins to form early in life in everyone's blood vessels. A number of factors affect the rate at which plaque buildups form. See 6-5.

As plaque increases, it hardens and narrows the arteries. This condition is called **atherosclerosis**, the most common form of heart disease. The heart has to work harder to pump blood through narrowed arteries. This strains the heart and causes blood pressure to rise.

Blood clots are more likely to form at the sites of plaque buildups. Blood clots can become lodged in narrowed arteries and cut off the blood supply to tissues fed by the arteries. A buildup of plaque in the arteries feeding the heart muscle can lead to a **heart attack**. A buildup of plaque in the arteries leading to the brain may result in a **stroke**. These conditions can be life threatening. In both cases, cells are destroyed because the blocked arteries cannot supply enough nutrients or oxygen to the tissue.

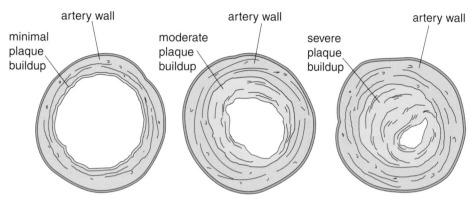

artery wall

minimal plaque buildup

artery wall

moderate plaque buildup

artery wall

severe plaque buildup

6-5 A heavy buildup of plaque in the arteries is the most common cause of coronary heart disease.

Scientists have identified a number of risk factors that contribute to CHD. The chances of developing CHD increase rapidly as more factors begin to apply to you. You can reduce the risks of factors beyond your control by carefully managing the factors within your control.

The Uncontrollable Heart-Health Risk Factors

Unfortunately, you cannot control some factors that greatly affect your state of health. Risks for CHD are associated with certain age, gender, and race groups. Certain inherited traits present risks, too. If any of these risks applies to you, getting regular medical checkups can help detect potential problems.

Age

The risk of heart attack increases with age. Most heart attacks occur after the age of 65. Following healthy lifestyle behaviors when you are young can help prevent heart disease later in life.

Gender

If you are male, you are at a greater risk of coronary heart disease than females. Female hormones tend to protect against CHD. Hormonal changes that occur during menopause reduce this protective factor in older

women. Therefore, if other factors are equal, women over age 50 have a risk for CHD equal to men. See 6-6.

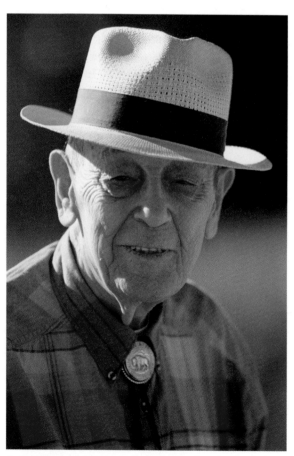

6-6 Advanced age and male gender are both factors that increase the risk of heart disease.

● Race

Some races are at greater risk of heart disease than others. For instance, African Americans are twice as likely to have heart attacks as members of some other races. African Americans also have a higher incidence of high blood pressure. The reasons for this are unclear. However, members of higher-risk racial groups should make an extra effort to manage controllable risk factors.

● Family History

If one or more of your blood relatives have had heart disease, your risk increases. Blood relatives include parents, grandparents, aunts, uncles, brothers, and sisters.

● The Controllable Heart-Health Risk Factors

Is it possible to do something to prevent heart attacks? People who have survived heart attacks will be the first to tell you that you can change lifestyle behaviors. Many heart attack victims have the motivation to make some drastic changes. They quit smoking. They start exercising more. They learn how to manage stress. They also lose weight and eat diets low in saturated fats and trans-fatty acids.

The biggest risk factors for CHD are smoking, high blood pressure, and high blood cholesterol. Diabetes mellitus, inactivity, stress, and overweight are risk factors, too. Through your lifestyle choices, you have some control over all these risk factors. Changing lifestyle behaviors to control these factors could reduce CHD risk for up to 95 percent of the population.

● Smoking

Heart attacks before age 55 can often be traced to cigarette smoking. Smokers have two to four times more risk of dying from a heart attack than nonsmokers. Smoking constricts blood vessels which might be narrowed with plaque. Therefore, a smoker's heart must work harder to get needed blood and oxygen to body cells. When the heart has to work harder, the risk of CHD increases.

By quitting, people can undo most of the damage caused by smoking. The best advice for a healthy heart is to never begin smoking. See 6-7.

Absence makes the heart grow stronger.

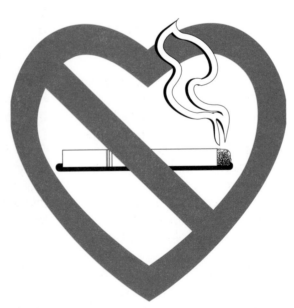

6-7 For a healthy heart, the best advice is to avoid smoking.

High Blood Pressure

Abnormally high blood pressure, or **hypertension**, is a heart-health risk factor. It involves an excess force on the walls of the arteries as blood is pumped from the heart. A normal blood pressure reading is 120/80 mm of mercury. The first number in this reading measures *systolic pressure.* This is the pressure on the arteries when the heart muscle contracts. The second number in a blood pressure reading measures *diastolic pressure.* This is the pressure on the arteries when the heart is between beats.

Hypertension affects 20 to 25 percent of the adult population in the United States. People with hypertension have a systolic value at or above 140. A diastolic reading at or above 90 also defines high blood pressure. High blood pressure is a strong indicator of coronary disease.

High blood pressure places added stress on the heart. It contributes to CHD by damaging the walls of the arteries. The walls then accumulate plaque more easily.

Doctors cannot cure high blood pressure. However, some people can control it through diet, exercise, and stress management. Doctors often prescribe medication for people who have trouble controlling their blood pressure.

High Blood Cholesterol

Blood serum refers to the watery portion of blood in which blood cells and other materials are suspended. One of these materials is cholesterol. This cholesterol is known as *serum cholesterol.* Do not confuse serum cholesterol with *dietary cholesterol,* which is the cholesterol found in food.

Artery-clogging plaques are made up largely of cholesterol. Therefore, a large amount of serum cholesterol is a risk factor for CHD.

You should know your blood cholesterol level. If you have a family history of high cholesterol or high blood pressure, you should have your cholesterol level checked. A **blood** *lipid profile* is a medical test that measures cholesterol, HDL, LDL, and triglycerides in the blood. Test results will identify the number of milligrams of each of these components found in a deciliter (0.1 liter) of blood. A cholesterol count of over 200 mg/dL is considered a risk factor for CHD. See 6-8.

The HDL and LDL measurements in a blood lipid profile are heart-health indicators. HDL are sometimes called "good cholesterol" because these lipoproteins carry excess cholesterol to the liver to be discarded. Therefore, a high level of HDL in the blood, greater than 35 mg/dL, indicates a low risk of CHD. LDL, on the other hand, are sometimes called "bad cholesterol." They carry cholesterol that is deposited in body tissues. A high level of LDL in the blood, greater than 130 mg/dL, indicates a high risk of CHD.

Notice the level of LDL that is considered high is a much higher number than the level of HDL that is considered high (130 versus 35). As you might guess from this, most people have a higher proportion of LDL in their blood than HDL. The ratio of these two lipoproteins is another risk indicator for CHD. The desirable ratio of LDL to HDL is less than 5 to 1 in men. It is less than 4.5 to 1 in women. A man with an LDL of 180 mg/dL and an HDL of 30 mg/dL would have a ratio of 6 to 1. He would be at increased risk of heart disease. On the other hand, suppose the man had an LDL of 120 mg/dL and an HDL of 40 mg/dL. His LDL to HDL ratio would be 3 to 1, indicating a reduced risk of CHD.

People who have other risk factors for CHD should also be aware of their blood triglyceride levels. High levels of blood triglycerides are usually associated with high levels of serum cholesterol. A triglyceride level of over 200 mg/dL may increase the risk of CHD for people with other risk factors.

Diabetes Mellitus

Diabetes mellitus causes blood vessels to become damaged or blocked with fat. This reduces blood circulation beyond the effects

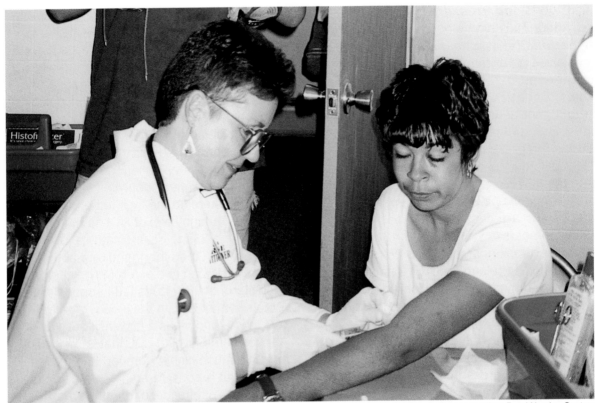

Penn State School of Nursing, Rural Nursing Centers

6-8 A blood lipid profile will reveal your blood cholesterol level.

of normal plaque buildups. Therefore, people with diabetes mellitus are at a higher risk of CHD.

People with Type I diabetes cannot view their disease as a controllable heart-health risk factor. They must take insulin injections to manage their condition. They cannot control it through lifestyle behaviors. However, about 80 percent of people who have diabetes mellitus have Type II. These people do have some control over this risk factor. This is because Type II diabetes can often be managed with diet and physical activity.

● Excess Weight

Because fats are such a concentrated source of energy, calories from fat mount up surprisingly fast. For example, a tablespoon of peanut butter adds 72 fat calories to a slice of bread. The body can easily convert excess calories from fat into adipose tissue. Excess calories from carbohydrates and proteins are stored as body fat, too.

Every pound of stored body fat is equal to 3,500 calories of energy. One way your body can get energy needed between meals is to break down these fat stores. However, many people regularly consume more calories than they need. Therefore, their fat stores continue to build rather than being burned for energy. This causes these people to become overweight.

As fat stores in the body increase, the number of blood vessels must increase to nourish the added tissue. This creates more work for the heart, which increases blood pressure. High blood pressure causes blood vessels to become stretched and injured. Points of injury attract cholesterol, adding to plaque buildups. If blood pressure remains high, blood vessels begin to lose their elasticity. This makes it harder to control blood pressure.

Overweight people, statistically, have a shorter life span. Being overweight increases a person's risk of diabetes mellitus and high blood cholesterol as well as high blood pressure. Each of these factors is also a risk factor for CHD. Therefore, an overweight person is more likely to have a combination of heart-health risk factors. Multiple risk factors place a person's heart health in greater danger than a single factor.

If you are like most people, you are concerned about how you feel. You want to keep your weight at a healthy level. Eating a nutritious diet and getting plenty of exercise will help you maintain a healthy weight. Reducing fat in your diet and increasing activity are two key steps for preventing excess weight gain.

Dieting to lose excess weight is not recommended for most teens. If teens fail to get enough nutrients, their growth can be impaired. Be sure to check with your physician or a registered dietitian before starting any weight loss program. See 6-9.

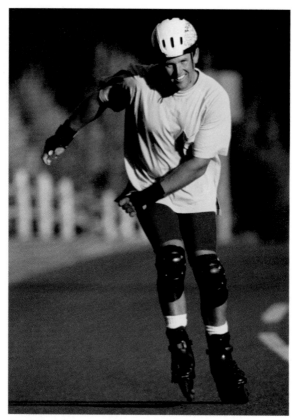

6-9 Exercising regularly will help you avoid becoming overweight.

● Inactivity

A lack of physical activity contributes to many people's excess weight problems. In addition, inactive people fail to give their heart the kind of regular workout it needs to remain healthy. People who spend much time sitting need to make a point of getting some exercise nearly every day. Exercise helps people manage weight, reduce stress, control cholesterol, and strengthen the heart muscle. All of these benefits have a positive impact on heart health.

● Stress and Personality

Research has linked stress and personality to a person's potential for developing heart disease. People who overreact to life's demands may suffer negative heart health. Those who are competitive, impatient, and irritable may also be at greater risk.

People can learn ways to develop emotional balance. They can acquire skills that will help them adapt to the stresses in life, too. For instance, eating right and getting enough rest and exercise can give people the strength they need to handle stress. Finding enjoyable hobbies can help them get their mind off stressful conditions. Setting priorities and using time effectively can keep some stressful situations from arising. Using these and other techniques can help people control this heart-health risk factor.

● Recommended Limits

Experts have linked too much cholesterol and fat in the diet with heart and blood vessel diseases. The National Cholesterol Education Program recommends a maximum intake of 300 mg of cholesterol per day. Many people in the United States include more cholesterol than this in their daily diets. Studies show that too much dietary cholesterol raises serum cholesterol for some people, increasing their risk of CHD. These people must strictly limit their intake of such high-cholesterol foods as egg yolks and organ meats.

People who have high serum cholesterol may also want to increase their intake of plant foods. In fact, all people can benefit from a diet high in plant foods. Plant foods provide fiber and other heart-protective substances that can help lower blood cholesterol.

For most people, dietary cholesterol does not affect serum cholesterol as much as total dietary fat, especially saturated fat. Nutrition experts recommend that no more than 35 percent of the total calories in your diet come from fats. No more than 10 percent of your total daily calories should come from saturated fats. A heart-healthy diet is one that reduces total fat calories from all food groups.

Active teenage boys should eat no more than 123 grams of fat per day. No more than 35 grams should be from saturated fats. Active teenage girls should eat no more than 92 grams of fat daily. Teen girls should limit saturated fats to 26 grams per day. However, many teens go beyond these recommendations.

Suppose a teen chooses a quarter-pound cheeseburger, French fries, and a milk shake for lunch. How much fat do you think would be in this meal? The answer is about 43 grams, 17 of which are saturated. This is nearly the fat equivalent of half a stick of butter! Now suppose the teen chooses a sausage and egg biscuit for breakfast. Dinner includes fried chicken, coleslaw, and ice cream. Throw in a bag of chips and a handful of cookies for snacks. The total for the day would be 147 grams of fat, with over 54 of those grams being saturated. Clearly, this is beyond the daily recommended limits. Keep in mind that these examples did not include all side dishes. Hash browns with the breakfast biscuit would add 8 more grams of fat.

By choosing other meals and snacks with care, however, a teen could include hamburgers and fries in a nutritious diet. For instance, the teen could select a bowl of cereal and fresh strawberries for breakfast. Roasted, skinless chicken and a tossed salad with lowfat dressing could be chosen for dinner. Popcorn and an apple would be lower in fat than the other snack choices. Now the day's meals would net 54 grams of total fat, with only 20 grams of saturated fat. See 6-10.

● Fish Oils and Heart Health

A number of years ago, the health community focused much attention on the effects of fish oils on heart health. The attention arose from the observation that the incidence of coronary heart disease was low among native Alaskans. When analyzing the diet of this culture, researchers found that the Alaskans ate high-fat, high-cholesterol foods from marine fish. This led the researchers to question why the high-fat diet did not cause the Alaskans to have clogged arteries.

The researchers discovered that fish oils contain a certain type of polyunsaturated fatty acids called ***omega-3 fatty acids***. Researchers found that omega-3 fatty acids lowered the risk of heart disease. This finding led people to ask if taking fish oil in pill form would improve their health.

The American Heart Association has found no conclusive evidence that fish oil pills lessen the risks of heart disease. In fact, including large amounts of fish oil supplements in the diet can cause health problems. Large amounts of fish oil have been found to thin the blood and may prevent clotting of the blood. Some fish oil, like cod liver oil, contains dangerously high amounts of vitamins A and D.

Fish contain high quality protein and a variety of vitamins and minerals as well as omega-3 fatty acids. You cannot get this

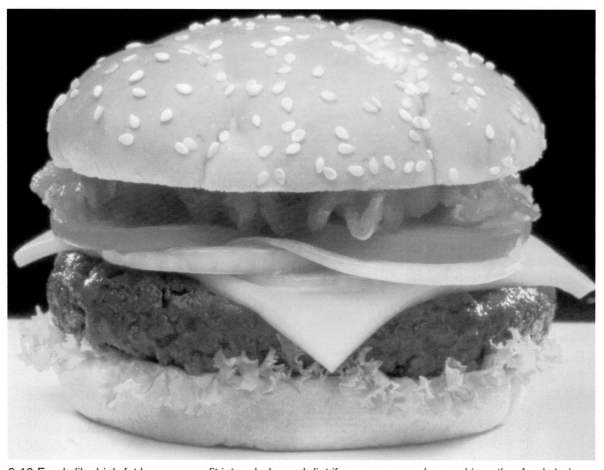

6-10 Foods like high-fat burgers can fit into a balanced diet if you use care when making other food choices.

range of nutrients from fish oil pills alone. Including fish in your diet at least once a week offers more benefits than taking fish oil supplements.

● Fats and Cancer

Cancer is a general term that refers to a number of diseases in which abnormal cells grow out of control. This is in sharp contrast to normal cell growth, which is highly regulated. Cancers can spread throughout the body. As a group, they are the second largest cause of death in the United States.

Scientists have spent years researching the causes and prevention of cancer. Much remains to be learned. However, researchers have determined that many factors increase your chances of developing cancer. Diet is among these factors. Up to half of all cancer cases appear to be related to diet.

The American Institute for Cancer Research reports that lifestyle choices have a great impact on cancer development. Lifestyle choices can be grouped as cancer promoting or cancer protective. Eating a high-fat diet may promote the development of colon, prostate, breast, and some other types of cancer. Choosing a diet that includes a variety of fruits, vegetables, and grains is a cancer-protective lifestyle choice. These foods contain fiber and certain chemicals that have anticancer effects. Maintaining a healthy weight is a cancer protective factor, too. This is because having a high percentage of body fat increases the risks of some types of cancer. See 6-11.

Factors Associated with Cancer Deaths

Diet	35 percent
Tobacco use	30 percent
Occupation	4 percent
Alcohol use	3 percent
Pollution	2 percent
Food additives*	1 percent

*Some food additives are also helpful in reducing cancer risk.

Source: American Institute for Cancer Research

6-11 Personally controlled lifestyle factors account for most cancer deaths.

Limiting Fats and Cholesterol in Your Diet

Selecting foods low in fats and cholesterol is important for most Americans over the age of two. By adolescence, most people already have some buildup of fat deposits on their arteries. To keep dietary fat at a recommended level, you need to know where fats are in foods. Then you need to be willing to select a diet that contains no more than 35 percent fat.

Be a Fat Detector

If you are going to limit fat and cholesterol in your diet, you need to be a fat detector. If you know where the fat is in foods, you can learn how to limit or avoid it.

Lipids can be deceiving to the eyes. Sometimes they are easy to see, but sometimes they are not. The *visible fats* are those that you can clearly see. Butter, fat on meats, and salad oil are visible fats. You know you need to limit your intake of these foods because you can see the fat.

Many times you cannot see the fat, but it is there. The *invisible fats* are those that are hidden in foods. Baked goods, snack foods, and luncheon meats are often sources of invisible fat. For instance, one hot dog has about 145 calories, and 117 of them come

from fat. You may be more likely to consume excess fat and calories when you cannot see the fat in foods.

Remember that fats, oils, and sweets form the tip of the Food Guide Pyramid. These foods include visible sources of fat, such as salad dressings, oils, butter, and margarine. Invisible sources of fat, such as high-fat desserts and snacks, are found at the tip of the Pyramid, too. You know you should use these foods sparingly because they are high in calories and low in other nutrients.

Keep in mind that the first three levels of the Food Guide Pyramid also include sources of dietary fat. Biscuits, muffins, and other baked goods are sources of fat from the grains group. Vegetables served with butter and fruits served with cream are sources of fat. Many foods in the milk group, including whole milk, cheese, milk shakes, and ice cream, are high in fats. Eggs, nuts, and many meat cuts are fat sources from the meat and beans group. You need to carefully choose the recommended number of daily servings from each group in the Food Guide Pyramid. This will help you limit fats and cholesterol in your diet.

When you buy prepared foods, read the Nutrition Facts panel on the product labels. This will help you analyze how many calories per serving come from fat. Remember the recommendation is that no more than 35 percent of your total daily calories should come from fat. The label will also tell you the percent Daily Value for fat, saturated fat, and cholesterol provided by a product. A product is considered low in any nutrient for which it provides five percent or less of the Daily Value. See 6-12.

Making Diet Changes

Old eating habits are not easy to change. As a teen, your habits are not so old. You are young and your body is strong. You are in a good position to make a fresh start. Forming a program of good nutrition will help you feel your physical and mental best.

Most people in the United States need to reduce fat and cholesterol in their diets to meet current recommendations. When making diet changes, where do you start? First, decide how you are doing right now. You need to keep a food diary for a few days,

---

Nutrition Facts

Serving Size 1 tbsp (14g)
Servings per Container about 32

Amount Per Serving	
Calories 70	Calories from Fat 70

	% Daily Value*
Total Fat 8g	**13%**
Saturated Fat 1.5g	**8%**
Polyunsaturated Fat 1.5g	
Monounsaturated Fat 2.5g	
Cholesterol 0mg	**0%**
Sodium 100mg	**4%**
Total Carbohydrate 0g	**0%**
Protein 0g	

Vitamin A 10% (30% as Beta Carotene)
Vitamin D 15%

Not a significant source of Dietary Fiber, Sugars, Vitamin C, Calcium or Iron.

* Percent Daily Values are based on a 2,000 calorie diet.

6-12 Information about fats and cholesterol on the Nutrition Facts panel can help you determine how foods fit into your total diet plan.

---

writing down everything you eat and drink. (Refer to Chapter 4, "Nutrition Guidelines," for more information about food diaries.) Use the information in your food diary to find out about the fats in your diet. Diet analysis software or a food composition table can help you.

Your analysis should help you determine which foods in your diet contribute most to elevated blood lipids. You should discover how many grams of fat you are consuming each day. You should be able to calculate the number and percentage of calories in your diet that are coming from fat. You may learn what percentage of your fat intake is coming from saturated, monounsaturated, and polyunsaturated fats. Your analysis should show you your daily cholesterol intake, too.

Decide what is good about your current diet. Then identify changes you can make to help reduce blood triglycerides and cholesterol. Set realistic goals for yourself to make these changes gradually. Then make choices that support your goals. For instance, you might decide to eat French fries no more than once a week. Sticking with this decision might mean ordering a salad with lowfat dressing instead of fries at your next meal.

Support from your family can affect your ability to reach your dietary goals. Talk to family members about your desire to make changes in your diet. See if they might be willing to make changes, too. If not, ask for their respect and encouragement as you work to change your eating habits. See 6-13.

Using Fat Replacers

Have you tasted the new foods with fat replacers in them? *Fat replacers* are used as ingredients in food products. They are designed to replace some or all the fat typically found in those products. Some fat replacers are made from egg whites and other common ingredients. They have a flavor and texture similar to fats and oils, but they have less fat and fewer calories. For example, a tablespoon of regular mayonnaise provides

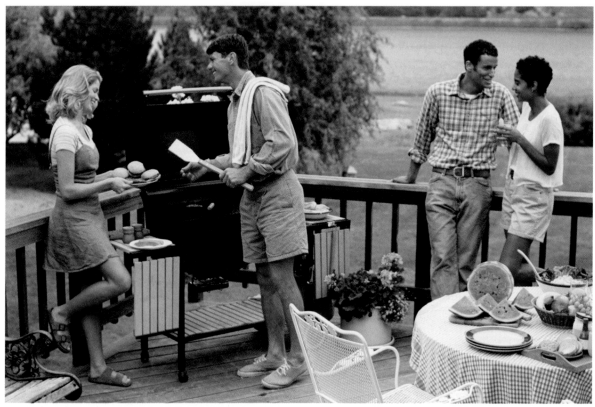

6-13 Support from family members and friends can improve success in making dietary changes.

11 grams of fat and 100 calories. A tablespoon of fat free mayonnaise, which is made with a fat replacer, provides no fat and only 10 calories. Some of the fat replacers can be used only in foods that are not cooked for a long time. You may find them in foods like salad dressings, cheese, and ice cream.

Scientific research on animals and human beings shows fat replacers are safe. However, some of them have drawbacks. For instance, some products containing fat replacers have an aftertaste. One type of fat replacer may cause digestive problems and inhibit absorption of some nutrients.

Fat replacers may allow you to more easily enjoy some traditionally high-fat foods as part of a nutritious diet. However, you need to be aware that some foods containing fat replacers have added sugar. Therefore, they may not be much lower in

calories than their high-fat counterparts. Read labels carefully when buying products to compare fat, calories, and sugars.

You have many choices available to help reduce fat in your diet. Foods containing fat replacers are not a simple answer to poor food habits. They are not a quick-fix substitute for lifestyle changes, either. You should check out all your options before deciding how often you will include foods that contain fat replacers.

● Guidelines for Food Choices

Most teens eat certain foods because of habit. You can break or modify habits to retrain your taste buds. Try to switch your food choices to reduce your consumption of total fats, especially saturated fats and cholesterol.

The American Heart Association recommends eating more fruits, vegetables, whole grain products, and fat free dairy products. They also recommend eating no more than 6 ounces of cooked fish, skinless poultry, or lean meat a day. Go easy on fried foods, such as potato chips and fried chicken. Limit visible fats, such as butter, cream, and salad dressing, too.

Drinking fat free milk makes a difference in fat intake. Whole milk contains 8 times more fat and 17 times more saturated fat than fat free milk. Some people do not enjoy drinking fat free milk because they miss the thick, rich flavor of whole milk. These people may find it easier to switch to reduced fat milk for a while before trying fat free milk.

A good percentage of the fat in many people's diets comes from meat products. You can reduce the amount of fat you get from meats by choosing lean cuts. Trim all visible fat before cooking. Use lowfat cooking methods, such as roasting, broiling, and grilling. Limit portion size to 3 ounces of cooked meat, which is about the size of a deck of playing cards. See 6-14.

People who make changes to reduce dietary fat generally see an improvement in their blood lipid profile within six months. Eating for good health does not just happen. You have to be informed about what will make your body strong and healthy for a full, productive life. Following through on your knowledge requires a commitment to a healthy lifestyle. Deciding to improve your diet is not just a goal for yourself. It will affect those around you, too. The better you feel, the more you are free to interact positively with others.

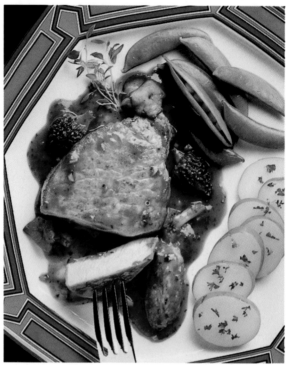

National Pork Producers Council

6-14 Choosing lean cuts, using lowfat cooking methods, and limiting portion sizes allow meats to fit easily into a healthy diet.

Chapter 6 Review

Summary

Lipids, which include all fats and oils, are made up of different types of fatty acids. Saturated fatty acids contain the maximum number of hydrogen atoms. Monounsaturated fatty acids have a double bond between just one pair of carbon atoms. Polyunsaturated fatty acids have double bonds between two or more pairs of carbon atoms. A high percentage of saturated fatty acids tends to make lipids solid at room temperature. A high percentage of unsaturated fatty acids tends to make lipids liquid at room temperature. When oils are hydrogenated, they become more solid at room temperature.

Most of the lipids in foods and in the body are triglycerides. Other classes of lipids are phospholipids and sterols.

Lipids are important to the diet for several reasons. They provide essential fatty acids. They provide a concentrated source of energy. Lipids carry the fat-soluble vitamins A, D, E, and K. They are needed to form cell membranes and various secretions in the body. They provide an internal blanket to hold in body heat. Lipids also cushion body organs.

Of course, the body must digest and absorb fats before using them as an energy source. Most fat digestion takes place in the small intestine where bile keeps fats emulsified while pancreatic enzymes break down triglycerides. Chylomicrons carry fats from foods into the bloodstream following digestion. Other types of lipoproteins help transport fats made in the body away from and back to the liver.

Fats in the body can form deposits in the arteries, which can lead to coronary heart disease. A number of factors contribute to a person's risk of CHD. Some of these factors, such as age, gender, race, and heredity, are beyond a person's control. However, people can control a number of lifestyle factors to help reduce their risk of CHD. Controllable heart-health risk factors include smoking, inactivity, stress and personality type, overweight, diabetes, high blood pressure, and high blood cholesterol.

Learn to identify sources of visible and invisible fats in your diet. Limit fat intake to 35 percent of your total calories, with less than 10 percent coming from saturated fats. Avoid too much cholesterol.

Your present eating habits were not formed in one day. Do not expect your fat consumption to drastically change in one day. With realistic goals and a determination to improve your state of wellness, you can succeed.

Check Your Knowledge

1. What are the three main classes of lipids?
2. Give two food sources that are high in each of the three types of fatty acids.
3. By what process is corn oil made into margarine?
4. How are trans-fatty acids formed?
5. What are three major food sources of cholesterol?
6. What are five major functions of lipids in the body?
7. How do lipoproteins play a role in moving lipids in the body?
8. What is the difference between a heart attack and a stroke?
9. What age and gender groups are at increased risk for CHD?
10. True or false. Changing lifestyle behaviors could reduce coronary heart disease risk for up to 95 percent of the population.
11. What does a blood lipid profile measure?
12. What is the recommended limit for cholesterol in the diet?

13. What is the food source of omega-3 fatty acids?

14. What effect does diet have on cancer development?

15. When should most people begin limiting fats and cholesterol in their diets?

16. Give five guidelines for making food choices to reduce fats, saturated fats, and cholesterol.

Put Learning into Action

1. Prepare a display showing examples of foods high in saturated, monounsaturated, or polyunsaturated lipids.

2. Design a poster or bulletin board illustrating the major functions of lipids in the body.

3. Write a set of survey questions to help determine people's awareness of their risk factors for coronary heart disease. Use your survey to interview three people in different age groups. Share your findings in class.

4. Prepare a brochure suggesting ways to improve heart health. Distribute it at a school health fair.

5. Develop a "heart-healthy" menu for a breakfast, lunch, or dinner. Using diet analysis software, determine how many grams of fat and saturated fat are in the meal. Also notice how many milligrams of cholesterol the meal provides. Share your meal plan and analysis results with others in your class.

Explore Further

1. Test several types of margarine, such as stick margarine, soft spreads, and reduced-calorie margarine. Compare their tastes and textures with butter. Compare Nutrition Facts panels for amounts of saturated and unsaturated fats. Also compare information on trans-fatty acids if it is available.

2. Research and compare the incidence of coronary heart disease in three countries, including the United States. Investigate typical diet patterns in each country. Write a summary of your conclusions about the link between diet and CHD based on this analysis.

3. Write a five-page research report on a recent study linking diet and cancer risk.

4. Collect nutritional information from three fast-food chains. Compare the fat content of the leading items from each restaurant. Identify which food items on each menu are lowest in saturated fats and cholesterol.

Chapter 7

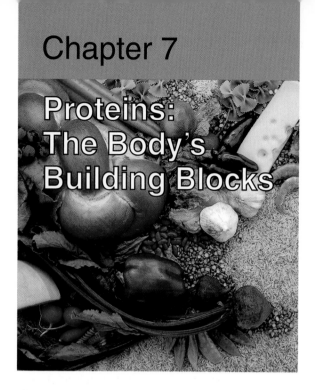

Proteins: The Body's Building Blocks

Mothers often tell children, "You have to eat your meat and drink your milk to get your protein." These mothers are right about meat and milk being good protein sources. However, they may not fully understand what protein does in the body and where protein can be found. They may not realize how much protein children really need, either. Although protein is an important nutrient, people often misunderstand it. Myths about how much you need and the power it has to build strong bodies abound. See 7-1.

Proteins make important contributions to your diet. You need to be sure to eat recommended amounts of protein each day. This chapter will help you determine your protein needs. It will also help you understand the effects of too little and too much protein in the diet.

● **Learn the Language**

protein	vegetarianism
amino acid	complete protein
denaturation	incomplete protein
nonessential amino acid	complementary proteins
essential amino acid	nitrogen balance
antibody	deficiency disease
acid-base balance	protein-energy malnutrition (PEM)
buffer	kwashiorkor
legume	marasmus

● **Objectives**

After studying this chapter, you will be able to

- explain the difference between essential and nonessential amino acids.
- discuss the functions of protein.
- identify animal and plant food sources of protein.
- calculate your daily protein needs.
- describe problems associated with protein deficiencies and excesses.

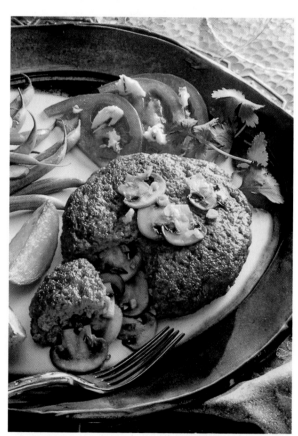

National Pork Producers Council

7-1 Meat is an excellent food source for meeting daily protein needs.

● What Is Protein?

Protein is an energy-yielding nutrient composed of carbon, hydrogen, oxygen, and nitrogen. The presence of nitrogen is what makes this nutrient different from carbohydrates and fats.

Amino acids are the building blocks of protein molecules. Most proteins are made up of different patterns and combinations of 20 amino acids, which are linked in strands. Most amino acids have the following basic chemical structure:

$$NH_2 \leftarrow \text{amino group}$$
$$\text{side chain} \rightarrow R - C - COOH \leftarrow \text{acidic carboxyl group}$$
$$| \\ H$$

The body probably has at least 30,000 types of protein. Each type performs a specific job. The number of amino acids and the order in which they are linked determine the type of protein.

Think of the 20 amino acids like letters in the alphabet. You can combine the different letters to make words. The words can contain any letter in any sequence. There is no limit to the number of letters in a word. That is why it is possible to have so many different words. In a similar way, amino acids are combined in different sequences to form different proteins. The amino acids can be arranged one after the other in a straight line. However, they may be stacked up and branched like a tree.

DNA (deoxyribonucleic acid) is found in the nucleus of every cell. It provides the instructions for how the amino acids will be linked to form the proteins in your body.

Protein molecules can change their shape and take on new characteristics. This is called **denaturation**. Heat, acids, bases, and alcohol are among the factors that can denature proteins. You can see the effects of denaturation when you cook an egg or marinate a roast—both high-protein foods. Applying heat to an egg changes it from a runny fluid to a solid mass. Soaking a roast in an acidic marinade makes the meat more tender. The shapes of the protein molecules in these foods have changed. Once proteins are denatured, they can never return to their original state. For example, once a fertilized egg is cooked, it will never hatch into a chick. See 7-2.

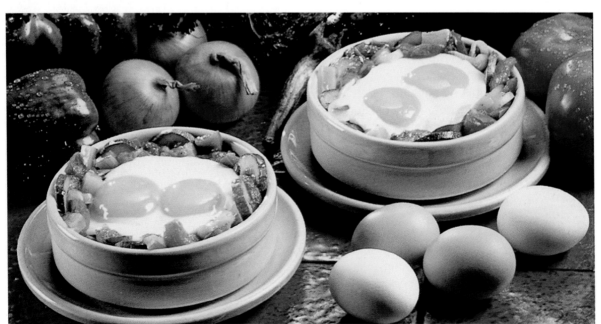

7-2 Heat denatures the proteins in eggs. This is why eggs become firm when they are cooked.

Types of Amino Acids

You need all 20 amino acids for good health. However, your body can synthesize 11 of the amino acids from the other amino acids. (*Synthesize* means your body can use one or more compounds to make a new and different compound.) The amino acids your body can make are called **nonessential amino acids**. Your body is not able to make the remaining 9 amino acids. These are called **essential amino acids**. You must get them from the foods you eat.

Protein in the Body

When you eat a protein food, stomach acids denature the proteins. This makes it easier for enzymes in the stomach to begin breaking down large protein molecules into smaller pieces. As these protein pieces move into the small intestine, other enzymes break them down into single amino acids. The amino acids are absorbed into the bloodstream. The blood then carries amino acids to body cells that need them.

Functions of Protein

Your cells can use amino acids from food proteins to build new proteins. Cells can also convert amino acids to other compounds, including other amino acids.

The proteins built by cells are custom designed to perform a wide variety of functions in the body. The roles proteins play depend on where they are located and how your body needs them. The following sections describe several key functions of proteins.

Build and Maintain Tissues

Protein is a necessary part of every cell. You need protein to form the structure of muscles, organs, skin, blood, hair, nails, and every other body part. As your body grows, it uses protein to help make new tissues. This is why it is important for people to get enough protein during the growth years. Otherwise, they will not grow as tall and strong as they should. See 7-3.

Protein makes up about 18 to 20 percent of your body. About three percent of this protein is broken down each day. Besides building new tissues, therefore, you need protein to maintain existing tissues. Each cell has a limited life span. Your body constantly makes new cells to replace those that have died.

When you eat a nutritious diet and exercise regularly, your body uses proteins to build lean muscle mass. Before you can build muscles, however, you must meet your protein needs for normal growth and repair of tissues. Growth and repair are possible only when your diet provides the necessary mix of amino acids.

Make Important Compounds

Your body uses proteins to make a number of important compounds. These compounds include enzymes, which cause

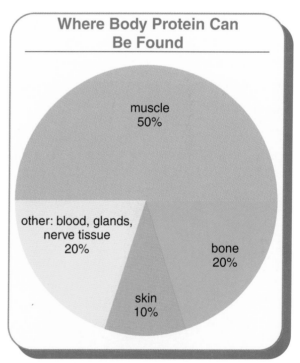

Where Body Protein Can Be Found

muscle
50%

other: blood, glands, nerve tissue
20%

bone
20%

skin
10%

7-3 The largest amount of body protein is stored in muscle tissue. Protein is also located in bone, skin, blood, and all other cell tissue.

specific chemical reactions in the body. For instance, digestive enzymes cause a chemical breakdown of carbohydrates, fats, and proteins from foods. Proteins are also used to make some hormones. Hormones are chemicals released into the bloodstream to control specific body processes. For example, the hormone insulin helps regulate the level of glucose in the blood. Your body's immune system uses proteins to make antibodies. **Antibodies** are proteins that defend the body against infection and disease. See 7-4.

● **Regulate Mineral and Fluid Balance**

Proteins help carry the minerals sodium and potassium from one side of cell walls to the other. These minerals and other proteins

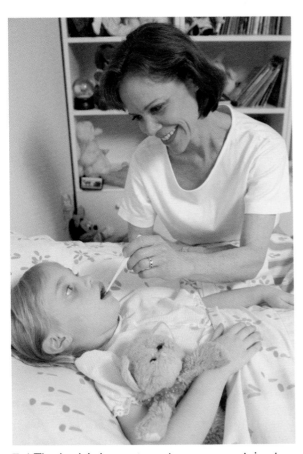

7-4 The body's immune system uses proteins to defend itself against infection and disease by making antibodies.

control the flow of water through cell membranes. A balance of fluid inside and outside the cells is crucial. This balance is needed for normal functioning of the heart, lungs, brain, and every other cell.

● **Maintain Acid-Base Balance**

Proteins help maintain the acid-base balance of the blood. **Acid-base balance** refers to the maintenance of the correct level of acidity of a body fluid. A life-threatening condition can result if the blood becomes too acidic. Proteins in the blood act as chemical buffers. A **buffer** is a compound that can counteract an excess of acid or base in a fluid. (You will read more about acid-base balance in Chapter 9, "Minerals: Regulators of Body Functions.")

● **Carry Vital Substances**

Proteins linked with fats form *lipoproteins,* the compounds used to carry fats in the bloodstream. (You read about lipoproteins in relation to blood lipids and heart disease in Chapter 6.) A protein is also used to transport iron and other nutrients. Oxygen transport in the blood depends on the presence of a protein, too. Health will suffer if proteins are not available to carry these vital substances to needed points throughout the body.

● **Provide Energy**

Only protein can perform the critical functions of cell growth and repair. However, the body's number one priority is to provide the cells with the energy they need to exist. Therefore, if carbohydrates and fats are lacking in the diet, the body will use proteins as an energy source. Protein can also be converted to glucose, which can be used as fuel. Proteins yield 4 calories of energy per gram. When proteins are used to provide energy, they cannot be used for other purposes, such as building cells.

A shortage of dietary carbohydrates and fats is not the only condition that causes the body to burn proteins for energy. The body will also use proteins as an energy source when there is an excess of protein in the diet.

Food Sources of Protein

Most people meet their protein needs by eating both animal and plant food sources. Many factors influence which protein foods people choose. Availability, cost, health concerns, food preferences, religious beliefs, and environmental factors all affect people's food choices.

Animal Sources of Protein

Animal flesh is by far the largest source of protein in a meat-eating culture, such as the United States. Animal foods include beef, veal, pork, lamb, poultry, and fish. Other animal sources of protein include eggs, milk, yogurt, cheese, and ice cream. See 7-5.

The USDA reports that U.S. citizens eat an average of 200 pounds of meat, poultry, and seafood annually. Over the last 100 years, meat consumption has increased dramatically. The fast-food chains, serving hamburgers, chicken, and fish sandwiches, provide much of the protein in teen diets.

Although meat is an excellent source of protein, some meat products are quite high in fat. The same is true of some dairy products. For instance, 57 percent of the calories in regular ground beef come from fat. Of the calories in whole milk, 48 percent come from fat. Much of the fat in foods from animal sources is saturated. These foods provide no dietary fiber, either.

The cost of protein from animal sources is high. For example, one ounce of cooked top round steak would provide about 8 grams

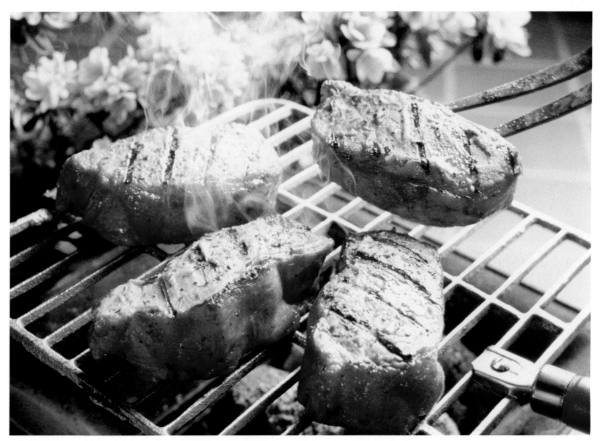

7-5 Pork is a popular source of animal protein.

of protein. One ounce of Cheddar cheese would provide about 7 grams of protein. The cost of the steak is about 23¢ and the cost of the cheese is about 21¢. In contrast, a ½-cup serving of cooked dried beans provides about 7 grams of protein and costs only about 6¢. High costs often limit the amount of animal protein low-income families can buy.

● Plant Sources of Protein

A plentiful supply of protein is available from plant foods. Protein is found in grains, nuts, seeds, and legumes. **Legumes** are plants that have a special ability to capture nitrogen from the air and transfer it to their protein-rich seeds. Examples include peanuts, black-eyed peas, kidney beans, black beans, lentils, chickpeas, and lima beans.

Soybeans are an especially rich source of plant protein. These legumes can be processed and modified to form a variety of food products. For example, *tofu* is a curd product made from soybeans. It is used as a meat alternative in some dishes. Other pastes and meatlike products can also be made from soybeans.

● Vegetarianism

Vegetarianism is the practice of eating a diet consisting entirely or largely of plant foods. Fruits, vegetables, grains, nuts, and seeds are the mainstays of a vegetarian diet.

Some vegetarians also eat dairy products and eggs.

Forms of vegetarianism have existed since history began. Today, as in the past, many people choose to avoid eating foods from animal sources. Interest in vegetarianism, especially among young people, seems to be growing. This may explain the increasing popularity of vegetarian cookbooks and restaurants.

The eating patterns of people who call themselves vegetarians vary greatly. Four main types of vegetarians are described in 7-6.

In recent years, health benefits of vegetarianism have received much attention. Most of the fats in plant protein foods are polyunsaturated. Plant foods contain no cholesterol, and the foods are generally high in fiber and low in saturated fat. These are positive factors in terms of heart health and cancer risk reduction.

Ask a vegetarian why he or she prefers not to eat meat. The answer may simply be that the person grew up in a vegetarian household. Other reasons, such as the following, may also be mentioned:

* *Religious reasons* for vegetarianism are cited by followers of many Eastern religions, such as Buddhists and Hindus. Seventh-Day Adventists and Trappist monks from the Roman Catholic church also choose a vegetarian diet.

Types of Vegetarians

Vegans, or strict vegetarians, eat no foods from animal sources. Their diet is limited to foods from plant sources.

Lacto-vegetarians eat animal protein in the form of milk, cheese, and other dairy products. They do not eat meat, fish, poultry, or eggs.

Lacto-ovo vegetarians eat animal protein in the form of dairy products and eggs. However, they do not eat meats, fish, or poultry.

Semivegetarians, or partial vegetarians, eat dairy products, eggs, poultry, and seafood. They eat little or no red meat—beef, veal, pork, and lamb.

7-6 Vegetarians are identified by the degree to which they refrain from eating animal foods.

- *Health reasons* are mentioned by people who want to avoid the fat and cholesterol in meat. They may also want to avoid certain hormones and chemicals used in raising livestock. Some people are concerned about illnesses that can be transmitted by animal foods, too. These people may claim some animal foods give them digestive problems. They say they feel better when they eat primarily fruits, vegetables, and cereals.

- *Socioeconomic reasons* are given by people who believe eating animals is wasteful. About 90 percent of the soybeans, corn, oats, and barley grown in the United States is fed to livestock. These crops would feed many more people directly than can be fed by the animals who eat the crops. See 7-7.

- *Environmental reasons* are given by people who say animal grazing is hard on land. These people may also mention that meat processing uses a tremendous amount of water and energy.

- *Humanitarian reasons* are stated by people who believe sacrificing the life of an animal for food is wrong.

● Protein Quality

Proteins in various food sources differ in their quality. The quality of the protein in meat, poultry, and fish is very high. Animal foods are sources of **complete proteins**. This means all the essential amino acids humans need are present in the proteins. Eggs, milk, cheese, and yogurt are excellent sources of high-quality protein, too.

The protein provided by plant sources is of lower quality than that provided by animal sources. Plants furnish **incomplete proteins**. These proteins are missing or short in one or more of the essential amino acids.

Your body needs the right balance of all 20 amino acids to build tissues and other compounds. If one or more essential amino acids are missing, your cells will not be able to make needed proteins. To understand this concept better, think about a group of students working on an election campaign. They want to make 10 large sets of signs of the individual letters in the word *vote*. One student volunteers to make the *V*s, *T*s, and *E*s. Another student volunteers to make the *O*s. However, through lack of communication,

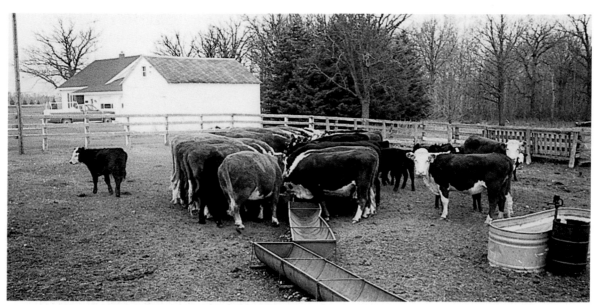

7-7 Large quantities of grain are fed to cattle to prepare them for market.

the second student makes only eight *O*s. Instead of having 10 good signs, 2 signs are incomplete and unusable. Now suppose each letter represents a different essential amino acid. You can see how not having enough of all the essential amino acids leaves some proteins incomplete and unusable.

● Complementary Proteins

You can get the amino acids missing from one incomplete protein source by combining it with another incomplete source. Eaten together, these two incomplete protein foods become a source of complete protein. Two or more incomplete proteins that can be combined to provide all the essential amino acids are called *complementary proteins*.

How do you know which plant foods complement each other? A general guideline is to combine grains, nuts, or seeds with legumes. For example, peanuts (legumes) and wheat (grain) are complementary proteins. They are both incomplete sources of protein. When peanut butter is combined with wheat bread, however, the sandwich becomes a source of complete protein. See 7-8.

People from all over the world combine complementary proteins. For example, Mexicans often serve corn tortillas with refried beans (grain plus legumes). People in the Middle East combine sesame seeds and chickpeas (seeds plus legumes) to make a dip called *hummus.* How many combination foods and meals can you think of that contain complementary protein food sources?

Another way to extend the quality of incomplete protein foods is to combine them with complete protein foods. For instance, you might add a small amount of pork (complete protein) to a large amount of rice (incomplete protein). This will extend the protein value of the rice.

Strict vegetarians must think carefully about using complementary proteins. High-quality protein is essential if normal growth and development are to occur. Diets that focus on only one source of incomplete protein, such as rice, are harmful to long-term good health.

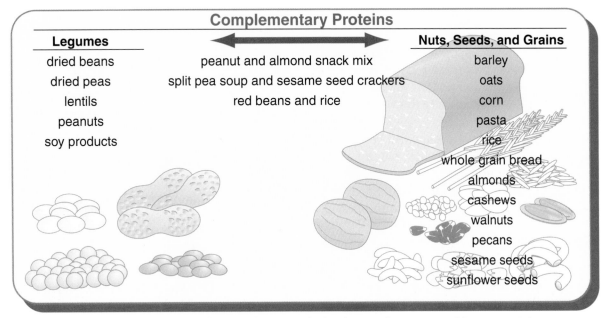

Complementary Proteins		
Legumes		**Nuts, Seeds, and Grains**
dried beans	peanut and almond snack mix	barley
dried peas	split pea soup and sesame seed crackers	oats
lentils	red beans and rice	corn
peanuts		pasta
soy products		rice
		whole grain bread
		almonds
		cashews
		walnuts
		pecans
		sesame seeds
		sunflower seeds

7-8 Eating the right combination of incomplete protein foods together can provide a complete source of protein.

How Much Protein Do You Need?

Your body does not store protein. Therefore, you need protein every day. The amount of protein you need is related to age, gender, and body size. It also depends on your state of health. If you are like most people in the United States, you need less protein than you are consuming.

As children and teens grow, their bodies are building new tissue as well as maintaining existing tissue. Therefore, children and teens have a higher proportional need for protein than people who are no longer growing. In other words, they need more protein per pound of body weight. Similarly, women who are pregnant need extra protein to support the growth of their babies. Women who are breast-feeding need extra protein, too. They need protein to produce milk.

Protein needs vary between males and females. The body needs protein to replace lean tissue that wears out and is lost on a daily basis. Men generally have a higher percentage of lean tissue than women. Therefore, teen and adult males usually require more protein than females of similar age and body size. See 7-9.

The more lean tissue a person has, the more protein will be needed to maintain it. Therefore, a large, tall person will have a slightly greater protein need than a small, short person.

Illness and injury increase the need for protein. When someone is sick, his or her immune system needs extra protein to build antibodies. When someone is injured, extra protein is needed to rebuild damaged tissue.

The RDA for Protein

The RDA for protein is 52 grams per day for 14- to 18-year-old males. The RDA is 46 grams of protein daily for females in the same age range. These are generous

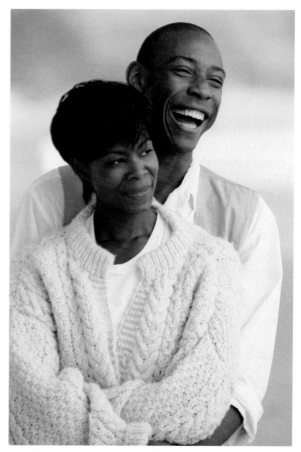

7-9 Because they have a larger proportion of lean muscle tissue, men typically need more protein than women.

allowances that include a margin of safety. RDAs are designed for healthy individuals who eat adequate amounts of carbohydrates and fats. They are also based on the assumption that people are choosing high-quality sources of protein.

To meet the RDA, 10 to 35 percent of your daily calories should come from protein. This means a young woman who needs 2,400 calories a day should include at least 240 calories from protein.

By reading the Nutrition Facts panel on food products, you can estimate how much protein you consume each day. A daily food diary will also help you analyze what percentage of calories in your diet is from protein.

How does your daily intake of protein compare with your calculated RDA? Are you eating more or less than the RDA for protein?

Do Athletes Need More Protein?

Some athletes associate eating a solid piece of meat with building body muscle for added strength. These athletes may wonder if they need more protein than less active people. People who exercise occasionally do not need extra protein. However, well-trained athletes do need a little more protein to build muscle and supply energy. An extra half glass of milk or a chicken wing will provide the extra protein needed. Protein supplements and big chunks of meat are not necessary. See 7-10.

Athletes should remember their primary need is for energy. (Athletes need to keep their need for extra water in mind, too.) They should focus on the high end of the calorie range for carbohydrates—about 55 to 65 percent of total calories. Athletes should stay at the low end of the range for fats—20 to 25 percent of total calories. If the remaining 10 to 25 percent of calories comes from protein, an athlete's needs will be adequately met.

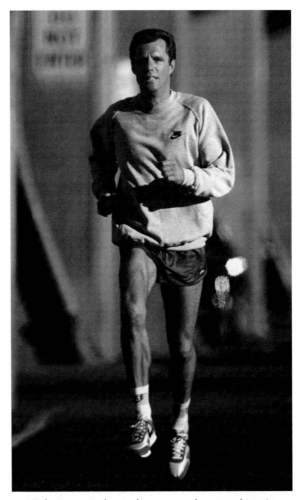

7-10 A runner who trains every day needs extra protein to build muscle and provide energy.

Meeting the Protein RDA

One of the simplest ways to meet protein needs is to follow the recommendations of the Food Guide Pyramid. The meat and milk groups are your primary food sources of protein.

Two to three daily servings are recommended from the milk, yogurt, and cheese group. A serving equals one cup of milk or yogurt. One and one-half ounces of cheese or two ounces of process cheese food are also considered a serving.

Two to three daily servings are also recommended from the meat, poultry, fish, dry beans, eggs, and nuts group. These servings should total only six to seven ounces of cooked meat, poultry, or fish. One-half cup of cooked legumes, one egg, or two tablespoons of peanut butter equal one ounce of meat.

When choosing protein sources, avoid the health risks of a diet high in saturated fats. Choose lowfat protein foods often. Fat free milk, lowfat cheese, most fish, and legumes are lowfat protein sources. Trim visible fat from meats and remove skin from poultry. Use lowfat cooking methods. Avoid adding high-fat cooking oils, sauces, and gravies to protein foods, too.

● The Risks of Too Little or Too Much Protein

As with all nutrients, you need to consume enough protein, but you should avoid getting too much. A lack of protein and a surplus of protein can both cause health problems.

Nitrogen balance is a comparison of the nitrogen a person consumes with the nitrogen he or she excretes. Protein is the only energy nutrient that provides nitrogen. Therefore, nitrogen balance is used to evaluate a person's protein status. Most healthy adults are in *nitrogen equilibrium.* This means they excrete the same amount of nitrogen they take in each day. A person who is building new tissue takes in more protein than he or she excretes. This person is said to be in *positive nitrogen balance.* A pregnant woman or a growing child would be in positive nitrogen balance. Someone whose tissues are deteriorating would be losing more nitrogen than he or she consumes. This person is said to be in *negative nitrogen balance.* A person whose body is wasting due to starvation would be in negative nitrogen balance.

● Protein Deficiency

A deficiency is a shortage. In nutrition, *deficiency* refers to an amount of a nutrient less than the body needs for optimum health. A *deficiency disease* is a sickness caused by a lack of an essential nutrient.

For a large portion of the U.S. population, protein is easy to get in amounts that exceed daily recommendations. Among people who are fighting poverty, however, protein deficiency is not uncommon. This is especially true in countries throughout the world where there is simply not enough food. If the only foods eaten are low in protein, a protein deficiency is likely to occur. See 7-11.

Protein-energy malnutrition (PEM) is a condition caused by a lack of calories and proteins in the diet. Symptoms of PEM include diarrhea and various nutrient deficiencies.

A form of PEM is *kwashiorkor,* which is a protein deficiency disease. This disease most frequently strikes a child when the next sibling is born. The disease is common in poor countries where mothers stop breast-feeding an older child to begin breast-feeding a newborn. The weaned older child is no

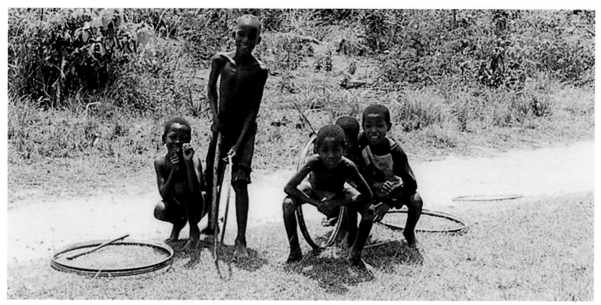

7-11 Protein deficiencies are common among the people in some African nations where high-quality sources of protein are scarce.

longer receiving protein-rich breast milk. He or she begins eating a diet that is much lower in protein.

A child suffering from kwashiorkor does not reach his or her full growth potential. The child develops a bloated abdomen and has skinny arms and legs. Lack of protein also affects the body's fluid balance and immune system. Many children die of such simple illnesses as a fever or the common measles.

Another PEM disease is marasmus. *Marasmus* is a wasting disease caused by a lack of calories and protein. It most often affects infants. The muscles and tissues of these children begin to waste away. The children become thin, weak, and susceptible to infection and disease. In short, they are suffering from starvation.

● Excess Proteins in the Diet

If you are like most people in the United States, you consume more than the RDA for protein. On the average, women in the United States eat almost one and one-half times the RDA for protein. Men eat nearly twice the RDA for protein.

Some people take protein or amino acid supplements, believing these products offer health benefits. Others simply enjoy eating diets rich in high-protein foods. These people should consider the problems associated with high-protein diets. Several health issues have been identified. See 7-12.

● Liver and Kidney Problems

A high-protein diet produces an overabundance of nitrogen waste. The body must excrete this waste before it builds up to toxic levels. The liver turns nitrogen waste into urea. The kidneys are responsible for excreting urea in urine. Therefore, excess protein creates extra work for the liver and kidneys. Stress on these organs can be a problem and may cause them to age prematurely. Extra work for the kidneys is a special problem for diabetics, who may already have problems with kidney disease.

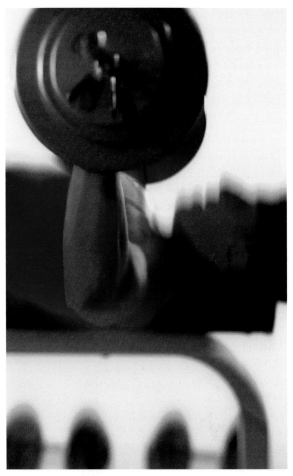

7-12 Body builders should be aware of the health risks of taking amino acid supplements and eating a high-protein diet.

● Calcium Loss

Several studies have shown diets high in protein from animal sources may contribute to calcium losses in the bones. A loss of calcium weakens the bones, which leads to a number of other health problems. A person whose diet is low in calcium is particularly at risk. (The effects of calcium loss on bones will be discussed further in Chapter 9, "Minerals: Regulators of Body Functions.")

● Excess Body Fat

Many common high-protein foods, such as whole milk, beef, cheese, and peanut butter, are also high-fat foods. Extra calories from fat can contribute to weight problems. Foods high in fat are also associated with heart-health and cancer risks. See 7-13.

The body cannot store excess amino acids as a protein source. However, it can store them as an energy source by converting them to body fat. Whether fat accompanies the protein in food or is manufactured from excess amino acids, the consequences are the same. Excess body fat is associated with a number of health problems, as discussed in Chapter 13, "Healthy Weight Management."

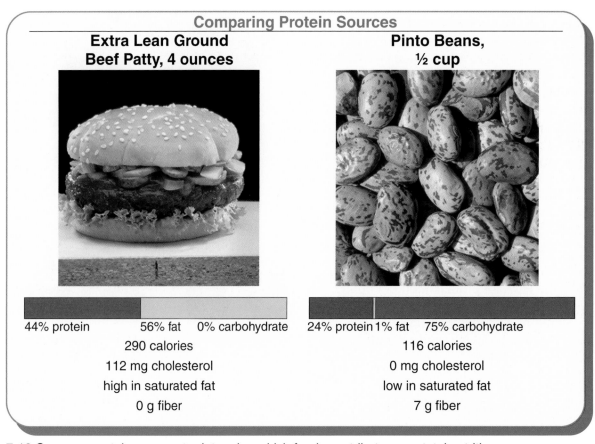

Comparing Protein Sources

Extra Lean Ground Beef Patty, 4 ounces	**Pinto Beans, ½ cup**
44% protein 56% fat 0% carbohydrate	24% protein 1% fat 75% carbohydrate
290 calories	116 calories
112 mg cholesterol	0 mg cholesterol
high in saturated fat	low in saturated fat
0 g fiber	7 g fiber

7-13 Compare protein sources to determine which foods contribute more total nutrition.

Summary

Protein is an energy-providing nutrient. Proteins in the diet are made of 20 amino acids. Nine of the amino acids are essential and cannot be manufactured by your body.

Proteins serve multiple functions. They provide for growth and maintenance of body tissues. Proteins are used to make important compounds, such as enzymes, hormones, and antibodies. They regulate fluid and acid-base balance. They carry vital substances, and they provide energy under special conditions.

Proteins come from animal food sources, including meat, fish, poultry, milk, and eggs. They also come from plant sources, such as cereals, legumes, seeds, and nuts. Animal sources of protein are complete; plant sources are incomplete. Complete proteins provide all the essential amino acids; incomplete proteins do not. Incomplete sources of protein can be combined to make a complete protein. This is important information for vegetarians, who eat little or no animal protein.

Protein needs depend on age, gender, body build, and state of health. Growing children need proportionally more protein than adults. Pregnant women need additional protein for building new tissue, and breast-feeding mothers need it to produce milk. Men tend to need more protein than women because they have a higher percentage of lean tissue. Individuals who are sick or injured need proteins to build body tissues. Athletes may have slightly higher protein needs than less active people. However, athletes can easily meet these needs by eating a nutritious diet.

Two to three daily servings from the milk and meat groups easily meet the RDA for protein. Most people in the United States consume more than the recommended amount of protein. Kwashiorkor and marasmus are two types of protein-energy malnutrition that are common in developing countries. These diseases especially affect young children, who then become susceptible to other life-threatening diseases and infections.

Check Your Knowledge

1. How does the chemical structure of protein differ from carbohydrates and fats?
2. What is the difference between an essential and a nonessential amino acid?
3. What role do stomach acids play in protein digestion?
4. Why is it important for people to get enough protein during the growth years?
5. How can a diet low in carbohydrates and fats affect the way the body uses proteins?
6. Name three specific animal sources and three specific plant sources of protein.
7. Describe two reasons vegetarians might give for eating little or no food from animal sources.
8. How can vegans meet their needs for complete sources of protein?
9. About what percentage of daily calories should come from protein?
10. Give three tips for limiting fat while meeting protein needs.
11. What type of nitrogen balance would describe the protein status of a healthy teen?
12. A disease brought on by a protein deficiency is _____.
13. True or false. On the average, men in the United States eat nearly twice the RDA for protein.
14. What are three problems associated with high-protein diets?

Put Learning into Action

1. Fry an egg in a moderately hot skillet containing a small amount of fat. Observe the egg carefully while it is cooking. Write a detailed description of how and why its consistency changes.

2. As a class, debate the pros and cons of eating meat versus following a vegetarian diet.

3. Keep a daily food diary for three days. Use diet analysis software to compare your actual daily protein consumption with the RDA.

4. Survey three teens and two adults to find out their favorite sources of protein. Compile your findings with those of your classmates. Work together to make a poster listing the calorie, fat, and protein content of the top 10 favorites.

5. For one day, eat a diet much like someone from a developing country might eat. Give an oral report describing the country and the typical diet of the population. State your opinion of the taste and nutritional quality of the diet.

Explore Further

1. Choose one of the functions of proteins. Write a three-page research report explaining how the body uses proteins to perform that function.

2. Find out how textured vegetable protein is used to make meat substitutes. Research the comparative costs and nutritional value of these substitutes with the foods they are intended to replace. Sample a product made from textured vegetable protein and evaluate its taste. Report your findings in class.

3. Make a videotape in which you play the role of an investigative news reporter. Investigate the foundation for claims made by manufacturers of protein and amino acid supplements. Determine whether the claims are valid. Relate how the cost and nutritional value of these supplements compare to whole food protein sources. Expose any dangers the use of these products might pose.

4. Research three possible solutions to the problem of protein-energy malnutrition in developing countries. Write an opinion paper or give an oral report on the solution you think is most viable. Give reasons for your choice.

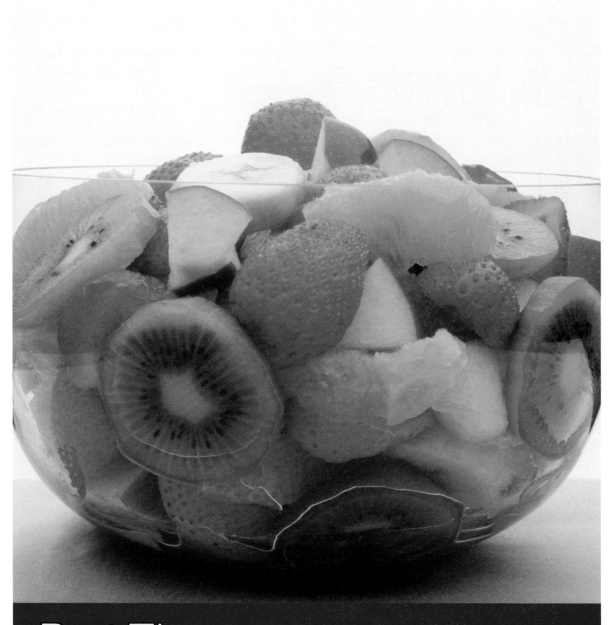

Part Three
The Work of
Noncaloric Nutrients

Chapter 8

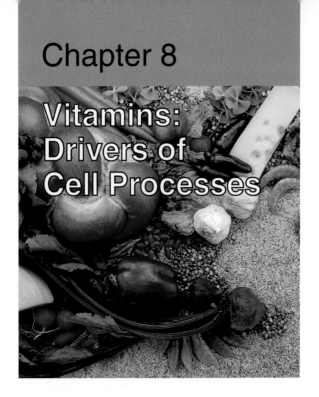

Vitamins: Drivers of Cell Processes

Although nutrition research began in the nineteenth century, vitamins were not identified until the beginning of the twentieth century. Scientists have learned much about vitamins. However, many questions concerning the roles of vitamins in the diet remain.

Will taking extra vitamin C help you prevent a cold? Should you take vitamin pills rather than trying to get vitamins from food? Will you get more vitamins if you eat fresh, raw vegetables instead of canned or cooked vegetables? These are among the questions for which researchers have already found answers. You will learn about these and other topics related to vitamins as you study this chapter.

● Learn the Language

vitamin
provitamin
fat-soluble vitamin
water-soluble vitamin
toxicity
epithelial cells
night blindness
fortified food
rickets
osteomalacia
antioxidant

free radical
erythrocyte hemolysis
coagulation
coenzyme
enriched food
beriberi
pellagra
pernicious anemia
scurvy
collagen
phytochemicals

● What Are Vitamins?

A *vitamin* is an essential nutrient needed in tiny amounts to regulate body processes. Vitamins have no calorie value because they yield no energy. However, the body needs vitamins for the chemical reactions involved in releasing energy from other nutrients. See 8-1.

Vitamins in the diet are vital to health and wellness. Each vitamin has specific functions. As a nutrient group, vitamins assist with the following functions:

- nutrient metabolism
- energy production and release
- tissue maintenance
- normal digestion
- infection resistance

Vitamin Names

In 1912, Casimir Funk coined the word *vitamine. Vita* means life; *amine* refers to a certain chemical structure that contains nitrogen. After years of research, it was discovered few vitamins had the amine structure in their chemical compounds. Therefore, the final *e* was dropped to avoid confusion with the amine groups found in the chemical structure of proteins.

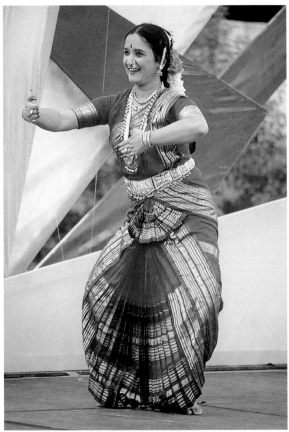

Photo courtesy of University Relations, MSU, Bruce A. Fox, photographer

8-1 Vitamins help the body release energy needed for physical activity.

Vitamins were named as they were discovered. The first vitamin discovered was named vitamin A. Logically, the next vitamin discovered was named vitamin B. However, it was later discovered that vitamin B was really several different vitamins. Also, some compounds originally thought to be vitamins turned out not to be. Therefore, the pattern to the naming of the vitamins became harder to recognize.

You may wonder how researchers prove whether a compound is a vitamin. Vitamins are essential for life for a specific species. A compound that is essential for humans may not be essential for earthworms. However, the compound is essential for all humans. This means removing the compound from the human diet will eventually cause all humans to develop deficiency symptoms. Conversely, if removing the compound does not result in deficiency symptoms, the compound is not a vitamin.

Today, there are 13 known vitamins. Some are most often referred to by a letter, such as vitamins A, C, D, E, and K. Most of the B vitamins are better known by a name, such as riboflavin, thiamin, and niacin.

Most vitamins have several *active forms,* or types that perform in the body. All the active forms have similar molecular structures. However, they may not all be able to do every function associated with the vitamin. The different active forms are like different car models. Some models have power windows and some do not, but they can all provide transportation. There are different names for each form of the same vitamin. For example, *pyridoxine, pyridoxal,* and *pyridoxamine* are all forms of vitamin B_6. You may have noticed some of these complex names on the ingredient lists of food labels. See 8-2.

The Chemistry of Vitamins

Unlike carbohydrates, fats, and proteins, the different vitamins do not share a typical molecular structure. Each is unique, but all

Morning Crunch

Whole Grain Cereal

Nutrition Facts

Serving Size	1 cup (56 g)
Servings Per Container	9

Amount Per Serving	
Calories	90
Calories from Fat	10

	% Daily Value
Total Fat 1g	2%
Saturated Fat 0g	0%
Cholesterol 0mg	0%
Sodium 180mg	8%
Total Carb. 15g	5%
Fiber 2g	
Sugars 1g	
Protein 2g	

Vitamin A 15%		Vitamin C 15%	
Calcium 2%		Iron 25%	

Percent Daily Values are based on a 2,000 calorie diet. Your daily values may be higher or lower depending on your calorie needs:

	Calories:	2,000	2,500
Total Fat	Less than	65g	80g
Sat Fat	Less than	20g	25g
Cholesterol	Less than	300mg	300mg
Sodium	Less than	2,400mg	2,400mg
Total Carbohydrate		300mg	375mg
Dietary Fiber		25g	30g

Calories per gram:
Fat 9   Carbohydrate 4   Protein 4

INGREDIENTS: WHOLE OAT FLOUR, WHEAT, BARLEY, BROWN SUGAR, CORN, RICE, SALT, MALT FLAVORING, RICE BRAN. VITAMINS AND MINERALS: IRON (FERRIC PHOSPHATE), VITAMIN E (ALPHA TOCOPHEROL ACETATE), NIACINAMIDE, ZINC (OXIDE), CALCIUM PANTOTHENATE, VITAMIN B_6 (PYRIDOXINE HYDROCHLORIDE), VITAMIN B_2 (RIBOFLAVIN), VITAMIN A (PALMITATE), VITAMIN B_1 (THIAMIN HYDROCHLORIDE), FOLIC ACID, BIOTIN, VITAMIN B_{12} AND VITAMIN D.

INGREDIENTS: WHOLE OAT FLOUR, WHEAT, BARLEY, BROWN SUGAR, CORN, RICE, SALT, MALT FLAVORING, RICE BRAN. VITAMINS AND MINERALS: IRON (FERRIC PHOSPHATE), VITAMIN E (ALPHA TOCOPHEROL ACETATE), NIACINAMIDE, ZINC (OXIDE), CALCIUM PANTOTHENATE, VITAMIN B_6 (PYRIDOXINE HYDROCHLORIDE), VITAMIN B_2 (RIBOFLAVIN), VITAMIN A (PALMITATE), VITAMIN B_1 (THIAMIN HYDROCHLORIDE), FOLIC ACID, BIOTIN, VITAMIN B_{12} AND VITAMIN D.

8-2 Ingredient lists on food labels often include the complex chemical names of added vitamins.

vitamins are *organic compounds,* which means they contain carbon. They also contain hydrogen and oxygen. Some contain nitrogen, sulfur, or cobalt in their structures, too.

Several vitamins have provitamin forms. **Provitamins** are compounds that are not vitamins, but the body can convert them into the active form of a vitamin. For example, *beta-carotene* is a provitamin for vitamin A. Beta-carotene is a deep yellow compound found in dark green and deep yellow fruits and vegetables, including carrots. When you eat this compound, your body can change the beta-carotene into vitamin A.

● How Much of the Vitamins Are Needed?

Long ago, doctors wondered why just small amounts of specific foods improved health problems like scurvy and night blindness. They learned the answer with the discovery of vitamins. They found the amounts of vitamins you need for growth, maintenance, and reproduction were tiny. In fact, you need only about one ounce of vitamins for every 150 pounds (2,400 ounces) of food you eat. All the vitamins you need in one day add up to only one-eighth of a teaspoon.

Nutrition experts have made recommendations stating how much of various vitamins people need each day for good health. Eating a nutritious diet that meets the AIs or RDAs is an important daily goal. However, if your intake of some vitamins is short now and then, there will be no serious harm. The first symptoms of a vitamin deficiency take a month or so to appear in most people.

There are two main causes of vitamin deficiency diseases. The first cause is an insufficient amount of a vitamin in the diet. In cases of poverty, people may lack the variety of foods that would provide all the vitamins they need. Even with a bounty of different foods, however, some people simply fail to choose rich sources of some vitamins.

Getting enough vitamins in the diet can be more of a challenge for people who have increased vitamin needs. Pregnant women need larger amounts of many nutrients, including most vitamins. Infants and adolescents need extra nutrients to aid in the growth of body tissues. See 8-3. People who are sick or recovering from injuries have greater needs, too. Lifestyle behaviors can also increase needs for certain vitamins. For instance, cigarette smokers need more vitamin C in their diets than nonsmokers.

The second cause of a vitamin deficiency disease is a failure of the body to absorb a vitamin. For instance, changes in the

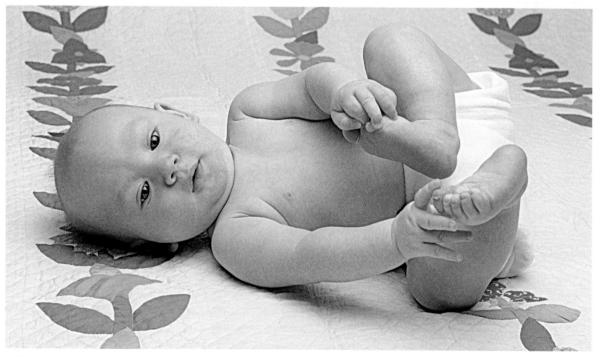

8-3 Infants need relatively large amounts of vitamins to support their rapid growth.

body that occur with age can affect a person's ability to absorb vitamin B_{12}. When food moves through the intestinal tract too quickly, vitamins do not have a chance to be absorbed adequately. Diarrhea or a very high-fiber diet may affect absorption in this way. Malabsorption of some nutrients can also be due to a lack of other nutrients.

Vitamin Classifications

All vitamins are grouped in two categories: fat-soluble or water-soluble. *Soluble* refers to a substance's ability to dissolve. Some vitamins dissolve in fats. The four **fat-soluble vitamins** are vitamins A, D, E, and K. Other vitamins dissolve in water. The nine **water-soluble vitamins** are the B-complex vitamins and vitamin C.

Your body stores excess fat-soluble vitamins when you take in more than you can use. An advantage of this is it is not crucial to consume the fat-soluble vitamins every day. A disadvantage is toxicity can result if amounts of these vitamins that are stored become too large. **Toxicity** is a poisonous condition. Vitamins A and D are especially toxic if consumed in large amounts over long periods. Toxicity does not occur from eating vitamin-rich foods. It occurs when people take large amounts of vitamin supplements.

Your body does not store water-soluble vitamins to any great extent. Excesses are normally excreted in the urine. Therefore, water-soluble vitamins do not readily build up to toxic levels in the body. Without large stores of these vitamins, however, deficiency symptoms may not take long to develop. Therefore, you need to be sure to consume enough of the water-soluble vitamins every day.

The Fat-Soluble Vitamins at Work

The fat-soluble vitamins, A, D, E, and K, are present in a wide range of foods in the diet. They are absorbed through the intestinal walls with fats from foods. Your body can draw on stored reserves of these vitamins when your intake is low.

Vitamin A

Vitamin A deficiency is the leading cause of blindness in children living in Africa, Asia, and South America. Up to 500,000 children go blind each year because their diets lack this vitamin.

Functions of Vitamin A

Vitamin A is necessary for the formation of healthy epithelial tissue. The **epithelial cells** are the surface cells that line the outside of the body. Epithelial tissue also covers the eyes and lines the passages of the lungs, intestines, and reproductive organs. Because of this function, vitamin A plays a role in keeping skin and hair healthy. Adequate amounts of vitamin A help keep the eyes free from dryness and infections. Vitamin A also helps the linings of the lungs and intestines stay moist and resistant to disease. See 8-4.

Maintaining healthy eyesight is another main function of vitamin A. Without sufficient vitamin A, the cells in the eyes cannot make the compounds needed by the eyes to see well in dim light. That means the eyes adapt slowly to darkness and night vision becomes poor. This condition is called **night blindness**.

Vitamin A is also crucial for the development of bone tissue. If bone formation is hampered, normal growth will not occur.

Meeting Vitamin A Needs

The RDA for vitamin A is 900 micrograms for males ages 14 and older. The RDA is 700 micrograms for females over age 14. (Males need more of many nutrients to support their higher percentage of lean body tissue.)

Another unit of measure for vitamin A is the *retinol activity equivalent (RAE)*. This unit is used to measure how strong various vitamin A compounds are and how easy they are for the body to use.

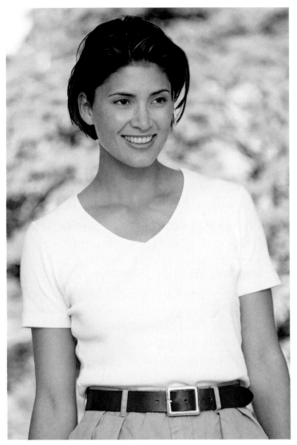

8-4 Vitamin A helps keep skin, hair, and eyes healthy.

Vitamin A in foods exists in two basic forms—one from animal sources and the other from plant sources. Animal foods usually provide vitamin A as a *preformed* vitamin. This is an active form the body can use. Plant foods provide vitamin A as provitamin *carotenes,* including alpha- and beta-carotene. The body can convert these compounds into the more usable form of vitamin A. However, they are not in an active form your body can use when you consume them. Therefore, they have a lower RAE value than preformed vitamin A.

Liver, fish oils, egg yolks, and whole milk dairy products are good sources of preformed vitamin A. Removing the fat from dairy products removes the fat-soluble vitamin A, too. Therefore, reduced-fat dairy products are fortified with vitamin A. **Fortified foods** are those that have one or more nutrients added during processing. Good sources of provitamin A carotenes include winter squash, carrots, broccoli, and apricots. See 8-5.

Eating a nutritious diet is the best way to meet vitamin A needs. Try to select rich sources each day.

● **Effects of Vitamin A Deficiencies and Excesses**

People who drink little milk or eat few vegetables may show signs of vitamin A deficiency. Symptoms of the deficiency may include night blindness; dry, scaly skin; and fatigue.

Vitamin A deficiency is one of the major causes of blindness in the world. It is a serious problem in underdeveloped nations. Without adequate vitamin A, the membrane covering the eyes becomes dry and hard. Infection and blindness can develop. If detected early enough, vision problems caused by deficiency can be reversed with large doses of vitamin A.

Getting enough vitamin A is important. However, getting too much can cause health problems. The body can store vitamin A to

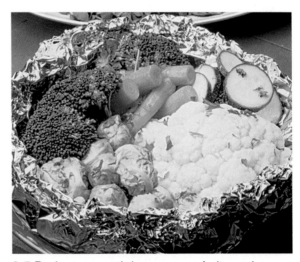

8-5 Dark green and deep orange fruits and vegetables, including broccoli and carrots, are good sources of beta-carotene. The body can convert beta-carotene into vitamin A.

toxic levels. Symptoms of vitamin A toxicity include severe headaches, bone pain, dry skin, hair loss, vomiting, and liver damage. Toxicity poses a greater risk for children. Very high vitamin A intakes are especially dangerous during pregnancy. Such intakes can cause babies to be born with disabilities.

● Vitamin D

Vitamin D is a unique fat-soluble vitamin. With direct exposure to sunlight, your body can make all the vitamin D it needs. Of course, you can also obtain vitamin D from your diet. See 8-6.

● Functions of Vitamin D

An important function of vitamin D is to help regulate the levels of calcium in the bloodstream. Normal amounts of calcium in the blood are needed for healthy nerve function, bone growth and maintenance, and other functions. Vitamin D performs this

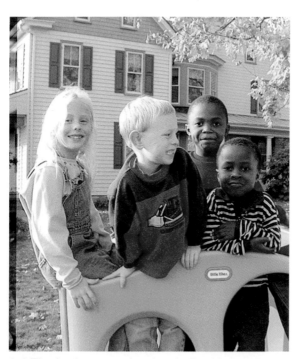

8-6 The body can make vitamin D with exposure to sunlight.

function by triggering the release of calcium from the bones. Vitamin D also controls blood calcium levels by enhancing the absorption of calcium from the intestines. When blood calcium levels are low, vitamin D also reduces the amount of calcium the kidneys excrete.

Bone tissue is the chief user of blood calcium. This mineral makes bones rigid and strong. However, nerve, muscle, and other cells also require calcium drawn from the bloodstream to function properly. Therefore, vitamin D plays a role in maintaining all body tissues.

● Meeting Vitamin D Needs

The Adequate Intake (AI) for vitamin D is 5 micrograms (200 IU) per day for all people through age 50. The AI is higher for older adults. This is to help older adults avoid developing porous, fragile bones—a condition that is more common in later life.

As mentioned, with exposure to sunshine, the body can make vitamin D. When sunlight shines on skin, a cholesterol-like compound in the skin forms a provitamin. The liver and kidneys then change the provitamin into vitamin D.

Spending too much time in the sun without protecting the skin increases the risk of skin cancer. Fortunately, the skin does not need prolonged sun exposure to make vitamin D. A light-skinned person can make enough vitamin D to meet the body's needs in 15 minutes of sun exposure. Dark-skinned people require a somewhat longer time to produce the same amount of vitamin D. Anything that filters sunlight, including clouds, smog, window glass, sunscreen, and heavy clothing, inhibits vitamin D production. Anyone who does not receive enough sunshine must get vitamin D from food sources.

Vitamin D occurs in a limited number of foods. Fatty fish and fish oils, eggs, butter, and vitamin D fortified milk and margarine are the best food sources. See 8-7.

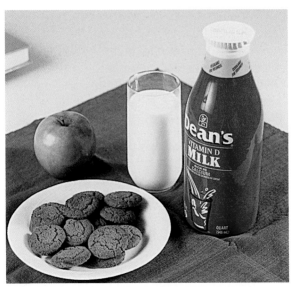

8-7 Fortified milk is an excellent source of vitamin D.

Effects of Vitamin D Deficiencies and Excesses

Rickets is a deficiency disease in children caused by lack of vitamin D. Without adequate vitamin D, not enough calcium is deposited in the bones. This causes the bones to be soft and misshapen. The leg bones may bow in or out. The chest bones may bulge outward.

A similar vitamin D deficiency disease in adults is called *osteomalacia*. It can cause the leg and spine bones to soften and bend. Osteomalacia is different from *osteoporosis,* which is a bone condition due to a calcium deficiency that affects older adults.

Too much vitamin D can be poisonous, and toxicity occurs most quickly in children. Too much sun exposure does not cause vitamin D toxicity. Getting an excessive amount of vitamin D from food would be difficult. Therefore, toxic intakes are usually the result of consuming supplements in amounts greater than the UL.

Excessive amounts of vitamin D cause too much calcium to be absorbed into the bloodstream. This surplus calcium is then deposited in the kidneys and other soft organs. This causes the organs to become hard and unable to perform their vital functions.

Vitamin E

Vitamin E may be the most advertised vitamin. Salespeople boost its popularity by making dramatic claims about its benefits. They have promoted vitamin E as an aid for enhancing athletic performance and reducing the signs of aging. However, research does not support such claims.

Functions of Vitamin E

Vitamin E helps maintain healthy immune and nervous systems. However, the main function of vitamin E in your body is as an antioxidant. *Antioxidants* are substances that react with oxygen to protect other substances from harmful effects of oxygen exposure. Vitamin C and provitamin A are also antioxidants. As an antioxidant, vitamin E ties up oxygen that could damage the membranes of white and red blood cells. It also protects the cells of the lungs.

Oxygen usually occurs as two oxygen molecules bonded together. When bound together, they are stable. However, when a single oxygen molecule is present, it is highly reactive. This molecule wants to react with other compounds as quickly as possible. Such a highly reactive, unstable single oxygen molecule is called a *free radical.* Free radicals regularly form in the body due to ordinary cell processes and environmental conditions. These single oxygen molecules can generate a harmful chain reaction that can damage tissue.

Vitamin E and other antioxidants help deactivate or transform free radicals. If vitamin E does not step in, tissue damage can lead to disease.

Meeting Vitamin E Needs

The RDA for vitamin E is 15 milligrams per day for males and females over the age of 14. Research provides no strong support for consuming large amounts of vitamin E. There is also no support for taking vitamin E supplements instead of getting it from food sources.

A varied diet includes many sources of vitamin E. The best sources are vegetable oils, some fruits and vegetables, and margarine. Wheat germ, multigrain cereals, and nuts are also good sources. See 8-8.

High temperatures destroy vitamin E. Therefore, foods that are prepared or processed with high heat lose their vitamin E value.

Effects of Vitamin E Deficiencies and Excesses

Because sources of vitamin E are widespread in the diet, deficiencies are not common. However, deficiencies have been seen in premature babies. This is because babies store vitamin E during the last few weeks of their mothers' pregnancies. If babies are born prematurely, they do not have vitamin E stores. These deficiencies cause red blood cells to break, a condition called **erythrocyte hemolysis**, which makes the babies weak and listless. Premature babies almost always receive a vitamin E supplement when they are born to prevent these problems. Vitamin E

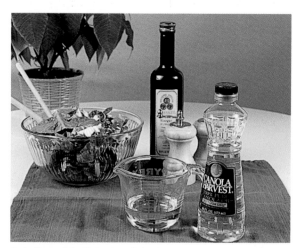

8-8 Canola oil and salad dressings made with it are rich sources of vitamin E.

deficiency in adults negatively affects speech, vision, and muscle coordination.

Vitamin E is less toxic than other fat-soluble vitamins. However, large doses have caused digestive problems and nausea. Excessive amounts of vitamin E may interfere with blood clotting.

Vitamin K

Few people look forward to surgery or welcome bleeding injuries. However, if you must face these plights, you will be glad for the action of vitamin K.

Functions of Vitamin K

The main function of vitamin K is to make proteins needed in the coagulation of blood. **Coagulation** means clotting. This is the process that stops bleeding. Vitamin K is also needed to make a protein that helps bones collect the minerals they need for strength.

Meeting Vitamin K Needs

The need for vitamin K increases throughout childhood, the teen years, and young adulthood. For 14- to 18-year-old males and females, the AI for vitamin K is 75 micrograms per day.

Bacteria in the intestinal tract help meet a significant part of your vitamin K needs. These bacteria can synthesize vitamin K.

A varied diet will help you meet the rest of your vitamin K needs. Good food sources of vitamin K include green leafy vegetables and liver. Fruits, milk, meat, eggs, and grain products also supply small amounts of this vitamin.

Effects of Vitamin K Deficiencies and Excesses

There are few cases of vitamin K deficiency. However, a deficiency can occur among people who take antibiotics that kill intestinal bacteria. Newborns can also be at risk for vitamin K deficiency. This is because

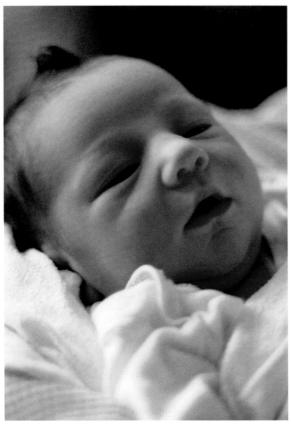

8-9 Newborns may lack vitamin K because they have not yet developed the intestinal bacteria that make it.

they do not yet have enough bacteria in their intestines to synthesize the vitamin. Newborns almost always receive a vitamin K supplement. This helps meet their needs until bacteria in their intestines can begin producing enough vitamin K. See 8-9.

Although vitamin K can be toxic, toxicity is rare. A symptom of toxicity is *jaundice,* which is a yellow coloring of the skin. Vitamin K toxicity can cause brain damage.

● The Water-Soluble Vitamins at Work

The water-soluble vitamins include all the B vitamins and vitamin C. Lean tissues may store surpluses of these vitamins for short

periods. However, excesses are generally excreted in the urine. Therefore, the accepted recommendation is that you include them in your diet every day.

● The Teamwork of B Vitamins

The B vitamins are thiamin, riboflavin, niacin, pantothenic acid, biotin, B_6, folate, and B_{12}. These vitamins work as a team. They are all parts of coenzymes.

A *coenzyme* is a nonprotein compound that combines with an inactive enzyme to form an active enzyme system. Think of an inactive enzyme as a car without wheels. The vitamin coenzyme is like the wheels. When you put the wheels on the car, the car can move. Just as a car will not work without wheels, an inactive enzyme will not work without the vitamin coenzyme.

The metabolism of energy nutrients is one critical area requiring the joint action of enzymes and coenzymes. Without coenzymes, the enzymes that release energy from carbohydrates, fats, and proteins could not do their jobs. As parts of the coenzymes, the B vitamins help provide the energy needed by every cell in the body.

The B vitamins are found in many of the same food sources. Therefore, deficiency symptoms are often due to a shortage of several vitamins rather than a single vitamin. Deficiencies of B vitamins can cause a broad range of symptoms. These symptoms include nausea and loss of weight and appetite. Severe exhaustion, irritability, depression, and forgetfulness may also occur. The heart, skin, and immune system may be affected, too.

Besides their roles as a group, each of the B vitamins has individual functions. These will be discussed in the following sections.

● Thiamin

Thiamin was named for its molecular structure. *Thi-* means sulfur, which is one of the elements in a thiamin molecule.

Functions of Thiamin

Thiamin plays a vital role in energy metabolism. It is also required for normal functioning of the nerves and the muscles they control.

Meeting Thiamin Needs

The more calories you burn, the more thiamin you need. Teens who are 14 to 18 years old have fairly high daily calorie needs. The thiamin RDA that corresponds with these needs is 1.2 milligrams per day for males. The RDA for females is 1.0 milligram per day.

Whole grain breads and cereals are sources of thiamin as well as several other B vitamins. Refined grain products are commonly enriched with these vitamins and iron. **Enriched foods** have had vitamins and minerals added back that were lost in the refining process. Enriched foods can be important sources of nutrients. See 8-10.

Other foods that are good sources of thiamin include pork products, dried beans, nuts, seeds, and liver. Because the body does not store much thiamin, you need to consume thiamin-rich foods daily.

Effects of Thiamin Deficiencies and Excesses

Beriberi is the thiamin deficiency disease. *Beriberi* means "I can't, I can't." Without enough thiamin, the body cannot perform the tasks required for everyday living. Symptoms include weakness, loss of appetite, and irritability. Poor arm and leg coordination and a nervous tingling throughout the body are also symptoms of thiamin deficiency. Some people develop edema and heart failure. *Edema* is an excess accumulation of fluid.

The disease of alcoholism increases the risk of thiamin deficiency because alcohol diminishes the body's ability to absorb and use thiamin. A diet in which a large percentage of calories comes from alcohol also lacks calories from nutritious food sources.

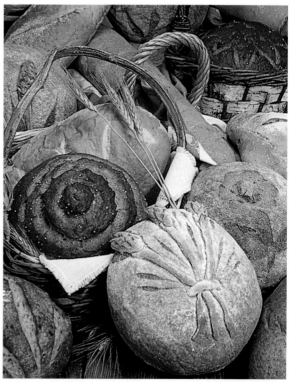

Wheat Foods Council

8-10 Enriched and whole grain breads and cereals are good sources of several B vitamins.

Symptoms of thiamin toxicity have not been identified. However, nutrition experts state there is no health benefit in consuming thiamin at levels higher than the RDA.

Riboflavin

The word *riboflavin* comes from the yellow color of this vitamin compound. *Flavus* means yellow in Latin.

Functions of Riboflavin

Riboflavin helps the body release energy from carbohydrates, fats, and proteins. You also need it for healthy skin and normal eyesight.

Meeting Riboflavin Needs

Daily riboflavin needs for males and females in their late teens are 1.8 and 1.3 milligrams, respectively. Milk and milk products are excellent food sources for meeting these needs. Enriched and whole grain cereals, meats, poultry, and fish are also good sources of riboflavin. See 8-11.

Healthy people who eat a nutritious diet generally get enough riboflavin. People who do not drink milk or eat milk products may be at risk for developing a deficiency.

Effects of Riboflavin Deficiencies and Excesses

Many symptoms are associated with riboflavin deficiency. They include an inflamed tongue and cracked skin around the corners of the mouth. Various eye disorders and mental confusion are symptoms, too.

Toxicity symptoms have not been reported. Extra riboflavin is excreted in the urine.

Niacin

There are several types of niacin. These include *nicotinic acid* and *nicotinamide.* All types of niacin are water-soluble.

Functions of Niacin

Like the other B vitamins, niacin is involved in energy metabolism. It also helps keep the skin and nervous system healthy. It promotes normal digestion, too.

Meeting Niacin Needs

Niacin in foods is available as a preformed vitamin. It is also available in a pro-vitamin form—*tryptophan,* which is one of the amino acids in many protein foods.

The RDA for niacin is stated in terms of *niacin equivalents (NE).* This unit accounts

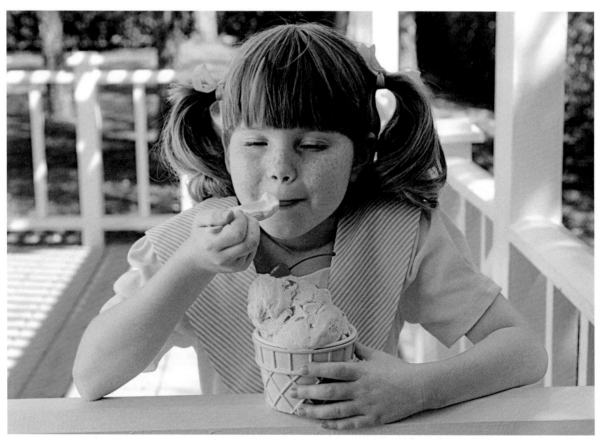

8-11 Ice cream, like other dairy products, is a source of riboflavin.

for both the provitamin and preformed forms of niacin. Males in the 14- to 18-year age range need the equivalent of 16 milligrams of niacin daily. Females in this age range need the equivalent of 14 milligrams.

Whole grain and enriched breads and cereals, meat, poultry, and nuts are popular sources of niacin. Tryptophan is found in protein foods, such as meats and dairy products. See 8-12.

Effects of Niacin Deficiencies and Excesses

Pellagra is the niacin deficiency disease. The symptoms of pellagra are often known as the *four D*s. These symptoms are diarrhea, dermatitis (dry, flaky skin), dementia (insanity), and death. Early disease symptoms include poor appetite, weight loss, and weakness.

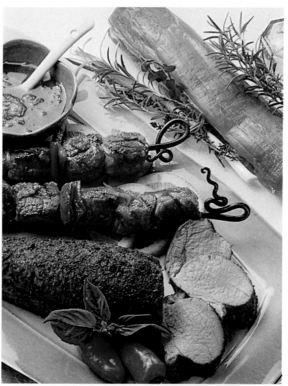

National Pork Producers Council

8-12 Meat and other protein foods are sources of tryptophan, which the body can convert to niacin.

Niacin can be toxic when too much is consumed through supplements. Toxicity is characterized by dilated blood vessels near the surface of the skin. The resulting painful rash is sometimes called *niacin flush.* Nausea, dizziness, and low blood pressure are also symptoms of too much niacin.

Pantothenic Acid

Pantothenic acid is another B-complex vitamin. It gets its name from the Greek word *pantothen,* which means from all sides. This name seems appropriate because pantothenic acid is found in all living tissues.

Functions of Pantothenic Acid

Pantothenic acid promotes growth. It is part of a coenzyme that is critical to the metabolism of the energy nutrients. It is also involved in synthesizing a number of vital substances in the body.

Meeting Pantothenic Acid Needs

Studies on pantothenic acid have not produced enough conclusive data to set an RDA. Therefore, an AI has been established as a guide for intake. For people ages 14 and over, the AI for pantothenic acid is 5 milligrams per day.

Effects of Pantothenic Acid Deficiencies and Excesses

Pantothenic acid is found in many food sources. Therefore, deficiency symptoms are rarely a problem. Toxicity is also rare.

Biotin

Biotin gets its name from the Greek word for *sustenance,* which means something that helps support life.

Functions of Biotin

Biotin helps activate several enzymes involved in the release of energy from carbohydrates, fats, and proteins. Biotin also helps the body make fats and glycogen.

● Meeting Biotin Needs

Like pantothenic acid, there is no RDA for biotin. The AI for males and females ages 14 to 18 is 25 micrograms per day.

Biotin is widespread in foods. Egg yolks, yeast, beans, nuts, cheese, and liver are especially good sources. See 8-13.

● Effects of Biotin Deficiencies and Excesses

Because biotin is widely available in foods, deficiencies among people who eat nutritious diets are uncommon. A biotin deficiency produces similar symptoms of the circulatory and muscular systems as a thiamin deficiency. These symptoms include abnormal heart rhythms, pain, weakness, fatigue, and depression. Nausea; loss of appetite; dry, scaly skin; and hair loss are other symptoms.

Nutrition researchers have found no evidence of biotin toxicity. Although there may be no health risk, there are no advantages to biotin intakes above the recommended range.

● Vitamin B_6

Remember from Chapter 7 that the diet must supply only 9 of the 20 amino acids that

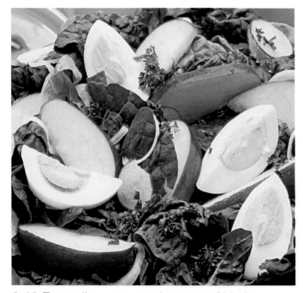

8-13 Egg yolks are a good source of biotin.

make up proteins. This is because the body can make sufficient amounts of the other 11 amino acids. However, the body could not do this without the help of vitamin B_6.

● Functions of Vitamin B_6

Vitamin B_6 plays a key role in synthesizing nonessential amino acids. It is needed to convert the amino acid tryptophan to niacin. Vitamin B_6 helps make the protein that allows red blood cells to carry oxygen. It also affects the health of the immune and nervous systems.

● Meeting Vitamin B_6 Needs

The RDA for vitamin B_6 for males ages 14 through 50 is 1.3 milligrams per day. Females ages 14 to 18 need 1.2 milligrams per day. Needs increase to 1.3 milligrams daily for adult females through age 50. Vitamin B_6 needs increase for people of both sexes after age 50.

Vitamin B_6 is found in meats, fish, and poultry. Dairy products and some fruits and vegetables, such as bananas, cantaloupe, broccoli, and spinach, are also good sources.

● Effects of Vitamin B_6 Deficiencies and Excesses

Vitamin B_6 deficiencies are rare. Symptoms of vitamin B_6 deficiencies are related to poor amino acid and protein metabolism. Symptoms include skin disorders, fatigue, irritability, and convulsions.

People who have taken large doses of vitamin B_6 have reported symptoms of toxicity. These symptoms include walking difficulties and numbness in the hands and feet. Irreversible nerve damage can also result from excessive intakes of this vitamin.

● Folate

Folate, which was also called *folacin* in the past, is another B vitamin. The term *folate* is derived from the Latin word *folium,* which means leaf. This is a logical name because leafy green vegetables are good sources of folate. *Folic acid* is a synthetic form of this vitamin found in nutrient supplements and fortified foods.

Functions of Folate

The main function of folate is to help synthesize DNA, the genetic material in every cell. Without folate, cells cannot divide to form new cells.

Another function of folate is especially important to any woman of childbearing age. Women who have inadequate folate intakes are more likely to give birth to babies with *neural tube damage.* Such damage affects the brain and spinal cord and can cause mental retardation, paralysis, and premature death. See 8-14.

Meeting Folate Needs

The RDA for folate is 400 micrograms per day for everyone age 14 and over. Pregnancy increases folate needs. Pregnant women need 600 micrograms of folate daily.

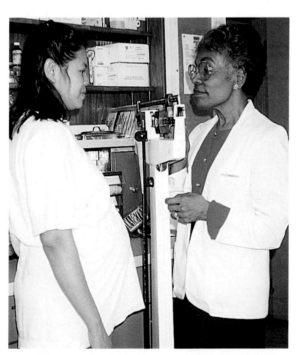

8-14 Women should be sure to meet their folate needs before and during pregnancy to help prevent neural tube damage in their babies.

Dark green leafy vegetables are excellent sources of folate. Liver, legumes, oranges, cantaloupe, and broccoli are also good sources. In addition, most enriched breads, flours, and other grain products are fortified with folic acid.

Meeting daily folate recommendations is especially important for women of childbearing age. This is because neural tube damage occurs during the first weeks of pregnancy, before many women realize they are pregnant. Fully meeting folate requirements before becoming pregnant reduces a woman's risk of having a baby with neural tube damage.

Research confirms that folic acid from fortified foods and supplements reduces the risk of neural tube damage. Researchers do not know if the folate that occurs naturally in foods has the same preventive effect. Therefore, they recommend all women of childbearing age consume 400 micrograms of folic acid daily from supplements or fortified foods. Eating a nutritious diet will provide additional folate from foods.

Effects of Folate Deficiencies and Excesses

You have already read about the increased risks of neural tube damage due to folate deficiency in pregnant women. Other population groups can also be affected by folate deficiencies.

Folate deficiencies are not uncommon. They usually result from low intakes of folate. Several medications, such as aspirin and oral contraceptives, can interfere with the body's ability to use folate.

The first signs of a folate deficiency appear in the red blood cells. Without sufficient folate, the red blood cells are fragile and cannot mature and carry oxygen. With a reduced number of mature red blood cells, a person feels tired and weak. Other symptoms of a folate deficiency include diarrhea and increased risk of infection.

Little information is available about folate toxicity. However, large intakes of folate can conceal symptoms of a vitamin B_{12} deficiency.

This reduces the likelihood that the vitamin B_{12} deficiency would be diagnosed and treated. Irreparable nerve damage could result.

Vitamin B_{12}

Vitamin B_{12} is a chemical compound that contains cobalt. That is why the vitamin is sometimes called *cyanocobalamin.*

Functions of Vitamin B_{12}

Vitamin B_{12} helps folate function. It is needed for growth, maintenance of healthy nerve tissue, and formation of normal red blood cells. It also is needed for the release of energy from fat.

Meeting Vitamin B_{12} Needs

The RDA for vitamin B_{12} for males and females ages 14 and over is 2.4 micrograms per day. People who eat foods from animal sources easily meet these needs. Meat, poultry, fish, eggs, and dairy products are all good sources. Vitamin B_{12} does not naturally occur in foods from plant sources. See 8-15.

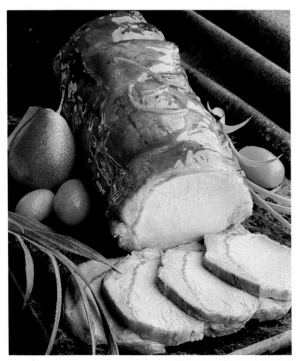

National Pork Producers Council

8-15 Meat and other animal foods are good sources of vitamin B_{12}.

Effects of Vitamin B_{12} Deficiencies and Excesses

Pernicious anemia, the deficiency disease associated with vitamin B_{12}, is actually caused by an inability to absorb the vitamin. Impaired absorption is due to the lack of a compound made in the stomach. An injury or a rare genetic disorder can cause the stomach to stop producing this important compound. As people grow older, they may lose their ability to make this compound. Pernicious anemia prevents red blood cells from maturing and dividing properly. This causes a person to feel tired and weak.

Symptoms of pernicious anemia also include a red, painful tongue and a tingling or burning in the skin. Nerve damage can eventually lead to walking difficulties and paralysis. Nerve damage can cause memory loss and mental slowness, too.

Fortunately, pernicious anemia can be treated. Injections of vitamin B_{12} periodically, perhaps throughout life, will allow red blood cells to mature normally. (The vitamin must be injected due to the body's inability to absorb a supplement taken by mouth.) With vitamin B_{12} present, the insulation remaining around nerve cells will be maintained. However, nerve damage that occurred before the deficiency was diagnosed usually cannot be reversed.

People who eat animal foods and can absorb vitamin B_{12} are unlikely to develop deficiencies. Strict vegetarians, who eat no animal products, must include alternative sources of vitamin B_{12} in their diets. Such sources might be vitamin supplements and fortified soy milk. Older adults are also at risk for developing pernicious anemia. Regular blood tests can help identify those people who need vitamin B_{12} injections.

The body can maintain long-term stores of vitamin B_{12}. However, no toxicity symptoms are known.

Vitamin C

Vitamin C is often referred to as *ascorbic acid.* Long before this vitamin was identified, sailors who went on lengthy voyages often developed the deadly disease scurvy. In a search for a cure, a British doctor, James Lind, carried out the first nutrition experiment using human subjects. He added different substances to the diets of each of several groups of sailors with scurvy. Lind found those sailors who ate citrus fruits were cured.

Nutritionists now know it was the vitamin C in the citrus fruits that helped cure the disease. **Scurvy** has been correctly identified as a disease caused by vitamin C deficiency.

● Functions of Vitamin C

Vitamin C performs a number of important functions in the body. It assists in the formation of collagen. **Collagen** is a protein substance in the connective tissue that holds cells together. Collagen is needed for healthy bones, cartilage, muscles, and blood vessels. Collagen helps wounds heal quickly. It also helps maintain capillaries and gums.

Vitamin C increases iron and calcium absorption. It plays a role in synthesizing thyroxine, the hormone that controls basal metabolic rate. Vitamin C is also vital to the body's immune system.

Vitamin C is an antioxidant. It works with vitamin E to protect body cells from free radicals. Some experts believe this may allow vitamin C to help prevent some cell damage. This may include the cell damage that leads to the development of some cancers, cataracts, and heart disease.

● Meeting Vitamin C Needs

The RDA for vitamin C for males ages 14 to 18 is 75 milligrams per day. After age 19, it increases to 90 milligrams per day. For females ages 14 to 18, the RDA is 65 milligrams per day. After age 19, it increases to 75 milligrams per day. The body does not store vitamin C, so a daily intake is necessary.

People exposed to cigarette smoke need extra vitamin C. This is because smoke hinders the body's use of vitamin C. Smokers and anyone exposed to smoke should include an extra 35 milligrams of vitamin C in their daily diets.

Vitamin C is found in many fruits and vegetables. Fruits rich in vitamin C include citrus fruits, cantaloupe, and strawberries, 8-16. Good vegetable sources include sweet peppers, broccoli, cabbage, and potatoes.

● Effects of Vitamin C Deficiencies and Excesses

Most people in the United States meet their daily needs for vitamin C through diet. However, low intakes of vitamin C are not unusual among older adults. As a group, they tend to eat diets that contain fewer fruits and vegetables.

What happens if there is inadequate vitamin C in the diet? Scurvy is the most severe form of vitamin C deficiency. It rarely occurs in developed countries because the causes and cure of the disease are known. In poorer countries where diets are inadequate, however, scurvy is not uncommon.

The symptoms of scurvy are many. They include tiredness, weakness, shortness of breath, aching bones and muscles, swollen and bleeding gums, and lack of appetite. Wounds heal slowly. The skin can become rough and covered with tiny red spots. The marks are small patches of bleeding just under the skin that appear as capillaries break.

Some extra vitamin C may not be harmful. Most excess vitamin C just ends up being excreted. However, large doses of one to three grams (1,000 to 3,000 milligrams) have had reported side effects. People taking large doses have complained of nausea, diarrhea, and stomach cramps. Large doses may also reduce the ability of vitamin B_{12} to function.

Many people believe that taking extra vitamin C can prevent or cure the common cold. Current research does not support this claim. However, adequate amounts of vitamin C do help protect the body against infections.

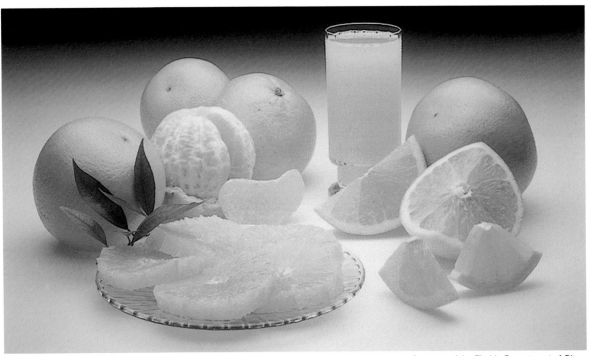

8-16 Citrus fruits and juices are excellent sources of vitamin C.

Nonvitamins and Other Nonnutrients

A number of substances have been discovered to have vitaminlike qualities. Examples include *choline* and *inositol,* which play roles in energy metabolism similar to B vitamins. These compounds are active in the body. However, research has not shown them to be vital for human life. Therefore, they are not currently regarded as vitamins. Future studies may lead researchers to add some of these substances to the list of essential nutrients.

Other compounds sometimes labeled as vitamins include *laetrile* (sometimes called vitamin B_{17}) and *pangamic acid* (sometimes called vitamin B_{15}). These substances have no vitamin value for humans. Some people use these compounds to treat diseases for which the compounds have not been proven effective. This may keep these people from seeking reliable medical care.

Health food fans promote the benefits of dietary supplements such as melatonin and ephedrine. Like the nonvitamins just described, many of these substances are active in the body. However, they are not essential to human nutrition. Therefore, they may be viewed as nonnutrients. Although these nonnutrients may be advertised and sold, claims made for many of them are unproven. Some of them have caused harmful reactions.

Phytochemicals

Although some nonnutrient substances seem to be of little value, scientific studies document the benefits of others. Among the helpful nonnutrients are some ***phytochemicals***. These are health-enhancing compounds in plant foods that are active in the body at the cellular level. Plants make hundreds of phytochemicals to protect themselves against such factors as ultraviolet light, oxidation, and insects. Scientists have just begun to learn about the useful roles some of these compounds play in the body.

Research has shown certain phytochemicals help prevent heart disease and some forms of cancer. They achieve this preventive effect through various chemical reactions in the body. Prompting the body to make enzymes, binding harmful substances, and acting as antioxidants are among the ways phytochemicals work.

Studies citing the value of certain phytochemicals have led many nutrition faddists to buy phytochemical supplements. Research has not proven these supplements to be safe and effective. The combinations of phytochemicals and nutrients found in foods cannot be duplicated in a supplement. Therefore, supplements cannot perform the same way foods can.

Eating plant foods is the best way to include phytochemicals in your diet. Fruits, vegetables, herbs, spices, legumes, and grains are all sources of helpful phytochemicals. See 8-17.

● Are Vitamin Supplements Needed?

In the United States, people spend billions of dollars on vitamin supplements each year. Why do they do it? Is it necessary? Many people worry they are not getting enough vitamins in their diets. Their schedules are busy and they may not take time to eat nutritiously.

Those who sell vitamins have profited from consumer concerns about health and nutrition. They promote numerous benefits of taking vitamin supplements to persuade people to spend more money. Contrary to some advertisements, vitamins are not "miracle cures" for everything from acne to AIDS. Vitamins cannot pep you up when you are feeling tired and run-down. They do not make you strong, attractive, or more popular. Supplements do not make up for poor eating habits, either. The only symptoms a vitamin supplement will relieve are those caused by a lack of that vitamin. For example, a thiamin supplement would relieve the symptoms of beriberi.

Some groups of people may need supplements to augment the vitamins provided by their diets. Doctors may advise pregnant and breast-feeding women to take supplements. Doctors may recommend supplements for infants, older adults, and patients who are ill or recovering from surgery. Doctors also occasionally prescribe large doses of vitamins for pharmaceutical purposes. For instance, large doses of vitamin A are sometimes prescribed for their drug effects in treating an incurable eye disease. Few people outside these groups need vitamin supplements. A diet including the recommended servings from all the food groups will supply most people with the vitamins they need. See 8-18.

Phytochemicals	
Family	**Major Food Sources**
Allyl sulfides	Chives, garlic, leeks, onions
Indoles	Broccoli, cabbage, cauliflower, kale
Isoflavones	Soybeans, soymilk, tofu
Phenolic acids	Carrots, citrus fruits, nuts, tomatoes, whole grains
Polyphenols	Grapes, green tea
Saponins	Beans, legumes
Terpenes	Cherries, citrus peel

8-17 Food choices that are rich in phytochemicals can improve health and decrease risks for certain diseases.

People who decide to use supplements have a number of choices available. They may choose products in pill, liquid, or powder form. They may also choose between natural and synthetic vitamins. *Natural vitamins* are extracted from foods. *Synthetic vitamins* are made in a laboratory. Advertisers may claim natural vitamins are superior. Chemically speaking, there is no advantage of a natural vitamin over a synthetic vitamin. The body uses both types of vitamins the same way. However, synthetic vitamins are less expensive and are usually purer than natural vitamins.

People who choose to use supplements should also be aware that some supplements provide large doses of vitamins. Amounts may be many times higher than the recommended daily levels. You know vitamins have specific functions and only very small amounts are needed for good health.

The Food and Drug Administration regulates the sale of vitamin supplements. They require scientific research to back up health claims made on product labels or in advertising. However, the FDA has little authority to regulate the amounts of vitamins supplements contain.

Taking several vitamin pills at a time, or several pills throughout the day, can cause health problems. The body can store toxic levels of fat-soluble vitamins. Excess water-soluble vitamins are normally excreted in the urine. However, large doses of some water-soluble vitamins produce negative effects for some people. For instance, too much vitamin C in the diet can irritate the gastrointestinal system. Also, an excess of one nutrient may affect how the body uses other nutrients.

Buying supplements is a costly way to get nutrients. In addition, vitamin tablets provide no fiber, energy, or taste. You cannot enjoy supplements as you do foods. Most nutritionists agree people benefit more from spending their money on a nutritious diet than on vitamin supplements.

● Preserving Vitamins in Foods

Eating vitamin-rich foods should ensure you are meeting your body's need for vitamins. Right? Wrong! Many vitamins are unstable. Careless food storage can destroy some vitamins. Cooking techniques can affect vitamin retention, too. This section will help you learn how to select foods high in vitamins. You will also learn how to preserve the vitamins that are present in foods.

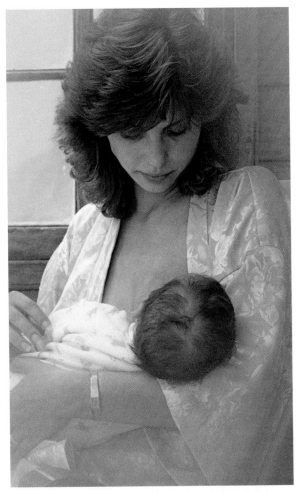

8-18 Doctors often recommend vitamin supplements for breast-feeding women to help meet the extra needs caused by producing milk.

● Selecting Foods High in Vitamins

Modern processing methods minimize nutrient losses. Therefore, canned, frozen, and dried foods are comparable to fresh in terms of vitamin content. Choose the form that is most convenient for you. However, be aware of products that contain large amounts of added fat, sugar, and sodium. Read Nutrition Facts panels to help you choose foods that are nutrient dense.

Knowing signs of quality can help you avoid foods that may have suffered excessive vitamin losses. When buying fresh fruits and vegetables, choose items that have bright colors and firm textures. Avoid pieces with wilted leaves, mold growth, or bruised spots. When selecting canned products, do not buy cans that are dented or bulging. These signs may indicate a broken seal and possible contamination of the food. Choose foods from the freezer case that are firmly frozen. Avoid frozen foods that have a layer of ice on the package. This indicates the food may not have been stored at a constant low temperature. Partial thawing can result in nutrient losses and a general decrease in quality. When buying dried foods, look for packages that are securely sealed. See 8-19.

● Storing Foods for Vitamin Retention

The way you handle food can affect its nutritional value. Exposing foods to air, light, and heat during transportation and storage causes vitamin losses. If fresh foods are not properly stored, they may have fewer vitamins than frozen or canned foods.

The following suggestions will help you minimize nutrient losses when handling and storing food:

- Keep freezer temperatures at zero degrees or lower to retain vitamin content of frozen foods. Try to use frozen foods within several months. Avoid thawing and refreezing foods, which causes some vitamin losses.

- Store canned foods in a cool, dry storage area. The liquid in which foods are canned contains nutrients. Serve the canning liquid with the food or use it in cooking.

- Store milk in opaque containers to protect its riboflavin content. Riboflavin is destroyed by light.

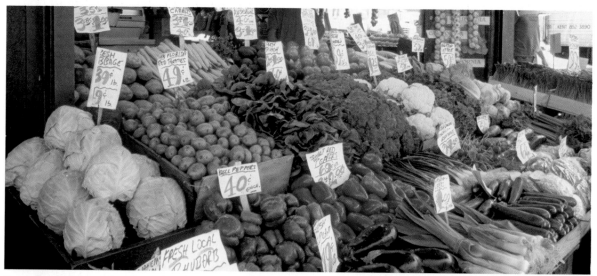

8-19 Buying fresh foods and eating them soon after they are purchased will help you get maximum vitamin value.

- Ripen fresh fruits and vegetables at room temperature away from direct sunlight.
- Store fresh vegetables promptly in a vegetable crisper in the refrigerator. The low temperature and high humidity of the crisper help preserve the vitamins in the vegetables.
- When storing cut foods, be sure to wrap them tightly. This will prevent vitamins from being destroyed by oxidation. Storing foods promptly in the refrigerator will reduce the action of enzymes that can break down vitamins.

Preparing Foods to Preserve Vitamins

Water, heat, acids, and alkalis used in cooking can all destroy vitamins. Knowing how vitamins respond to different cooking methods can help you preserve vitamins when preparing foods. The following guidelines may be helpful:

- To preserve water-soluble vitamins, do not soak fruits or vegetables in water.
- Many vitamins are located just under the skin of fresh produce. Therefore, avoid paring and peeling fruits and vegetables, if possible. Eat the whole food.
- Keep foods in large pieces to avoid exposing large amounts of surface area to light, air, and water.
- Cut up fruits and vegetables just before you are ready to cook or eat them. This reduces air and light exposure, which can damage vitamins. See 8-20.
- Choose steaming over boiling to help retain water-soluble vitamins. If you do boil vegetables, do not add them to cooking water until the water begins to boil. Use

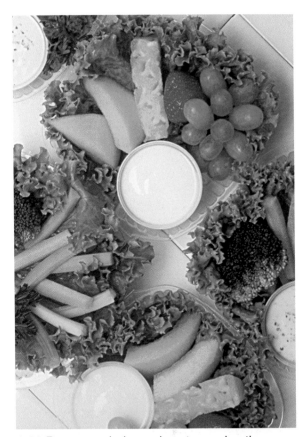

8-20 Prepare salads as close to serving time as possible to avoid exposing vitamins to air and light for long periods.

only a small amount of water and cook the vegetables just until tender. Avoid adding baking soda, which is an alkali, to vegetables. It can destroy some vitamins. Use cooking water in soups, gravies, or sauces.
- Use a pressure cooker or microwave oven to help preserve nutrients by reducing cooking times.

In general, keep cooking times short and use little water. Overcooking will destroy heat-sensitive vitamins. Water-soluble vitamins leach into cooking water.

Chapter 8 Review

Summary

Vitamins are essential nutrients. No one food supplies all the vitamins needed. Choosing a variety of foods is likely to supply all the vitamins most people need.

Vitamins perform a number of major roles in the diet. They are needed to release energy from carbohydrates, fats, and proteins. They help maintain healthy body tissues. They are required for the normal operation of all body processes. They also help the body's immune system resist infection.

The fat-soluble vitamins are vitamins A, D, E, and K. They dissolve in fats and are found in foods containing fats. Fat-soluble vitamins can be stored in body tissues to toxic levels.

The water-soluble vitamins include the B vitamins (thiamin, riboflavin, niacin, pantothenic acid, biotin, vitamin B_6, folate, and vitamin B_{12}) and vitamin C. Excess water-soluble vitamins are generally lost through the urine. However, large doses of some water-soluble vitamin supplements, especially niacin and vitamins B_6 and C, can produce toxic symptoms.

Doctors may advise extra vitamin supplements for some people with special health or dietary needs. However, most people who use vitamin supplements should choose those that provide no more than the RDA or AI for each vitamin. Most nutritionists agree foods are the preferred source of vitamins.

Storing and preparing foods carefully will help preserve vitamins. Avoid exposing foods to excess heat, light, water, and alkalis, all of which can destroy vitamins. Cooking with low temperatures for short periods using a small amount of water also saves vitamins.

Check Your Knowledge

1. List five basic functions vitamins assist with in the body.
2. True or false. Most vitamins have several active forms, which have similar molecular structures.
3. What are two main causes of vitamin deficiency diseases?
4. List three differences between fat-soluble vitamins and water-soluble vitamins.
5. What form of vitamin A is provided by plant foods?
6. Why do some people *not* need vitamin D in their diets?
7. What is the main function of vitamin E in the body?
8. What is the main function of vitamin K in the body?
9. Name three deficiency symptoms shared by all the B-complex vitamins.
10. What is the name of the thiamin deficiency disease?
11. List three food sources of riboflavin.
12. True or false. Because niacin is water-soluble, it cannot build up to toxic levels in the body.
13. What is the RDA for pantothenic acid?
14. Why is adequate folate intake especially important to women of childbearing age?
15. What group of people has an increased need for vitamin C and why?
16. List two ways phytochemicals help prevent heart disease and some cancers.
17. Name three groups of people for whom doctors might recommend vitamin supplements.
18. What is the difference between the sources of natural vitamins and the sources of synthetic vitamins?
19. Give three tips for selecting foods high in vitamins.
20. List five ways to prevent vitamin losses when storing and preparing foods.

Put Learning into Action

1. Prepare a chart that will help you review information from the chapter. Headings on the chart should include *Name of Vitamin,*

Functions, Deficiency Symptoms, Toxicity Symptoms, Recommended Daily Need, and *Common Food Sources.*

2. Collect pictures of foods high in each of the fat-soluble and water-soluble vitamins. Prepare posters or bulletin boards for other classes to see. Emphasize that eating a variety of foods is the best way to get all the vitamins you need each day.

3. Examine how well your diet meets vitamin needs. Complete a food diary listing all the foods you eat for a three-day period. Use diet analysis computer software to analyze your vitamin intake for each day. Compare your daily vitamin intakes with the recommended amounts given in the text. Which vitamin needs have you met and which are low? Identify foods you could add to your diet to increase intakes of needed vitamins.

4. Visit a health food store to find a supplement for a "vitamin" that was not discussed in the chapter. What functions is this product supposed to perform? Write to the manufacturer to request evidence that supports claims made on the product label or in advertising. Share your findings in class.

5. Prepare a poster showing pictures of foods high in phytochemicals. Attach a summary of the roles of phytochemicals in the diet to your poster. Display the poster in your school cafeteria.

Explore Further

1. Use library references to make a list of the alternative names for each of the vitamins. Read the labels of 25 food products to see how many of these names you can find on ingredient lists. Choose one of the alternatives on your list and investigate how it differs from other forms of the same vitamin. Make a poster to illustrate your findings.

2. Write a research report on how alcohol and other drugs affect the body's need for and use of vitamins.

3. Interview a food scientist to learn more about how vitamins are destroyed through food handling, storage, and cooking. Research the best ways to preserve the vitamins in foods. Present your findings to the class in an oral report.

Chapter 9

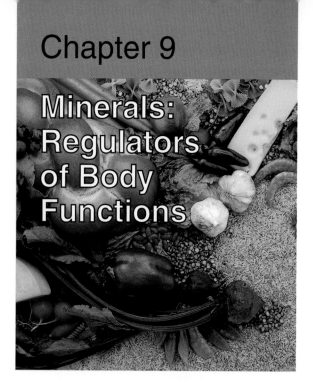

Minerals: Regulators of Body Functions

Like vitamins, **minerals** are nutrients needed in small amounts to perform various functions in the body. Also like vitamins, minerals provide no calories. In Chapter 8, you learned that vitamins are organic compounds. This means they are made of different elements bonded together, and one of the elements is carbon. In contrast, minerals are *inorganic elements.* This means they are not compounds, and they do not contain carbon.

Minerals in nutrition are the same as those listed on the periodic table of elements found in most chemistry classrooms. Nutritionists know a number of minerals, including calcium, phosphorus, and iron, are vital to good health. However, they are still studying the roles and functions of other minerals, such as tin, lead, and lithium. This chapter will discuss the minerals most researchers believe to be essential in the diet. See 9-1.

How Minerals Are Classified

At least 16 minerals are known to be important in your diet. These minerals can be classified into two groups. The first group is **macrominerals**, which are also called *major minerals.* These are minerals required in the diet in amounts of 100 or more milligrams per day. The second group is **microminerals**, or *trace minerals.* These are minerals required in amounts of less than 100 milligrams per day. Microminerals are just as important for health as macrominerals. See 9-2.

All the minerals in your body combined make up only about four percent of your weight. Although your mineral needs are small, meeting those needs is critical to good health. Minerals serve a variety of complex functions, including

- helping enzymes complete chemical reactions

● Learn the Language

mineral	hemoglobin
macromineral	myoglobin
micromineral	iron-deficiency
osteoporosis	anemia
menopause	cofactor
amenorrhea	thyroxine
osmosis	goiter
pH	cretinism
acid	fluorosis
base	

● Objectives

After studying this chapter, you will be able to

- list the major roles of minerals in the diet.
- identify functions and sources of specific macrominerals and microminerals.
- describe symptoms of various mineral deficiencies and excesses.
- write guidelines for maximizing mineral absorption and availability in the body.

Minerals in Food

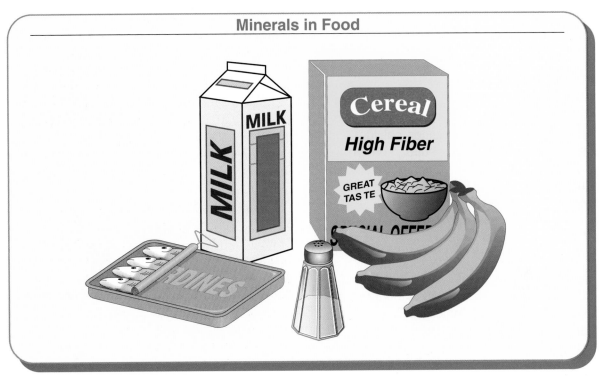

9-1 Can you identify the minerals that are in each of these foods?

Classification of Minerals

Macrominerals (Major Minerals)	Microminerals (Trace Minerals)
Calcium	Iron
Phosphorus	Zinc
Magnesium	Iodine
Sulfur	Fluoride
Sodium	Selenium
Potassium	Copper
Chlorine	Chromium
	Manganese
	Molybdenum

9-2 Minerals are classified as macrominerals or microminerals based on the amount that is recommended every day for good health.

- becoming part of body components
- aiding normal nerve functioning and muscle contraction
- promoting growth
- regulating acid-base balance in the body
- maintaining body fluid balance

Studying key minerals will help you understand their specific, individual functions.

The Macrominerals at Work

The macrominerals include calcium, phosphorus, magnesium, sulfur, sodium, potassium, and chlorine. Each of these minerals serves specific functions in the body. Learning about food sources and daily needs will help you plan diets rich in minerals.

Calcium

The macromineral found in the largest amount in the body is calcium. Calcium represents about two percent of body weight. This means the body of a 150 pound person contains about 3 pounds of calcium.

You may have heard a parent say to a child, "Drink your milk." There is good reason for parents to be concerned about their children's milk intake. Milk is a great source of calcium for people of all ages. Informed parents know how important calcium is for normal growth. See 9-3.

Functions of Calcium

Nearly all the calcium in your body is stored in your bones. Calcium from your diet is absorbed from your small intestine into your bloodstream. The blood then carries the calcium to your bones. Bones are always being rebuilt. Calcium in the blood is added to and removed from bones as needed throughout life.

Bone mass refers to the extent to which the bone tissue is filled up with minerals. Bone tissue at the ends of long bones looks something like a sponge covered by a shell layer. Healthy bone tissue is dense. The cells of the sponge are small, and the walls of the cells are thick. The shell layer is hard. When bones lose calcium, they become less dense. The cells of the sponge become larger, and the walls of the cells become

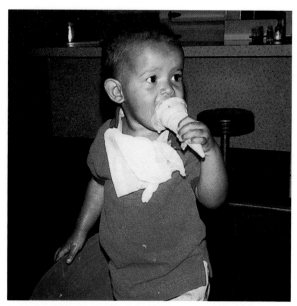

9-3 Frozen yogurt, like milk and other dairy products, is a good source of calcium.

thinner. The outer layer of the bone becomes brittle.

During the growing years, calcium from your diet is deposited in your bones to build and strengthen them. Through this process you achieve your full body height. In a similar way, calcium is used to build strong teeth.

Many people associate calcium with bones and teeth. However, they often overlook the fact that a tiny amount of calcium is found in every cell of the body. This calcium plays many vital roles. It helps muscles contract and assists in blood-clotting processes. Calcium also helps transmit nerve impulses.

Amount of Calcium Needed

The Adequate Intake (AI) for calcium for males and females ages 14 through 18 is 1,300 milligrams per day. After age 19, the recommended amount decreases to 1,000 milligrams per day. The AI increases again for people over age 50. Consuming the recommended amount of calcium will help protect bones and teeth over a lifetime.

During the preteen, teen, and young adult years, your body uses calcium to build bone mass and strengthen bone tissue. At around age 35, your body stops adding to bone mass. By age 40, many people begin to gradually lose bone density if they are inactive and consume too little calcium. A gradual loss of bone tissue that continues for many years may lead to osteoporosis. **Osteoporosis** is a condition that causes the bones to become porous and fragile due to a loss of calcium. The signs of this bone loss usually appear only after many years as the bones lose their strength.

You should note that a loss of bone mass is not necessarily age related. It is largely related to diet and exercise. People who eat calcium-rich diets and engage in weight-bearing exercise do not lose much bone mass as they age. On the other hand, even teens can lose bone mass if they follow extreme diet and exercise practices. Also, people who have lost bone mass can restore it, at least partly, through calcium supplementation and exercise.

The effects of bone loss will depend partly on the amount of calcium you store in your bones now. Many teens and young adults fail to recognize the importance of eating good sources of calcium. This gives them a hedge against future bone loss. One study reported only 15 percent of 12- to 16-year-old females met their daily need for calcium. Males in this age group fared better, with 53 percent meeting their need for calcium.

Teenage males may get more calcium than teenage females simply because the males eat more food. Many teen women limit their food intake to lose weight. Some consume less than 300 milligrams of calcium per day. Anyone watching calories should remember fat free milk and leafy greens are low in calories *and* rich in calcium.

● Sources of Calcium

The milk, yogurt, and cheese group of the Food Guide Pyramid is your primary source of calcium. Consuming the recommended number of daily servings will help you meet your calcium needs.

Relying on the milk, yogurt, and cheese group is difficult for people who are lactose intolerant. However, they still have a number of options for meeting their calcium needs. They can add the enzyme lactase to fluid milk to aid digestion. They may be able to eat cheese and yogurt as calcium sources. Most of the lactose in these products is in the form of lactic acid. They can also choose calcium-rich foods from other food groups.

A variety of nondairy foods supply calcium. Leafy green vegetables, legumes, and sardines eaten with the bones all provide calcium. Some foods are processed with added calcium. For instance, orange juice is sometimes fortified with calcium, making it a good mineral source. Read food labels to identify calcium-fortified products. See 9-4.

● Effects of Calcium Deficiencies and Excesses

Cells get the calcium they need from a supply found in the blood. Your life depends on the maintenance of normal blood calcium levels at all times. If your diet is calcium deficient, your blood will pull calcium from your bones. Eating a nutritious diet containing rich sources of calcium will help you avoid depleting bone calcium and developing weak bones.

Obtaining enough calcium from the diet is especially important for certain groups of people. Infants and adolescents are in peak growth periods. If their calcium needs are not met, their bones and teeth may not develop normally. Pregnant and breast-feeding women need calcium to meet their babies' needs. If these women do not consume enough calcium, the calcium stored in their bones will be used. This will increase the women's chances of developing osteoporosis later in life.

People who fail to eat a calcium-rich diet through their young adult years will not attain maximum bone mass. This will increase their risk of problems due to bone loss in old age. Conversely, people who achieve a higher bone density in their youth are less likely to

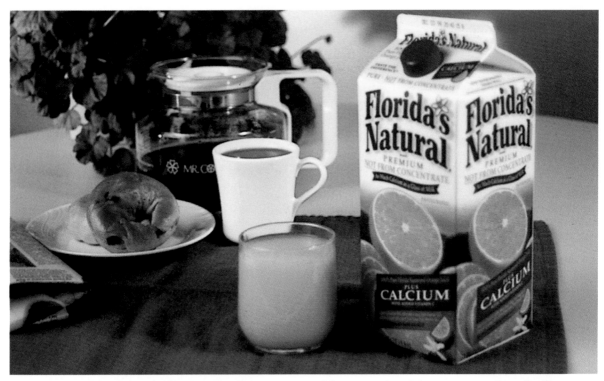

9-4 A serving of calcium-fortified orange juice may provide as much calcium as a serving of milk.

experience problems as they age. To illustrate this point, think about a bone that lacks mass as a toothpick. Think about a bone that has reached maximum mass as a 2" × 4" board. Suppose both bones lose the same amount of calcium. The one that started out as a toothpick is much more likely to break.

Although low calcium intakes are fairly common, calcium excesses from dietary sources are relatively rare. Excesses are generally the result of taking too many supplements. Possible problems include kidney stones, constipation, and gas.

● Osteoporosis

Breaks of wrist and hip bones in older adults are frequently the result of osteoporosis. A loss of calcium causes the bones to be less strong. Tooth loss may occur due to weakening of the jaw bone. Bones in the spinal area can compress, causing height to decrease by several inches. See 9-5.

Osteoporosis affects more than half the female population age 60 and older. Although osteoporosis occurs most often in women, it can occur in men as well. Women are at greater risk for osteoporosis for several reasons. First, their bones are smaller and loss of mass makes the bones more fragile at an earlier age. During pregnancy and breast-feeding, extra demands may be placed on the calcium stored in their bones. Women also have a longer life expectancy than men and, therefore, have more time to experience bone mass losses.

Hormonal changes are another factor that place women at greater risk of osteoporosis than men. At around age 50, women go through menopause. **Menopause** is the time of life when menstruation ends due to a decrease in production of the hormone *estrogen*. Among other functions, estrogen plays a role in maintaining bone tissue. Therefore, bone density loss occurs more rapidly in women after menopause due to the drop in estrogen levels.

Middle-aged women are not the only ones at risk of bone losses due to

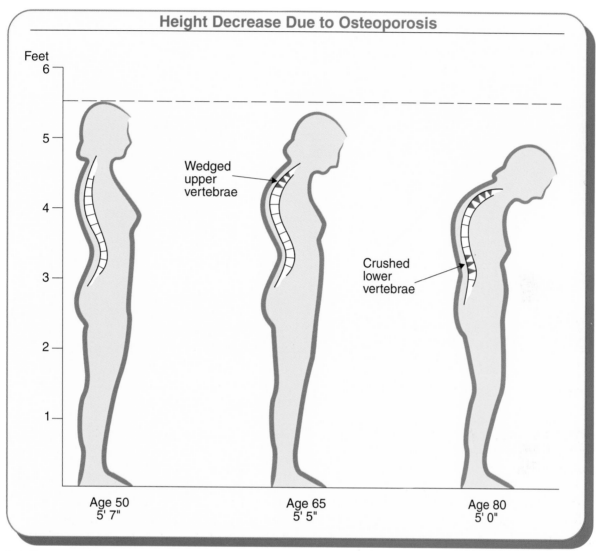

Height Decrease Due to Osteoporosis

Feet

Wedged upper vertebrae

Crushed lower vertebrae

Age 50
5' 7"

Age 65
5' 5"

Age 80
5' 0"

9-5 Compression of bones in the spinal column due to osteoporosis results in a decrease in height.

hormonal changes. A number of teenage and young adult women develop ***amenorrhea***. This means they stop having menstrual periods. This condition is fairly common among females who have eating disorders. It also occurs among female athletes who exercise excessively. The hormonal changes caused by amenorrhea are just like those that occur during menopause. They have the same effect on bone tissue, causing a loss of bone mass that can lead to osteoporosis.

Eating a diet rich in calcium can help reduce the rate of bone loss. Moderate exercise that places weight on the bones can also help keep bones dense and strong over a lifetime. Good choices of physical activity to reduce bone loss include walking, dancing, and jogging. See 9-6.

● **Calcium Supplements**
With poor calcium intakes being so common, you may wonder about the value of calcium supplements. Calcium supplements

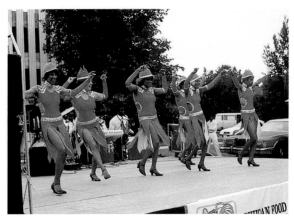

Photo courtesy of University Relations, MSU,
Bruce A. Fox, photographer

9-6 Weight-bearing exercise, such as dancing, helps increase bone density.

can benefit some people, especially those who cannot consume dairy products.

A number of types of calcium supplements are available. The body can absorb some types better than others. For instance, compounds of concentrated calcium, such as calcium carbonate, calcium phosphate, and calcium citrate are the best choices. Supplements made from powdered calcium-containing materials, such as bones and oyster shells, are not recommended. They are often contaminated with lead. Taking supplements in small doses between meals will help improve absorption. This is because acid, such as stomach acid, helps improve calcium absorption. People (usually older adults) who produce little stomach acid, should take supplements with meals. This is so any acid produced during digestion can aid calcium absorption.

Calcium supplements help reduce the risk of osteoporosis. Along with this advantage, taking calcium supplements can have some disadvantages, as mentioned earlier. Calcium supplements can also hinder the absorption of some other nutrients, such as iron and zinc. Most nutritionists agree getting calcium from food sources is preferred to using supplements.

Phosphorus

Phosphorus is the mineral found in the second largest amount in the body. It makes up one to one and one-half percent of your body weight. Phosphorus and calcium together represent more than half of all the mineral weight in your body.

Functions of Phosphorus

Phosphorus works with calcium to help form strong bones and teeth. It helps maintain an acid-base balance in the blood. It is part of ATP (adenosine tri*phosphate*), which is the source of immediate energy found in muscle tissue. Phosphorus is also in cell membranes and is part of some enzymes. Like calcium, it is part of every cell.

Meeting Phosphorus Needs

The Recommended Dietary Allowance (RDA) for phosphorus for males and females ages 14 through 18 is 1,250 milligrams daily. Phosphorus is easily found in the diet, and it is absorbed efficiently. Therefore, typical U.S. diets supply adequate amounts of phosphorus.

Phosphorus is found in protein-rich foods, including milk, cheese, meats, legumes, and eggs. Peas, potatoes, raisins, and avocados are good sources, too. Baked products, chocolate, and carbonated soft drinks are also sources of phosphorus. See 9-7.

Effects of Phosphorus Deficiencies and Excesses

Phosphorus deficiencies are virtually unknown. However, too much phosphorus in the diet can hinder the absorption of other minerals. For example, excess phosphorus can reduce calcium absorption.

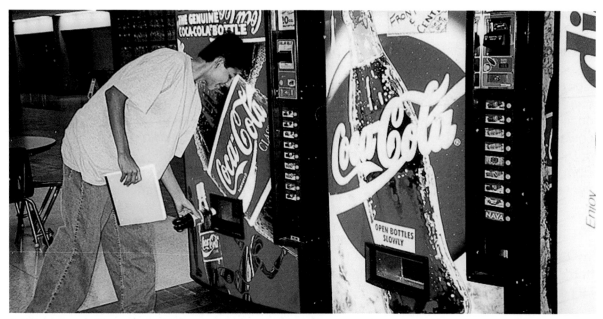

9-7 Beverages like milk and juice provide a much wider range of nutrients than soft drinks. However, carbonated soft drinks can serve as a source of phosphorus.

For best absorption, the diet should never provide more than twice as much phosphorus as calcium. This ratio is not maintained in a diet that is low in milk and high in soft drinks. This type of diet is common among teens. Such a diet greatly increases the risk of not building optimal bone density.

Magnesium

Like calcium and phosphorus, most of the magnesium in the body is in the bones. However, the amount of magnesium is much smaller than the amounts of the other two minerals. The magnesium content in the body of an adult is less than two ounces.

Functions of Magnesium

Magnesium is involved in over 300 enzymatic reactions in the body. Magnesium makes the enzymes active and lets them work more efficiently. Magnesium also activates the ATP in your body so it can release energy. It helps the lungs, nerves, and heart function properly. Magnesium is also tied to your body's use of calcium and phosphorus.

Meeting Magnesium Needs

The RDA for magnesium is 360 milligrams per day for women ages 14 through 18 years. For men in the same age group, the RDA is 410 milligrams per day. Many people in the United States consume less than the RDA for magnesium.

Good sources of magnesium include leafy green vegetables, potatoes, legumes, seafood, nuts, dairy foods, and whole grain products. Hard water, which has a high concentration of minerals, is also a source of magnesium.

Effects of Magnesium Deficiencies and Excesses

The body can store magnesium, so deficiency symptoms develop slowly in most people. Magnesium deficiencies are often the result of other health problems. For instance, starvation or extended periods of vomiting or diarrhea can cause low magnesium levels. Alcohol increases magnesium excretion. Therefore, alcoholics are at an increased risk of magnesium deficiency. Deficiency symptoms include weakness, heart irregularities, disorientation, and seizures.

Too much magnesium in the blood occurs mainly when the kidneys are not working properly. Excess magnesium from food sources is not considered a health concern. However, daily intakes of over 350 milligrams of magnesium from supplements may produce toxicity symptoms in teens and adults. Lower intakes from supplements may produce toxicity symptoms in children. Magnesium toxicity can cause weakness and nausea.

Sulfur

Sulfur is present in every cell in your body. Sulfur is in high concentrations in your hair, nails, and skin. If you have ever burned your hair, you may have recognized the sulfur smell.

Functions of Sulfur

Sulfur is part of the protein in your tissues. It is also part of the vitamins thiamin and biotin. It helps maintain a normal acid-base balance in the body. It also helps the liver change toxins into harmless substances.

Meeting Sulfur Needs

There is no RDA for sulfur. You can easily meet your sulfur needs through diet. You get sulfur from protein foods and sources of thiamin and biotin. See 9-8.

Effects of Sulfur Deficiencies and Excesses

Sulfur presents no known deficiency symptoms. There is no danger of toxicity associated with sulfur from food sources.

Sodium, Potassium, and Chloride

Sodium, potassium, and chloride are grouped together because they work as a team to perform similar functions. (Chloride is the form of the mineral chlorine that is found in the body.)

Functions of Sodium, Potassium, and Chloride

Water makes up a large percentage of your body weight. There is water inside every type of cell, from muscle to bone. There is also water in the spaces surrounding the cells. Most sodium is found in fluids outside the cells. Most potassium is found within the cells. Chloride is found both inside and outside cells.

If all body compartments do not contain the right amount and type of fluid, they cannot function properly. If a continuous fluid imbalance occurs, it can cause a serious medical condition and may lead to heart failure. Sodium, potassium, and chloride help regulate the fluid balance in cells and body compartments.

The membrane that encloses each cell in your body is *semipermeable*. This means water can flow freely through the membrane but particles, such as minerals, cannot.

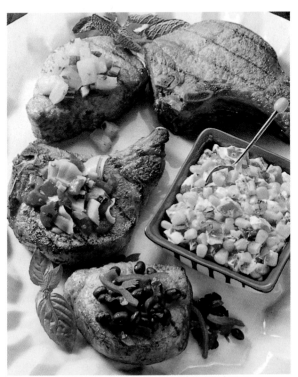

National Pork Producers Council

9-8 Meat and other protein foods are good sources of sulfur.

When the mineral concentrations on each side of the membrane are different, water is drawn across the membrane. Water moves from the side with fewer particles to the side with more particles. This helps equalize the concentrations of mineral particles on each side of the membrane. This movement of water across cell membranes is known as *osmosis.* See 9-9.

The Process of Osmosis

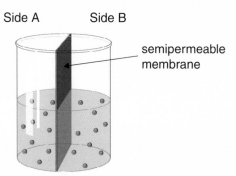

A container is divided with a semipermeable membrane. Side A and side B contain equal amounts of an equally concentrated solution. The volume of water and the concentration of mineral particles is equal on both sides of the membrane.

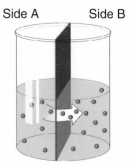

Particles are pumped across the membrane from side A to side B. The concentration of mineral particles becomes unequal.

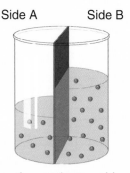

Water follows the particles across the semipermeable membrane from side A to side B to dilute the concentrated solution. The volume of water on either side of the membrane becomes unequal as the concentration of mineral particles becomes equal.

9-9 Osmosis helps balance the concentration of fluids that are inside and outside body cells.

Pumping mechanisms help draw potassium into body cells and sodium out of body cells. This controls the flow of water in and out of cells as the water moves to balance mineral concentrations.

Controlling osmosis is not the only function of sodium, potassium, and chloride. They also play an important role in maintaining the acid-base balance in the body. The term *pH* is used to express the measure of a substance's acidity or alkalinity. This measure is expressed on a scale from 0 to 14. Water and other neutral substances have a pH of 7. Compounds that have a pH lower than 7 are *acidic* and are called **acids**. Compounds that have a pH greater than 7 are *alkaline* and are called *alkalis* or **bases**. The more acidic a solution is, the lower its pH will be. Conversely, the more basic a solution is, the higher its pH will be. See 9-10.

All body fluids must remain within a narrow pH range for essential life processes to occur. For instance, blood must maintain a near-neutral pH of 7.4. Gastric juice is a strong acid with a pH of about 1.5. Pancreatic juice, with a pH of 8, is a weak base. Sodium and potassium combine with other elements to form alkaline compounds. This helps maintain the proper pH levels of body fluids by neutralizing acid-forming elements in your body. Chloride combines with other elements to form acids.

Sodium, potassium, and chloride play other important roles in the body. They aid in the transmission of nerve impulses. Potassium helps maintain a normal heartbeat. Chloride is a component of the hydrochloric acid in your stomach.

● Meeting Sodium, Potassium, and Chloride Needs

The estimated safe and adequate intake of sodium for adolescents and adults is 500 milligrams a day. The estimated minimum daily requirement of chloride for these age groups is 750 milligrams.

Sodium occurs naturally in many foods. However, the primary dietary source of both of these minerals is table salt, which is chemically known as *sodium chloride.* One teaspoon of salt equals roughly 5,000 milligrams: 2,000 milligrams of sodium and 3,000 milligrams of chloride.

Much salt in the typical U.S. diet is added to food during cooking and at the table. However, you may not realize the majority of salt in the diet comes from processed foods. Many people in the United States consume well over 3,000 milligrams of sodium per day. Some

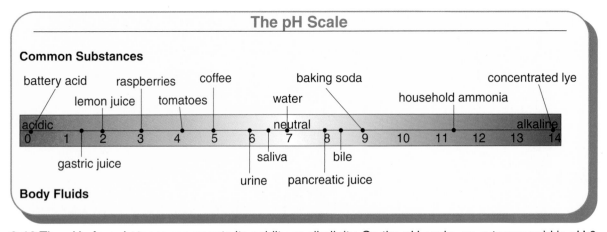

9-10 The pH of a substance represents its acidity or alkalinity. On the pH scale, an extreme acid is pH 0 and an extreme alkali is pH 14. The neutral point is 7.

experts estimate as much as 75 percent of this sodium comes from processed foods.

Salt is often added during processing to enhance flavors and preserve foods. Pickles, cured meats, canned soups, frozen dinners, and snack items are among the foods that are often high in sodium. Because salt contains chloride as well as sodium, foods containing added salt are also sources of chloride. See 9-11.

The Nutrition Facts panel on food labels states that your sodium intake should be less than 2,400 milligrams per day. Reading nutrition labels can help make you aware of sources of sodium in your diet.

The estimated minimum requirement for potassium for adolescents and adults is 2,000 milligrams per day. Fresh fruits and vegetables are rich sources of potassium. Milk and many kinds of fish are also good sources.

● Effects of Sodium, Potassium, and Chloride Deficiencies and Excesses

Deficiencies are rarely the result of too little sodium in the diet. More often, fluid losses, such as vomiting or diarrhea, cause a drop in the body's sodium level. The kidneys respond to these losses by increasing retention of sodium and water. A typical diet will soon more than make up for sodium losses. Increased fluid intake is needed to replace missing water. Sodium deficiency can cause muscle cramps, nausea, vomiting, and perhaps even death.

Sodium losses through perspiration during normal exercise are usually negligible. If you lose more than three percent of body weight through perspiration, however, you may need to replace sodium. Adding salt to your food can restore your sodium needs. There is no need to take salt tablets.

The average person in the United States consumes several times the estimated minimum requirement for sodium each day. In most healthy people, the kidneys filter excess sodium from the blood and excrete it in the urine. However, about 10 to 15 percent of the population is *sodium sensitive.* In these people, the kidneys have trouble getting rid of extra sodium.

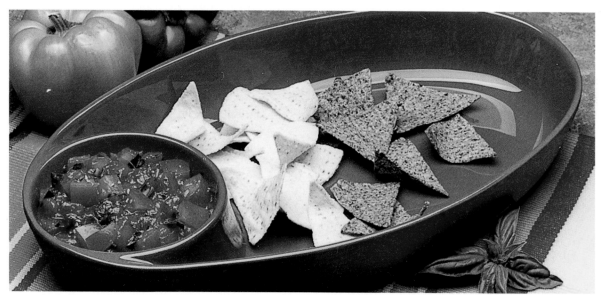

Progressive International Corp.

9-11 Many snack foods and condiment sauces are high in sodium.

Too much sodium in the blood can provoke hypertension in sodium-sensitive people. Someone who has hypertension has excess force on the walls of his or her arteries. Sodium draws water into blood vessels, causing the volume of blood to expand. Arteries are elastic. They stretch as blood volume expands. However, an excess of sodium causes blood volume to expand too much. This puts increased pressure on the arteries. If arteries are overstretched too much, they weaken, lose their elasticity, and may become damaged. If left untreated, hypertension can lead to heart attack or stroke.

Factors other than eating habits, including heredity, overweight, smoking, inactivity, and stress, affect the development of hypertension. You cannot prevent high blood pressure by reducing sodium in your diet. However, sodium-sensitive people can reduce their blood pressure by decreasing their salt intake. Also, the chance of becoming sodium sensitive increases with age. Therefore, experts recommend all people in the United States choose and prepare foods with less salt. Experts recommend people have their blood pressure checked yearly, too. See 9-12.

Potassium needs must be kept in balance for a healthy heart. Too little potassium can cause the heart to malfunction. Other symptoms of potassium deficiency include muscle cramps, loss of appetite, constipation, and confusion. Like sodium, potassium can be lost with body fluids during bouts of vomiting and diarrhea. Fluid losses that happen with the use of some high blood pressure medications can also lead to potassium deficiencies.

Due to the quantity of chloride provided by salt in the typical diet, chloride deficiencies are rare. Deficiency symptoms are similar to those for sodium and are likely to appear under the same circumstances. Excess chloride in the diet does not normally produce toxicity symptoms.

● The Microminerals at Work

There are at least nine microminerals needed by the body. These include iron, zinc, iodine, fluorine, selenium, copper, chromium, manganese, and molybdenum. Several other trace minerals may also play a role in human nutrition. A pile containing all the microminerals from your body would fit in the palm of your hand. However, these tiny amounts perform a variety of important functions.

Ways to Reduce Sodium in Your Diet

- Taste foods before adding salt to them during cooking or at the table.
- Use pepper, lemon juice, and herbs and spices instead of salt to flavor foods.
- Choose fresh fruits, vegetables, meats, fish, and poultry often. They generally contain less sodium than processed products.
- Check the Nutrition Facts panel on processed foods. Choose those products that provide the least amount of sodium per serving.
- Use cured and processed meats, such as hot dogs, sausage, and luncheon meats, sparingly.
- Use condiments, such as soy sauce, catsup, mustard, chili sauce, pickles, and olives, sparingly.
- Choose low- or reduced-sodium versions of foods when they are available.
- Limit use of salty snack foods.

9-12 Following these tips can help you reduce the amount of sodium in your diet.

Trace mineral research is one of the newest areas in the science of nutrition. Much of what nutritionists know about trace minerals has been identified in just the last 30 years. Many questions about trace minerals still remain. Could the average diet be low in some essential, yet unidentified, mineral? Are trace minerals that occur naturally in foods removed when foods are refined and processed? Can trace mineral supplements serve as a safety net for people who fail to eat nutritious diets? Researchers will continue to seek the answers to these and other questions about how microminerals can affect wellness. See 9-13.

Iron

The total amount of iron in your body is about one teaspoon. This may seem to be a trivial amount. However, iron plays a critical role in maintaining your health.

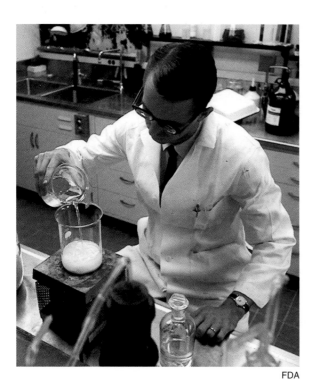

FDA

9-13 Nutrition researchers conduct studies to learn more about the roles microminerals play in the diet.

Functions of Iron

Most of the iron in your body is found in your blood. It is part of **hemoglobin**. This is a protein that helps red blood cells carry oxygen from the lungs to cells throughout the body. It is what makes blood red. Hemoglobin also carries carbon dioxide from body tissues back to the lungs for excretion.

Another iron-containing protein is **myoglobin**. This protein carries oxygen and carbon dioxide in muscle tissue.

Bone marrow stores some iron in the body, which is used to build red blood cells. The liver releases new red blood cells into the bloodstream. Red blood cells perform their oxygen delivery and carbon dioxide removal duties for three to four months before they die. Then the liver and spleen harvest the iron from the dead red blood cells. They send the iron back to the bone marrow for storage until it is recycled into new hemoglobin molecules.

Besides carrying oxygen, iron helps the body release energy from macronutrients. It is also needed to help make new cells and several compounds in the body.

Meeting Iron Needs

The RDA for iron for 14- through 18-year-old males is 11 milligrams per day. During these growth years, males have a significant increase in muscle mass. Extra iron is needed as myoglobin carries more oxygen and carbon dioxide in growing muscles. After age 19, the body is no longer growing, so the iron RDA for males drops to 8 milligrams daily. Maintaining muscle does not require as much iron as building new muscle.

Because iron is part of red blood cells, whenever blood is lost, iron is lost. Females lose blood every month through menstruation. Therefore, the RDA for iron for females ages 14 through 18 is 15 milligrams per day. Iron needs increase to 18 milligrams per day for females ages 19 to 50. Iron needs drop to 8 milligrams daily for women over 50, who are assumed postmenopausal.

Iron in foods is found in two forms: *heme* and *nonheme.* Heme iron is found in the hemoglobin and myoglobin of animal foods. Nonheme iron is found in plant and animal foods. The body can absorb heme iron more easily than nonheme iron.

Red meat, clams, oysters, duck, and goose are excellent sources of iron. Legumes, dark green leafy vegetables, and whole grains are good iron sources, too. Many bread and cereal products are enriched with iron. Acidic foods, such as tomatoes, also become good sources when they are cooked in iron pans. The acid helps liberate some of the iron from the cookware. This liberated iron remains in the food. Consuming good sources of vitamin C along with iron-rich foods will increase iron absorption. This is because vitamin C helps the body absorb iron. See 9-14.

Milk is a very poor source of iron. This is why infant formulas and cereals are fortified with iron. The addition of iron has helped reduce the number of iron deficiencies among young children.

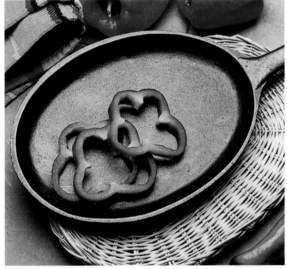

Progressive International Corp.

9-14 Cooking some foods in iron cookware can help increase their iron content.

Effects of Iron Deficiencies and Excesses

When the body's iron stores become depleted and the diet does not provide enough iron, an iron deficiency occurs. The body will make fewer red blood cells, and each cell will contain less hemoglobin. The smaller number of red blood cells means the blood has a decreased ability to carry oxygen to body tissues. Symptoms of this condition include pale skin, fatigue, loss of appetite, and a tendency to feel cold. A person who has this condition has **iron-deficiency anemia.** This is the most common type of anemia found worldwide.

Iron-deficiency anemia is common during the teen years, especially among females. One reason for this is iron needs increase during the teenage growth spurt. In addition, females are beginning their menstrual cycles and losing iron supplies that must be replaced. Females also tend to eat less than males and, therefore, have trouble getting enough iron in their diets.

The problem of low iron stores persists into adulthood for many women. In times of illness or pregnancy, the likelihood of an iron shortage increases. Doctors advise some women to take an iron supplement to help meet their daily needs.

Some people have an inherited disorder that causes them to absorb too much iron. This results in a condition called *iron overload.* The consequent buildup of iron is toxic and can damage the liver. Iron toxicity can also result from overdoses of iron supplements. This is a leading cause of accidental poisoning among children in the United States. Besides liver damage, iron toxicity can cause infections and bloody stools.

Zinc

Zinc is an amazing trace mineral that plays many important roles in the body.

Functions of Zinc

Zinc serves a wide variety of functions. It aids in body growth and sexual development. It serves as a cofactor for many enzymes. A *cofactor* is a substance that acts with enzymes to increase enzyme activity. Zinc is also necessary for the successful healing of wounds and acid-base balance. It affects the body's storage and use of insulin. Zinc helps with the metabolism of protein and alcohol. Zinc performs an important role in the body's resistance to infections, too. See 9-15.

Meeting Zinc Needs

Zinc is particularly important during periods of rapid growth and sexual development. The RDA for zinc is 9 milligrams per day for females ages 14 through 18. The RDA is 8 milligrams per day for all females over age 19. The RDA for zinc for all males over age 14 is 11 milligrams per day.

A protein-rich diet, including seafood and red meats, is rich in zinc. Good plant sources include whole grains, legumes, and nuts.

Effects of Zinc Deficiencies and Excesses

A zinc deficiency will hinder a child's growth and sexual development. A number of other deficiency symptoms may appear. These include loss of appetite, reduced resistance to infections, and a decreased sense of taste and smell.

People are unlikely to get too much zinc from a nutritious diet. Excess zinc, resulting in toxicity, is most often due to the use of supplements. Excess zinc will reduce the body's ability to absorb iron and copper.

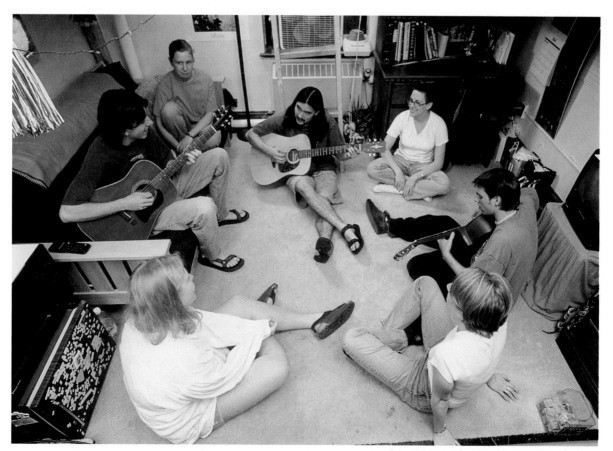

Photo courtesy of University Relations, MSU, Bruce A. Fox, photographer

9-15 Zinc is especially important during the teen years and other periods of rapid growth.

Toxicity symptoms include diarrhea, nausea, vomiting, and impaired functioning of the immune system.

Iodine

The percentage of children with mental retardation is greater in countries where malnutrition is widespread. This is because women in these countries are often unable to obtain adequate sources of an essential mineral during pregnancy. This mineral is iodine.

Function of Iodine

Most of the iodine in your body is concentrated in one area, the thyroid gland. The thyroid produces a hormone called **thyroxine**. This hormone helps control your body's metabolism. As part of thyroxine, iodine plays a role in metabolic functions.

Meeting Iodine Needs

How much iodine do you need in your diet? The RDA is 150 micrograms per day for most people over age 14. However, many people in the United States consume more than this amount.

Iodine is present in food as the compound iodide. Lobster, shrimp, oysters, and other types of seafood are rich sources of iodide. In addition, *iodized* salt is a common source. Milk and bakery products also contain iodide, which is a result of processing. See 9-16.

Effects of Iodine Deficiencies and Excesses

Iodine must be available for the thyroid gland to make thyroxine. When iodine levels are low, the thyroid gland works harder to produce the hormone. This causes an enlargement of the thyroid gland called a **goiter**. Other symptoms of iodine deficiency include weight gain and slowed mental and physical response.

If a woman's diet is iodine-deficient during pregnancy, the development of the fetus may be impaired. The child may have severe

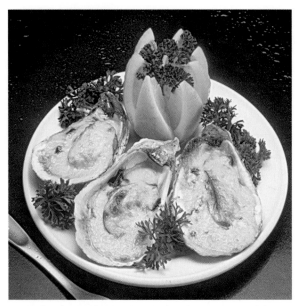

9-16 Oysters, like most seafood, are a good source of iodine.

mental retardation and dwarfed physical features. This condition is called **cretinism**.

A goiter is not only a symptom of iodine deficiency, it is also a symptom of iodine excess. Iodine is toxic in large amounts.

Fluoride

Fluoride is important for strong, healthy bones and teeth. Some scientists suggest it may help prevent the onset or decrease the severity of osteoporosis. Fluoride also helps prevent tooth decay. Children who drink fluoridated water have a much lower incidence of dental caries.

The AI for fluoride is 3 milligrams per day for all females over age 14. For males ages 14 to 18, the daily recommendation for fluoride is 3 milligrams. Adult males should consume 4 milligrams per day.

Tea, seaweed, and seafood are the only significant food sources of fluoride. Fluoride occurs naturally in some water. In the United States, most people get fluoride from fluoridated water. Many communities add fluoride to their drinking water. See 9-17.

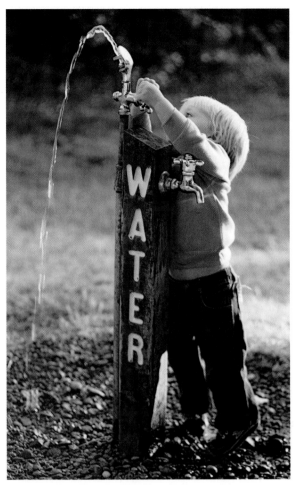

9-17 Fluoridated drinking water is a primary source of fluoride for many people in the United States.

There is no evidence fluoridating water is harmful. A very high fluoride intake can cause teeth to develop a spotty discoloration called *fluorosis*.

Selenium

Selenium works with vitamin E in an antioxidant capacity. It assists an enzyme that helps reduce damage to cell membranes due to exposure to oxygen. Antioxidants have been shown to play a role in the prevention of certain cancers. However, there is no clear evidence selenium will reduce the production of cancer cells.

The RDA for selenium is 50 micrograms daily for all males and females 14 years and older. Most teens in the United States have little trouble getting this amount.

Selenium is found in meats, eggs, fish, and shellfish. Grains and vegetables grown in selenium-rich soil are also good sources of the mineral.

A deficiency of selenium causes heart disease. Too much selenium is toxic, producing such symptoms as nausea, hair loss, and nerve damage.

Other Microminerals

Several other minerals have been identified as having important roles in the body. Each has varying and specific functions. Without them, health suffers.

The two values used for daily micromineral recommendations are based on scientific knowledge that is available at this time. When research is inconclusive, daily recommendations are given as AIs. RDAs are given when research is more conclusive.

Copper helps the body make hemoglobin and collagen. It also helps many enzymes work. The RDA for copper is 890 micrograms daily for all teens ages 14 to 18. Rich sources are organ meats, seafood, seeds, nuts, and beans. Deficiencies are uncommon but can result in anemia. Excesses can cause liver damage.

Chromium works with insulin in glucose metabolism. The AI for chromium is 35 micrograms daily for 14- to 18-year-old males. The AI is 24 micrograms daily for females in this age group. Chromium is found in meat, poultry, fish, and some cereals. Deficiencies lead to impaired glucose metabolism. Excesses can cause kidney failure.

Manganese helps many enzymes work. It plays a role in carbohydrate metabolism and in normal skeletal development. The AI for manganese is 2.2 milligrams for 14- to 18-year-old males and 1.6 milligrams for 14- to 18-year-old females. Excesses of this mineral can be toxic.

Molybdenum is an essential part of several enzymes. The RDA for males and females ages 14 through 18 years is 43 micrograms daily. Beans, whole grains, and nuts are good food sources. Excess molybdenum in the diet may affect the reproductive system.

Do not attempt to self-diagnose mineral deficiencies. If you have symptoms you suspect are due to a mineral deficiency, discuss them with a doctor. If he or she diagnoses a deficiency, a registered dietitian can help you evaluate your diet for good mineral sources.

Minerals and Healthful Food Choices

Information from this chapter can help you make healthful decisions about foods. You can put the facts you have read about minerals and their functions into practice at a personal level.

Mineral Values of Foods

The mineral content of plant foods depends on the soil, water, and fertilizers used to grow them. Thus, it is difficult to determine exactly how much of a mineral a given plant food will provide. Because animals eat plants, the mineral content of foods from animal sources is also hard to determine. See 9-18.

Most minerals in grains are located in the outer layers of the grain kernel. Most minerals in fruits and vegetables are located near the skin. Therefore, for maximum mineral value, choose whole grains and avoid peeling fruits and vegetables.

Generally, the most concentrated food sources of minerals are meat, fish, and poultry. Plant foods are rich in minerals, however they provide a less concentrated source of minerals. People who eat no animal foods may be low in some minerals. They need to carefully plan their diets to include mineral-rich foods of plant origin.

Processing tends to decrease the mineral value of many foods. You are likely to find more minerals in whole foods than in processed foods. Fresh fruits and vegetables, whole grains, meat, poultry, and dairy products are rich sources of minerals. Fats, sugars, and refined flour are low in essential minerals.

Mineral Absorption and Availability

You take in minerals when you consume food and beverages. These minerals are absorbed into the bloodstream mostly through the small intestine. Your body does not absorb all the minerals you consume. In fact, most

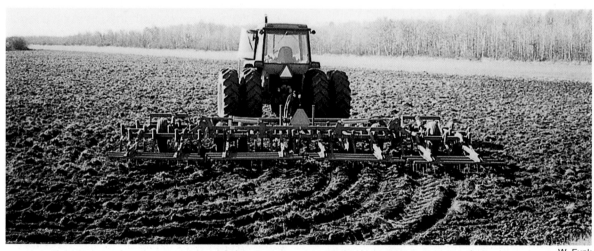

W. Funk

9-18 The mineral content of soil will affect the mineral content of foods grown in it.

adults absorb less than half of the minerals in their diets. Only the amounts of minerals your body absorbs are available to perform important functions. Unabsorbed minerals will be excreted with other body wastes.

What can you do to maximize absorption of minerals needed for growth and regulation of body processes? You should learn what dietary factors decrease and increase the availability of minerals for absorption.

Aside from being toxic, an excess of some minerals can interfere with the absorption of others. For instance, excess zinc can hinder the absorption of iron and copper. Absorption problems usually occur only when people take supplements. Therefore, avoid taking mineral supplements unless a doctor or registered dietitian advises you to do so.

High-fiber diets can decrease absorption of some minerals, including iron, zinc, and magnesium. Fiber binds these minerals and the minerals are excreted with body wastes. Although getting adequate fiber in the diet is important, exceeding daily recommendations is not advisable.

Drugs and caffeine can affect the availability of minerals in many complex ways. If you are taking prescription drugs, ask your doctor about any effects they may have on mineral absorption. Caffeine is a diuretic, which increases urine output. It thereby increases the loss of certain minerals excreted in urine. Avoid unneeded medications and excess caffeine.

The presence of certain vitamins can promote the absorption of some minerals. For example, the presence of vitamin D improves calcium and phosphorus absorption. Also, foods high in vitamin C increase iron absorption.

Your body's ability to absorb many minerals increases with your need for those minerals. This is a lifesaving defense in times of starvation or illness. It also helps the body meet increased mineral demands, such as those that occur during growth spurts and pregnancy. See 9-19.

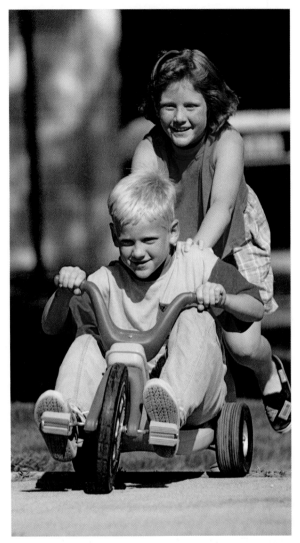

9-19 The body absorbs many nutrients very efficiently during the childhood years when growth is occurring rapidly.

Conserving Minerals in Food During Cooking

Minerals are not as fragile as vitamins. Minerals are not affected by heat or enzyme activity. However, minerals can be lost when foods are washed or cooked in liquid. Therefore, to preserve mineral content, avoid soaking foods when cleaning them. Also, cook foods using the smallest amount of water possible. Retain the minerals that have leached into cooking liquid by using it to make sauces, soups, and gravies.

Chapter 9 Review

Summary

Minerals are inorganic elements that can be divided into two classes. The macrominerals, or major minerals, include calcium, phosphorus, magnesium, sulfur, sodium, potassium, and chloride. The microminerals, or trace minerals, include iron, zinc, iodine, fluoride, selenium, copper, chromium, manganese, and molybdenum.

Although you need only small quantities of minerals, getting the right amounts is a key to good health. Without adequate intakes, deficiency symptoms can occur. At the same time, you need to avoid mineral excesses, which can be toxic.

Each mineral plays specific roles in the body. The vital functions of minerals include becoming part of body tissues. Many minerals help enzymes do their jobs. Some minerals help nerves work and muscles contract. Minerals also promote growth and control acid-base balance in the body. They help maintain fluid balance, too.

Minerals are widely found throughout the food supply. Choose a variety of plant and animal foods. Limit your use of highly processed foods. Eat the recommended number of daily servings from each group in the Food Guide Pyramid. Following this basic nutrition advice should provide you with most of your mineral needs.

Check Your Knowledge

1. True or false. Because they are needed in larger amounts, macrominerals are more important for health than microminerals.
2. Where is nearly all the calcium in the body stored?
3. Which group of the Food Guide Pyramid is the primary source of calcium?
4. Give two reasons women are at greater risk than men for developing osteoporosis.
5. What are three functions of phosphorus?
6. What are five dietary sources of magnesium?
7. Where are high concentrations of sulfur found in the body?
8. What process helps equalize the fluid balance inside and outside of body cells?
9. What is the pH of a neutral substance, such as water?
10. What minerals are contributed by salt, and what is the primary source of salt in the diet?
11. What organ is affected by potassium deficiencies and excesses?
12. What mineral is part of a protein that helps red blood cells carry oxygen?
13. Give two reasons why iron-deficiency anemia is common among teenage females.
14. What is the most common source of excess zinc resulting in toxicity?
15. Where is most of the iodine in the body concentrated?
16. Where do most people in the United States get fluoride?
17. What is the main function of selenium?
18. Name two microminerals other than iron, zinc, iodine, fluoride, and selenium and give a function of each.
19. What are three factors that affect the mineral content of plant foods?
20. True or false. An excess of some minerals can interfere with the absorption of others.

Put Learning into Action

1. Select any one of the minerals identified in this chapter. Prepare a "Nutrition News" report identifying functions, daily requirements, sources, and symptoms of deficiencies and excesses. Show the class a videotape of your report or present a "live broadcast."

2. Write menus for one day to meet the RDA for calcium for a friend who refuses to drink milk. Your friend is not lactose-intolerant, and he or she likes cheese and other dairy products.

3. Design a showcase or bulletin board display titled "Tracking the Sodium in Your Diet." Mount labels illustrating the high sodium content of popular snack foods and convenience products. Beside each label, identify the sodium content of a low-sodium alternative.

4. Prepare a brochure describing factors that increase and decrease mineral absorption and availability.

5. Prepare a demonstration illustrating a technique for choosing, preparing, and/or storing foods carefully to maximize the mineral content of your diet.

⬤ Explore Further

1. Complete a food diary for three days. Use food composition tables or diet analysis software to compare your intakes of calcium, sodium, and iron with the AIs and RDAs. Describe adjustments you can make in your diet to improve outcomes.

2. Use litmus paper to identify the pH of 10 food items and record your findings in a chart. Then investigate why eating foods that are acidic does not drastically affect the pH of your digestive tract. Share what you learn in a brief oral report.

3. Investigate nutrition research being conducted on arsenic, nickel, silicon, boron, cobalt, or some other mineral not discussed in this chapter. Write a three-page report describing the health implications scientists are studying.

4. Use the Internet to research the relationship between calcium consumption and a health concern. You might look into a link between calcium and heart disease, stroke, cancer, osteoporosis, arthritis, depression, or oral problems. Prepare a chart to illustrate your findings.

Chapter 10

Water: The Forgotten Nutrient

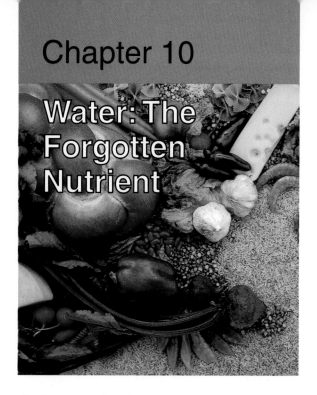

Carbohydrates, fats, proteins, vitamins, minerals, and water are the six major nutrients you need for survival. Of these, water is the one that is most often overlooked. This seems odd considering you could make a good argument for viewing water as the most critical nutrient.

Water is an essential nutrient that must be replaced every day. Depending on your state of health, you may be able to survive 8 to 10 weeks without food. Without water, however, you can survive only a few days. This chapter will highlight the vital role water plays in promoting health and wellness. See 10-1.

● Learn the Language

reactant
solvent
lubricant
intracellular water

extracellular water
water intoxication
diuretic
dehydration

● Objectives

After studying this chapter, you will be able to
- identify four main functions of water in the body.
- list sources of the body's water supply.
- describe effects of water loss on the body.
- determine whether your water intake is adequate.

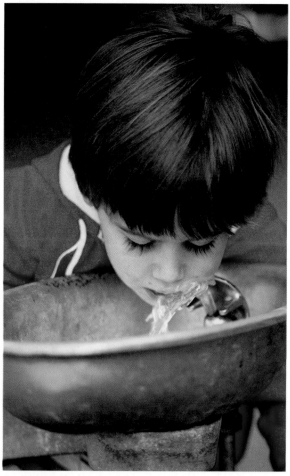

10-1 Much more than a thirst quencher—water is a vital nutrient.

● The Vital Functions of Water

Water is in every body cell. In fact, the presence of water determines the shape, size, and firmness of cells.

For most adults, body weight is about 50 to 70 percent water. That equals roughly 10 to 12 gallons (38 to 46 L). Fat tissue is about 20 to 35 percent water whereas muscle tissue is about 75 percent water. Therefore, the total percentage of body weight from water depends on the ratio of fat to lean body tissue. This ratio varies from person to person. People who have a higher percentage of lean tissue have a higher percentage of water weight. Men typically have a higher percentage of lean tissue and, thereby, water weight than women. Young people usually have a higher percentage of lean tissue and water weight than older people.

Body fluids include saliva, blood, lymph, digestive juices, urine, and perspiration. Water is the main component in each of these fluids. Your diet must include adequate amounts of water to allow your body to form enough fluids. Otherwise, body fluids will not be able to perform their functions normally. For example, without enough water intake, you will not be able to produce enough sweat to cool your body. A buildup of heat in the body can cause such symptoms as headache, nausea, dizziness, and loss of consciousness. If body temperature is not lowered, death can result.

Water performs a number of functions in the body. It helps chemical reactions take place. It carries nutrients to and waste products from cells throughout the body. It reduces friction between surfaces. It also controls body temperature.

● Facilitates Chemical Reactions

Most chemical reactions in the body need water to take place. This includes the reactions involved in breaking down carbohydrates, fats, and proteins for energy. It also includes reactions that result in the formation of new compounds, such as the making of nonessential amino acids. Water seems to help some enzymes perform their functions. It dilutes concentrated substances in the body, too.

Water is a reactant in many chemical reactions in the body. A **reactant** is a substance that enters into a chemical reaction and is changed by it. For example, water is needed during digestion to break down starches into glucose. Remember that starch is a chain of glucose molecules bonded together. Water is needed to split the bonds in the starch chain. The elements of the water molecules, hydrogen and oxygen, become part of the separate glucose molecules. See 10-2.

● Transports Nutrients and Waste Products

Water is a solvent. **Solvents** are liquids in which substances can be dissolved. Water can dissolve most substances, including amino acids from proteins, glucose from carbohydrates, minerals, and water-soluble vitamins. These nutrients are dissolved in the water of digestive fluids. Then they are absorbed from the small intestine and transported through the blood to the cells. Blood is primarily made of water. Water-soluble proteins are attached to fatty acids and fat-soluble vitamins so the water-based blood can transport them, too.

The blood carries dissolved wastes away from the cells. Your kidneys filter wastes from your blood and form urine. Water also plays a role in removing wastes from the body through perspiration, exhaled water vapor, and feces.

● Lubricates Surfaces

A **lubricant** is a substance that reduces friction between surfaces. Water is an excellent lubricant in your body. The water in saliva lubricates food as you swallow it.

Water as a Reactant

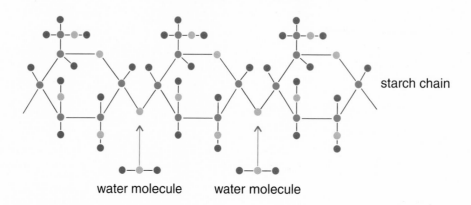

water molecule   water molecule

This small part of a starch chain shows three glucose molecules bonded together. Water serves as a reactant in the chemical reaction required to split the bonds between the glucose molecules.

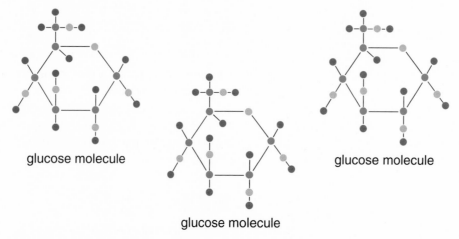

glucose molecule

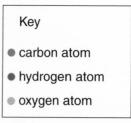

glucose molecule

glucose molecule

Through the course of the chemical reaction, the atoms of the water molecules have become part of the separate glucose molecules.

Key

● carbon atom
● hydrogen atom
● oxygen atom

10-2 Water serves as a reactant in many chemical reactions that take place in the body.

Throughout the digestive system, water acts like a lubricant to assist the easy passage of nutrients. Tears lubricate your eyes. Fluids surround your joints to keep bones from rubbing against each other. Water also cushions vital tissues and organs to protect them from injury.

Regulates Body Temperature

Another key function of water is to regulate your body temperature. Blood and perspiration are the body fluids responsible for this task.

Normal body temperature is near 98.6°F (37°C). Temperatures that are above or below this by 5°F (3°C) or more can cause serious health problems. For instance, the heat of high body temperatures can denature enzymes, which are proteins. This means when the body overheats, there is a slowdown in the chemical reactions promoted by enzymes in the body. Extremely high or low body temperatures can result in death.

Imagine you are riding a stationary bicycle. Although you are using only your leg muscles, your whole body becomes hot. This is because blood distributes body heat. Your body uses this distribution system to regulate body temperature.

Heat from your body is released into the air when blood flows near the surface of your skin. When you become warm, the blood vessels near your skin surface expand. This happens when you are exercising or have a fever. The expanded blood vessels allow more blood to flow near the skin surface, releasing heat into the air.

At the same time, your sweat glands begin producing perspiration. The perspiration transmits heat from your body through pores in your skin surface. The evaporation of water in perspiration helps cool your body. The slowed evaporation of perspiration is what causes you to feel uncomfortable when the humidity level is high. See 10-3.

When your body temperature drops, your body takes steps to conserve heat. It constricts the blood vessels near the surface

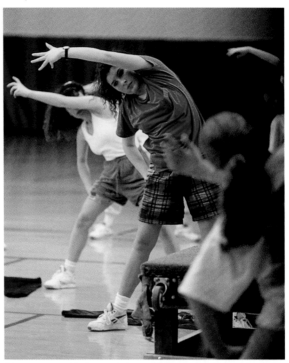

Photo courtesy of University Relations, MSU, Bruce A. Fox, photographer

10-3 Perspiring during exercise helps reduce body temperature.

of your skin. This restricts the amount of blood flowing near your skin surface, so less heat is lost.

Keeping Fluids in Balance

You can think of fluid balance at two levels. In the cells, there needs to be a balance between the water inside cells and the water outside cells. Throughout the body, there needs to be a balance between water intake and water excretion.

Cellular Fluid Balance

Cells are like balloons that maintain their shapes. Like balloons, cells do not have an infinite ability to expand. If too much water flowed into a cell, it could burst. Conversely, if a cell did not contain enough water, it would collapse. However, the body has mechanisms that keep the balance of water inside and outside the cells fairly constant. These mechanisms keep cells from bursting and collapsing.

There are two categories of water in the body. **Intracellular water** is the water inside the cells. **Extracellular water** is the water outside the cells. Water can move freely across cell membranes. The concentration of sodium, potassium, and chloride particles inside and outside the cells determines the movement of water. Health experts call these minerals *electrolytes*. (Review Chapter 9, "Minerals: Regulators of Body Functions," for more information about cellular fluid balance.)

The Source of the Body's Water Supply

Most people need 2 to 3 quarts of water per day to replace body fluids. You meet these needs through the liquids you drink and foods you eat. You also get some water as a by-product of nutrient metabolism.

Drinking liquids generally supplies the greatest amount of body fluids. Of course, plain water is a pure source of this vital nutrient. However, milk, soft drinks, juices, broth, tea, and other liquids also have a high water content.

You may be surprised to learn foods supply almost as much of your daily water needs as liquids. Most foods contain some water. Some foods are higher in water content than beverages. As an example, summer squash is 96 percent water, whereas orange juice is only 87 percent water. Even foods that look solid are a source of water. For instance, bread is 36 percent water. Butter and margarine contain water, but cooking oils and meat fats do not. See 10-4.

Roughly 12 percent of your water needs are met through metabolism. When carbohydrates, fats, and proteins are broken down in the body, some water is released. Your body can then use this water in other chemical reactions.

Your sources of water replacement may vary greatly from day to day. When you eat many water-loaded fruits and vegetables, you may not drink as much liquid. When you eat dry foods, you are likely to consume more liquids.

Bottled Water Versus Tap Water

As a source of water, you may be curious about whether bottled water is better for you than tap water. In recent years, sales of bottled water have shot upwards. The cost of bottled water can be several hundred times higher than the cost of tap water. However, bottled water is no healthier than safe, clean, pure tap water.

Why do people buy bottled water? The reasons vary. Some think bottled water contains miracle minerals that promote health. Research does not confirm this.

Many people claim bottled water tastes better than local water supplies. Dissolved minerals give water its taste. Depending on where you live, the water from the tap may taste of iron deposits, sulfur, or other minerals. People who object to such mineral tastes may buy bottled water even though tap water is safe and clean.

Some bottled-water drinkers are concerned tap water contains contaminants. Purity of tap water depends on the area in which you live. Public drinking water is treated to meet federal health standards. Water from private wells is more likely to contain microorganisms. People who are concerned about the safety of their water can have it tested for the presence of contaminants.

Water sold in bottles is not always safer, cleaner, or purer than tap water. In fact, bottled water comes from the same sources as water from the faucet. The FDA requires bottled water to meet the same federal standards for purity as public drinking water.

Some people choose to use filtration systems to treat their tap water at home. These systems vary in cost and require upkeep or filter replacement from time to time. They also vary in terms of what they filter from the

Water Content of Common Foods

Food	Percent Water Content*
Lettuce	96
Salsa	92
Fat free milk	91
Cola	89
Orange juice	87
Tomato soup	85
Apple	84
Potato	80
Egg	75
Milk shake	74
Tuna, water pack	74
Pasta, cooked	66
Chicken breast, roasted, skinless	65
Hot dog	54
Ground beef, lean	53
Pizza	48
Whole wheat bread	38
Cheddar cheese	37
Butter	16
Chocolate chip cookie, homemade	6
Jellybeans	6
Corn flakes	3
Peanut butter	1
White sugar	<1
Corn oil	0

*percent of total weight

10-4 Nearly every food contains some water.

water. Some systems remove certain harmful contaminants. Others may do little more than make water taste better. See 10-5.

Can You Drink Too Much Water?

Whether bottled or from the tap, you may wonder if it is possible to drink too much water. The answer is yes. The result is a rare condition called *water intoxication*. People who regularly drink excessive amounts of water usually do so because of a psychological disorder.

Drinking very large quantities of plain water can dilute the concentration of electrolytes in the extracellular fluid. If electrolyte levels stay low, symptoms such as headache and muscle weakness may appear. Severe cases of water intoxication can cause death.

The greatest danger of water intoxication is when infants with diarrhea and/or vomiting

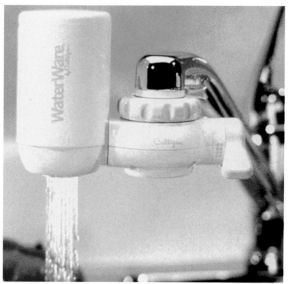

Culligan

10-5 A water filtration system can help improve the taste and quality of tap water.

are given plain water. Diarrhea and vomiting pull electrolytes as well as water from the body. When fluid losses are excessive, electrolytes as well as fluids must be replaced. Electrolyte imbalance can happen to people of all ages. However, infants are at greater risk. They can lose body fluids more easily than people in other age groups.

How Is Body Water Lost?

Water losses occur naturally as you carry on regular activities throughout the day. On the average, you will lose about two to three quarts of fluid each day.

How does water leave the body? There are several paths. Most body fluids are lost through urine. Your kidneys regulate the amount of urine lost. Kidneys can retain some water, but they must also produce urine to rid the body of wastes.

You lose body water through three vehicles other than urine. Fluids are lost through your skin as you sweat. You lose moisture in your breath as you breathe. You have small losses through bowel wastes, too.

Factors That Increase Water Losses

A number of factors can greatly increase water losses. Being aware of these factors can help you determine your fluid replacement needs. Hot weather as well as warm work or living environments can cause larger losses through sweating. Dry climates increase water losses through quick skin evaporation. Such climates include the atmosphere on airplanes and in buildings when heating systems are operating. The low oxygen pressure at high altitudes increases water losses for people not used to these altitudes. By breathing harder to draw more oxygen into their bodies, they have a greater output of water vapor. See 10-6.

Using diuretics promotes water losses. **Diuretics** are substances that increase urine production. Doctors often prescribe diuretics for patients with high blood pressure or body fluid imbalances. However, caffeine and alcohol are diuretics, too. For this reason, you need to use care when choosing liquids to replace body fluids. Coffee or soft drinks that contain caffeine may not be the best options for fluid replacement. Liquids that do not contain caffeine, such as water or fruit juices, may be better choices for restoring fluid losses.

Illness

Vomiting, diarrhea, bleeding, and high fever are all conditions that can cause fluid losses. Tissue damage caused by burns also affects the body's fluid balance. The more severe these conditions are, the greater the fluid losses will be. Medical supervision and treatment may be necessary to correct these fluid losses.

During illness, you may not always feel thirsty. However, drinking plenty of liquids is important to replace increased losses. Consuming fluids also helps flush the products of drug metabolism from your body.

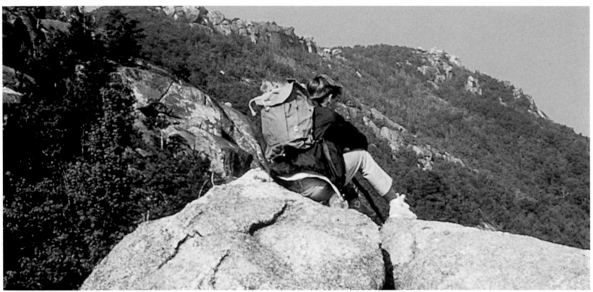

USDA

10-6 Water losses increase in high altitudes where harder breathing causes a greater output of water in the breath.

Exercise

Exercise causes increased water losses. The body's energy production takes place in the fluid environment of the blood and muscles. The release of chemical energy in food generates much heat. The heat must be removed by sweating to avoid dangerous increases in body temperature. The more energy you expend, the more you will sweat, and the more water you will need. A marathon runner can lose up to 13 pounds of water weight during a 26-mile race. See 10-7.

Effects of Water Loss

Because fluids make up a high percentage of your body weight, when you lose water, you lose weight. Someone who wants to drop a few pounds may think this is good news. However, the weight you want to lose is fat, not water. Water weight is quickly regained when body fluids are replenished.

Even a small percentage weight drop due to water loss will make you feel uncomfortable. When you lose two percent of body weight in fluids, you will become aware of the sensation of thirst. Both the brain and the stomach play a role in making you aware there is a water imbalance. If you do not replace water losses, you may become dehydrated. **Dehydration** is a state in which the body contains a lower-than-normal amount of body fluids.

When dehydration occurs, the body takes steps to help conserve water. Hormones signal the kidneys to decrease urine output. Sweat production also declines. As the volume of fluid in the bloodstream drops, the concentration of sodium in the blood increases. The kidneys respond to the higher blood sodium level by retaining more water. These water-conserving efforts cannot prevent all fluid losses from the body. If fluids are not replaced, the damaging effects of dehydration will begin to take their toll.

Replacing lost water is important for peak athletic performance. Athletic performance levels will go down after a 3 percent loss in water weight. When water is lost from working muscles, blood volume decreases. The heart

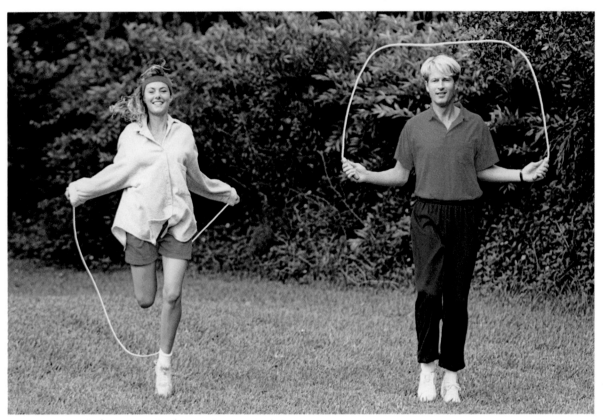

10-7 Exercise increases water losses as the body sweats to remove excess heat.

must pump harder to supply the same amount of energy. Mental concentration is affected as fluid losses increase. A 10- to 11-percent drop in body weight due to water losses can result in serious organ malfunctions.

● Guidelines for Fluid Replacement

Deciding how much to drink is a lifestyle choice you can make that affects your state of wellness. To keep your body in top condition, drink six to eight 8-ounce glasses of water or liquids daily. If you are like most people, you need to increase your fluid intake.

Thirst is the body's first signal that it needs water. Therefore, if you feel thirsty you should drink liquids. Thirst goes away automatically when you consume liquids.

The thirst mechanism is not always a reliable indicator of fluid needs. During hot weather or heavy exercise, the body may lose a fair amount of fluid before signaling thirst. Some older adults do not always recognize the thirst sensation. In cases such as these, it is important not to wait for the thirst signal to begin consuming liquids. When the weather is hot, you should make an effort to increase your fluid intake. You should also begin drinking before you start to exercise. Older adults may need to make a point of drinking even when they do not feel thirsty.

Some groups of people have above-average needs for water. An infant's immature kidneys are not as efficient as an adult's kidneys at filtering waste from the bloodstream. Therefore, infants excrete proportionately more water than adults to rid their bodies of waste. This increases their fluid needs, 10-8.

Other groups who have above-average water needs include older adults, who lose some of their water-conserving abilities.

Pregnant women need extra liquids because they have an increased volume of body fluids to support their developing babies. Lactating women need fluids to produce breast milk. People on high-protein diets require extra water to rid their bodies of the waste products of protein metabolism. A buildup of these waste products can cause kidney damage.

The volume of your urine will help you determine if you are drinking enough water. If you produce less than 2½ cups (625 mL) of urine per day, the urine will be concentrated with wastes. This increases the risk of kidney stones. *Kidney stones* are hard particles of mineral deposits that form in the kidneys. They can cause tremendous pain when they pass from the kidneys to the bladder and out of the body. A healthy urine output is one to two quarts per day or more.

Be aware of the color of your urine, too. Dark yellow urine indicates a high concentration of wastes. This is stressful to your kidneys. When fluid intake is too low, the kidneys must work harder to eliminate wastes. Light-colored urine shows you are drinking

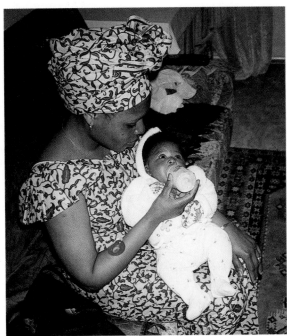

10-8 Infants need more water per unit of body weight than children and adults.

enough to keep wastes flushed out of your body. Drinking plenty of water while you are young may lessen your chances of kidney problems in later years.

Chapter 10 Review

Summary

Water is a vital nutrient you must replace daily. It is in every cell in your body and is the main component in all body fluids. Water makes up over half of your body weight.

Water performs a number of functions in the body. It plays a role in chemical reactions. It transports nutrients to cells and carries wastes away from cells. Water acts as a lubricant and helps regulate your body temperature, too.

The fluids in your body need to remain in balance. There needs to be a balance between intracellular and extracellular water. There also needs to be a balance between your total water input and output. You receive water through the liquids you drink and the foods you eat. You also get water as a by-product of metabolism. You lose body fluids through urine, sweat, vapor in your breath, and bowel wastes. Hot weather, warm environments, dry climates, high altitudes, and use of diuretics can all increase water losses. Illnesses and exercise increase water losses, too.

When you do not replace water losses, you can become dehydrated. Greater levels of fluid loss can cause a decrease in physical performance and a lack of mental concentration. An excessive drop in body fluids can result in serious organ malfunctions.

As a general guideline, you should drink at least six to eight glasses of liquids daily. Responding to your thirst and factors that increase fluid requirements can help you meet your water needs. Noting the volume and color of your urine will also help you determine if you are drinking enough water.

Check Your Knowledge

1. Name five body fluids composed mainly of water.
2. How does water's function as a solvent play a role in human nutrition?
3. How does water help the body release excess heat?
4. What three minerals control cellular fluid balance?
5. Name three foods that are more than 50 percent water.
6. True or false. Bottled water is safer to drink than tap water.
7. Why is plain water not the recommended liquid for replacing an infant's fluid losses due to vomiting or diarrhea?
8. Why is a caffeinated soft drink not the best choice for replacing body fluids?
9. Why does a loss of body fluids affect weight?
10. Name three groups of people who have increased water needs.

Put Learning into Action

1. For one day, avoid all beverages except water. Evaluate your satisfaction with water as your primary source of fluids. Include your personal evaluation in a written report on the advantages and disadvantages of water as a beverage.
2. Interview a sports coach. Find out what advice he or she gives athletes regarding fluid intake before, during, and after a game or competition. Share your findings with the class.

Explore Further

1. Choose five food substances. Place a tablespoon (15 mL) of each food in a cup (250 mL) of water. Stir briefly. Then record a description of each food's appearance after 5 minutes, 30 minutes, 1 hour, 3 hours, and 24 hours. In a written report, summarize your observations of water's effects as a solvent on the food substances you chose.
2. Collect samples of drinking water from taps at home and at school and from three bottled sources. Send the samples to a community-based health laboratory for an analysis of mineral content and contaminant levels. Discuss what the results mean regarding the quality of drinking water.

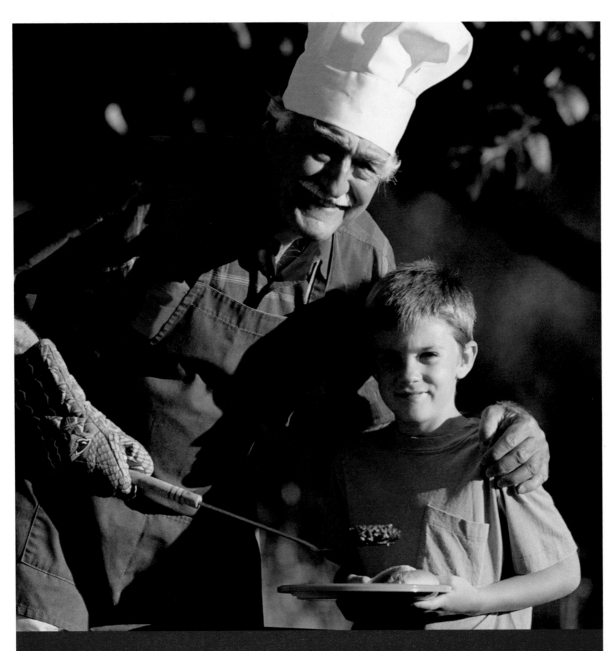

Part Four
Nutrition Management: A Lifelong Activity

Chapter 11

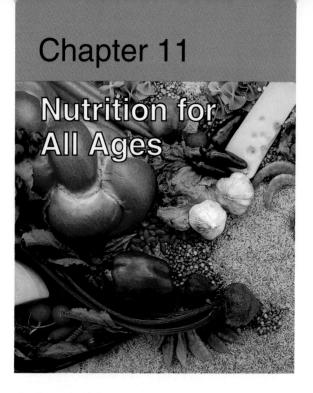

Nutrition for All Ages

The *life cycle* is a series of five main stages through which people pass between birth and death. These stages are infancy, toddlerhood, childhood, adolescence, and adulthood. Human beings in each stage need all the same basic nutrients. However, each life stage is associated with special nutritional concerns. Nutrition experts have subdivided the stages of the life cycle to address differing nutritional needs in various *life-stage groups.* These groups are defined by age ranges. Separate recommendations are made for women who are pregnant or producing breast milk. This chapter will help you look more closely at nutritional needs throughout the life cycle. See 11-1.

● **Learn the Language**

life cycle
fetus
lactation
low-birthweight
  baby
premature baby
trimester
placenta

congenital disability
fetal alcohol
  syndrome (FAS)
infant
toddler
adolescence
puberty
growth spurt

● **Objectives**

After studying this chapter, you will be able to
- list the five stages of the life cycle.
- describe factors that affect nutritional needs at each stage of the life cycle.
- discuss nutritional problems associated with each stage of the life cycle.
- use nutrient recommendation tables to find the suggested daily intake of specific nutrients for a given person.

● **Changing Nutritional Needs**

At the beginning of your life, you were smaller than the period at the end of this sentence. Then you grew. As an adult, you will be several million times bigger than you were at the start of your life. What allows you to grow? One answer is food.

Throughout life, people need adequate amounts of nutritious foods to build, repair, and maintain body tissues. The need for nutrients begins before birth. From the moment pregnancy begins, an unborn child's development depends on nutrients from the mother's bloodstream.

Each child's development is unique. Different parts of the body grow at different times and at different rates. However, there are predictable growth patterns. For instance, bone and muscle growth are most rapid in infancy and adolescence. Nutritional requirements are especially high during these periods. Rapid bone growth increases the need for calcium. Rapid muscle growth increases the need for protein.

Nutrient needs for adults decrease to a maintenance level. During the later years of

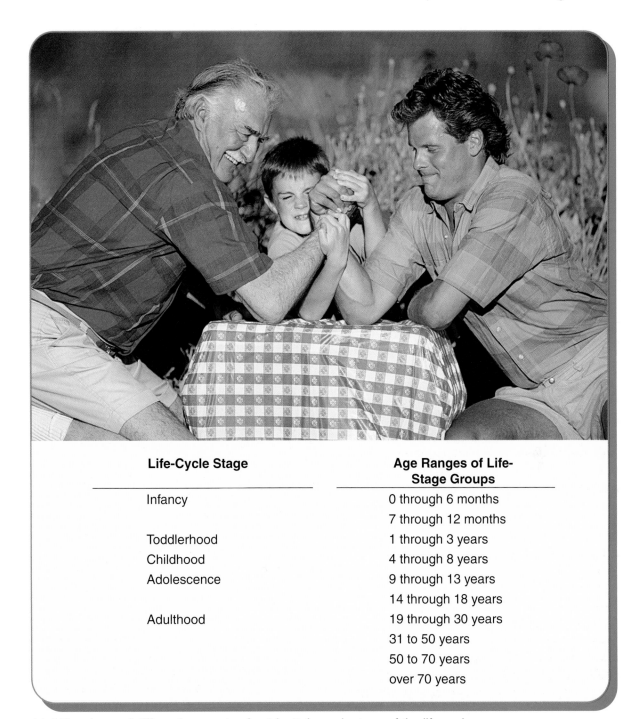

Life-Cycle Stage	Age Ranges of Life-Stage Groups
Infancy	0 through 6 months
	7 through 12 months
Toddlerhood	1 through 3 years
Childhood	4 through 8 years
Adolescence	9 through 13 years
	14 through 18 years
Adulthood	19 through 30 years
	31 to 50 years
	50 to 70 years
	over 70 years

11-1 People need different amounts of nutrients in each stage of the life cycle.

life, the aging process affects nutritional status. Consuming a nutritious diet increases the chance of being able to enjoy good health throughout life.

As you can see, the nutritional needs of people vary during the life cycle. A number of factors influence the amounts of nutrients needed. These factors include body size and composition, age, gender, activity level, and state of health.

The following sections will focus on the foods the body needs during the various stages of life, beginning with pregnancy. You will read about which components in foods are of greatest concern for infants, toddlers, and young children. You will discover what nutritional needs you have in common with other teens. You will also learn how your nutrient requirements will change in early and later adulthood.

● Pregnancy and Lactation

The life cycle begins in a woman's body. During pregnancy, a woman's normal body functions change to take care of the developing baby. During the first eight weeks after conception, a developing human is called an *embryo.* From eight weeks after conception until birth, a developing human is called a **fetus**. Following the birth of the baby, the mother's body begins producing breast milk. This is called **lactation**. The demands pregnancy and lactation place on a woman's body affect her nutritional needs.

● Health Needs Before Pregnancy

Women should be in good health before becoming pregnant. When planning a pregnancy, a woman should see a medical professional who can evaluate the woman's health. The woman should visit a doctor again as soon as she thinks she is pregnant. The doctor needs to monitor the woman's health throughout the pregnancy. This type of *prenatal* (before birth) care helps reduce the risk of health problems for the mother and the fetus. Prenatal care also increases a woman's chances of delivering a healthy baby.

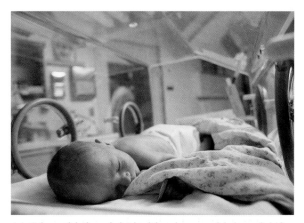

11-2 Low-birthweight babies have a higher risk for health problems at birth and throughout their lives.

A woman's weight before pregnancy should be appropriate for her height. Obstetricians advise underweight and overweight women to attain a healthy weight before becoming pregnant. This helps ensure good health for the women and their babies.

Women who enter pregnancy 10 percent or more below healthy weight face a greater risk of having a **low-birthweight baby**. This is a baby that weighs less than 5½ pounds (2,500 g) at birth. Low-birthweight babies have an increased risk of illness and death in early life. They are also more likely to have health problems that could affect them throughout life. See 11-2.

Women who are 20 percent or more above healthy weight are also more likely to experience problems during pregnancy. However, pregnancy is not an appropriate time for a woman to try to lose or maintain weight. A woman needs to gain a certain amount of weight for a healthy pregnancy and a healthy baby. A special diet plan can help an overweight woman achieve a healthful weight gain during pregnancy.

Both underweight and overweight women are at greater risk of giving birth to a premature infant. A **premature baby** is a baby born before the 35th week of pregnancy.

Premature birth is the leading cause of death among babies. Most premature babies have a low birthweight and are at risk for related health problems. Premature babies also have underdeveloped lungs. This increases their risk of respiratory problems throughout life.

● Nutrient Needs During Pregnancy

You may know a normal pregnancy lasts about nine months. When describing prenatal development, doctors refer to trimesters. A *trimester* is one-third of the pregnancy period and lasts about 13 to 14 weeks. A pregnant woman's nutritional needs vary a bit from one trimester to the next. This is because nutrients are critical in varying proportions for different aspects of a baby's development.

A woman needs extra amounts of many nutrients during pregnancy. One of the best ways to prepare for these increased needs is to form healthful eating habits before pregnancy. This approach will benefit a woman in two key ways. First, a well-nourished female builds reserves of some nutrients. These reserves will help her meet the increased nutrient demands of pregnancy and avoid deficiencies. Second, a woman who chooses a nutrient-dense diet knows which foods will increase her nutrient intake during pregnancy.

Pregnant women need extra protein to help build fetal tissue. They also need extra protein to support changes in their bodies, such as increasing their blood supply and uterine tissue. Many women already consume more than enough protein. Therefore, most women do not need to adjust their diets to meet the protein needs of pregnancy.

A pregnant woman needs increased amounts of most vitamins. Folate is especially important at the beginning of the first trimester. This vitamin aids the normal development of the baby's brain and spinal cord during the first few weeks of pregnancy. This is before most women know they are pregnant. Therefore, health experts recommend all women of childbearing age consume 400 micrograms of folic acid from fortified foods and supplements daily. Meeting this recommendation will reduce the number of babies born with damage to the brain and spinal cord. See 11-3.

Pregnant women have an increased need for vitamin B_{12}. This vitamin works with folate to make red blood cells. It occurs naturally only in animal foods. Therefore, women following strict vegetarian diets need to eat fortified foods or take supplements containing vitamin B_{12}.

Women have some increased mineral needs during pregnancy. They need extra zinc to support the growth and development of the fetus. They need more magnesium to promote healthy fetal bones and tissues. Pregnant women require increased amounts of iron to provide reserves the infant will need after birth. They also need iron because their growing bodies are making

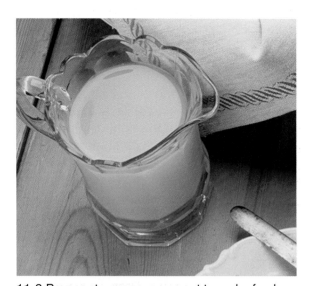

11-3 Pregnant women may want to make fresh orange juice part of their daily diets. It is a good source of folate.

more red blood cells. Pregnant women need extra iodine, too. This mineral supports thyroid activity as basal metabolic rate increases in the second trimester.

The recommended daily intake for calcium does not increase during pregnancy. However, the calcium needed to form the baby's bones is pulled from the mother's bones. Therefore, it is critical that pregnant women consume the recommended 1,000 mg of calcium per day. This will help reduce the loss of minerals from their bones. Pregnant teens need 1,300 mg of calcium daily.

Hormonal changes affect the way a pregnant woman's body uses certain nutrients. For instance, when a woman is pregnant, her body absorbs and stores more calcium and iron. These changes help provide for some of an expectant woman's additional nutrient needs. However, many pregnant women have trouble meeting all their needs through diet alone. This is especially true for iron. Therefore, health professionals often prescribe vitamin and mineral supplements to help pregnant women meet their increased needs. Pregnant women should take supplements only with their doctor's recommendation.

A woman who fails to meet added nutrient needs during pregnancy can affect her health. She can affect the health of her baby, too. The woman may experience iron deficiency anemia. She is more susceptible to disease. She is even at an increased risk of death. Her baby is more likely to be born early or have a low birthweight. The newborn may not have the necessary nutrient reserves to draw on for growth. The baby may also be more susceptible to illnesses.

Along with extra nutrients, a pregnant woman needs extra calories to support fetal development. In the second trimester, an expectant woman needs to begin eating an extra 340 calories per day. In the third trimester, she needs to add another 110 calories to her daily diet.

For the healthiest pregnancy and baby, adult women of normal weight need to gain about 25 to 35 pounds (11 to 16 kg). Underweight women need to gain 28 to 40 pounds (13 to 18 kg). This is also the recommended weight gain for pregnant teens because their bodies have not yet finished growing. Overweight women need to gain about 15 to 25 pounds (7 to 11 kg) during pregnancy.

Gaining enough but not too much weight during pregnancy is very important. The recommended weight gains result in the best chances of having a healthy baby. This weight reflects the weight of the developing fetus. It also allows for the growth of tissue and increase of body fluids in the mother. Most weight gain occurs during the second and third trimesters. With good eating habits and exercise, most women lose the majority of this weight within a few months after delivery. See 11-4.

A woman should follow a plan of regular exercise before, during, and after pregnancy. Having a fit body may help ease her delivery and speed her recovery afterward. Following a daily exercise program will also smooth the transition to active parenthood. A woman needs to ask her doctor what types of exercise to do during pregnancy.

● Nutrient Needs During Lactation

After giving birth, a mother must feed her baby frequently to help it grow and develop. Nearly all health and nutrition experts strongly urge most mothers to choose breast-feeding over formula-feeding. Breast-feeding benefits the health of the baby and the mother. Breast milk is perfectly designed to meet the nutritional needs of a baby. Formula has a different nutrient composition that is harder for babies to digest. Babies who are breast-fed develop fewer allergies and infections than formula-fed babies. Mothers who breast-feed lose their pregnancy weight faster, and they have a reduced risk of some forms of cancer. Breast-feeding also promotes family bonding. It saves

Normal Weight Gains During Pregnancy	
Component	**Weight Gain**
Fetus	7–8 pounds (3.2–3.7 kg)
Amniotic fluid	2 pounds (.9 kg)
Placenta	1–2 pounds (.5–.9 kg)
Growth of uterus	2 pounds (.9 kg)
Extra blood volume	3–5 pounds (1.4–2.3 kg)
Growth of breast tissue	1–2 pounds (.5–.9 kg)
Other body fluids	3–5 pounds (1.4–2.3 kg)
Fat stores and other body tissues	6–9 pounds (2.7–4.1 kg)
Total	**25–35 pounds (11.5–16.1 kg)**

11-4 The average woman gains about 25 to 35 pounds during pregnancy.

the expense of formula and the environmental waste created by formula bottles and cans.

Mothers who choose to breast-feed will need even greater amounts of some nutrients than they needed when they were pregnant. Their doctors may prescribe vitamin and mineral supplements to augment a nutritious diet. Besides vitamins and minerals, lactating women need increased amounts of protein. They also need generous amounts of fluids and extra calories to produce the milk that will nourish their babies. Lactating women should drink at least two quarts of liquids per day and consume an extra 500 calories. Recommended daily nutrient intakes during lactation and pregnancy are shown in Appendix A.

Meals to Meet Nutritional Needs

Pregnant and lactating women are advised not to skip meals, especially breakfast. Eating regular meals and snacks provides them and their infants with a steady supply of needed nutrients. They are also advised to drink six to eight glasses of water a day to help meet their fluid needs.

Meals should offer a variety of nutritious foods. Whole grain and enriched breads and cereals supply B vitamins and iron. Whole

grain products provide dietary fiber, too. Fruits and vegetables are good sources of vitamins, including the folate needed before and during early pregnancy. Fat free and lowfat milk, yogurt, and cheese provide protein and calcium while limiting fat. Lean meats, poultry, fish, and meat alternates furnish protein, iron, B vitamins, and zinc. See 11-5.

When planning meals, lactating women can include soups and fruit juices to help meet their fluid needs. Both during and after pregnancy, women can select fruits, vegetables, peanut butter, and lowfat yogurt and cheese as nutritious snacks. However, these women should limit foods that provide little more than fats and sugars.

Special Dietary Concerns

Certain conditions can create special dietary concerns during pregnancy. Women who follow vegetarian diets, experience nausea, or develop diabetes during pregnancy may have specific needs. These women may want to discuss their concerns with a registered dietitian.

Pregnant or lactating women who follow vegetarian diets have an extra challenge when meeting nutrient needs. They should discuss their food patterns with a doctor or

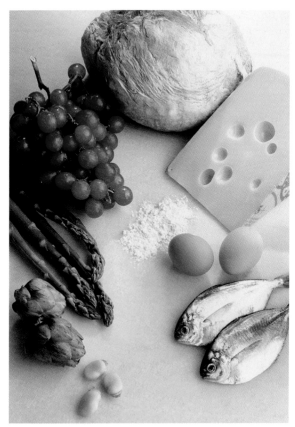

11-5 Eating a variety of nutritious foods will help a woman meet the extra nutrient needs of pregnancy.

registered dietitian. Vegetarians must plan carefully to get enough iron, calcium, and vitamin B$_{12}$. They may require supplements to meet their needs for iron. They will need to meet vitamin B$_{12}$ needs by consuming supplements or fortified foods. Women who do not use dairy products may need a calcium supplement, too.

Nausea, often called *morning sickness,* may be a problem during the first months of pregnancy. Some women have morning sickness throughout their pregnancies. Many women feel nauseated at times other than morning. To relieve nausea, pregnant women are advised to eat whatever they believe will make them feel better. For some women, this may mean salty foods; for others it may mean bland foods. Eating frequent small meals may also help ease this condition.

Constipation becomes a problem for many pregnant women, especially later in pregnancy. Hormones cause the intestinal muscles to relax, and the expanding uterus crowds the intestines. These factors decrease the rate at which the intestines are able to move waste through the body. The longer feces remain in the large intestine, the more water is absorbed from them. As feces lose water, they become hard, making bowel movements painful. Straining during bowel movements can increase the likelihood of developing hemorrhoids during pregnancy.

To avoid problems with constipation and hemorrhoids, pregnant women should be sure to drink plenty of fluids. Consuming an ample amount of fiber by choosing foods such as whole grains, fruits, and vegetables will help, too. Getting moderate daily exercise will also promote regular elimination.

Some women develop a form of diabetes or high blood pressure during pregnancy. These conditions can be serious and require careful monitoring by a doctor. They may also call for some dietary changes. Fortunately, these conditions often go away after delivery.

● Concerns Related to Teen Pregnancy

Pregnancy places extra stress on the body of a teenager. The adolescent body is still growing and, therefore, has large nutrient requirements. The nutrient needs of the fetus are then added to the teen's needs. Meeting these combined nutrient needs is very difficult for most teens. See 11-6.

Many adolescent women have poor diets. They fail to get enough calories, iron, and calcium to help them grow to their optimum height and muscle development. Teens with poor nutritional status do not have the nutrient reserves needed to meet the demands of a developing fetus. If these teens have had an inactive lifestyle, they will not be at an ideal level of physical fitness, either.

These factors place teens at a much higher risk of complications during pregnancy

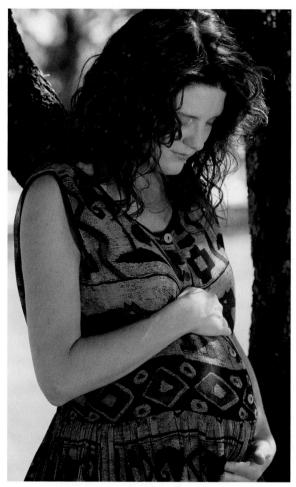

11-6 Pregnancy creates especially great nutrient needs for teenage women.

than adult women. Teens are more likely to have miscarriages and stillbirths. They are also more likely to have premature and low-birthweight babies. Their babies are at higher risk for health problems and death.

To help reduce risks, a teen needs to visit her doctor as soon as she thinks she is pregnant. Being aware of the first signs of pregnancy can help teens determine when to seek prenatal care. These signs include a missed menstrual period, fatigue, nausea, swelling and soreness in the breasts, and frequent urination.

A pregnant teen must carefully follow the advice of her doctor. She needs to select an adequate number of servings of nutrient-dense foods each day. She must also take any nutrient supplements her doctor prescribes. This type of diet will provide the nutrients needed by the teen and her developing baby. It will help her gain the recommended 28 to 40 pounds (13 to 18 kg) during her pregnancy. Taking these steps will improve a teen's chances of avoiding complications and delivering a healthy baby.

Drug Use During Pregnancy and Lactation

During pregnancy, an organ called the **placenta** forms inside the uterus. In the placenta, blood vessels from the mother and the fetus are entwined. Materials carried in the blood can be transferred between the mother and the fetus through the placenta. Oxygen and nutrients from the mother's bloodstream are delivered to the fetus. Waste products and carbon dioxide from the fetus are transported to the mother for elimination. Harmful substances like alcohol and drugs from the mother's bloodstream can also be passed to the fetus through the placenta.

The term *drug* describes a broad range of substances. These include caffeine in coffee and soft drinks and nicotine in tobacco. They also include alcohol, over-the-counter and prescription medications, and illegal drugs. You will read more about these substances in Chapter 19, "The Use and Abuse of Drugs." However, it is worthwhile to note here how these substances can affect pregnancy and lactation.

When a woman uses a drug, it enters her bloodstream. If she is pregnant, it can pass through the placenta to her unborn child. If she is lactating, the drug may be secreted in her breast milk. Therefore, any drug a woman uses affects not only her but also her baby.

Fetuses and infants have such little bodies that even a small amount of a drug can be harmful. They also have immature organs that cannot break down drugs efficiently.

Therefore, the effects of drugs will last longer in fetuses and infants.

Drugs present dangers to a fetus throughout pregnancy. However, they are of special concern during the first trimester of the pregnancy. This is the period when the vital organs and systems of the fetus are developing. Some drugs can also cause excessive bleeding during the last trimester of pregnancy. Some over-the-counter and prescription drugs are known to cause congenital disabilities. ***Congenital disabilities*** are conditions existing from birth that limit a person's ability to use his or her body or mind.

Doctors discourage pregnant women from using any types of drugs, even common nonprescription drugs, such as aspirin. Over-the-counter drug labels warn pregnant women to seek the advice of a health professional before using the product. A physician can recommend which over-the-counter drugs might be safe during pregnancy.

Caffeine is a stimulant found in colas and many other soft drinks, coffee, tea, and chocolate. Caffeine is in many over-the-counter and prescription drugs, too. Studies about the effects of caffeine on fetuses have led researchers to various conclusions. Further study is needed to settle the debate. However, many health professionals recommend that women limit foods and beverages containing caffeine during pregnancy. Health professionals also recommend limiting caffeine during lactation. This is because caffeine passes into breast milk and has been shown to cause irritability and restlessness in nursing babies. See 11-7.

Smoking is not healthy for anyone. However, health care providers especially caution pregnant women against smoking. A pregnant woman who smokes is more likely to have a low-birthweight baby. Cigarette smoking decreases the oxygen delivered to the fetus and can endanger its health. Also, smoking causes

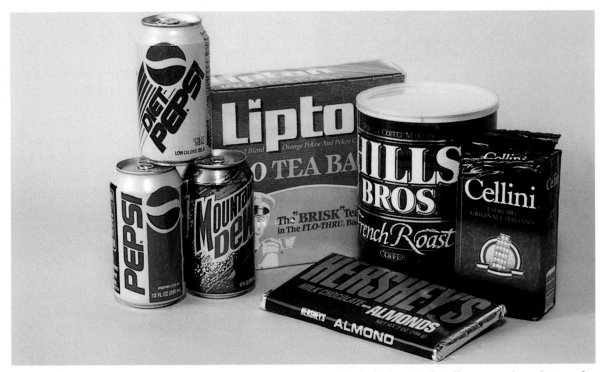

11-7 Many health professionals advise pregnant women to limit their use of coffee, tea, chocolate, soft drinks, and other products containing caffeine.

nicotine to circulate in the mother's bloodstream. The fetus can absorb this nicotine, which increases the risk of the fetus developing certain types of cancer in childhood.

Pregnant women should not drink alcohol, including beer and wine. Drinking even a small amount of alcohol during pregnancy can cause permanent damage to the fetus. A miscarriage or stillbirth may occur. Alcohol may damage the baby's developing organs like the brain and heart. The head may not grow properly. The baby may die in early infancy or be mentally retarded. The baby may have sight and hearing problems, slow growth, and poor coordination.

Fetal alcohol syndrome (FAS) is a set of symptoms that can occur in newborns whose mothers drink alcohol while pregnant. Babies born with FAS will suffer its effects throughout their lives. A baby born with FAS could have some or all the following symptoms:

- brain damage and below-average intelligence
- slowed physical growth
- facial disfigurement, including a flattened nose bridge, small eyes with drooping eyelids, and receding forehead
- short attention span
- irritability
- heart problems

Mothers should continue to refrain from drinking alcohol during lactation. If a lactating mother drinks alcohol, the alcohol can reach the baby through the breast milk. This may cause the baby to have developmental problems.

● Infancy and Toddlerhood

Infants and toddlers have special nutritional needs and problems. An ***infant*** is a child in the first year of life. Children who are one to three years old are often called ***toddlers***. Nutritional care is very important during these periods.

Many parents receive nutritional advice from their children's doctors. Some doctors suggest parents consult a registered dietitian to better understand their children's unique nutritional needs.

● Growth Patterns of Infants and Toddlers

Growth is more rapid during infancy than at any other time in the life cycle. The muscles, bones, and other tissues grow and develop at dramatic rates. A healthy baby's weight will triple during the first year. The baby's length will increase by one-half. That means a 7-pound, 20-inch newborn will be at least a 21-pound, 30-inch 12-month-old. See 11-8.

The pattern of growth changes during the toddler years. The muscles of the legs and arms begin to develop more fully. Bone growth slows, but minerals are deposited in the bones at a rapid rate. This helps make the bones stronger to support the increasing weight of the toddler.

● Nutrient Needs of Infants and Toddlers

Infants and toddlers need the same variety of nutrients as adults. However, growing, active children have *proportionately* greater nutritional needs than adults. This means children require more of each nutrient per pound of body weight. For example, the AI for calcium for a four-month-old infant is 210 milligrams per day. A 35-year-old adult needs 1,000 milligrams of calcium daily. Suppose the infant weighs 15 pounds and the adult weighs 150 pounds. This means the infant needs approximately 14 milligrams of calcium per pound of body weight. However, the adult requires only about 6.7 milligrams per pound of body weight. Proportionately, the infant needs more than twice as much calcium as the adult.

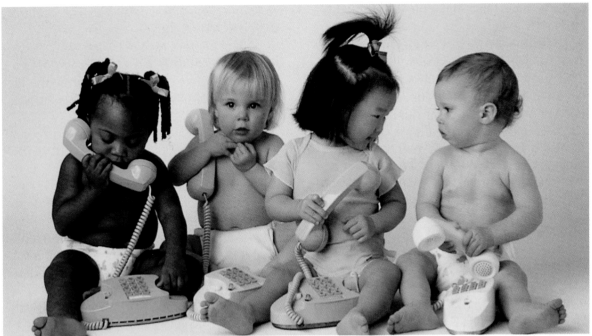

Gerber Products Company

11-8 Babies grow and change rapidly during the first year of life.

Infants born to healthy women who consumed adequate amounts of iron during pregnancy should have iron stored in their bodies. This stored iron should be enough to last until the infants are able to begin eating iron-fortified cereals. Infants also need high-quality protein to support the growth of muscles and other body tissues. An ample supply of calcium and phosphorous is essential for the development of teeth and bones. Breast milk or infant formula is designed to meet infants' needs for these and other nutrients.

Infants grow fastest in the first six months or so of life. Growth slows during the second six months, and it continues to slow through the toddler years. Toddlers still need proportionately more nutrients than adults, 11-9. However, their proportional needs are smaller than those of an infant. Daily nutrient requirements for infants and toddlers are listed in Appendix A.

● Meals for Infants

Proper feeding of an infant is critical to ensure normal growth. During the first few

weeks, babies need to be fed every two to three hours. They are just learning how to eat, and their digestive tracts are immature. Therefore, newborns can handle only small

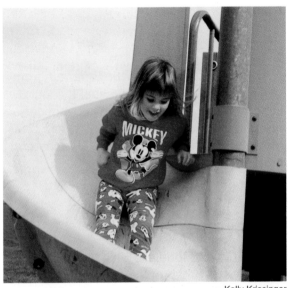

Kally Krissinger

11-9 A toddler's diet must supply enough calories to support the toddler's high level of activity.

amounts of breast milk or infant formula at each feeding.

After the first few weeks, babies usually want to be fed at fairly regular times. Most babies require six feedings a day. Caregivers can plan a schedule to space feedings at four-hour intervals. Caregivers usually can reduce the number of daily feedings to five when the infant is around two months old. At around seven or eight months, four daily feedings usually are sufficient. By a child's first birthday, he or she can be joining family members for three daily meals.

Caregivers need to be flexible in following a feeding schedule. They need to remember a baby may be hungry at irregular times. Caregivers need to respect an infant's signs of hunger or lack of appetite. They need to feed the infant when he or she cries to indicate hunger. However, they should avoid forcing the infant to eat when signs of satisfaction appear. These signs include spitting out food or turning the head away from food.

● Foods for Infants

Many nutrition experts view breast milk as the ideal food for infants. Human breast milk has a nutrient composition that is specifically designed to nourish humans. This composition is quite different from cow's milk and from infant formulas. Formulas include more of some nutrients than breast milk. However, more is not necessarily better. The smaller amount of protein in breast milk is easier for babies' immature systems to digest. Babies absorb the smaller amount of iron in breast milk more fully than they absorb the iron in formula. Breast milk also contains antibodies not found in formula. These antibodies help protect babies against diseases.

The only alternative to breast milk recommended by the American Academy of Pediatrics (AAP) is iron-fortified infant formula. The nutrient composition of infant formula must meet AAP standards. Iron fortification is important because an infant's iron stores at birth are enough to last only four to six months. A variety of formulas are sold in

liquid or powder form. A doctor can help parents find a suitable formula. See 11-10.

Babies should receive breast milk or iron-fortified formula for at least one year. Caregivers should not give babies cow's milk until they are a year old. It does not have enough iron and it has too much calcium.

Caregivers should not add solid foods to infants' diets until they are four to six months of age. Before four months, infants have trouble swallowing such foods. In addition, their immature GI tracts can absorb whole proteins instead of just amino acids. This can greatly increase infants' risks of developing allergies. Also, infants' kidneys are immature and cannot handle the increased load of excreting wastes generated by solid foods. These wastes include sodium and certain other minerals. To rid their bodies of these extra wastes, infants must excrete more urine. Thus, eating solid foods before four to six months can cause dehydration.

Caregivers can watch for several signs to tell if infants are ready for solid foods. Infants should be able to sit with support. This provides a straight passage for solids to travel from the mouth to the stomach. Infants should no longer drool. This indicates they can control their mouths and tongues in a way that will permit swallowing of solids. Infants should double their birthweight. They should also show interest in eating solids by practicing chewing when they see others eating.

Infant cereals are usually the first solid foods added to a baby's diet. These cereals provide iron in a form babies can easily absorb. After cereals, infants are usually given strained vegetables then fruits. Many parents introduce fortified apple juice at this time as a source of vitamin C. Meats are generally introduced last. By the end of the first year, a baby's diet should include a variety of foods.

Caregivers should introduce only one food at a time. They should wait four to five days before introducing another food. This will help them identify food allergies and sensitivities. Pediatricians usually recommend

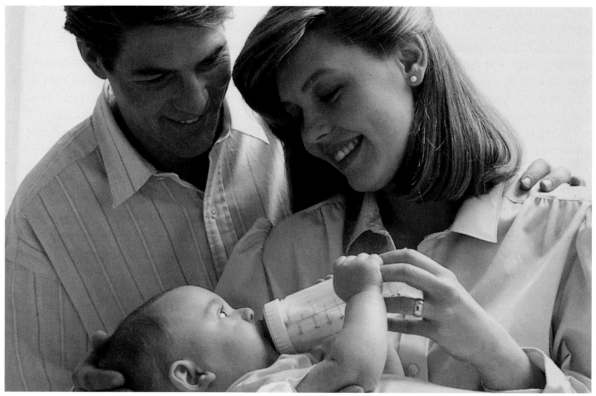

Gerber Products Company

11-10 Iron-fortified formula is a suitable alternative to breast milk for meeting the nutritional needs of infants.

introducing infants to rice cereal first. It is the least allergenic. Wheat cereal is more likely to cause an allergic reaction. Therefore, it is usually introduced later. Egg white and orange juice can also cause allergic reactions if they are introduced too early. Pediatricians advise waiting until after a baby's first birthday to introduce these foods.

Caregivers should repeatedly serve new foods. This allows the baby to learn to accept the foods by growing used to their new flavors and textures.

Caregivers should avoid overfeeding infants to prevent the development of excess fat tissue. The amount of food infants willingly accept varies. The quantity consumed depends on age, sex, size, state of health, and characteristics of the food.

As infants develop teeth and the muscle coordination to chew, they can begin to eat mashed and chopped foods. They enjoy chewing crusts of hard bread, especially if they are teething. By the age of six or seven months, infants can pick up foods with their fingers. Holding foods with their hands helps prepare infants to hold spoons.

● Feeding Problems During Infancy

Though their nutrient needs are high, infants have small stomachs. This is why they need frequent feedings.

Premature infants need special attention. They have greater needs for calories and all the nutrients. Premature infants do not have the iron reserves full-term babies have. They may also have trouble sucking and swallowing.

Problems can arise when caregivers have inappropriate expectations about when and how babies should eat. For instance, it is unrealistic to expect an infant to consume every last drop of milk or spoonful of cereal. Infants will start eating less as their growth slows and their weight gain begins to taper off. Caregivers must be patient and understanding about such normal infant behaviors.

Caregivers should not be upset when a child rejects a food. Rejecting a food is one of the few ways a baby has of showing independence. The child may accept the food if caregivers offer it again a few days later. Pediatricians do not recommend forcing children to eat. Pleasant, happy eating conditions help children form positive feelings toward food and eating.

Babies are not born with food dislikes—they learn them. Caregivers must be aware of how they communicate their likes and dislikes to an infant. When a caregiver acts negatively toward a food, a child will notice this response. As a result, the child may learn to reject that particular food. See 11-11.

● Foods for Toddlers

Foods for toddlers should be cut into bite-sized pieces. Toddlers like foods they can pick up with their fingers. They also like colorful foods and soft textures that are easy to chew.

Milk continues to be one of the most important foods in the toddler's diet. Three or four half-cup servings of milk per day are recommended. Some of this milk may be served as cream soups, pudding, yogurt, and cheese. Milk provides calcium as well as needed protein and phosphorus. It also supplies vitamins A and D, riboflavin, and some of the other B vitamins. Fat free or lowfat milk is not recommended during the first two years of life. This is because fat is needed for calories and the normal development of organs like the brain. These milk products can be given to children over two years of age to help them limit fat intake.

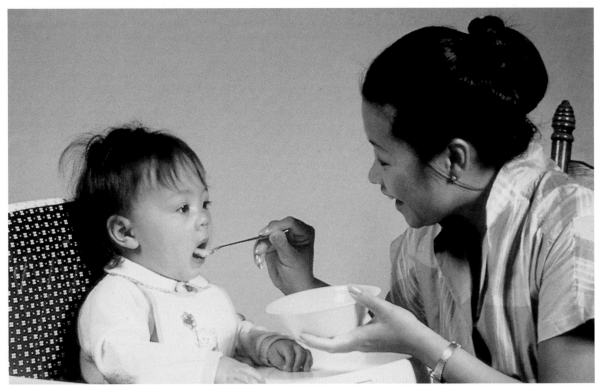

Gerber Products Company

11-11 A caregiver's attitude when feeding a baby can affect the baby's response to the food.

Eggs; meats; peanut butter; and mashed, cooked dried beans and peas contribute protein to a child's diet. Two to three tablespoons of these foods is an appropriate serving size for a toddler. Caregivers can grind meat for children who have only a few teeth. Toddlers who have more teeth can eat meat that is cut into small pieces.

A toddler needs a minimum of two servings of fruits and three servings of vegetables every day. At least one of these servings should be a good source of vitamin C. Foods rich in vitamin C include orange juice, strawberries, cantaloupe, and tomatoes. Dark green and deep yellow fruits and vegetables are important for vitamin A. Potatoes and other starchy vegetables provide carbohydrates. A toddler-sized serving is two to three tablespoons of fruits or vegetables or four ounces of juice.

Toddlers need at least six servings of cereal or bread a day. These foods add carbohydrates, iron, and B vitamins to a toddler's diet. Half a slice of bread or two to three tablespoons of cereal equals one serving for a toddler. See 11-12.

Toddlers can be served three meals a day with some between-meal snacks. Snacks are very important for toddlers. They have small stomachs and cannot eat enough at mealtime to carry them through to the next meal. Caregivers may choose the kind and

Comparing Adult and Toddler Serving Sizes

Food Group	Toddler Serving Size	Adult Serving Size
Breads, cereals, rice, and pasta	• ½ slice bread • ½ ounce ready-to-eat cereal • 2–3 tablespoons cooked cereal, rice, or pasta	• 1 slice bread • 1 ounce ready-to-eat cereal • ½ cup cooked cereal, rice, or pasta
Vegetables	• 2–3 tablespoons cooked vegetables • ½ cup vegetable juice	• ½ cup cooked vegetables • ¾ cup vegetable juice
Fruits	• 2–3 tablespoons chopped, cooked, or canned fruit • ½ cup fruit juice	• ½ cup chopped, cooked, or canned fruit • ¾ cup fruit juice
Milk, yogurt, and cheese	• ½ cup milk or yogurt • 1 ounce process cheese	• 1 cup milk or yogurt • 2 ounces process cheese
Meat, poultry, fish, dry beans, eggs, and nuts	• 1–2 ounces cooked lean meat, poultry, or fish • 2–3 tablespoons cooked dry beans, ½ egg, or 1 tablespoon peanut butter	• 2–3 ounces cooked lean meat, poultry, or fish • ½ cup cooked dry beans, 1 egg, or 2 tablespoons peanut butter

11-12 When planning meals for toddlers, caregivers need to remember that toddler servings are smaller than adult servings.

amount of snack food to complement the foods a toddler eats at mealtime. Snack foods should contribute nutrients, not just calories from sugar and fat. Caregivers should avoid giving toddlers cookies, candy, and soft drinks as regular snacks. Instead caregivers can offer fresh fruits, juices, milk, toast, and graham crackers. If snacks are eaten about two hours before a meal, they will not interfere with a child's appetite at mealtime.

● Eating Problems of Toddlers

Several factors can lead to eating problems during the toddler stage. However, being aware of normal patterns of growth and development can help caregivers avoid many of these problems. Caregivers can help toddlers form food habits that will promote good health and nutritional status.

Lack of teeth can be a source of eating problems for young toddlers. A one-year-old child may have only six to eight teeth. This can make chewing difficult and may lead to problems with choking. To make chewing easier, foods like fresh ripe fruit may be mashed into pulp or chopped into bite-sized pieces. To prevent choking, caregivers should avoid feeding toddlers foods that contain seeds. Toddlers can also choke on nuts, corn, raisins, gristle in meat, and round slices of hot dogs and carrots.

Some caregivers view toddlers' messy eating habits as a problem. Toddlers learn by using their senses to explore their environment, and food is part of that environment. Toddlers may involve their whole bodies in the eating process. They mash food with their hands to see how it feels. They place food in their mouths to taste it and feel the texture. They drop food on the floor to see what happens when they let go of it. By the end of a meal, toddlers may have applesauce in their hair and peanut butter on their elbows. Understanding about how toddlers learn will help caregivers develop patience during this stage.

A toddler's developing sense of independence can sometimes lead to eating problems. When toddlers become physically able to use a spoon, they usually want to feed themselves. This can be time-consuming and messy. When toddlers learn to talk, they begin to ask for the foods they want. They may not always ask for the most healthful foods. Caregivers should encourage these steps toward independence. Allowing toddlers to feed themselves helps them develop hand-eye coordination. Allowing toddlers to choose between two nutritious foods helps them learn decision-making skills. See 11-13.

A toddler's short attention span can be another eating problem. Toddlers are often easily distracted from eating. They may find it difficult to sit through a meal with their families. They may want to get down on the floor to play. Children need to have regular mealtimes with few distractions. Turning off the television and keeping toys out of the eating area will help children focus on enjoying their food.

Picky eating is a common problem among toddlers. A child may not want to eat a certain food for many reasons. The food might be too hot, cold, spicy, or bland. The toddler may want a special plate or cup and will not eat without it. The child may be tired or excited about something. He or she may not be hungry because of eating a snack

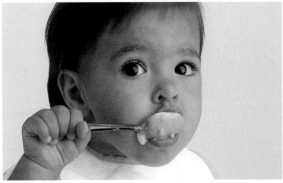

Gerber Products Company

11-13 Young toddlers may make a mess when they feed themselves, but they are learning important skills.

too close to mealtime. The toddler may be coming down with an illness. Sometimes a toddler will simply reject food because of the attention he or she can gain from the rejection.

At times, a toddler may eat all the food on his or her plate and want more. At other times, the toddler may eat only part of the food. Children's appetites vary. Appetite tends to increase during a growth spurt and slow when growth slows.

Parents often worry their toddler is not eating enough. Two indicators can assure parents a child is getting adequate calories and nutrients. These are normal growth and infrequent infections.

Caregivers need to make mealtimes pleasant experiences for toddlers. Caregivers should offer familiar foods children like in small, attractive servings. They can help children develop interest in new foods by expressing positive attitudes toward new tastes. Caregivers should not force children to eat or fuss over whether they are eating. After a reasonable amount of time, caregivers can simply remove any uneaten food.

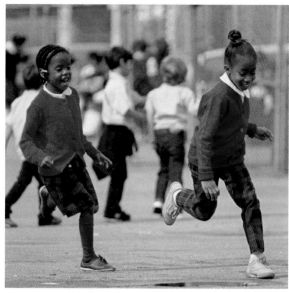

11-14 Growing, active children need a healthful diet to meet their nutrient and calorie requirements.

● Childhood

Nutritional needs change for children ages four to eight. Preschool and school-age children continue to eat the same basic foods they ate as toddlers. However, they need larger quantities to meet increasing energy needs. See 11-14.

● Growth Patterns During Childhood

Growth rates vary among children. Every year brings unique changes. Illness, emotional stress, poor eating habits, and genetics can all affect growth patterns.

Growth is generally slower during childhood than it was in the first years of life. The chubby toddler becomes a taller, thinner preschool child. The child continues to grow

and develop muscle control throughout the early school years.

Children are active during these years. Parents should encourage children to exercise through play activities. Exercise promotes wellness and helps children develop strong muscles and bones.

● Nutrient Needs During Childhood

Preschool and school-age children need more total calories than infants and toddlers due to their larger body size. Activity level also affects calorie needs. Boys and girls 3 to 8 years of age have an average requirement of about 1,700 calories per day. Average calorie needs increase to nearly 2,300 calorie per day for boys and 2,100 calories per day for girls ages 9 to 13.

The daily requirements for high-quality protein and many vitamins and minerals increase for children ages four and over. An adequate supply of nutrients allows for growth and maintenance of new body tissue. Children should eat a variety of nutritious foods to meet their nutrient needs. Children's diets should contain enough calories from carbohydrates like cereals, breads, and pasta to spare protein for tissue building.

Meals for Children

Good meal plans for children include eating meals throughout the day. One important meal is breakfast. It should contain carbohydrates and a small amount of fat. It should provide at least one-fourth of the daily requirements for calories and protein. Children who skip breakfast may have trouble concentrating and performing well in school. They may also have trouble meeting their daily nutrient needs. A nutrient-dense lunch will help improve performance in school and provide energy for after-school activities. See 11-15.

Children can supplement meals with snacks to help meet nutrient needs. Healthful snacking is easier if the kitchen is stocked with nutritious foods. Parents should keep such items as fruits, yogurt, raisins, carrot sticks, and fat free milk on hand. They should limit snack foods that have a high salt, sugar, or fat content.

Too much snacking at the wrong times can spoil a child's appetite for regular meals. Caregivers can help children learn good snacking habits by offering appropriate amounts of snack foods. For example, caregivers can serve two graham crackers instead of offering children the whole box of crackers. They can give children a cup of plain popcorn rather than the bag.

Nutrition and Fitness Problems of Childhood

On the average, children today grow taller than children years ago. One reason for this is the availability of a healthful diet. However, children today are also more likely to be overweight than their ancestors. Poor

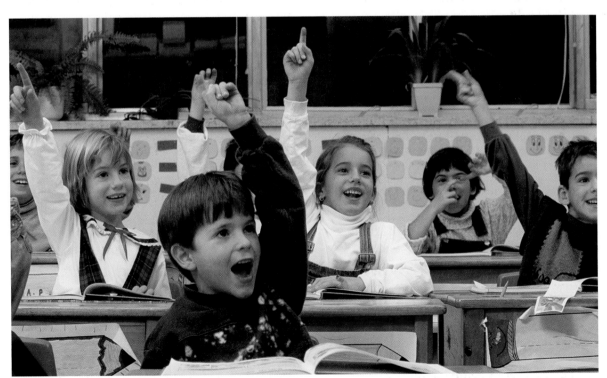

11-15 Eating a nutritious breakfast and lunch helps children stay alert and perform well in school.

eating habits and lack of exercise are the main causes of childhood weight problems.

Caregivers play an important role in preventing weight problems among children. By providing healthful options, caregivers can help children learn to make wise food choices. Caregivers can also limit the amount of time children spend in sedentary activities like watching television. They can encourage children to spend more time doing physical activities, such as riding bicycles or playing ball.

Dental caries is another problem related to nutrition that is common in childhood. The type of food and when it is eaten greatly affect the risk of dental caries. Sticky, carbohydrate-rich foods eaten between meals are the chief promoters of this problem. However, sound nutrition and dental health practices help develop and maintain healthy teeth and oral tissues. Caregivers can help children prevent tooth decay by teaching them about good eating and dental care habits. See 11-16.

● Adolescence

Adolescence is the period of life between childhood and adulthood. You and others who are in this part of the life cycle are called *adolescents*. Adolescence is an important transition period. The body undergoes many changes during this time. Good food habits started in childhood need continued emphasis as your body continues to develop.

● Growth Patterns During Adolescence

Puberty marks the beginning of adolescence. **Puberty** is the time during which a person develops sexual maturity. This is the time when females begin menstruating. Hormonal changes cause secondary sexual characteristics to appear. For males, these characteristics include a deeper voice, broader shoulders, and the appearance of facial and body hair. Breast development and the growth of body hair are among the

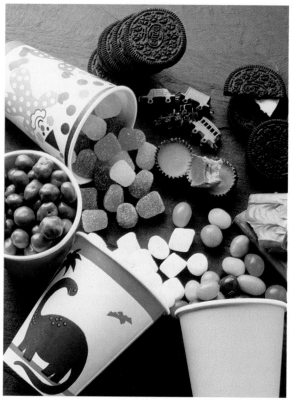

11-16 Caregivers can help children prevent dental caries by limiting sweet, sticky snack foods and encouraging children to brush after eating.

changes that occur in females. The onset of puberty occurs between the ages of 10 and 12 years for most girls. It occurs between the ages of 12 and 14 years for most boys.

Growth rates vary from person to person during adolescence. However, most adolescents experience a **growth spurt**. This is a period of rapid physical growth. Adolescents become taller as their bones grow. This increase in height is accompanied by muscle development and an increase in weight.

Body composition changes during adolescence. Well-nourished females develop a layer of fatty tissue that remains throughout life. Well-nourished males have an increase in lean body mass, which gives them a muscular appearance. When fully grown, males will have two times the muscle tissue and two-thirds as much fat tissue as females.

Nutrient Needs During Adolescence

Daily calorie needs in adolescence are higher than they are in late childhood. Specific needs vary with an adolescent's growth rate, gender, and activity level. The average caloric requirement for active 14- to 18-year-old females is roughly 2,300 calories a day. Males need more calories than females. This is partly because males have a higher percentage of lean body mass. The average daily requirement for active males 14 to 18 years old is about 3,100 calories. Teens of both sexes who are involved in intense physical activity have greater calorie needs. Likewise, teens who are less active have lower calorie needs. See 11-17.

Needs for most nutrients increase significantly for young people in the 9- to 13-year-old age group. Nutrient needs increase again for teens who are 14 to 18 years old. Teens in this group have needs equal to or greater than the needs of adults for most nutrients. Females need slightly smaller amounts of some nutrients than males.

Teens must consume adequate calories and nutrients to fulfill their growth potential. Daily nutrient recommendations for adolescence are stated in Appendix A.

Meals for Adolescents

The body functions better when it receives supplies of energy and nutrients at regular intervals throughout the day. A busy school, work, and social schedule may make you feel you do not always have time for regular meals. Some days you may skip breakfast. When you are in a hurry, you may be tempted to grab a candy bar instead of stopping for lunch.

You need to be aware of how irregular eating patterns can affect your overall wellness. Young people who skip meals tend to have more difficulty concentrating in school.

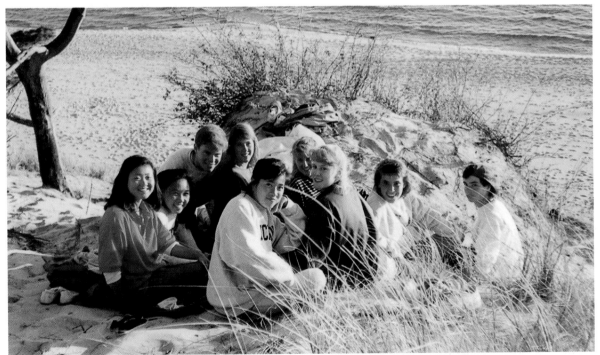

11-17 Growth is more rapid during adolescence than at any other life stage except infancy.

They also become tired and irritable more easily and report suffering from more headaches and infections.

Eating a good breakfast replenishes your energy supplies after a night of sleep. Breakfast should provide about one-fourth of your daily nutrient and calorie needs. Any nutritious food will help get your body off to a good start in the morning. If you do not like cereal or eggs, try eating a peanut butter sandwich, yogurt, fresh fruit, or even pizza.

Eating at least two other meals throughout the day should allow you to meet your remaining calorie needs. Carefully choosing the recommended number of daily servings from the Food Guide Pyramid should supply you with your nutrient requirements. Between-meal snacks can help provide some of these servings.

If you are like most teens, you probably eat some of your meals at fast-food restaurants.

Foods like pizza, hamburgers, and milk shakes provide nutrients. However, they also tend to be high in calories, sugar, fat, and sodium. Therefore, choose these foods in moderation. Balance them with other nutritious food choices throughout the day. Also consider ordering the salads, pastas, and fruits and juices many fast-food restaurants now offer. See 11-18.

● Nutritional and Fitness Problems of Adolescence

Teens often have a reputation for having poor eating habits. Many young people do not deserve this reputation. Surveys suggest many adolescents get enough of most nutrients. However, some adolescent nutritional problems exist.

Anemia is an iron-deficiency disease that often occurs during the teen years. Adolescents

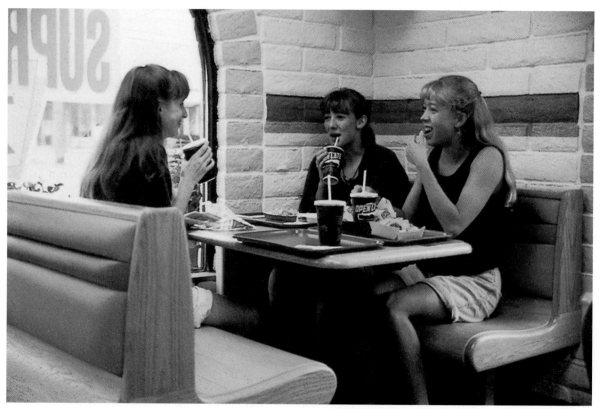

11-18 With careful selection and planning, fast foods can be part of a nutritious diet.

need increased amounts of iron to support growth of body tissues. After age 14, females require more iron than males due to losses through menstruation. Some doctors prescribe iron supplements to help adolescent females make up for a lack of dietary iron. Red meat, legumes, dark green leafy vegetables, and whole grain and enriched breads and cereals are good iron sources.

Weight problems are common among adolescents. Teens who are overweight need to adjust their food intake and increase their activity level. Teens who are underweight are at the other end of the weight management spectrum. These teens need to consume excess calories and exercise to build muscle. Eating disorders are also a common weight problem among adolescents. (Weight management and eating disorders will be discussed in detail in Chapters 13 and 14.)

Smoking, consuming alcohol, and abusing drugs are habits that sometimes begin in adolescence. The effects of these lifestyle behaviors on nutritional status will be discussed in Chapter 19, "The Use and Abuse of Drugs."

You need to be aware of the relationship between your diet during adolescence and your health as an adult. If your diet does not include enough calcium and vitamin D, your bones will not achieve maximum density. This lack of bone density will increase your risk of osteoporosis later in life. If you eat a diet high in sugar without proper dental hygiene, you are more likely to have dental caries. This increases your risk of gum disease and tooth loss in your later years. Eating a high-fat diet raises your chances of developing heart disease and some forms of cancer as an adult. Eating a healthful diet now can help prevent future health problems. See 11-19.

● Adulthood

Young men and women move from adolescence into adulthood. This phase of the life cycle lasts until death. It covers the largest number of years.

Menu Plan for an Adolescent Male	
Meal	**Sample Menu**
Breakfast	¾ cup orange juice 1 cup oatmeal 1 slice wheat toast
Snack	carrot sticks cottage cheese
Lunch	turkey sandwich sliced tomatoes coleslaw banana 1 cup fat free milk
Snack	peanut butter sandwich
Dinner	pork chop noodles broccoli tossed salad 2 dinner rolls pear halves 1 cup fat free milk
Snack	applesauce graham crackers

11-19 This is a nutritious meal plan for a 15- to 18-year-old male. How does your daily diet compare with this meal plan?

Nutritionists often divide adulthood into four stages. Early adulthood is the time from 19 through 30 years. By this stage, the rapid growth of adolescence has ceased and people's bodies have reached mature size. However, the bones are still storing calcium and increasing their density. Early middle adulthood describes the years from ages 31 through 50. Some visible signs of aging begin to appear during this stage of life. Late middle adulthood includes people who are ages 51 through 70. Signs of aging become more apparent during these years. Late adulthood is over 70 years of age. People in this age group are more likely to develop special health and nutrition needs.

Signs of aging include graying hair, wrinkling skin, deteriorating vision, and slowing reflexes. These are natural changes that occur as the body gets older. However, many health problems that are more common among older people are not a natural result of aging. Research shows following a nutritious diet and exercising can help prevent such problems as heart disease and high blood pressure. This information has spurred many middle-aged adults to adopt good health habits. The earlier people make these habits part of their lifestyles, the more benefits they gain.

Nutrient Needs During Adulthood

Good nutrition is as important as ever during adulthood. The nutritional needs of adults are similar to those of adolescents. Adults need nutrients mainly to support vital body functions. Adult males need a bit more protein than adolescents. Because bones are no longer growing, adults need less calcium and phosphorus than adolescents. However, the AIs for calcium and vitamin D increase for adults over age 50. In addition, doctors often recommend calcium supplements for older women to help maintain strong bones. The RDA for vitamin B_6 increases for older adults as well. Iron requirements drop for women following menopause. Nutrient recommendations for adulthood are stated in Appendix B.

Calorie needs gradually decrease in adulthood. For many adults, this is due to a decrease in the basal metabolic rate. However, BMR can remain at the levels seen in early adulthood if a person exercises and maintains lean body mass. Older adults require fewer calories to maintain their body weight. Some older people become less active, which causes physical abilities to change. This lowers the need for calories even more. Many adults gain weight as they age because they fail to stay active and match their calorie intake to their calorie output. See 11-20.

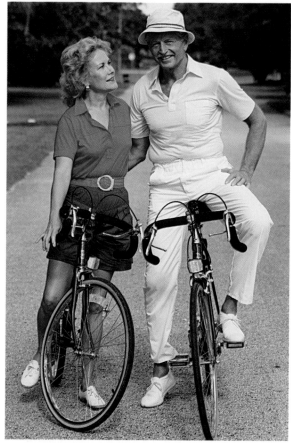

11-20 Remaining active can help adults over age 50 avoid weight gain.

Adult Food Choices

Some adults find it hard to change eating habits they established during childhood and continued in adolescence. In earlier life stages, people have high energy needs for growth. Some less nutritious food choices can fit more easily into diets at these stages. In adulthood, however, food choices need to be more nutrient-dense to meet nutrient requirements without exceeding calorie needs.

Many adults claim busy schedules and time pressures keep them from eating a nutritious diet. When they eat in a hurry, adults often choose foods that are high in fat, sugar, and sodium.

Menu Plan for an Adult Male

Meal	Sample Menu
Breakfast	¾ cup grapefruit juice 1 ounce cereal 1 slice wheat toast
Snack	carrot sticks melba toast
Lunch	tuna sandwich sliced tomatoes banana 1 cup fat free milk
Snack	yogurt
Dinner	broiled chicken breast rice zucchini tossed salad 2 whole wheat rolls sliced peaches iced tea
Snack	popcorn

11-21 Adults need to choose foods that are rich in nutrients without being too high in calories.

The meal plan in 11-21 would provide a nutritious diet for a healthy adult male. Foods recommended in this food plan are nutrient dense. Adults who require more calories to maintain a healthy weight can increase the number and size of portions. Adults who need fewer calories to maintain a healthy weight are encouraged to increase their activity levels.

● Nutritional and Fitness Problems During Adulthood

Maintaining a healthy body weight may be the biggest diet-related problem affecting adults today. Overweight has been linked with Type II diabetes, heart disease, and gall bladder disease. Avoiding overweight is wise because losing weight is hard for most adults. Adopting a healthy lifestyle including a nutritious diet and regular, moderate physical activity can help older people avoid becoming overweight.

Constipation is a problem for some adults. Getting regular exercise and choosing fiber-rich foods can help prevent this problem. Fruits, vegetables, legumes, and whole grains supply dietary fiber. Drinking at least six glasses of water a day can help prevent constipation, too.

Many adult women fail to get enough calcium and vitamin D in their diets. This, along with hormonal changes of menopause and lack of weight-bearing exercise, increases their risk of developing osteoporosis. Eating the recommended number of daily servings of milk, yogurt, and cheese can help women meet their calcium needs. Some women may also need calcium supplements.

As people age, their ability to absorb some nutrients decreases. In addition, they may fail to get enough nutrients in their diets. Vitamin D, folate, and vitamin B_{12} are of special concern in the later years. Some physicians recommend supplements for people in this age group.

● Special Problems of Older Adults

You may have friends or relatives who are in their later years. Some of these older people may be healthy and active. Others may have serious health problems and be confined to their homes. Health status is just one of several factors that affect nutritional needs in late adulthood.

Doctors recommend modified diets to help treat many diseases, including heart disease and diabetes. However, many other health problems can affect nutrient needs. For instance, recovering from surgery and some illnesses increases the need for protein. Recovery also increases the need for some vitamins and minerals, especially vitamin C and zinc. Medications can affect a person's nutritional status, too. As an example, taking large daily doses of aspirin increases the rate of blood loss from the stomach. This can increase the need for iron. Older adults may want to consult a registered dietitian about how health problems and medications affect their nutrient requirements.

A number of factors can affect an older adult's desire and ability to eat. This, in turn, has an impact on the adult's nutritional status. A diminished sense of taste causes foods to seem bland to some older adults. Tooth loss may make chewing difficult. Digestive problems may result in stomach upset after eating.

Isolation is another factor that affects the appetites of some older adults. A number of older adults live alone. They may be separated from family members and friends. Living alone may decrease their motivation to prepare and eat nutritious meals.

Limited income and lack of mobility can have an impact on food intake for some older people. Some older adults have low incomes that limit their food expenditures. Others may have trouble getting to a food market and carrying home bags of groceries. Buying, preparing, and serving a pleasing variety of foods for one or two persons may be a difficult task.

Some senior citizens' centers offer meals to help older people who are troubled by loneliness. Home meal delivery services assist those who have difficulty getting out to shop for food. Programs such as these help older adults meet their nutrient needs. See 11-22.

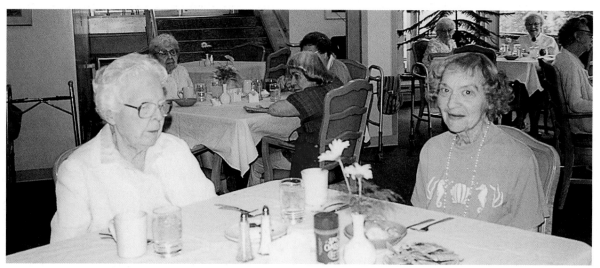

11-22 Eating with others makes mealtime a more pleasant experience for many older adults.

Chapter 11 Review

Summary

The life cycle is divided into stages. People in each of these stages require the same basic nutrients. However, the amounts needed vary due to special nutritional needs associated with each stage.

Good health and nutritional status before pregnancy helps ensure the health of mothers and their babies. Women require extra calories and nutrients during pregnancy to meet the needs of the developing fetus. Pregnant teens have especially high nutrient needs to support their development as well as their babies' development. Women who choose to breast-feed their babies have increased nutrient needs, too. Eating a variety of nutritious foods is the best way to meet these needs. Smoking and using alcohol and other drugs during pregnancy may harm a developing fetus. These habits may also harm infants during breast-feeding.

Healthy babies grow rapidly during the first year of life. Toddlers, who are one to three years of age, grow more slowly. Infants and toddlers both need nutritious foods to support rapid growth. Breast milk or formula is the only food infants need for the first few months. Then a variety of strained foods are gradually added to the diet. Toddlers can eat small portions of most table foods. Being aware of normal infant and toddler development helps caregivers know what to expect when feeding young children.

Preschool and school-age children need more calories and nutrients each day than infants and toddlers. Healthful snacks can be an important source of nutrients for children at this age.

Bone and muscle growth are rapid during the adolescent growth spurt. Nutritional requirements are especially high during this period. Teens need to avoid poor eating habits, such as skipping meals or eating too many high-fat foods from fast-food restaurants. Such habits can cause nutritional deficiencies that may lead to health problems later in life.

By adulthood, the body has reached its mature size. Nutrient and energy recommendations for this age group are set at a maintenance level. However, many adults exceed these recommendations. This makes overweight the biggest diet-related problem affecting adults. A number of physical, emotional, and social factors can place an older adult's nutritional status at risk. Consuming a good diet throughout the life span contributes to a state of wellness.

Check Your Knowledge

1. What are the five stages of the life cycle?
2. What five factors influence the amounts of nutrients needed by people at each stage of the life cycle?
3. In what two ways will forming healthful eating habits before pregnancy help a woman during pregnancy?
4. True or false. Mothers who choose to breast-feed will need even greater amounts of some nutrients than they needed when they were pregnant.
5. What are two factors that place teens at a higher risk of complications during pregnancy than mature women?
6. What are three symptoms that might occur in a baby born with fetal alcohol syndrome?
7. Explain the statement "Children have *proportionately* greater nutritional needs than adults."
8. Why should caregivers introduce only one food at a time to an infant's diet?
9. Describe two factors that can lead to eating problems during the toddler years. Give a suggestion for dealing with each factor.

10. What are four examples of healthful snacks for children?

11. What are two problems related to nutrition that are common in childhood?

12. Give one reason adolescent males usually need more calories than adolescent females.

13. Give two examples of how diet during adolescence can affect health in adulthood.

14. Give two reasons calorie needs decrease after age 50.

15. What are four factors that can affect an older adult's desire and ability to eat?

Put Learning into Action

1. Interview a pregnant woman to find out what nutritional advice she has received from health care professionals. Report your findings in class.

2. Research the average gains in height and weight that occur each month during the first year of life. Prepare a graph illustrating your findings.

3. Prepare two healthful snacks that would appeal to young children. Serve the snacks to a group of preschoolers and evaluate their reactions.

4. Use the nutrient recommendation tables in Appendix B to find the suggested intakes of nutrients for your life-stage group. List these in a chart with a food source of each nutrient.

5. Investigate meal service and delivery programs that are available for older adults in your community. Design a brochure describing these programs.

6. Interview a healthy older adult about his or her diet and lifestyle. Ask what eating and activity patterns he or she believes have contributed to his or her well-being.

7. Prepare a poster on aging that shows a figure of an older adult in the center. Place boxes around the figure with arrows pointing to the following body parts: ears, skin, hair, teeth, eyes, reproductive organs, muscles, bones, heart, and brain. In each box, describe what happens to the corresponding body part as a result of aging.

Explore Further

1. Use Appendix B to compare the recommended daily intakes of nutrients for people in two life-stage groups. Write a report describing factors that would account for differences in nutritional needs between the two groups.

2. Choose one of the stages of the life cycle. Research one of the nutritional problems associated with that stage. Prepare a presentation describing the age-related factors that contribute to the problem. Discuss how people in that life-cycle stage can avoid the problem. Also explain how the problem is treated, focusing on nutrition-based therapies.

Chapter 12

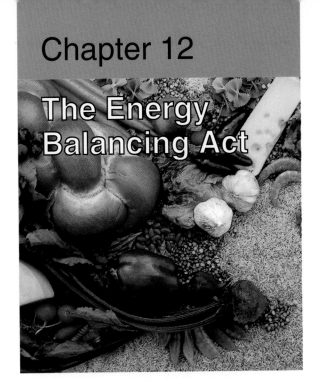

The Energy Balancing Act

Energy is the ability to do work. There are many different forms of energy. You cannot create or destroy energy. However, you can change energy from one form to another. When you eat, you take in chemical energy stored in food. Your body changes this energy into mechanical energy when you move. Through various activities, your body also generates heat, which is another form of energy. See 12-1.

Understanding energy balance is the key to weight management. Balancing energy involves equating the amount of energy you take in with the amount of energy you use. The energy in foods is measured in calories. Therefore, the energy balance equation could be expressed as "calories in equal calories out." When energy in and energy out are in balance, body weight does not change.

● **Learn the Language**

energy
calorie density
basal metabolism
basal metabolic rate
  (BMR)
body composition
sedentary activity
thermic effect of
  food
ketone bodies
ketosis

body mass index
  (BMI)
healthy weight
overweight
obese
underweight
skinfold test
subcutaneous fat
bioelectrical
  impedance

● **Objectives**

After studying this chapter, you will be able to
● describe how the amount of energy in food is measured.
● calculate the three components of your energy expenditure.
● identify the outcomes of energy deficiency and energy excess.
● use various tools to determine your healthy weight.

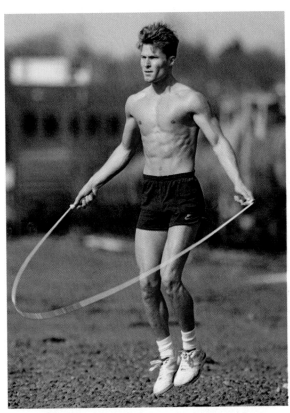

12-1 The body converts chemical energy from food into the heat and mechanical energy of physical activity.

211

Balancing energy does not have to be complicated. This chapter will help you understand the relationships between calorie intake, use of energy, and weight gains or losses.

● Energy Input

One side of the energy balance equation looks at the foods you consume. Three nutrient groups provide food energy: carbohydrates, fats, and proteins. (Although alcohol provides calories, it is not considered a nutrient. Alcohol is a drug.) For most people in the United States, approximately 43 to 58 percent of daily calories comes from carbohydrates. About 30 to 45 percent comes from fats, and about 12 percent comes from proteins. The metabolism of these nutrients is the source of chemical energy in your body.

● Measuring the Amount of Energy in Food

Did you ever wonder how people know how many calories are in a spoonful of sugar? Researchers have determined the energy value of foods by burning them and measuring the amount of heat they produce. This technique for measuring energy is called *direct calorimetry* because it measures the heat produced directly by the food. To take this measurement, a piece of food is first precisely weighed. Then it is placed in a closed, insulated device called a *bomb calorimeter*. The chamber holding the food is surrounded by a container holding a kilogram of water. After the food is burned completely, the change in water temperature is accurately measured. Each degree of increase on a Celsius thermometer equals one calorie of energy given off by the food. See 12-2.

Through direct calorimetry, researchers have measured the calories in the wide range of foods listed in food composition tables. They have also determined the energy yield of one gram of a pure nutrient. As you have

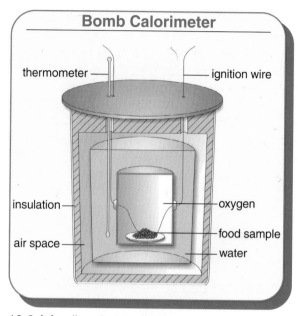

12-2 A food's calorie value is a measure of the heat it gives off when it is burned in a bomb calorimeter.

already learned, one gram of pure carbohydrate or protein yields 4 calories. One gram of pure fat yields 9 calories. This means fats produce more than twice the energy of the other two nutrients.

Being aware of the calorie density of foods can help you balance energy. **Calorie density** refers to the concentration of energy in a food. Fats are a concentrated source of energy. Therefore, foods that are high in fat are calorie dense. On the other hand, foods that are high in water lack calorie density because water yields no energy. Comparing 100 grams of two foods will help you see the relationship between fat content and calorie density. Lettuce, which is high in water and contains no fat, provides 13 calories per 100 grams. Mayonnaise, which is low in water and high in fat, provides 714 calories per 100 grams. Mayonnaise is clearly the more calorie dense food.

Review the information in Chapter 4, "Nutrition Guidelines," about keeping a food diary and analyzing your diet. Keeping a food diary can help you evaluate your daily energy intake as well as your nutrient intake. Examine the number of calories per serving of foods listed in your diary. Those high in calories are energy dense.

The RDA for energy for people of both sexes and different ages is listed in Appendix B. You can compare your energy intake with the recommendations in the chart. Remember, the chart serves only as a guideline. It does not take into account your height, weight, or level of energy expenditure.

● Energy Output

The other side of the energy balance equation looks at the calories you burn throughout the day. Researchers have determined you need energy for basal metabolism, physical activity, and the thermic effect of food. Together, these three factors account for the calories you expend each day.

● Basal Metabolism

No matter how still your body is, even during sleep, internal activity continues. Your brain and liver use about 40 percent of your body energy when you are resting. *Basal metabolism* is the amount of energy required to support the operation of all internal body systems except digestion. Basal metabolism keeps your body alive when it is at rest. It includes the energy your body uses every day to breathe, circulate blood, and maintain nerve activity. Secreting hormones, maintaining body temperature, and making new cells are also part of basal metabolism. See 12-3.

The *basal metabolic rate (BMR)* is the rate at which the body uses energy for basal metabolism. In general, women require 0.4 calorie per pound (0.9 calorie per kilogram) of body weight per hour to support basal metabolism. Men require 0.5 calorie per pound (1.0 calorie per kilogram) of body weight per hour.

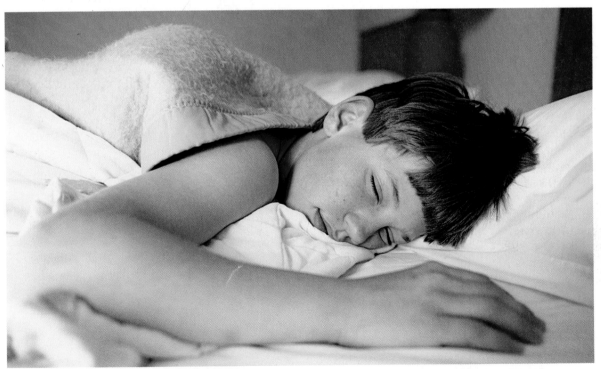

12-3 Even during sleep, the body needs energy to maintain the functions of its various systems.

A man would use the following formula to calculate his basal metabolic energy needs:

weight in pounds × 0.5 calorie per pound = basal energy needs per hour

(weight in kilograms × 1.0 calorie per kilogram = basal energy needs per hour)

basal energy needs per hour × 24 hours = basal energy needs per day

A woman would use the same formula, substituting 0.4 calorie for the BMR in the first equation. A 120-pound (55-kilogram) woman using this formula would calculate her daily basal energy needs to equal 1,152 calories. You may be surprised the amount is so large. However, basal metabolism is the largest part of energy output for most people.

What Affects Your BMR?

A person's BMR is affected by many factors. Body structure, body composition, and gender affect BMR. A tall person will have a higher BMR than a shorter person. This is because the taller person has more body surface area through which heat is lost. **Body composition** refers to the percentage of different tissues in the body, such as fat, muscle, and bone. A person with a larger proportion of muscle tissue will have a higher BMR than someone with more fat tissue. This is because it takes more calories to maintain muscle tissue than fat. Males generally have a higher BMR than females because males have more lean body mass.

Temperature, both inside and outside the body, can affect BMR. Fever increases the BMR. Adjusting to cold or hot temperatures in the environment increases BMR, too.

The thyroid gland secretes the hormone *thyroxine,* which regulates basal metabolism. An overactive thyroid produces too much thyroxine and increases the BMR. Conversely, an underactive thyroid secretes less thyroxine and decreases the BMR. This is why a thyroid disease can affect a person's body weight.

The BMR tends to decline with age. There is an approximate five percent decrease in BMR every 10 years past age 30. People over age 50 must reduce their energy intake up to 200 calories per day to avoid weight gain. Older people who remain active and maintain lean body mass do not experience as much of a decline in BMR. See 12-4.

A diet that is very low in calories decreases the BMR about 10 to 20 percent. This is because the body is responding as it would during a famine. It makes adjustments to preserve life as long as possible. By lowering the BMR, vital functions can be maintained even when fewer calories are available. Someone restricting calories to lose weight will have a harder time reaching his or her goal because of this factor.

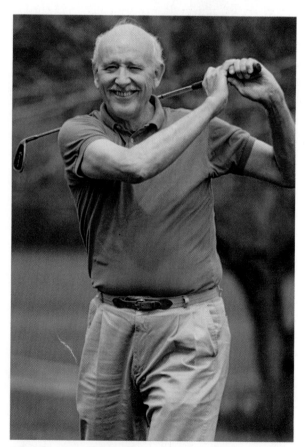

12-4 Staying physically active helps older people maintain a higher BMR.

The BMR is higher during periods of growth. Therefore, infants, children, and teens have a higher BMR than adults. Women have a higher BMR during pregnancy. Meeting the basal energy needs for growth and maintenance of cells is critical for body development. This is why infants, children, teens, and pregnant women should not reduce their calorie intake unless advised by a doctor. These groups of people need the nutrients provided by a variety of foods. If children and teens are having trouble balancing energy, increasing physical activity is a more healthful choice than reducing calories.

Some of the factors described above are temporary. Fever and pregnancy temporarily increase BMR. When these conditions end, BMR will drop back to its normal level.

You will notice you cannot change many of the above factors. Therefore, you cannot change the impact of these factors on your BMR. There is one way, however, you might change your basal metabolic rate. Adding a regular exercise program to your lifestyle will help you develop more muscle tissue. Generally, the greater the proportion of lean tissue in your body, the higher your BMR will be.

● Physical Activity

The second category of energy needs is the energy you use for physical activity. You need energy to move your muscles. You also need energy for the extra work of breathing harder and pumping more blood.

Energy output varies depending on body size. The larger the body size, the greater the amount of energy needed to make the muscles work. In other words, a 180-pound (82-kilogram) person burns more calories while walking than a 120-pound (55-kilogram) person walking at the same pace.

The actual amount of muscle movement also affects energy output. Therefore, you will burn more calories if you swing your arms while walking than if you keep your arms still.

Sedentary activities are activities that require much sitting. Watching television, studying, working in an office, driving, and using a computer are all sedentary activities. People who do many sedentary activities need to make a point of including physical motion in their daily lives.

If you want to burn more calories, try looking for more energy-intensive ways of completing your daily tasks. For instance, you might take the stairs instead of riding in an elevator. Swing your arms when walking. Stand rather than sit when you are waiting for someone. Walk or ride a bicycle instead of riding in a car. When you do drive, park the car away from your destination and walk the last block or two. See 12-5.

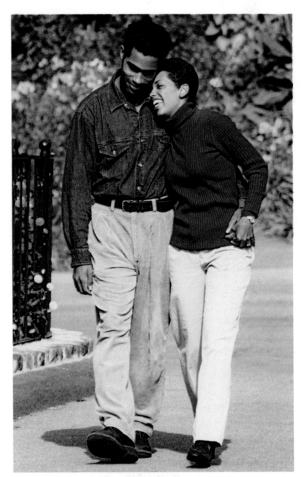

12-5 Walking instead of riding in a car can add more physical activity to your daily routine.

Determining Your Calorie Needs for Physical Activity

Researchers commonly measure the number of calories burned as a result of physical activity through *indirect calorimetry*. This measurement technique requires a person to wear an apparatus while performing a specific activity. The apparatus measures the person's oxygen intake and carbon dioxide output. (Oxygen consumption is required to burn calories. That is why you breathe harder when running or working hard.) The researchers then use mathematical formulas to convert the gas exchange into calories used.

Chart 12-6 lists ranges of calories used per hour for various common activities. These ranges include energy expended for basal metabolism as well as energy used for the activities. By comparing activities, you will soon know which ones are high energy users and which ones demand little energy. For instance, studying may seem like hard work. Unfortunately, studying burns no more calories per hour than watching television.

You can use Chart 12-6 to estimate how many calories you burn as a result of physical activity. Begin by keeping an accurate record of all your activities for one typical 24-hour period. Note the amount of time spent on each activity. Use the following formula to compute your approximate energy use for each activity:

calories used per hour × hours of activity = energy expended

Using this equation, you can calculate that you burn about 480 calories during 8 hours of sleep. You can also estimate that you use about 150 calories when you ride your bicycle for 30 minutes. Add the figures for all your activities in a 24-hour period to determine the total energy expended for the day. See 12-7.

Thermic Effect of Food

Your third need for energy is due to the thermic effect of food. The ***thermic effect of food*** is the energy required to complete the processes of digestion, absorption, and

Energy Cost for Various Physical Activities

Activity	Calories Used per Hour
Sleep	60
Sedentary activities—reading, eating, watching television, sewing, playing cards, using a computer, studying, other sitting activities	80 to 100 (average 90)
Light activities—cooking, doing dishes, ironing, grooming, walking slowly, more strenuous sitting activities	110 to 160 (average 135)
Moderate activities—walking moderately fast, making beds, light gardening, standing activities requiring arm movement	170 to 240 (average 205)
Vigorous activities—walking fast, bowling, golfing, yard work	250 to 350 (average 300)
Strenuous activities—running, dancing, bicycling, playing football, playing tennis, cheerleading, swimming, skiing, playing active games	350 or more

12-6 Body size and degree of muscle movement affect the specific number of calories a person burns through physical activity.

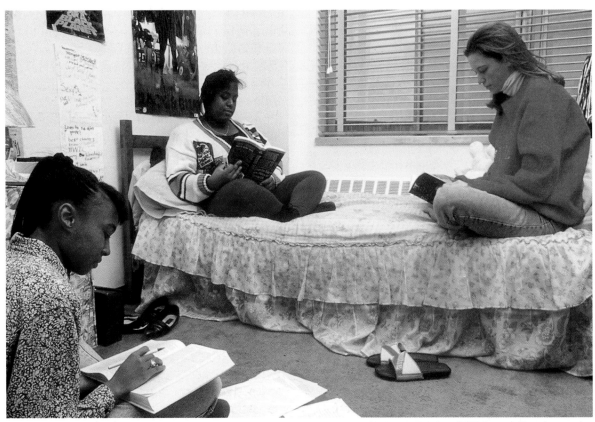

Photo courtesy of University Relations, MSU, Bruce A. Fox, photographer

12-7 Studying burns only about 90 calories per hour. Balancing sedentary activities with activities that are more vigorous will help burn the calories consumed from food.

metabolism. Think of it as the energy required to extract the energy from food.

The thermic effect of food may depend slightly on the types and amounts of foods eaten. However, it generally equals 5 to 10 percent of your combined basal metabolism and physical activity energy needs. Remember the calorie ranges you used to calculate your energy needs for physical activity included basal metabolism. Therefore, simply multiply your calculated total energy expenditure for the day by 0.1 (10 percent). This will give you a reasonable estimate of energy used for the thermic effect of food. Someone burning 2,200 calories for physical activity and basal metabolism would spend about 220 calories for the thermic effect of food.

For most people, approximately 60 to 65 percent of energy output is for basal metabolism. About 25 to 35 percent is for physical activity. For athletes, a lower percentage of energy output is for basal metabolism and a higher percentage is for physical activity. Five to 10 percent of energy output is for the thermic effect of food. See 12-8.

Calculating exact total energy needs is difficult for a layperson. However, your estimates can help you determine whether you are balancing your energy input and output. If you are neither gaining nor losing weight, you are in energy balance. Maintaining weight means the calories you eat are balancing the calories you need for energy.

● Energy Imbalance

Because of many factors, the two sides of the energy equation are not always in balance. *Energy imbalance* occurs when a person consumes too few or too many calories

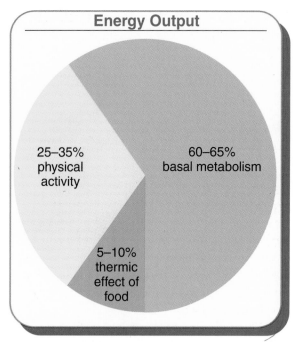

Energy Output

25–35% physical activity

60–65% basal metabolism

5–10% thermic effect of food

12-8 The majority of energy needs support basal metabolism, with a significant amount of energy also needed for physical activity.

for his or her energy needs. Over time, either of these conditions can lead to negative health consequences.

A regularly occurring energy imbalance will cause a change in body weight. People who are trying to lose or gain weight intentionally create an energy imbalance in their bodies. People who pay little attention to their eating and activity habits may unintentionally create an energy imbalance.

● Energy Deficiency

Energy deficiency occurs when energy intake is less than energy output. Several factors can result in an energy deficiency. In cases of poverty and famine, food sources may be too scarce to meet energy needs. Illness may depress appetite or hinder energy metabolism. Someone who eats a low-calorie diet purposely creates an energy deficiency.

The body responds to an energy deficiency in a number of ways. The body first uses energy from carbohydrates, fats, and proteins in food to meet its energy needs. If there is not enough food energy available, the body draws on stores of energy. The first store the body turns to is liver glycogen. This is the stored form of glucose from carbohydrates for use by nonmuscle tissue.

After about four to six hours, when glycogen stores are depleted, the body will draw on fatty tissue for energy. Weight loss will occur as fat is used. Unfortunately, the nervous system cannot use fat as a fuel source. It requires glucose, which cannot be obtained from fat.

The body can use amino acids from proteins in lean body tissues to make glucose to feed the nervous system. In order for the body to use this protein, however, it has to break down muscle and organ tissues. Muscle tissue is 75 percent water. Therefore, breaking down muscle proteins causes a rapid weight loss due to loss of body fluids. It also causes muscle weakness and can eventually lead to a number of dangerous health consequences.

When carbohydrates are not available, the body will take steps to limit muscle deterioration. It will slowly begin to use another method to feed the nervous system. The body will change fatty acids into compounds called ***ketone bodies***. The nervous system can use ketone bodies to meet some of its energy needs. Ketone bodies reach the nervous system through the bloodstream. An abnormal buildup of ketone bodies in the bloodstream is a condition known as ***ketosis***. This condition can be harmful because it changes the acid-base balance of the blood.

Carbohydrates are always important in the diet because they are the preferred fuel for nerve and brain cells to function. Nutritionists do not recommend high-protein or low-carbohydrate diets. These diets cause muscle tissue to be broken down and large amounts of ketones to form. Instead, nutritionists suggest including enough carbohydrates in the diet to fuel the brain and central nervous system. Carbohydrate intake should also be sufficient to preserve muscle tissue.

This will cause the body to use fat stores, not muscle, for energy. Weight loss will result from the loss of fat, not protein. See 12-9.

Energy Excess

Energy excess occurs when energy intake is greater than energy output. Excess calories from carbohydrates, fats, proteins, and alcohol can all be stored in adipose tissue. The body can use this stored energy when there is not enough food intake to meet immediate energy needs.

If energy excess occurs on a regular basis, weight gain will result. An excess of 3,500 calories in the diet leads to 1 pound (0.45 kg) of stored body fat. The amount of weight and the speed with which it is gained depend on the degree of energy excess.

Most overweight people have gained weight slowly over a period of years. Consuming an extra 25 calories each day adds approximately 2½ pounds (1.2 kg) each year. Just this small energy excess could cause a healthy-weight 20-year-old to be 25 pounds overweight by age 30.

Excess adipose tissue is a health concern. The greater the amount of fat carried on the body, the greater the risks for related health problems. (Chapter 13, "Healthy Weight Management," discusses risks of excess weight.)

Determining Healthy Weight

In the next chapter, you will read about health risks associated with too little and too much body fat. To avoid both sets of risks, you need to maintain a healthy weight. This may not be the weight at which you match the media image of a "perfect body." Instead, it is a weight at which your body fat is in an appropriate proportion to your lean tissue. Having a healthy weight reduces your risk of a number of serious medical problems.

There are several ways to determine whether your weight is healthy. You can use a mathematical calculation based on your weight and height. You can look at tables that give healthy weight ranges for people of your height. You can take measurements of your body fat, too. Each of these methods has advantages and disadvantages. However, they can all be useful tools in helping you evaluate your weight status.

Using Body Mass Index

Federal guidelines define weight groups by ***body mass index (BMI)***. This is a calculation of body weight and height. You can figure your BMI by dividing your weight in pounds by the square of your height in inches. Then multiply this figure by the constant 705. (When working in metric units, divide weight in kilograms by the square of height in meters. The result is the BMI. It does not have to be multiplied by a constant.) Someone who is 5 feet 9 inches (1.75 meters) tall and weighs 145 pounds (65.25 kilograms) would calculate BMI as follows:

$$(145 \text{ pounds} \div 69^2 \text{ inches}) \times 705$$
$$(145 \div 4{,}761) \times 705$$
$$0.0305 \times 705 = 21.5 \text{ (rounded) BMI}$$

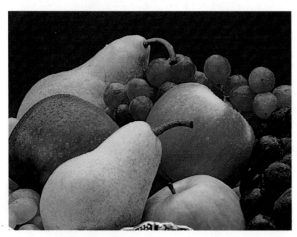

12-9 Including lowfat sources of carbohydrates in an energy deficient diet will result in weight loss without damage to body protein tissues.

A chart that can help you easily find your BMI is shown in 12-10.

For adults, *healthy weight* is defined as a BMI of 18.5 to 24.9. An adult who has a BMI of 25 to 29.9 is said to be *overweight*. If an adult's BMI is 30 or more, he or she is identified as *obese*. Any adult with a BMI below 18.5 is considered *underweight*.

BMI is not an appropriate weight evaluation tool for everyone. For example, body builders have excess muscle weight. For them, BMI is not an accurate gauge of overweight and obesity.

Definitions of weight categories based on BMI are less clear-cut for children and adolescents, whose bodies are still growing. Recommended BMI cutoffs to identify children and adolescents who are overweight vary according to age and sex. See 12-11.

Using Height-Weight Tables

You can estimate healthy weight using a standard height-weight table. The table lists a weight range for each height. Weights near the high end of each range apply to people with a greater proportion of muscle and bone tissue. (Muscle and bone are denser than body fat.) Most men fall into this group. See 12-12.

One drawback of height-weight tables is they are not precise and not designed for people under age 19. They do not take into account body composition or individual health risks. For instance, some athletes may appear to have excess weight due to their large muscle mass. Remember, unit for unit, muscle weighs more than fat. For most people, however, weighing above the healthy weight range increases health risks.

Body Mass Index

Weight in Pounds

Height	90	95	100	105	110	115	120	125	130	135	140	145	150	155	160	165	170	175	180	185	190	195	200	205
4' 11"	18	19	20	21	22	23	24	25	26	27	28	29	30	31	32	33	34	35	36	37	38	39	41	42
5' 0"	18	19	20	21	22	23	23	24	25	26	27	28	29	30	31	32	33	34	35	36	37	38	39	40
5' 1"	17	18	19	20	21	22	23	24	25	26	26	27	28	29	30	31	32	33	34	35	36	37	38	39
5' 2"	17	17	18	19	20	21	22	23	24	25	26	27	28	28	29	30	31	32	33	34	35	36	37	37
5' 3"	16	17	18	19	20	20	21	22	23	24	25	26	27	28	28	29	30	31	32	33	34	35	36	36
5' 4"	15	16	17	18	19	20	21	22	22	23	24	25	26	27	28	28	29	30	31	32	33	34	34	35
5' 5"	15	16	17	18	18	19	20	21	22	22	23	24	25	26	27	28	28	29	30	31	32	33	33	34
5' 6"	15	15	16	17	18	19	19	20	21	22	23	24	24	25	26	27	28	28	29	30	31	32	32	33
5' 7"	14	15	16	17	17	18	19	20	20	21	22	23	24	24	25	26	27	28	28	29	30	31	31	32
5' 8"	14	14	15	16	17	18	18	19	20	21	21	22	23	24	24	25	26	27	27	28	29	30	31	31
5' 9"	13	14	15	16	16	17	18	19	19	20	21	22	22	23	24	24	25	26	27	27	28	29	30	30
5' 10"	13	14	14	15	16	17	17	18	19	19	20	21	22	22	23	24	24	25	26	27	27	28	29	30
5' 11"	13	13	14	15	15	16	17	18	18	19	20	20	21	22	22	23	24	25	25	26	26	27	28	29
6' 0"	12	13	14	14	15	16	16	17	18	18	19	20	20	21	22	22	23	24	25	25	26	26	27	28
6' 1"	12	13	13	14	15	15	16	17	17	18	19	19	20	21	21	22	23	23	24	25	25	26	26	27
6' 2"	12	12	13	14	14	15	15	16	17	17	18	19	19	20	21	21	22	23	23	24	24	25	26	26

12-10 This chart can help you determine your BMI.

Age	BMI for Males		BMI for Females	
	At Risk	*Overweight*	*At Risk*	*Overweight*
14	23	27	24	28
15	24	28	24	29
16	24	29	25	29
17	25	29	25	30
18	26	30	26	30
19	26	30	26	30

Adolescent Overweight

12-11 Many teens can use their BMI to evaluate whether they are at risk of being overweight.

Healthy Weight Ranges

Height[1]	Weight in Pounds[2]
4'10"	91-119
4'11"	94-124
5'0"	97-128
5'1"	101-132
5'2"	104-137
5'3"	107-141
5'4"	111-146
5'5"	114-150
5'6"	118-155
5'7"	121-160
5'8"	125-164
5'9"	129-169
5'10"	132-174
5'11"	136-179
6'0"	140-184
6'1"	144-189
6'2"	148-195
6'3"	152-200
6'4"	156-205
6'5"	160-211
6'6"	164-216

[1]without shoes

[2]without clothes

12-12 Height-weight tables provide an easy way for most people to see if their weight is in a healthy range.

Weighing a little less than a height-weight table suggests is not always a cause for concern. Most health researchers agree it is better to veer to the lean side than to the heavy side. However, weighing significantly less than shown in a standard height-weight table may indicate a serious health problem.

● Using Body Fat Measuring Methods

Analyzing the percentage of fat in your body is another way to judge your weight status. For men, over 25 percent body fat is considered excessive. A more desirable range is 15 to 18 percent. For women, over 30 percent body fat is excessive. A range of 20 to 25 percent is more healthful.

How is percentage of body fat determined? One way is to do a *skinfold test*. This test uses a special tool called a *caliper* to measure the thickness of a fold of skin. An estimate is made about how much of the thickness is due to *subcutaneous fat*. This is the fat that lies underneath the skin, and it accounts for about half the fat in the body. Skinfold measurements are often taken on the thigh, upper arm, abdomen, and/or back. The amount of subcutaneous fat in these areas reflects the total amount of fat throughout the body.

A simple version of a skinfold test you can do at home is called the "pinch test."

Grasp the skin on the back of your upper arm halfway between your shoulder and elbow. Pinch this fold of skin between your thumb and forefinger. Be sure to grasp only the fat, not the muscle. A distance between your thumb and forefinger of more than one inch (2.5 centimeters) may indicate a high percentage of body fat.

Another method for measuring body fat is *bioelectrical impedance*. This process measures the body's resistance to a low-energy electrical current. Lean tissue conducts electrical energy, whereas fat does not. The more fat a person has, the more resistance there is to the flow of the electrical current. The measure of resistance is then converted to a percentage of body fat.

● Location of Body Fat

Recent evidence suggests the location as well as the amount of body fat affects health. Fat stored in the abdomen seems to pose a greater risk than fat stored in the buttocks, hips, and thighs. Fat around the waist increases the liver's production of low-density lipoproteins, which is a risk factor for heart disease.

Men and older women are more likely to accumulate fat in the abdominal area. They have what is sometimes referred to as "apple-shaped" bodies. Younger women more often store excess fat in the hips and thighs. They have what may be called "pear-shaped" bodies. You may have limited control over where your body stores excess fat. However, if you maintain a healthy weight, your fat stores should not pose a health problem.

When you evaluate your weight, avoid media-promoted stereotypes of how you should look. Try not to be concerned about every pound on your body. Eat a nutritious diet and follow a program of regular exercise. These lifestyle choices will help you maintain your energy balance and support wellness. See 12-13.

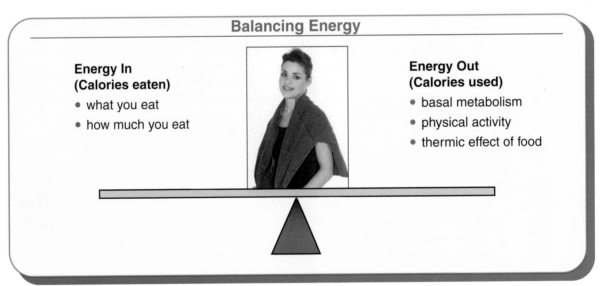

Balancing Energy

Energy In (Calories eaten)
- what you eat
- how much you eat

Energy Out (Calories used)
- basal metabolism
- physical activity
- thermic effect of food

12-13 To balance the energy equation, the calories in the foods you eat must equal the calories you use each day.

Summary

Balancing energy means matching the calories you take in from food with the calories you expend each day. You get food energy from carbohydrates, fats, and proteins. Knowing the calorie density of foods can help you balance energy.

You use energy for basal metabolism, physical activity, and the thermic effect of food. Basal metabolism is the energy needed to support basic body functions, such as breathing, blood circulation, and nerve activity. The rate at which the body uses energy for basal metabolism (BMR) is affected by many factors. Of the three basic energy need areas, you have the most control over physical activity. The longer and harder you exercise, the more calories you burn. The thermic effect of food is the energy needed for digestion, absorption, and metabolism.

If you consume too few or too many calories for your energy needs, you will be in energy imbalance. Energy deficiency occurs when there is not enough food energy available to meet the body's needs. Energy excess occurs when there is more food energy available than the body needs. Both energy deficiency and energy excess can lead to negative health consequences.

To avoid risks from too little or too much body fat, you need to maintain a healthy weight. You can estimate healthy weight using body mass index (BMI), height-weight tables, or fat measuring techniques. A desirable range of body fat is 15 to 18 percent for men and 20 to 25 percent for women. Excess fat in the abdomen seems to pose a greater health risk than fat in the buttocks, hips, and thighs. You can maintain a healthy weight by balancing energy through wise food choices and regular exercise.

Check Your Knowledge

1. True or false. When a person eats food, his or her body uses it to create energy.

2. How much energy does a pure gram of each of the energy nutrients yield?

3. What are three internal body functions, other than breathing, blood circulation, and nerve activity, supported by the energy of basal metabolism?

4. What are six factors that affect a person's BMR?

5. Give three examples of ways to increase energy expenditure while completing daily tasks.

6. Explain how to estimate how many calories a person burns as a result of physical activity.

7. Which of the three areas of energy expenditure accounts for the smallest percentage of calories burned?

8. Why do nutritionists avoid recommending low-carbohydrate diets?

9. How many excess calories are stored in 1 pound (0.45 kilogram) of body fat?

10. What do federal guidelines use to define adult underweight, healthy weight, overweight, and obesity?

11. What percentage of body fat is considered excessive for men and for women?

12. Why does fat stored in the abdomen pose a greater health risk than fat stored in the buttocks, hips, and thighs?

Put Learning into Action

1. Collect Nutrition Facts panels from five food product labels. Calculate the percentage of calories in each product coming from carbohydrates, fats, and proteins. Remember fats provide 9 calories per gram and carbohydrates and proteins each provide 4 calories per gram. Determine which nutrient is providing the greatest source of energy.

2. Use the formula given in the chapter to compute your basal energy needs for one 24-hour period. Also keep an accurate

record of all your activities for one 24-hour period. Note the amount of time spent on each activity. Use the formula given in the chapter and Chart 12-6 to compute your approximate energy use for each activity. (Remember the ranges in the chart include energy expended for basal metabolism as well as for the activities.) Figure your total energy expenditure for the day. Then calculate your energy needs for the thermic effect of food. Finally, compute the percentages of your total energy expenditure used for basal metabolism, physical activity, and thermic effect of food.

3. Make a poster or bulletin board display illustrating how the body responds to an energy deficiency.

4. Calculate your body mass index. Find your healthy weight range on a height-weight table. Do a pinch test to evaluate your percentage of body fat. Then write a two-page summary of your self-analysis. State whether you think your weight is healthy and explain why or why not.

Explore Further

1. Some experts believe the thermic effects of food play an insignificant role in total energy expenditure. Others believe the calories used for thermic effect can add up and contribute to leanness over a lifetime. Take part in a debate over these two theories using research to support your view.

2. Read a research article on the impact location of body fat can have on health. Summarize your findings in a brief oral report.

Chapter 13

Healthy Weight Management

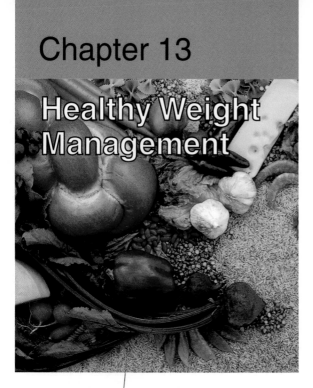

Learn the Language

weight management	crash diet
habit	fasting
environmental cue	weight cycling
fad diet	

Objectives

After studying this chapter, you will be able to

- describe health risks of obesity and underweight.
- recognize factors that influence a person's weight status.
- estimate your daily calorie needs and your daily calorie intake.
- state why some rapid weight-loss plans are dangerous and ineffective.
- explain guidelines for safe loss of body fat.
- list tips for safe weight gain.

Have you ever tried to lose or gain weight? If you have, you have much company. Millions of people every year take steps to try to adjust their weight. **Weight management** means attaining healthy weight and keeping it throughout life.

In this chapter you will be examining health risks associated with too much and too little body fat. You will identify factors that affect your weight status. You will also learn to follow the guidelines of good nutrition as you manage your weight.

Healthy People Need a Healthy Weight

Reaching a healthy weight and maintaining it throughout life are important wellness goals. Having a healthy weight can improve your total sense of well-being and reduce your risk of many diseases.

Instead of discussing *weight* management, it may make more sense to discuss *body fat* management. Not everyone who is overweight has excess body fat. Overweight can also be due to muscle development. Athletes, for example, often have high weights for their heights. However, the weight is due to muscle, not fat. This type of excess weight is not a health problem. Problems associated with overweight and obesity arise when the weight is due to excess fat rather than excess muscle. See 13-1.

With so much attention focused on overweight, problems associated with underweight are often overlooked. In the United States, the number of people who are underweight is much smaller than the number who are overweight. However, both groups are at increased risk of health problems.

Health Risks of Obesity

In the United States, overweight and obesity have become more common in recent years. As you read in the last chapter, an *overweight* adult has a body mass index

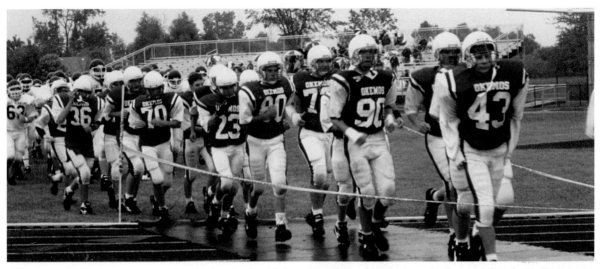

13-1 Many athletes are overweight due to the high proportion of lean muscle tissue in their bodies.

(BMI) of 25 to 29.9. An *obese* adult has a BMI of 30 or more. Currently, over 50 percent of the people in the United States meet one or both of these definitions.

Reducing the occurrence of obesity in the United States is a national health goal. This is because obesity is a risk factor for high blood pressure, heart disease, and stroke. Obesity is also linked to increased risks of Type II diabetes, arthritis, respiratory problems, and certain cancers. Obese people have a greater risk of accidents and problems during surgery and pregnancy, too. The more excess fat a person carries, the greater the risks.

● **Social and Emotional Health Risks**

Obesity can be a source of social and emotional problems as well as physical ones. For years, mass media have overvalued a thin body as a standard of beauty. Obese people are sometimes portrayed negatively simply because they are obese.

Some people can be very cruel to those who are overweight or obese. Obese people may face discrimination in school, work, and other social settings.

Faulty media images and ill treatment from others add to stress among obese people. These factors can also cause obese people to form low opinions of themselves.

Obese people often have the mistaken belief they are less worthy than people who have healthy body weights. Some weight management programs work to dispute this misconception. They use counselors to help clients realize that personal value is not based on body weight.

● **Health Risks of Underweight**

Having too little body fat can have serious effects on health. Underweight people may lack nutrient stores. Thus when stores are needed, such as during pregnancy or after surgery, underweight people may have problems. Underweight people may also feel fatigued and have trouble staying warm. Females with low body fat may stop menstruating. A number of other health risks result from underweight due to eating disorders. (Eating disorders will be more fully discussed in Chapter 14, "Eating Disorders.")

● **Factors Affecting Your Weight Status**

Weight status refers not only to how much you weigh but to your ability to gain and lose weight. Your weight status is the sum of many factors. Heredity is one factor known to influence what the scale says about you. Your eating habits and physical activity level also have a major impact on your weight.

Heredity

Genes set the stage for body shape. The size of bones and the location of fat stores in the body are inherited traits. Fortunately, healthy body weight can be found in a variety of body shapes. Heredity also affects basal metabolic rate. See 13-2.

A family history of obesity does not necessarily destine a person to be obese. However, weight management may be harder for people who inherited genes that lean toward obesity. They may need to watch their eating habits more closely than others. They will also need to be sure to get enough physical activity.

Similarly, someone who has numerous thin relatives has no guarantee of a thin body. However, some people are genetically prone toward thinness. Their bodies store fat less readily than others. People who inherit this trait may find it hard to gain weight.

Eating Habits

Eating habits affect weight status by influencing the "calories in" side of the energy balance equation. A **habit** is a routine behavior

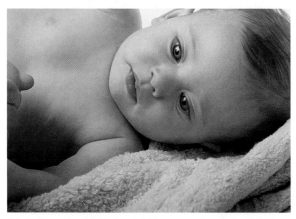

13-2 People are born with a genetic code that affects how their bodies will store fat throughout their lives.

that is often difficult to break. For example, eating buttered popcorn at the movies can become a habit.

People begin to form eating habits early in life based largely on the foods parents or guardians offer them. They develop patterns in the kinds and amounts of foods they choose. They form habits related to when and why they eat, too.

Parents need to be aware that obese children and teens have an increased risk of becoming obese adults. Parents can plan meals and snacks around appropriate portions of nutritious foods. This will help children establish healthful eating habits that promote weight management. Children who develop eating behaviors based on good nutrition are more likely to practice healthful eating habits throughout life.

As children grow up, some of their eating habits are likely to change. During the teen years, people begin to have more control over what foods they eat. Busy schedules, peers, and weight concerns often influence food choices. Many teens form habits of eating a lot of fast foods that are high in fat and calories. Others adopt patterns of skipping meals.

Eating habits continue to change through adulthood. Work and family obligations often impact food choices and eating behaviors. Adults who commute to work may eat on the go. Adults with children sometimes develop the habit of finishing leftovers from their children's plates. These habits may lead to excess calories.

Environmental Cues

Some eating habits are responses to environmental cues. An **environmental cue** is an event or situation around you that triggers you to eat. The sight, taste, and smells of foods are common cues that stimulate eating. The time of day, such as lunchtime, is an environmental cue for many people. Social settings, such as parties, can be environmental cues, too. See 13-3.

Appetite and hunger usually work to make sure people eat enough to supply the

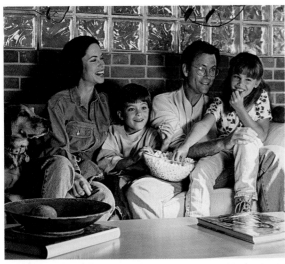

13-3 For many people, watching television is an environmental cue to eat.

fuel their bodies need. However, sometimes cues in the environment cause people to eat even when they are not hungry. For example, a vendor calling "Hot dogs!" may prompt you to eat at a ball game. This type of eating behavior often causes people to consume more calories than they need.

Being aware of when and why you eat is important. This will help you realize when you are responding to environmental cues rather than hunger. Developing this awareness of your eating habits can help you avoid overeating. When a cue triggers eating, replace your eating response with a response that makes you feel good about yourself. For example, coming home from school may be an environmental cue to have a snack. You could change your response to this cue and go in-line skating instead.

Psychological Factors

Have you ever noticed your emotions influencing when and how much you eat? Eating habits are sometimes responses to psychological factors. Boredom, depression, tension, fear, and loneliness may all lead to erratic eating patterns. Some people respond to such feelings by overeating; others respond by failing to eat.

Good nutrition can help you maintain good health, which is an important tool in handling emotional challenges. Try to notice which emotions affect your eating behaviors. Look for appropriate ways to deal with these emotions while following a nutritious diet. For instance, if you find yourself reaching for food when you are bored, consider going for a walk instead. This will promote your total state of wellness.

Activity Level

Physical activity levels affect weight status by influencing the "calories out" side of the energy balance equation. If you burn the same number of calories you consume, you will maintain your present weight. If you burn fewer calories than you consume, you will gain weight. If you burn more calories than you consume, you will lose weight.

One of the ways your body burns calories is through physical activity. The more active you are, the more calories you need for energy.

For some people, an energy excess is the result of overeating. For many people, however, an energy excess is due to physical inactivity. Many people in today's society spend much time doing sedentary activities. They ride in a car instead of walking. They watch television or surf the Internet instead of taking part in sports. See 13-4.

Losing Excess Body Fat

People who are overweight due to excess body fat would improve their health by reducing their fat stores. Numerous strategies for accomplishing this goal are promoted in books and magazines. Some of these strategies are safe and effective; others are dangerous. Knowing some basic information can help overweight people make sound weight management decisions.

People should consider several factors when thinking about beginning a weight-loss

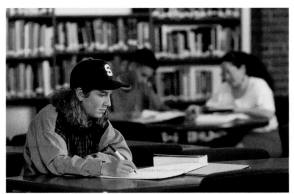

Photo courtesy of University Relations, MSU, Bruce A. Fox, photographer

13-4 Students need to balance time spent in sedentary study with time spent in physical activity.

program. One factor is health status. Women should not try to lose weight during pregnancy. A minimum weight gain is required to ensure the health of a developing fetus. People who are ill should avoid restricting calories to lose weight. The body needs an adequate supply of nutrients to restore health. Meeting these nutrient needs is difficult when calories are severely restricted.

Age is another issue to keep in mind when considering a plan to reduce body fat. Weight loss is not recommended for children and teens, who are still growing. Losing weight could permanently stunt their growth. The recommendation for children and teens is to hold weight steady and grow into it.

People need to evaluate their motivation and body structure when considering weight loss. The main goal of weight management is good health. People who try to lose weight to achieve an unrealistically slim appearance may put their health at risk. Remember, weight above a standard range is a health risk only if it is due to excess body fat. Weight due to muscle mass is not a cause for concern and does not indicate a need for weight loss.

People planning a weight-loss program should also consider how much emotional support they will have. Adopting new eating patterns is difficult. People who are most likely to succeed in a weight management plan are those who receive encouragement. You may want to join a class or program to help with weight management efforts. Some people choose a partner to help support and encourage them. Talking to family members and friends before beginning a weight-loss program can help gain their support.

The Math of Losing a Pound of Fat

One pound (0.45 kg) of body fat stores 3,500 calories of energy. To lose one pound (0.45 kg) of body fat, therefore, a person must create an energy deficit of 3,500 calories. Studies show weight maintenance is easier for people who spread this calorie deficit over one to two weeks. This means creating a calorie deficit of 250 to 500 calories per day.

You can create a calorie deficit by reducing calorie intake or increasing calorie needs. Before you can determine how to adjust your diet and exercise plan, you need to know your current energy needs. You also need to know how many calories you regularly consume.

Estimating Calorie Needs

Chapter 12 described how to estimate daily energy needs based on BMR, physical activity, and the thermic effect of food. Another way to estimate your body's calorie needs is by using the formulas shown in Chart 13-5. Simple calculations are made considering your gender and typical activity level.

When applying the formulas, you will see a lightly active male teen who weighs 140 pounds needs about 1,850 calories per day (1,080 + [5.5 × 140] = 1,850). Suppose this teen has a moderately active lifestyle that includes mowing the lawn, playing tennis, or walking regularly. His energy needs would increase to 2,156 calories (1,260 + [6.4 × 140] = 2,156). If this young man participates daily in strenuous activities, he must consume 2,462 calories to maintain weight (1,440 + [7.3 × 140 pounds] = 2,462).

Computing Approximate Daily Energy Needs

Activity Level	Men	Women
Light		
Sitting most of the day with some walking and light activities, such as cooking, doing dishes, and ironing	1,080 + (5.5 × weight)	960 + (3.8 × weight)
Moderate		
Sitting some of the day with some moderate activities, such as walking moderately fast, making beds, light gardening, and standing activities requiring arm movement	1,260 + (6.4 × weight)	1,120 + (4.5 × weight)
Active		
Heavy labor throughout the day or regular strenuous exercise, such as running, dancing, bicycling, swimming, skiing, and playing active games	1,440 + (7.3 × weight)	1,280 + (5.1 × weight)

13-5 Use the formula for your activity level to compute your daily energy needs.

Estimating Calorie Intake

Several chapters in this book have mentioned the value of keeping a food diary. You recall this is a record of the kinds and amounts of all foods and beverages you consume. Your food diary can help you figure the number of calories you consume during an average day. Use food composition tables or diet analysis software to find the calorie values of each food you consume. Add your totals for each day. Then add your daily totals and divide by the number of days to find the average.

Comparing Calorie Needs with Calorie Intake

You can figure what your daily calorie limit must be to achieve your weight management goals. Compare your estimated energy needs to your average daily intake. If your intake is greater than your estimated needs, you probably have been gaining weight. Reducing daily calorie intake to make the numbers match will allow you to maintain your present weight. Reducing intake even further will result in weight loss. See 13-6.

Some people should avoid diets that restrict calories below the number needed to maintain a healthy weight. A lactating woman's body requires a high level of energy to produce milk. Children and teenagers need energy to support growth. Older adults will have trouble meeting their nutrient needs if calories are restricted. See 13-7.

Unsafe Weight-Loss Practices

People who do not like what the scale tells them become prime targets for "quick and easy" weight-loss schemes. It seems to be human nature to want to tackle weight problems with fast solutions that require minimal effort. Unfortunately, no magic tricks exist for healthful weight loss.

Fad Diets and Other Weight-Loss Gimmicks

New weight-loss schemes turn up every day. Just turn the pages of any teen magazine.

A Case of Weight Loss

Carl is 25 years old. He is 5'10" and weighs 195 pounds. A skinfold test confirms Carl's excess weight is due to excess body fat. To bring his body mass index into a healthy range, he should weigh no more than 170 pounds.

Carl can use the formulas for estimating energy needs to figure his daily calorie limit. Instead of using his present weight in the formula, he uses his weight goal of 170 pounds. At a light activity level, Carl would need 2,015 calories per day to maintain his goal weight ($1,080 + [5.5 \times 170] = 2,015$).

Carl's food diary tells him he has been eating about 2,300 calories per day. He knows he needs to cut about 300 calories out of his daily diet. At first this sounds like a lot. Then Carl realizes 300 calories is about the amount in 20 French fries or two cans of soda. Carl figures that by making some healthier food choices, he can easily stick to a lower calorie limit. By cutting 300 calories from his daily diet, Carl would gradually lose weight until he reached his weight goal.

At the rate of 300 calories per day, Carl's weight loss may seem rather slow. It will take him about 12 days to create the 3,500-calorie deficit required to lose one pound. If Carl increases his physical activity to a moderate level, he will burn about 350 more calories per day. This will speed Carl's weight loss to about one pound every 5 days.

Once Carl reaches his weight goal of 170 pounds, he can return to a daily intake of 2,300 calories. However, he must maintain his moderate activity level ($1,260 + [6.4 \times 170] = 2,348$).

13-6 This story illustrates how to apply the math involved in creating a calorie deficit to lose weight.

You will likely find descriptions of eating plans promising rapid weight loss. Such plans that are popular for a short time are often referred to as **fad diets**.

Pills, body wraps, and other weight-loss gimmicks are also widely available. These products are often advertised with words like *fast-working, inexpensive, painless,* and *guaranteed.* However, the advertising is often more effective than the products. Consumers spend millions of dollars on dubious weight-loss products every year.

You may read advice such as, "Eat all the protein you want, but avoid fattening carbohydrates." You might hear a plan like, "Eat only rice for 10 days, and you will lose a pound a day." With all the slick advertising, separating dieting truths from fallacies can be difficult.

The truth is, anyone can make a claim about how to lose weight. Many people who promote dieting schemes lack medical or nutrition training. These people may be more interested in your money than they are in your health.

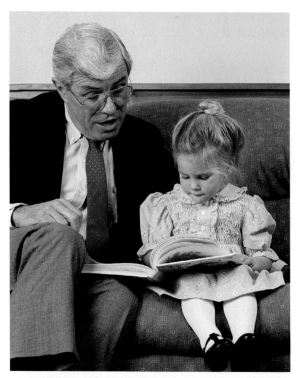

13-7 Older adults and children should not restrict calorie intake below the amount needed to maintain a healthy weight.

You may assume federal agencies will protect you from weight-loss frauds and the hucksters who promote them. However, the FDA and FTC take action only when false claims are made about particular products or foods.

The best way to deal with diet fads is to arm yourself with nutrition knowledge. Consult a registered dietitian or qualified nutrition educator if you have questions about the claims of a particular dieting scheme.

Dangers of Rapid Weight-Loss Plans

Weight-loss diets that provide fewer than 1,200 calories per day are sometimes referred to as **crash diets**. Such diets lack essential nutrients. It takes a minimum of about 1,300 calories to provide all the recommended servings from the Food Guide Pyramid. See 13-8.

Fasting is a form of crash dieting. **Fasting** means to refrain from consuming most or all sources of calories. Fasting over an extended period can create health problems. Within 24 hours of beginning a fast, the body's carbohydrate stores will be depleted. After this, the body will slowly begin breaking down lean

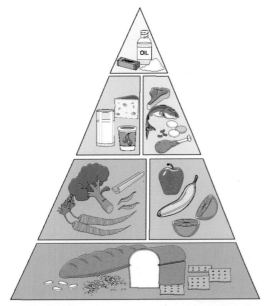

13-8 A weight-loss plan that does not follow the Food Guide Pyramid will be low in some nutrients.

tissues, including muscles and organs, to produce energy. The body will also convert fatty acids from body fat into ketone bodies that can fuel the nervous system. An abnormal buildup of ketone bodies in the bloodstream, which is known as *ketosis,* can be dangerous. Ketosis affects the acid-base balance of the blood.

Ineffectiveness of Rapid Weight-Loss Plans

Crash diets seldom have long-lasting positive weight-loss results. Crash dieting may produce some dramatic initial weight loss. Most of this weight loss is due to fluid loss. When the diet ends, fluid levels in the body readjust and water weight is quickly regained.

Fad diets often have several key drawbacks that keep them from being effective ways to lose weight. Very low calorie diets trigger the body to lower BMR, which makes it harder to lose weight. Fad diet plans usually tell people exactly how much and what they can eat. This gives people no control over their food choices. Fad diets require eating patterns that are radically different from most people's normal eating habits. This causes many people to give up on the diet because they miss the foods they are used to eating. Fad diets teach people nothing about better eating behaviors. These diets are not designed to help people maintain their new weights. After completing the diet, most people return to their old eating habits and the weight they lost quickly returns.

For some people, crash dieting leads to **weight cycling**, which is a lifelong pattern of weight gain and loss. Weight cycling is sometimes referred to as the *yo-yo diet syndrome.* Following the diet, people begin to eat more than ever simply because they feel starved and deprived of food. Some people gain more weight than they lost by dieting. Discouragement over the lack of success in maintaining weight loss causes them to try another crash diet. This dieting cycle may be repeated many times throughout life. See 13-9.

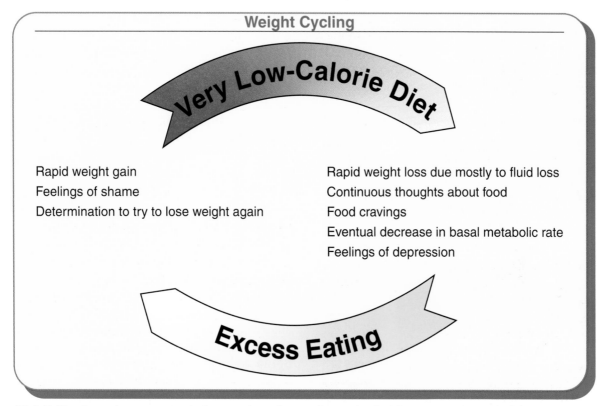

Weight Cycling

Very Low-Calorie Diet

Rapid weight gain

Feelings of shame

Determination to try to lose weight again

Rapid weight loss due mostly to fluid loss

Continuous thoughts about food

Food cravings

Eventual decrease in basal metabolic rate

Feelings of depression

Excess Eating

13-9 Failing to make permanent changes in eating and exercise habits causes some people to repeatedly lose and regain weight.

Research indicates weight ups and downs from year to year may be harmful to health. Emotional stress, physical fatigue, and food deprivation may create a greater chance of developing some diseases. Quality of life may be threatened.

● **Safe Fat-Loss Guidelines**

Weight management experts often advise people not to think of losing weight as "dieting." Likewise, they suggest not viewing food as an enemy to fight. Instead, they recommend thinking of losing weight as managing calorie and fat intake. Experts also remind people that food is meant to be *enjoyed*. It just needs to be enjoyed in moderation.

People with health problems should talk to a doctor before beginning a weight-loss program. A medical checkup is always recommended before children and teens

go on a weight-loss diet. A checkup is also advised for people in other age groups who are trying to lose more than five pounds.

Having correct information can help people be sure their weight-loss efforts will be safe and effective. The following guidelines for reducing calories and changing eating habits promote wellness through the loss of excess body fat.

● **Evaluate Weight-Loss Plans Carefully**

Evaluating a diet plan's effectiveness and related risks can be rather confusing. If a weight-loss plan sounds good to you, be sure to read the information carefully. Always be wary of diet schemes that encourage unsound eating patterns. Registered dietitians can counsel people about sensible weight loss.

Choose a weight management plan that is nutritionally sound. For greatest success, it should allow you to take off pounds slowly. It should also include a component of moderate exercise. According to the American Dietetic Association, a well-managed weight-loss program should include the following characteristics:

- The diet provides all the nutrients your body needs.
- The diet is as close to your tastes and habits as possible.
- The diet keeps you from being hungry or unusually tired.
- The diet allows you to eat away from home without feeling like a social outcast, 13-10.
- The diet offers you a change in eating habits you can follow for the rest of your life.

Avoid weight-loss plans that stress the eating of single food items. For instance, a diet that suggests eating only bananas does not reflect normal eating behaviors. Such a diet may be dangerous because it is not nutritionally balanced. Remember, a nutritious diet includes foods from all the major food groups in the Food Guide Pyramid.

Beware of programs that restrict which foods you can eat. This includes diet plans that stress eating mostly one macronutrient, usually protein. These eating plans cause you to miss important vitamins and minerals. In addition, high-protein diets may cause weakness, dizziness, and digestive disturbances. High-fat diets increase blood cholesterol levels and add to the risks of heart disease.

Avoid diet plans that require the use of pills. Many diet pills are ineffective and the long-term effects are unknown. No known pill can burn off body fat. Some pills can help suppress appetite or prevent fat absorption, but they cannot correct poor eating habits. Some diet pills may be addictive; others produce a variety of side effects.

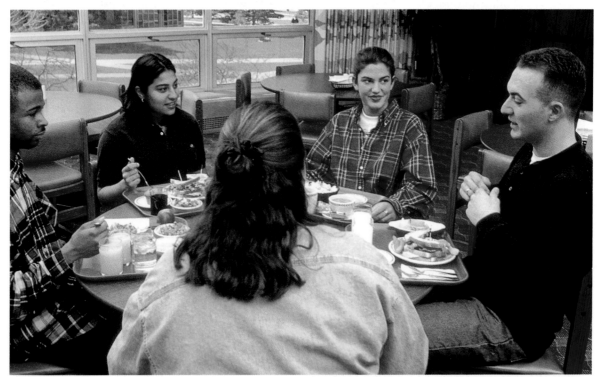

Photo courtesy of University Relations, MSU, Bruce A. Fox, photographer

13-10 An effective weight-loss plan will allow people to feel comfortable in social settings while following it.

Avoid weight-loss programs that suggest fasting or modified fasting. Liquid diets and other programs that are very low in calories may cause fatigue, irritability, nausea, and digestive upsets. They can also affect heartbeat rhythm and the acid level of the blood.

Be wary of weight-loss plans that promise large weight losses in a short time. Dieters who constantly follow the latest and greatest diet scheme often find only short-term successes. People who lose weight slowly are more likely to maintain a healthy weight once they reach it. Losing weight slowly also reduces health risks.

Through a combined eating and exercise plan, a person should attempt to lose no more than one to two pounds a week. Teens who are growing taller can modify this advice by maintaining weight throughout their growth. Gradual weight loss gives the body time to adjust. Remember, it takes time to gain excess weight. It will also take time to lose it without jeopardizing health.

● **Control Calorie Intake Through Planned Food Choices**

The foods you choose will directly relate to the number of calories you consume. The following suggestions for selecting foods may help you manage calories:

- Substitute foods lower in fat for those higher in fat. Fat has the highest number of calories per gram. Therefore, cutting fat is a key way to reduce excess calories. For example, low-fat dairy products are lower in fat and calories than whole milk dairy products. See 13-11 for other lowfat food substitutions.

- Eat more vegetables and whole grain foods. Make them the main dishes instead of the side dishes in your menus.

- Choose fresh fruits as an alternative to high-fat snack foods and desserts.

- When eating out, choose steamed, baked, or broiled foods rather than fried items. Ask for sauces and salad dressings on the side. Consider splitting an entree with a friend, or take part of your food home for a later meal.

- Select recipes carefully. Choose those that are low in fats most often. Substitute low-calorie ingredients when possible. For instance, you might sauté vegetables in broth instead of butter. You might also change the preparation method.

Substitutions to Reduce Fat

Consider selecting:	Rather than:
nonfat yogurt	sour cream
evaporated fat free milk	cream or nondairy creamers
fat free or 1% lowfat milk	whole or 2% reduced fat milk
reduced fat cheese	regular cheese
lowfat or nonfat dairy desserts	ice cream
two egg whites	one whole egg
angel food cake, sponge cake, gelatin dessert, or fresh fruits	butter cake, mousse, or fruit pie
broth-based soups	cream soups
jams, jellies, or reduced fat margarine in tubs	butter, lard, or stick margarine
bagels, English muffins, or toasted bread	doughnuts, pastries
pretzels, air-popped popcorn, or saltines	chips or other fried snacks
graham crackers, vanilla wafers, or gingersnaps	buttery cookies

13-11 Substituting lowfat foods for high-fat foods is an easy way to cut excess calories from the diet.

Microwaving or steaming vegetables instead of sautéing is another way to reduce fat and calories.

If you do not want to bother counting calories, concentrate on eating lowfat grains, fruits, and vegetables. Eat your favorite high-fat foods in moderation. Following these basic guidelines will help you maintain good health and a healthy weight while enjoying a delicious diet.

● **Change Eating Habits**

A food diary is a key self-monitoring weight management tool. It can help you identify eating habits shaped by environmental cues and psychological factors. When completing your diary, list the time of day and where you eat. Also note who you are with and what you are doing. Jot down how you are feeling at the time, too. This information can tell you as much as the list of what you consumed. See 13-12.

Analyze your completed food diary to see what you can learn about yourself. Do you snack while watching television? Do you eat after school? Do you skip any meals? Do you tend to eat more when you are alone or with friends? Answering questions like these may help you learn where and why you might be consuming excess calories.

Once you recognize problem eating behaviors, you can explore ways to change them. For example, you may realize the snack counter at the movies tempts you to eat. As a solution, you may decide not to bring along extra money for snacks when you go to the movies. Your new habits should not be temporary adjustments until you lose a few pounds. View your eating and exercise habits as permanent changes that will help you maintain a healthy weight throughout your life.

Knowing how emotions affect your eating behaviors can help you manage these

			Food Diary				
Meal	Amount	Food	Time	Location	People Present	Activity	Mood
breakfast	1 medium	banana	7:00 a.m.	kitchen	Mom, T.J.	getting ready for school	grumpy
	2 slices	toast					
	2 tsp.	raspberry jam					
	1 cup	lowfat milk					
lunch	1 slice	cheese pizza	11:45 a.m.	cafeteria	Carla, Darnell	studying for test	nervous
	1 cup	tossed salad					
	2 tbsp.	French dressing					
	1 cup	lowfat milk					
	½ cup	chocolate pudding					
snack	8 oz.	apple juice	3:00 p.m.	locker room	Carla, Lilly, Cecilia	getting ready for basketball practice	excited
	1	granola bar					

13-12 Keeping track of the circumstances in which you consume food can help you identify problem eating habits.

behaviors. You may find you eat when you feel lonely or bored. If so, prepare a list of activities you can do instead of eating when these feelings hit you. For instance, when you feel lonely, call a friend. If you are bored, try working on a hobby. See 13-13.

Modifying your behavior involves finding ways to change your response when overeating is a concern. For instance, suppose a friend invites you to an after-school study session at his home. The friend sets out a bowl of potato chips and dip. How can you change this environmental cue so you will not overeat? You could move away from the bowl of chips. This may prevent you from responding to their sight and smell. You might also bring some fruit or cut vegetables to share with your friend while you study. Eating a low-calorie snack can help satisfy your desire to nibble.

One way to change an eating habit is to write a habit change contract. This is an agreement with yourself about the methods you will use to reach a personal goal. Written contracts seem to work better than mental or verbal contracts. In the contract, write what you plan to do. You might write, "I will limit myself to no more than one soft drink each day." Your food diary can quickly show you if you are achieving your goal. After you reach one goal, you can celebrate success and move on to another goal.

Do not be discouraged if you fail to live up to your contract. You may have set a goal that was unrealistic. Evaluate the methods you are using and your ability to reach your goals. Rewrite your contract if necessary. With practice, you will be able to use habit change contracts to improve your eating habits.

Another technique some people find helpful for modifying eating habits is a point system. Give yourself a set number of points for healthful eating behaviors. For example, snacking on carrot sticks instead of corn chips might be worth a point. Skipping a rich dessert might be worth two points. After collecting a set number of points, treat yourself to a reward, like a movie or a new CD. Avoid giving yourself food rewards.

● **Increase Levels of Daily Activity**

Besides making careful food choices, you need to focus on your level of activity. Many studies show people lose weight faster and maintain weight loss longer when they become more active. Exercise speeds the body's metabolism as body composition changes to a higher proportion of muscle. Exercise also curbs short-term hunger for some people. Tips for increasing your activity level are provided in Chapter 15, "Physical Activity: A Way of Life."

Physical activity is an especially important weight loss strategy for children and teens. Young people need energy from food to support their growth. With moderate daily activity, they can lose weight without reducing their intake of nutritious foods. See 13-14.

● **Tips for Weight Loss**

If you have trouble achieving or maintaining a healthy weight, try the following tips:

- Avoid eating a large amount of food at any one time of the day. Spread the day's calories over all your meals.

- Eat three to six planned meals throughout the day rather than eating haphazardly.

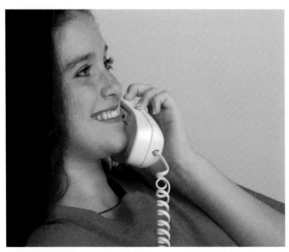

13-13 Calling a friend can be a fun way to take your mind off food when you are bored or lonely.

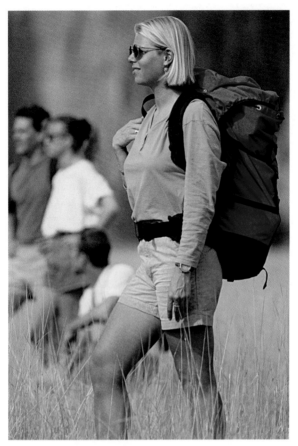

13-14 Physical activity plays a key role in reaching and maintaining a healthy weight.

Be sure to keep portion sizes at each meal moderate. This will help you avoid snacking binges.

- Make breakfast a habit. It gets you through the morning without experiencing extreme hunger. If you become exceedingly hungry, you are more likely to overeat.
- Keep a lean refrigerator and cupboard. Focus on stocking nutritious foods that are lower in calories. Keep foods that are high in calories and low in nutrients out of sight most of the time.
- Eat slowly. Lay your fork down between bites of food. You will feel full with less food.
- Avoid talking on the phone or watching TV while eating. This will keep you from associating these activities with wanting to eat.

- Before a meal begins, drink a glass of water. This may help you feel a little fuller, so you will eat less.
- Avoid feeling the need to finish leftover foods. Store leftovers promptly and eat them at another meal.
- Use a smaller plate so moderate portions do not look so small.
- Avoid taking second helpings of foods.
- When eating out, try to decide what you will have before other people order. Then stick with your decision. This will keep you from being swayed by the power of suggestion if other people order high-fat, high-calorie foods.
- Avoid weighing yourself more than once or twice a week. If you are following a healthful weight-loss plan, you will be losing no more than two pounds per week. Therefore, frequent weight checks are unlikely to show much progress and may result in discouragement.
- Reward yourself for small successes. Use nonfood rewards, such as seeing a movie or visiting a friend. See 13-15.

Most health professionals would agree maintaining a healthy weight is much easier than reducing weight. This is important information for young people who are establishing healthful eating habits. You can learn to maintain a healthy weight now. This will help you avoid the difficult task of taking off excess pounds at midlife.

Gaining Weight

For some people, managing weight means wanting to add pounds to body weight. Health issues are not as severe for moderately thin people as for obese people. However, being underweight may hamper a person's ability to feel strong and healthy. Underweight may also increase a person's susceptibility to infectious diseases like colds and flu. Anyone who has had an unexpected

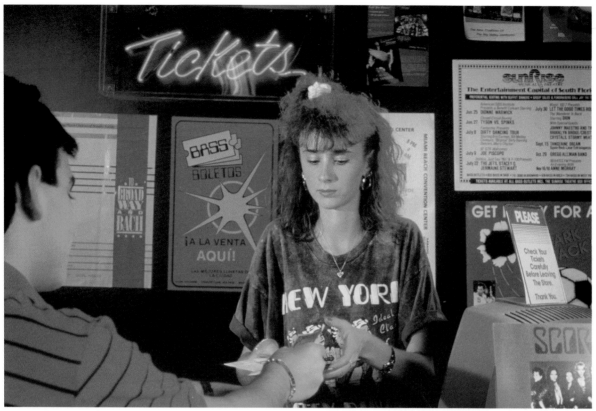

13-15 Show tickets can serve as a reward for achieving weight management goals.

weight loss should have a physical exam. A doctor can make sure there are no health problems causing the weight loss.

Gaining weight is as hard for someone who is underweight as losing weight is for someone who is overweight. Healthy weight gain should be due to a combination of added fat and muscle. Some people seem to inherit a tendency to be thin. They have difficulty storing body fat. However, they can add muscle mass through strength training exercises, such as weight lifting. See 13-16.

Like weight loss, weight gain requires a management plan. Gaining weight means consuming more calories than the body expends. It also means exercising to build muscle. Registered dietitians often recommend that people trying to gain weight consume 700 to 1,000 extra calories per day. Of course, the source of these calories should be nutritious foods. This will create an energy excess over what is needed for the increased level of activity.

People who are trying to gain weight need to avoid fads and gimmicks. Many body builder magazines have ads for products that promise to help people bulk up fast. These products may not provide a proper balance of nutrients. They will not help people establish long-term healthful eating habits. Some of these products may also have harmful side effects. Using a slow, steady approach to weight gain is the safest, most effective way to put on pounds.

● Tips for Weight Gain

People who are trying to gain weight can follow several suggestions for shifting their energy balance.

- Consume extra calories by choosing more calorie-dense foods that are low in saturated

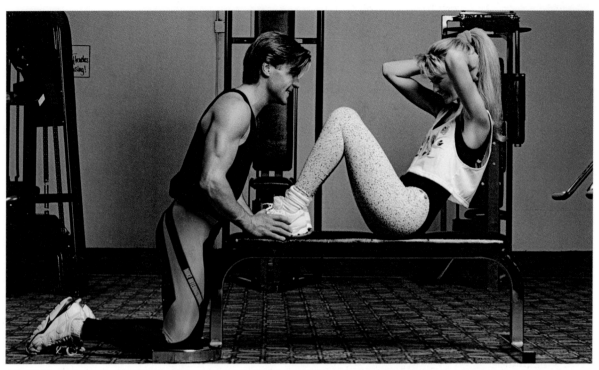

13-16 Exercises that build muscle are a required part of the formula for gaining weight.

fats. Peanut butter, olives, nuts, and raisins are a few good choices.

- Add small amounts of calorie-dense toppings, such as salad dressings and dessert sauces. See 13-17.
- Try eating bigger, more frequent meals.
- Consume snacks between meals, like sandwiches, puddings, and thick soups. Drink plenty of juices, milk, and milk shakes as fluid sources that are higher in calories than water.
- Limit bulky, low-calorie foods, such as leafy vegetable salads and clear soups.
- Avoid drinking extra fluids before eating or during your meal.

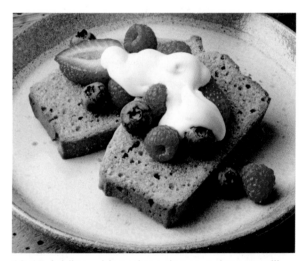

13-17 Adding whipped topping to a dessert will help build extra calories into a weight-gain diet.

Summary

Weight management means reaching a healthy weight and maintaining it throughout life. Obese and underweight people are both at increased risk of health problems.

Several factors affect your weight and your ability to put on and take off pounds. These factors include your heredity, eating habits, and level of physical activity. Environmental cues and psychological factors can influence your eating habits.

People who want to lose weight should first evaluate their health and consider their motivation. They need to estimate their current daily calorie needs. They also need to use a food diary to estimate their daily calorie intake. Comparing these two calorie figures can help them determine an appropriate daily calorie limit to maintain or lose weight.

To lose weight safely, people should avoid fad diets and other weight-loss gimmicks, which can be dangerous and ineffective. People trying to lose weight should carefully evaluate the nutritional quality of any weight-loss plan they are considering. Healthful weight loss involves controlling calorie intake through planned food choices. This may require modifying some eating habits. Effective weight loss also demands a plan of daily physical activity.

Weight gain can be just as difficult as weight loss. People who are trying to gain weight need to include more calorie-dense foods in their diets. They also need to follow a program of muscle-building exercise.

Managing weight does not mean losing or gaining weight quickly. It does not mean following a special diet formula that magically makes fat appear or disappear. The real secret to weight management is patience. You need the desire to improve daily eating and exercise habits to achieve a long life of optimum wellness.

Check Your Knowledge

1. True or false. A person who is overweight may not have excess body fat.
2. What are five physical health problems for which obese people are at a greater risk?
3. What are two health problems associated with being underweight?
4. How does heredity affect a person's weight status?
5. Who has the greatest influence on eating habits formed early in life?
6. How many calories does an active, 160-pound male need to maintain his current weight?
7. How can a person estimate his or her average daily calorie intake?
8. How can fasting be dangerous?
9. What are two reasons fad diets may be ineffective?
10. What is a basic weight management recommendation for an obese teenager who is still growing?
11. What information should be included in a food diary to help people identify factors that prompt them to eat?
12. What are five tips that might help someone lose body fat safely?
13. How many extra calories should a person who is trying to gain weight consume each day?
14. What are three tips for safe weight gain?

Put Learning into Action

1. Survey two adults about their weight management experiences. Find out if they have ever tried to lose or gain weight. Ask them to describe the diet plans they followed. Find out how they felt while following the plans. Also ask them if they achieved their weight goals

and, if so, how long they maintained their goal weights. Compile your findings with those of your classmates. Write an article for the school newspaper about successful weight management.

2. Prepare a showcase illustrating guidelines for safe loss of body fat. List important questions a person should ask before beginning a weight-loss program.

3. Design a weight management brochure. Include tips for safe weight loss and safe weight gain. Also include a list pairing similar low-calorie and high-calorie foods people might choose to meet weight management goals. For instance, you might pair a broiled chicken sandwich with a double cheeseburger or zucchini with avocado. Compare calorie density of each pair.

Explore Further

1. Use library and/or Internet resources to research a specific health risk associated with obesity or underweight. In an oral report, explain how unhealthy body weight increases this particular health risk.

2. Use the formulas in Chart 13-5 to estimate your daily calorie needs based on your activity level. Keep a food diary for three days. Be sure to record when, where, and with whom you eat; what you are doing; and how you are feeling. Use food composition tables or diet analysis software to figure your average daily calorie intake. Compare your daily calorie needs with your average daily intake. Identify any environmental cues and psychological factors that seem to influence your eating habits. Write a summary of what you learn from studying your food diary.

3. Find a description of a weight-loss plan in a magazine. Write an analysis explaining why the plan sounds appealing. Evaluate how well it follows the American Dietetic Association guidelines for a well-managed weight-loss program. Identify any characteristics that might cause the plan to be dangerous and/or ineffective. Write a brief summary stating how much potential you think the program has for long-term weight-loss success. Attach a copy of the weight-loss plan to your report.

Chapter 14

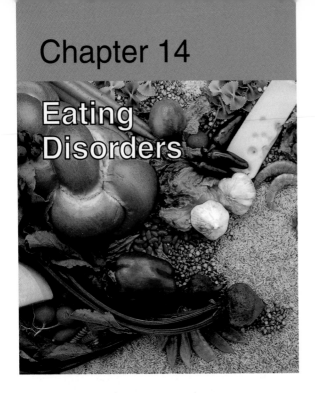

Eating Disorders

● Learn the Language

eating disorder
anorexia nervosa
bulimia nervosa
bingeing
purging

binge eating
  disorder
female athlete triad
outpatient treatment
antidepressant

● Objectives

After studying this chapter, you will be able to

- identify characteristics and health risks associated with three common eating disorders.
- analyze possible causes of eating disorders.
- describe sources of help for people with eating disorders.

Have you ever overeaten at a buffet or skipped lunch to finish a school project? Neither of these behaviors may be the wisest choice from a nutritional standpoint. However, making an occasional unwise choice is not likely to risk your health. This is especially true if you balance such a choice with wiser choices throughout the day. By contrast, an *eating disorder* is an abnormal eating pattern that endangers physical and mental health.

● Characteristics of Eating Disorders

The three most common eating disorders are anorexia nervosa, bulimia nervosa, and binge eating disorder. Certain behaviors are typical of each disorder. Each can be harmful to health. As you study these disorders, you will note they are alike in a number of ways.

Eating disorders are most common among teenage and young adult women. However, people of both genders and other age groups can develop these disorders, too. Many people who develop eating disorders share certain traits, 14-1.

● Anorexia Nervosa

Anorexia nervosa is an eating disorder typified by an intense fear of weight gain. This fear leads to self-starvation. A person with anorexia nervosa is called an *anorexic*.

The term *nervosa* indicates this illness has a psychological origin. Anorexics often have serious social and emotional problems. Signs of these problems may include a tendency to withdraw from social events and a quiet, serious personality. Anorexics view losing weight as a way to solve their problems. The ability to control their weight gives them a sense of power they lack in other areas of their lives.

Anorexics place excessive emphasis on the shape and weight of their bodies. They

Common Characteristics of People with Eating Disorders

- Fear of becoming overweight
- Poor body image (see self as overweight)
- Low sense of self-worth
- Preoccupation with food
- Distorted feelings about hunger and satiety (fullness)
- Emotionally withdrawn from friends
- High achievement orientation
- High stress levels
- Secretive eating behaviors

14-1 Being familiar with these common characteristics may help you identify someone who is at risk of developing an eating disorder.

may become consumed by unreasonable expectations about what they should look like and how much weight they should lose. They see themselves as fat even though they may be gravely underweight.

The onset of anorexia nervosa commonly begins in adolescence or during the early twenties, 14-2. Less frequently, it may occur in the adult years. Anorexics may start with a diet plan to lose a few pounds. People with this disorder tend to be highly achievement oriented. They feel a sense of control and pride when they reach their weight goals. They enjoy compliments from others about how nice they look. This inspires them to diet further to reach new, lower weight goals. As this dieting pattern continues, anorexics become more intent on losing weight. Feelings of pride turn into strong self-criticism. "I feel good about reaching my weight goal" becomes "I'm too fat. I have to

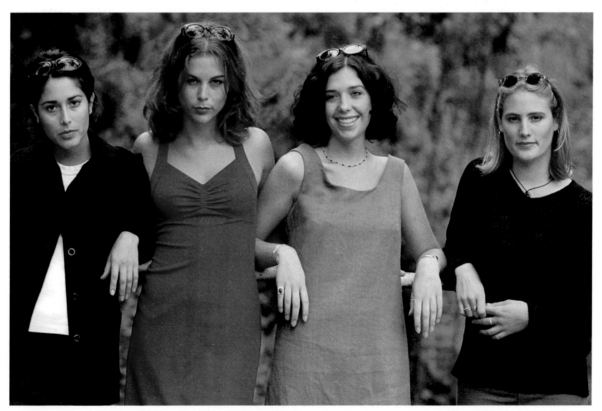

14-2 Young women are the population group most likely to develop anorexia nervosa.

lose more weight." Dieting becomes a life-threatening obsession. However, anorexics are usually unaware they have an eating disorder. Thus, denial becomes a serious obstacle to treatment.

Specific behaviors may vary from person to person. Anorexics often skip meals. When they do sit down for a meal, they are likely to eat very little. Instead they might simply move the food around on their plates. Others will eat only in private. Some anorexics choose to take laxatives or diet pills to lose weight. Besides dieting, many anorexics exercise excessively to control their weight and body shape. They may jog, swim, or do aerobics for hours each day. However, the desire to be thin rather than the desire to maintain good health is what motivates their workouts. Anorexics often wear baggy clothes to hide their overly thin bodies.

As anorexia nervosa develops, physical symptoms appear. A very low caloric intake leads to a large drop in weight as a key symptom. Low body weight and low body fat cause females to develop amenorrhea, or the cessation of menstrual periods. The disease causes stress, which may take the form of restlessness or irritability. Loss of insulation from the layer of body fat under the skin causes anorexics to feel cold. The body adapts to this loss of insulation by growing a covering of fine hair to trap heat. Rough, dry skin and hair loss are two other symptoms resulting from poor nutrient intake.

Anorexia nervosa takes a toll on health in many ways. Normal growth and development will slow down or halt. Muscle tissue wastes away along with body fat. Blood pressure and pulse rate drop and the body organs begin to shrivel. Bone density decreases and symptoms of osteoporosis may occur. (See Chapter 9, "Minerals: Regulators of Body Functions," for more information on osteoporosis.) Some anorexics die from starvation. Others fall into a deep depression, and the risk of suicide increases.

Bulimia Nervosa

Bulimics are people with an eating disorder known as **bulimia nervosa**. This disorder involves two key behaviors. The first is **bingeing,** which is uncontrollable eating of huge amounts of food. The second is an inappropriate behavior to prevent weight gain. For many people with this disorder, the second behavior is **purging**. This means clearing the food from the digestive system. Bulimics may purge by forcing themselves to vomit. Some abuse laxatives, diuretics, or enemas to rid their bodies of the food. Instead of purging, some bulimics use excessive exercise or periods of fasting to prevent weight gain. Some people alternate between bulimic and anorexic behaviors. See 14-3.

Bulimics repeat the cycle of bingeing and purging at least twice a week. Some repeat the cycle several times a day. Once the cycle begins, it is hard for many people to stop.

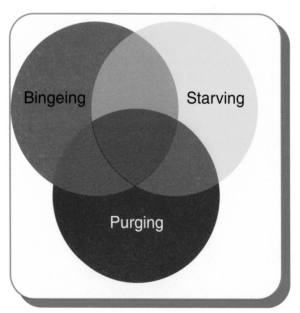

14-3 Patterns of behavior may overlap for people with eating disorders. A person may be involved in one, two, or all forms of disordered eating behavior.

A person with bulimia often comes from a family and social group where weight and appearance are important. He or she usually possesses a low self-esteem.

Like anorexics, bulimics are always thinking about food. When bingeing, bulimics consume thousands of calories in a few hours. Binge foods are often high in fats and carbohydrates. During a binge, a bulimic might eat a whole cake, a dozen donuts, and an entire carton of ice cream. Choices about which foods and how much to eat are not related to hunger and satiety. Eating behaviors are out of control.

People who have the bulimia disorder realize their eating patterns are not normal. They binge and purge in secret because they do not want others to be aware of their behavior. If a bulimic has a fairly average body size, others may not notice the problem for a long time.

Serious health problems are associated with bulimia nervosa. As the disorder becomes established, damage to the body becomes more severe and more difficult to reverse. Repeated vomiting can cause glands in the throat to swell. Acids from the stomach burn the esophagus. In addition, the acid can destroy tooth enamel. Vomiting can also cause a loss of water and minerals from the body. This can result in dangerous fluid and electrolyte imbalances. Bulimics can have problems with heart and liver damage. The disease can be fatal.

Binge Eating Disorder

Binge eating disorder is another eating disorder that involves repeatedly eating very large amounts of food. Binge eaters rapidly overeat until they are uncomfortably full. However, they do not engage in a follow-up behavior to prevent weight gain.

Binge eaters are likely to have problems with excess weight as their eating gets out of control. They tend to feel guilty about overeating. They may also have ongoing feelings of frustration and rejection.

Binge eaters are likely to drop out of weight-loss programs due to emotional stress. While in a program, they might lose weight. Without specific treatment for their disorder, however, they are apt to begin bingeing again after completing the program. This usually causes binge eaters to quickly regain lost weight.

Other Eating Disorders

Many forms of eating disorders exist. Not all fit the definition of anorexia nervosa, bulimia nervosa, or binge eating disorder. Disordered eating behaviors may show up in people who are too concerned about their body shapes. People with eating disorders may strictly limit their food choices to only a few foods. They may binge, purge, and/or fast from time to time. These behaviors can be harmful to health and may develop into specific eating disorders.

Probable Causes of Eating Disorders

The probable causes of eating disorders are complex and may be intertwined. A single factor may not lead to problem eating patterns. However, when several factors occur together, an eating disorder may be triggered. Exact reasons people develop eating disorders remain a puzzle. Some probable causes are listed in 14-4.

Theories

One theory of eating disorders says social pressure to be thin prompts people to form unhealthful dieting patterns. Much of this pressure comes from the media. Most of the models and stars on television and in movies and magazines are thin. The few overweight people that appear in the media are often portrayed as dull and dowdy. Thin celebrities shape society's concept of beauty. Many people feel they must be thin to be attractive and successful. They measure their self-worth by

Probable Causes of Eating Disorders

Social Influences
- Media emphasis on thinness
- Changing role expectations for women - career, success, and family

Psychological Influences
- A need for control
- Poor self-esteem
- Need for acceptance and approval
- Unrealistic self-expectations
- Inability to cope
- Family stresses

Genetic Influences
- Hormonal imbalance
- Depression
- Other medical causes

14-4 The probable causes of eating disorders might be social, psychological, or genetic in nature.

their body weight. This compels them to diet. However, they do not grasp the reality that most body types can never fit the model image. They may not realize photos of models are often retouched to look picture perfect. When one diet program fails to produce the unrealistic body size they desire, many people try other diets. This pattern eventually leads some people to develop eating disorders.

Another theory about what causes eating disorders suggests there may be a genetic link. Studies indicate certain chemicals produced in the brain may prompt people to overeat sweet, high-fat foods.

Evidence suggests typical family patterns may be involved in the development of eating disorders, too. Family members of eating disorder patients often show overt concern with appearances and high achievement. They may lack communication skills. They may also show a tendency to avoid conflicts within the family.

Risk Among Teens

The theory about social pressure to be thin points to emotional factors that may trigger eating disorders. Teens are especially vulnerable to such feelings as rejection, worthlessness, and guilt. Their lives are in a state of physical, social, and emotional change as they approach adulthood. They seek reassurance from others. Some teens assume their appearance is the reason for any feelings of rejection they sense from others. They may feel worthless if they are overweight. They develop feelings of guilt because they cannot achieve society's standard of beauty. See 14-5.

Emotional change during the teen years may also create out-of-control eating patterns. Facing the challenges of physically growing up and separating from family and friends creates much stress for many teens. They may feel powerless over their lives. Such feelings lead some teens to become emotionally dependent on food. They use food as a source of comfort. They may also see food as one aspect of their lives over which they can have control. Such views of food can be harmful.

Not measuring up to society's body image makes some teens reluctant to eat in public. Simply enjoying a piece of pizza with a friend may result in feelings of low self-esteem. These teens may fear their friends will think they lack self-control for not turning down the pizza. Such fears may prompt these teens to eat alone. This can lead to a pattern of secretive eating, which is part of disordered eating behavior.

Risk Among Athletes

Some groups of teens are more susceptible to eating disorders than others. Athletes are often at risk because many coaches focus on body weight during training. For instance, a wrestler knows he or she must compete within a weight class. A gymnast is told his or her body size will affect balance.

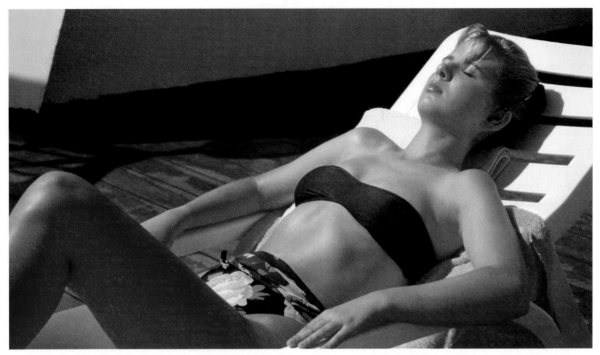

14-5 Teens feel social and emotional pressure to maintain a desired body shape and image.

Constantly trying to achieve and maintain weight goals for their sports may lead athletes to develop eating disorders.

Disordered eating among female athletes has become quite common. In fact, it is one of a trio of health problems many female athletes face. The second problem is amenorrhea. Amenorrhea has been linked with mineral losses from bone tissue. This leads to the development of the third health problem—osteoporosis. This set of medical problems has been given the name *female athlete triad*.

One part of female athlete triad leads to another. The combination of the three disorders poses a greater threat to health than each of the individual disorders. A female athlete trains hard and eats little to maintain a weight goal. This causes her to stop menstruating. The resulting hormonal imbalances cause her to lose bone mass. This puts her at greater risk of training and performance fractures. Lack of nutrients in the diet and minerals in the bones slows healing of

fractures. This causes sports performance to deteriorate, which may foster feelings of low self-esteem and perpetuate the disordered eating behaviors. If this cycle of health problems continues, the young woman is at risk of death. See 14-6.

● What Help Is Available?

People need professional help to overcome eating disorders. Without medical care, people with eating disorders can suffer long-term health problems or even death. Treatment programs vary depending on the factors that led to the eating disorder. However, treatment must focus on the psychological roots of the disorder as well as its physical symptoms. The treatment becomes highly personalized. It is designed to meet the needs of each anorexic, bulimic, or binge eater.

The recovery rate for people with eating disorders is much higher if they get early

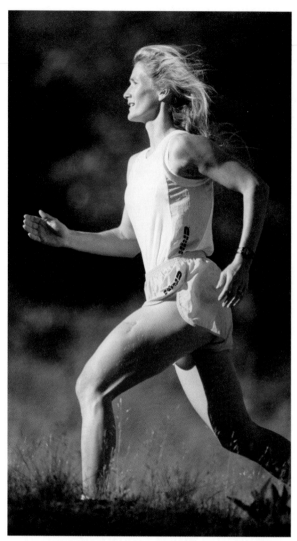

14-6 A female athlete must maintain a nutritious diet to avoid health problems associated with female athlete triad.

treatment. Family and friends can help get someone with an eating disorder into a treatment program. However, they must recognize that an eating disorder is not just a passing phase.

● Treatment for Anorexia Nervosa

Treatment for anorexia nervosa is neither quick nor simple. Therapy for this eating disorder can take many years.

Several approaches are used to treat anorexia. In some treatment programs, only the client is treated. In other programs, the family also becomes involved in the treatment. Sometimes programs require clients to stay in a hospital or treatment facility.

The first step in treatment is to attend to the physical health problems the disorder has caused. Care should be provided by a doctor trained in treating eating disorders. National help organizations can refer clients to treatment programs in their region. See 14-7.

Resources for Helping People with Eating Disorders

Anorexia Nervosa and Related Eating Disorders, Inc. (ANRED)
PO Box 5102
Eugene, OR 97405
(541) 344-1144
www.anred.com

Eating Disorder Referral and Information Center
2923 Sandy Pointe, Suite 6
Del Mar, CA 92014-2052
www.edreferral.com

National Association of Anorexia Nervosa and Associated Disorders
PO Box 7
Highland Park, IL 60035
(847) 831-3438
www.anad.org

National Eating Disorders Association
603 Stewart Street, Suite 803
Seattle, WA 98101
(800) 931-2237
www.nationaleatingdisorders.org

Addresses, telephone numbers, and Web sites may have changed since publication.

14-7 These organizations can provide information about eating disorders.

Once a patient's physical condition has been stabilized, he or she can begin to accept psychological help. Clients explore attitudes about weight, food, and body image. They learn to think about and accept what a healthy body weight means. They receive nutrition counseling to help them gain weight and form healthful eating habits. They find out how to view their body shapes more realistically. They develop suitable exercise programs. As patients receive help to improve their self-images, their overall health also improves.

Clients are taught to build new controls into their lives. They practice verbal skills that help them relate better to their family members and friends. They learn stress management techniques to use when responding to their emotions.

Family support helps ensure a patient will stick with a recovery program. Many professionals advise family therapy to improve relationships among all the members of an anorexic's family.

An anorexic's best chance for improved health lies in getting early treatment. Some people recover fully from anorexia nervosa. Most who recover do well in school and work. However, some anorexics continue to have problems. Studies show about 20 percent of adults who have a history of anorexia nervosa remain underweight. They may still struggle with bouts of low self-esteem and weight image distortion.

● Treatment for Bulimia Nervosa

Like anorexics, bulimics should be treated by health care professionals with specialized training. These professionals know how to fit treatment programs to the needs of the individual. Treatment for young patients often includes family members. Therapy for older patients may involve only the individual. In both cases, support from family members and friends is vital to the success of the treatment.

Unless a case is severe, bulimics usually receive **outpatient treatment**. This is medical care that does not require a hospital stay. Sometimes physicians prescribe **antidepressants** as part of a treatment program. These are a group of drugs that alter the nervous system and relieve depression. They may be used to help the client control mood swings and avoid bingeing. Drugs can help control behavior. However, they cannot cure the mental problems at the root of an eating disorder. The use of antidepressants also involves risks and side effects. Doctors should discuss these issues openly with clients before prescribing medications. See 14-8.

Support groups can provide recovering bulimics with information and encouragement. However, these groups cannot replace therapy.

Some studies show treatment helps about 25 percent of bulimics stop bingeing and purging. With or without treatment, however, many bulimics have relapses. Relapses most frequently take place during periods of stress or change. Counseling can help bulimics prepare for and manage stressful events and thus avoid a relapse.

● Treatment for Binge Eating Disorder

Like other eating disorders, binge eating disorder requires treatment that focuses on emotional issues as well as eating problems. Counseling usually involves helping binge eaters learn how to like themselves as people. It helps the clients analyze how their personal beliefs affect their actions. It gives clients the emotional tools to take control of their eating behaviors.

Treatment programs teach binge eaters weight management facts. They encourage binge eaters to seek a healthier weight and form better eating habits. Therapy and the support of friends can help binge eaters make sound lifestyle choices in many areas.

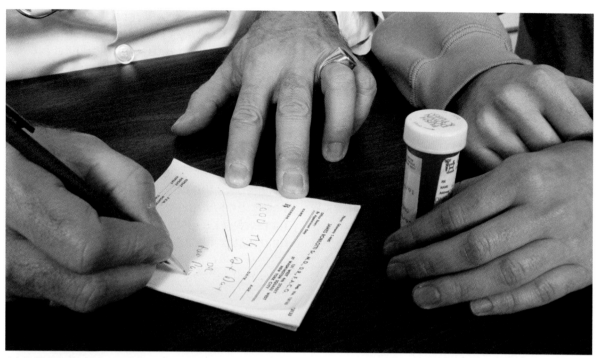

14-8 Prescription medication cannot cure bulimia nervosa, but it is sometimes helpful in the treatment of this eating disorder.

Seeking Professional Services

Treatment for an eating disorder is likely to require the services of a team of health care professionals. If the disorder has affected physical health, a medical doctor will be part of this team. A psychologist can help a patient deal with the emotional issues at the root of the disorder. In most instances, a registered dietitian will become part of the team. He or she can help the patient form healthful eating habits. An exercise specialist may help the patient plan a moderate exercise program.

All these professionals should have special training in handling eating disorders. Some regions may not have many qualified professionals. However, most health care providers can refer patients to specialists or clinics that are equipped to address eating disorders.

For treatment to be effective, a client needs to feel comfortable with the members of the health care team. A concerned friend or family member can help someone with an eating disorder find out about a treatment program. He or she can call to ask about treatment methods, fees, and insurance coverage. If everything sounds agreeable, the friend or family member can schedule an appointment. He or she can go with the client to a screening interview. This face-to-face meeting will help the client decide if he or she feels at ease with the health professionals. Having a positive feeling about the treatment program will help the client recover from his or her disorder. See 14-9.

Helping a Friend with an Eating Disorder

What can you do if you suspect a friend has an eating disorder? The person may not admit he or she has a problem. Your friend may even get angry if you suggest he or she has a disorder.

Questions to Ask a Therapist Before Treatment Begins

1. How long have you been working with clients who have eating disorders?

2. What is your treatment philosophy?

3. What types of treatment have you found most effective in treating eating disorders?

4. What is your success rate in treating people who have eating disorders?

5. What type of affiliations do you have with other support services, such as registered dietitians, physicians, hospitals, clinics, educational programs, and community-based support groups?

6. Do you provide family as well as individual counseling?

7. How long does treatment generally last?

8. Are you available for consultation if an emergency should occur?

14-9 Asking a professional counselor these questions can help someone with an eating disorder evaluate a treatment program before beginning therapy.

Do not give up on your friend. Tell the person you are very concerned about him or her. If your friend is not receptive to your concern, you can seek help. Talk to a counselor or to your friend's parents. Tell them about the symptoms you have spotted that concern you. See 14-10.

You can also take steps to help prevent people from developing eating disorders. Be careful when encouraging someone to lose weight. Emphasize your acceptance of the person regardless of his or her weight. Show concern for the person's health and well-being. Encouragement, support, and acceptance may be just what your friend needs to help him or her reach healthy weight goals.

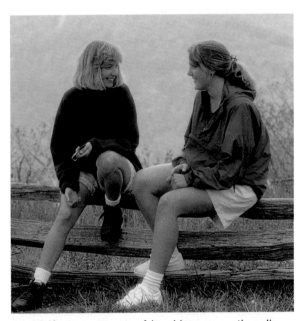

14-10 If you suspect a friend has an eating disorder, talk with him or her. Your concern may motivate your friend to seek help.

Chapter 14 Review

Summary

A person with anorexia nervosa starves himself or herself. Someone with bulimia nervosa engages in out-of-control eating. He or she then takes drastic steps to avoid weight gain. Binge eaters also go on uncontrollable eating sprees. These disorders all have psychological aspects. They can all lead to severe health consequences.

The causes of eating disorders are complex. Theories propose a range of explanations. Eating disorders are most common among teens and young adults. People who take part in sports or other activities where weight goals are rigid are most at risk.

Treatment for an eating disorder should be sought as soon as a problem is identified. Treatment must focus on the needs of the individual. It must address both psychological and physical characteristics of the disorder. This type of treatment generally requires the help of several professionals. Physicians, registered dietitians, and psychologists may all be part of the clinical team.

Check Your Knowledge

1. What are five physical symptoms of anorexia nervosa?
2. True or false. People who have bulimia nervosa realize their eating patterns are abnormal.
3. What is the main difference between bulimia nervosa and binge eating disorder?
4. What are five possible causes of eating disorders?
5. Why are many athletes at risk of developing eating disorders?
6. What factor improves the recovery rate for people with eating disorders?
7. What is the first step in treatment of anorexia nervosa?
8. What factors are likely to trigger a bulimic relapse?
9. Name three health professionals who might be part of a treatment team for someone with an eating disorder. Explain the role each professional would play in the treatment.
10. How can a person help prevent people from developing eating disorders?

Put Learning into Action

1. Write a journal entry answering the following questions about your feelings toward food:
   a. How do I use food to reward or punish myself?
   b. What strong emotions might cause me to eat when I am not hungry?
   c. How do I feel about being hungry?
   d. How do I feel about myself when I eat too much at a meal?
   e. How do I feel about myself when I turn down a snack or dessert?
   f. How do I feel about eating in front of other people?
   g. How do I feel about other people who eat too much food?
2. Use the Yellow Pages to make a list of resources in your community for people with eating disorders. Then contact the resources listed in 14-7 and request information about eating disorders. Organize the materials you receive along with your list into a resource folder. Distribute resource folders to the nurse and counselors at your school.

Explore Further

1. Choose a year in history. Research how thin and overweight people were portrayed in the media that year. Find out what movie and television stars were popular. Investigate how models were

used to advertise products in magazines and newspapers. Compile examples on a poster or presentation board. Prepare an opinion paper about the media's role in shaping society's concept of beauty.

2. Interview a person who is recovering from an eating disorder. If you are unable to interview someone, read a case history of a person with an eating disorder from the Internet or a library resource. Write a summary of your interview or reading describing how the eating disorder affected the person's life.

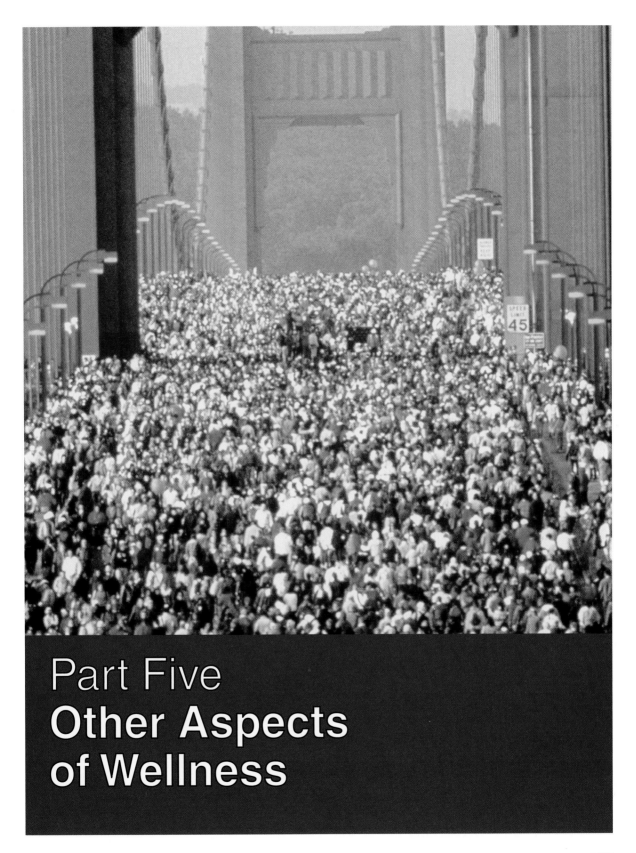

Part Five
Other Aspects
of Wellness

Chapter 15

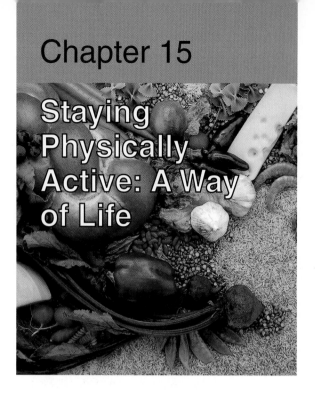

Staying Physically Active: A Way of Life

What is your daily routine like? Do you ride in a bus or car to get to and from school? After school, do you spend time studying and talking to friends on the phone? Do you watch television or surf the net for relaxation? Many teens would answer yes to these questions, indicating they may have formed a pattern of inactivity. If this pattern describes your life, this chapter will help you learn why and how you can make some changes.

Physical inactivity, especially among teens and adults, is a national health concern in the United States. It is a main reason many people lack physical fitness. *Physical fitness* is a state in which all body systems function together efficiently. See 15-1.

Learn the Language

physical fitness	agility
posture	balance
cardiorespiratory	coordination
fitness	speed
aerobic activity	reaction time
anaerobic activity	heart rate
muscular endurance	resting heart rate
strength	maximum heart rate
flexibility	target heart rate
power	zone

Objectives

After studying this chapter, you will be able to

- choose your goal for physical activity.
- describe the benefits of physical activity.
- list the health and skill components of physical fitness.
- determine your target heart rate zone.
- identify four keys to a successful exercise program.
- plan a personal exercise program.

Goals for Physical Activity

Most people who are active or who want to become active have one of three main goals for physical activity. They want to achieve either good health, total fitness, or peak athletic performance. The kinds of activities you do and the way you do them will be affected by which goal you choose.

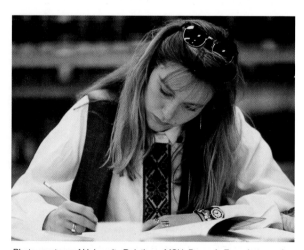

Photo courtesy of University Relations, MSU, Bruce A. Fox, photographer

15-1 A physically inactive lifestyle causes many teens to lack physical fitness.

Good Health

Most experts agree physical activity plays a key role in achieving and maintaining good health. Nearly everyone can be at least moderately active, regardless of age or physical limitations. Many activities that promote good health are free and require no special equipment. If you have been relatively inactive, this moderate level of activity would be a good place for you to start. You may be surprised how easy it is to include more activity in your lifestyle.

To achieve the goal of good health during your teen years, try to accumulate at least 60 minutes of moderate activity daily. Plan to accumulate this much activity nearly every day. Notice you do not have to set aside a 60-minute exercise period. You can accomplish this goal through lifestyle physical activities that are part of your daily routine. You could spend 15 minutes riding your bicycle to school and another 15 minutes riding home. Then take your dog for a 15-minute walk and spend 15 minutes shooting baskets in the driveway with friends. By the end of the day, you have accumulated a total of 60 minutes of activity.

Many household tasks can count as part of your daily physical activity. Pushing the lawn mower, shoveling snow, and raking leaves all require a moderate amount of physical effort. Sweeping the floor, washing the car, and using the vacuum cleaner will get your body moving, too. Even carrying laundry and groceries call for you to use your muscles. If you have been inactive, becoming active is more important than the type of activity you choose. See 15-2.

Total Fitness

Once you start feeling the benefits of being more active, you may become like a rolling wheel picking up speed. The better you feel, the more active you will want to be. After a while, you may want to change your goal to try to achieve total fitness. You may also

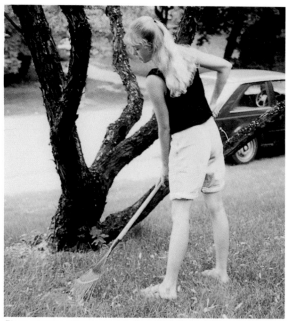

Photo courtesy of University Relations, MSU, Bruce A. Fox, photographer

15-2 Like many routine tasks, raking can count toward a daily goal of 60 accumulated minutes of moderate activity.

become more interested in other aspects of your health. Many people who start exercise programs develop an interest in nutritious eating and other healthful lifestyle behaviors.

Most of this chapter focuses on the goal of developing total fitness. You will learn what total fitness means. You will learn the benefits an exercise program can have for your body and your life. You will also study about what makes a good exercise program. If you follow the ideas discussed here, you can look forward to enjoying an improved sense of well-being.

Peak Athletic Performance

A third goal for some physically active people is to reach their highest potential in sports performance. Achieving this goal requires a good level of overall fitness. It also requires intense training designed to develop specific sports skills. For instance, the football team does drills to build speed. A gymnast does exercises intended to develop balance. A tennis player's workouts are devised to strengthen coordination.

Athletes who truly want to be the best in their sport spend many hours each week in training. They know there is always room for improvement. They also know they will not continue to improve if they do not practice nearly every day.

The Benefits of Physical Activity

Becoming physically active at any level can positively affect your total health and performance. Not only will you feel physical benefits, but your mental health will improve, too.

Improved Appearance

One benefit of physical activity that inspires many people to exercise is improved appearance. Exercise can positively affect your appearance by altering your posture, movements, and weight.

Exercise can help you develop strong back and abdominal muscles, which are necessary for maintaining good posture. **Posture** is the position of your body when you are standing or sitting. Having erect posture when standing helps your clothes hang properly so you will look your best. Having erect posture when sitting helps you look and feel more alert. Having good posture also helps you avoid back problems.

Many teens go through a stage when they feel clumsy and awkward. You will find exercise can help you move more gracefully. Agility, balance, and coordination developed through exercise will be reflected in all your movements. See 15-3.

Exercise burns calories. This is good news for people who are overweight. Thirty minutes of moderately intense activities will burn about 200 extra calories. This may not seem like much. When you multiply the calories burned over an extended period, however, the results are impressive. For instance, doing 30 minutes of moderate

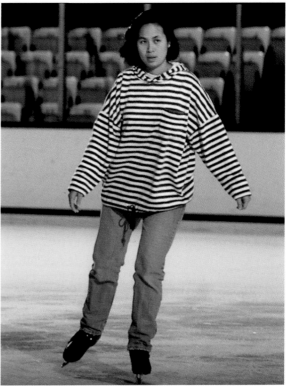

Photo courtesy of University Relations, MSU, Bruce A. Fox, photographer

15-3 The balance and agility you develop through activities like ice skating will be reflected in all your movements.

exercise five days a week will burn about 52,000 extra calories per year. That is nearly 15 pounds of body fat. Those who combine their exercise program with a lowfat diet that is moderate in calories can lose even more weight.

People who do not have weight problems should not overlook the benefits exercise can have for them. Over a lifetime, many people experience a slow weight gain by eating an extra 75 to 150 calories per day. An exercise program could easily burn up these excess calories and help keep weight at a healthy level throughout life.

Disease Prevention

Exercise can help reduce the risk of developing several diseases. These include osteoporosis, coronary heart disease (CHD), some cancers, diabetes mellitus, and stroke.

Exercise is not guaranteed to increase your life span, but it can improve your quality of life. It can help you have the energy you need for daily work and leisure activities.

Improved Mental Outlook

For many people, exercise creates a feeling of well-being. Adolescents who exercise regularly state they have improved self-control, self-esteem, and body image. They also report greater alertness and better school performance.

Although exercise does not solve problems, it helps relieve tension. When exercising, your thoughts focus on the physical activity rather than school or family pressures. Following a workout, you are likely to feel mentally refreshed. You will be more prepared to cope with day-to-day problems. See 15-4.

What Is Total Fitness?

Is a weight lifter who has difficulty running a mile physically fit? How would you rate the fitness of a distance runner who can only manage two push-ups? Total fitness involves more than being strong or fast. There are many aspects to physical fitness. Someone who has athletic skill will not necessarily be fit in all areas. However, striving for at least a moderate level of fitness in each area will promote good health and athletic performance.

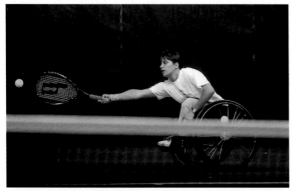

Photo courtesy of University Relations, MSU, Bruce A. Fox, photographer

15-4 Exercise can relieve tension and improve mental outlook.

Health Components of Physical Fitness

Five major components are used to measure the impact of physical fitness on your health. They are cardiorespiratory fitness, muscular endurance, strength, flexibility, and body composition. Being fit in each of these areas reduces your risk for certain health problems, including heart disease and certain cancers. It also improves your body's ability to perform its various functions.

Cardiorespiratory Fitness

The greatest sign of good health is cardiorespiratory fitness. *Cardiorespiratory fitness* is measured by the body's ability to take in adequate amounts of oxygen. It is also evaluated by the body's ability to carry oxygen efficiently through the blood to body cells. It involves the efficiency of your lungs, heart, and blood vessels.

Aerobic activities are especially good for building cardiorespiratory fitness. *Aerobic activities* use large muscles and are activities done at a moderate, steady pace for fairly long periods. *Aerobic* means with oxygen. Throughout an aerobic activity, your heart and lungs should be able to supply all the oxygen your muscles need. The goal of aerobic exercise is to increase your heart and breathing rates to safe levels for an extended time. Most fitness experts recommend holding these raised levels for 20 to 60 minutes to get the most cardiorespiratory benefits. Walking, jogging, in-line skating, bicycling, and swimming laps are aerobic activities. See 15-5.

Anaerobic activities are activities in which your muscles are using oxygen faster than your heart and lungs can deliver it. Anaerobic activities use short, intense bursts of energy. For example, sprint events and sports such as football, baseball, and tennis are anaerobic activities. They cannot be sustained long enough to help you increase cardiorespiratory fitness. This is because you have to stop often during anaerobic activities

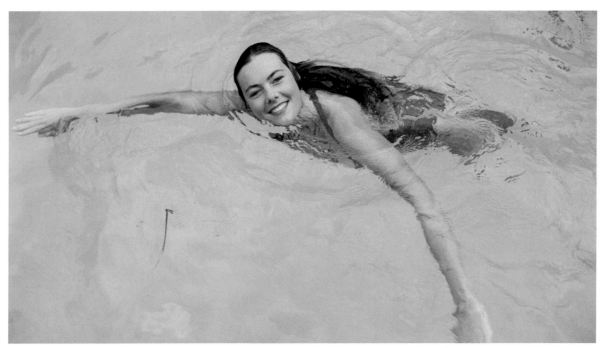

15-5 Using the muscles of the arms and legs while breathing rhythmically makes swimming an excellent aerobic activity.

to catch your breath. Anaerobic activities can help you build power and speed.

● **Muscular Endurance**

Muscular endurance refers to your ability to use a group of muscles over and over without becoming tired. For instance, muscular endurance allows you to use your leg muscles to continuously pedal a bicycle throughout an hour-long ride. Muscular endurance helps you perform physical activities comfortably. It also enables you to remain active for extended periods.

Some people have more endurance in one muscle group than in another. For instance, people trained as runners are bound to have developed endurance in their leg muscles. However, they may find it hard to swim several laps without their arms tiring. This is why it is important to work on developing all your muscle groups. Hiking, rowing, skating, and gymnastics can help you develop muscular endurance.

● **Strength**

Strength is the ability of the muscles to move objects. It is usually measured in terms of how much weight you can lift. You move your body by contracting your muscles. Having strong muscles will allow you to move your body more efficiently. Developing strength can also help you avoid some sports injuries. Obviously, weight training is an excellent activity for developing strength and lean muscle mass. See 15-6.

● **Flexibility**

Flexibility is the ability to move your joints through a full range of motion. *Joints* are the places in your body where two bones meet. Elbows, knees, shoulders, hips, and ankles are all examples of joints. A high degree of flexibility helps prevent injury to muscles that control movement of the joints. Females generally have the potential for greater flexibility than males. Stretching exercises can help increase flexibility.

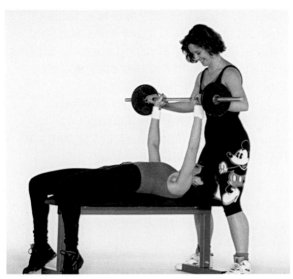

15-6 Using the muscles to lift weights helps develop strength.

● Body Composition

As you read in Chapter 12, *body composition* is the percentage of different types of tissues in the body. You recall having too high a percentage of body fat is a risk factor for a number of diseases. Therefore, body composition is a component of total physical fitness.

If you are at or below a healthy weight, you may ask, "Do I really need to exercise?" The answer is yes. Everyone at all ages needs to be physically active. As described earlier, physical activity has many benefits besides helping people maintain a healthy weight. It is an essential component in maintaining overall good health and fitness.

Remember, weight is not a reliable indicator of body composition. Someone who has a large percentage of lean body tissue may be overweight according to height-weight tables. However, he or she is not overfat.

Exercise helps the body burn fat and build muscle. Glucose is the body's chief source of energy. After about 20 minutes of aerobic activity, however, the body begins to use fat for energy. Doing activities that increase muscular endurance and strength help build muscle tissue. Increasing the proportion of muscle mass in the body will raise the BMR, thus helping to burn even more calories. Along with a lowfat diet, exercise is a key factor in achieving and maintaining a healthy body composition.

You will not see changes in body composition after a single workout. Over time, however, you will notice an increase in lean body tissue and a decrease in body fat. Cross-country skiing, racquetball, soccer, and other aerobic exercises are among the sports that are especially good for controlling body fatness. See 15-7.

● Skill Components of Physical Fitness

There are six skill components of physical fitness. They are power, agility, balance, coordination, speed, and reaction time. For some people, strength in these components seems to come naturally. However, most people can work to improve their ability in these areas.

Having a high level of the various skill components can improve your performance

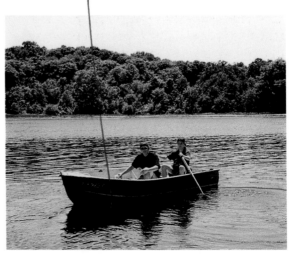

15-7 Rowing helps maintain a healthy body composition because it builds muscle while burning fat.

in certain sports. You are more likely to take part in activities when you are confident in your performance. Therefore, developing your skill components can motivate you to be active. This, in turn, can bring you the benefits that come from an active lifestyle.

Skill-related fitness can benefit you in everyday activities as well as sports. For instance, having good balance, agility, and coordination can help you avoid accidents. Older people who have these skills are less likely to fall and experience the problems of injury.

If you lack some of the skill components, keep in mind many activities do not require all of them. Such activities include walking, bicycling, and swimming laps. Maintaining an active lifestyle, regardless of the type of activity, is the key to a positive health status.

● Power

Power is your ability to do maximum work in a short time. It requires a combination of strength and speed. People need power to excel in some sports activities, such as football and many track and field events. Lifting and stacking boxes or pushing a child on a swing are everyday activities that require power.

As muscles get stronger, they also become more powerful. Joining a softball league or shooting baskets in the gym can help you develop power.

● Agility

Agility is your ability to change the position of your body with speed and control. Agility is an advantage in many sports. It is important to everyday living, too. An agile player can easily move down a sports field in and among other players. Agility can also help you weave through a crowded shopping mall. Downhill skiing, soccer, modern dance, and rope jumping can help develop agility. See 15-8.

● Balance

Balance is your ability to keep your body in an upright position while standing still or

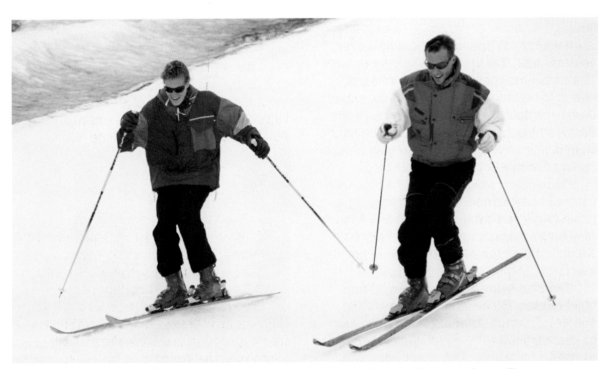

15-8 Controlling their bodies as they speed down a slope helps these skiers develop agility.

moving. Some sports, such as gymnastics and dancing, require athletes to have sensitive balance to excel. A good sense of balance can also help anyone avoid falls and feel more graceful. Ice skating and bicycling can help you develop balance.

● **Coordination**

Coordination is your ability to integrate the use of two or more parts of your body. Many sports require coordination of the eyes and hands or the eyes and feet. Many daily tasks require these types of coordination, too. A football player needs good coordination to catch a pass. You need coordination when chopping vegetables for a salad to avoid cutting off your fingers. A soccer player needs coordination to maintain possession of the ball when dribbling down the field. You need coordination to avoid tripping over objects and stepping in puddles. Bowling, golf, volleyball, and tennis are all activities that help develop coordination.

● **Speed**

Speed is the quickness with which you are able to complete a motion. Obviously, athletes who compete in sprint events need speed. You use speed in daily tasks when you hurry through chores or run to catch a bus. You might consider a class in judo or karate to help you develop speed. Handball, table tennis, and roller skating are also activities that will help you build speed.

● **Reaction Time**

Reaction time is the amount of time it takes you to respond to a signal once you receive the signal. In most physical activities, your response will be some type of movement. A soccer goalie needs good reaction time to block a ball headed for the net. A driver needs to be able to react to changes in traffic. Playing baseball, basketball, football, or softball can help you strengthen your reaction time. See 15-9.

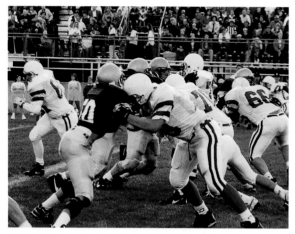

15-9 Responding to their opponents' movements requires football players to have good reaction time.

● **How Fit Are You?**

You can assess yourself in each health and skill component of physical fitness through a variety of simple tests. You are likely to find you are strong in some components but weak in others. To be totally fit, you should be moderately strong in all the health components. You can set goals to improve in your weaker areas. Building strength in each of the health areas will also help you develop more of the skill components.

Later in the chapter you will read about how to plan an exercise program and stay motivated to follow it. Following the guidelines outlined there will help you plot a strategy for improving your total fitness.

● Exercise and Heart Health

Physical inactivity is a risk factor for coronary heart disease (CHD). As higher levels of physical fitness are achieved, the risks of death from heart disease decline.

Exercise affects the *cardiovascular system* (the heart and blood vessels) in several complex ways to improve overall heart health. Remember that exercise helps develop cardiorespiratory fitness. One indication of this type of fitness is a slower heartbeat. The heart beats slower because it is able to work more efficiently. It pumps more blood with each beat. This improved efficiency puts less strain on the heart muscle. See 15-10.

Another way exercise affects heart health is through its impact on blood lipids. In Chapter 6, you learned a high level of LDL cholesterol indicates a high risk of CHD. You also learned a high level of HDL cholesterol indicates a low risk of CHD. Regular exercise, especially when combined with a diet low in fat, saturated fat, and cholesterol, reduces LDL and increases HDL. These changes in blood lipid levels lower the risks of coronary heart disease.

Exercise improves heart health by lowering blood pressure. Exercise also encourages the formation of extra branches in the arteries of the heart. This increases blood flow and allows the heart to work more efficiently.

● Measuring Your Heart Rate

Your heart rate is an indication of the effect physical activity is having on your heart.

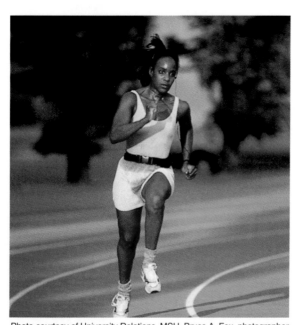

Photo courtesy of University Relations, MSU, Bruce A. Fox, photographer

15-10 Developing cardiorespiratory fitness helps reduce the risks of heart disease.

Your **heart rate**, or pulse rate, is the number of times your heart beats per minute. You can measure your heart rate by finding your pulse and counting the beats. When measuring your heart rate, always use your index and middle fingers, never your thumb. Heart rate is usually measured in one of two places: the wrist or the neck. At your wrist, slide the fingers of one hand along the thumb of your other hand to your wrist. You should feel your blood pulsating when you apply gentle pressure. You should be able to feel a similar pulsating in your neck. Put your two fingers just to the left or right of your Adam's apple. Using the second hand on a watch or clock, count the beats for 15 seconds. Then multiply the number of beats by four to find the number of beats per minute.

Another way to count your heart rate is to count the number of beats in six seconds. Then add a zero to the number to figure the number of beats per minute. In other words, 7 beats in six seconds equals a heart rate of 70 beats per minute.

Your heart rate will vary depending on your level of activity. The harder you work out, the faster your heart will beat.

A **resting heart rate** is the speed at which your heart muscle contracts when you are sitting quietly. An average resting heart rate for a moderately fit teen or adult is about 70 beats per minute. As mentioned above, improved cardiorespiratory fitness results in a slower heartbeat. Someone who has been training for several months may have a resting heart rate of about 60 beats per minute. See 15-11.

Maximum heart rate is the highest speed at which your heart muscle is able to contract. Maximum heart rate is related to age. It is higher for a younger person than for an older person. You can calculate your maximum heart rate using the following formula:

220 – your age = maximum heart rate

A 16-year-old using this formula would calculate his or her maximum heart rate to be 204 beats per minute (220 – 16 = 204).

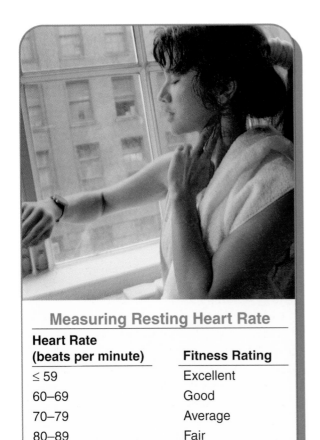

Measuring Resting Heart Rate

Heart Rate (beats per minute)	Fitness Rating
≤ 59	Excellent
60–69	Good
70–79	Average
80–89	Fair
≥ 90	Poor

15-11 As cardiorespiratory fitness improves, resting heart rate will drop because the heart is working more efficiently.

A 50-year-old would calculate his or her maximum heart rate to be just 170 beats per minute (220 − 50 = 170).

● Exercising Your Heart

The heart is a strong muscle. Like your other muscles, your heart needs exercise. Measuring your heart rate can help you see if you are giving your heart enough exercise.

For good exercise, your heart needs to beat faster than its resting rate. However, it should not beat so fast that it is unsafe. You should never try to reach your maximum heart rate. Instead, you should try to exercise within a safe *target heart rate zone*. This is the range of heartbeats per minute at

which the heart muscle receives the best workout. Your target heart rate zone is 60 to 90 percent of your maximum heart rate. A 16-year-old would calculate target heart rate zone as follows:

maximum heart rate: 220 − 16 = 204 beats per minute

204 × 0.6 = 122 beats per minute

204 × 0.9 = 184 beats per minute

target heart rate zone: 122 to 184 beats per minute

When you begin an exercise program, count your heart rate frequently during your workouts. This will help you decide whether you are pushing yourself too little or too much. Your initial goal should be to keep your heart rate at the low end of your target zone. As your fitness improves, you should be keeping your heart rate closer to the high end of your target zone. See 15-12.

● Keys to a Successful Exercise Program

Beginning an exercise program can be hard for some people. You have to feel sure rewards will follow. Talk with people who exercise regularly. Ask them what benefits they have noticed as a result of being physically active. Their answers may inspire you to begin an exercise program that includes more than just daily lifestyle activities.

Researchers have identified some factors that help people stick with their exercise programs. These factors include written goals, enjoyable activities, a convenient exercise schedule, and knowledge of personal fitness level. Consider these factors as you plan a program for yourself.

● Put Fitness Goals in Writing

Your physical fitness efforts are most likely to be effective if you set some specific goals for them. Your long-term goal may be

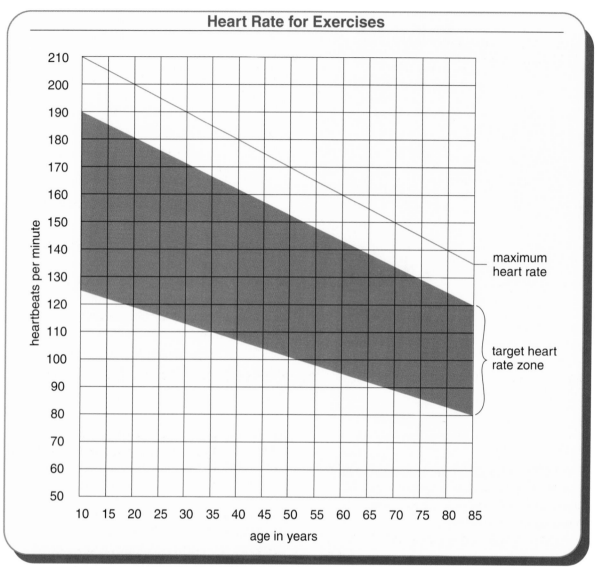

15-12 For a good cardiorespiratory workout, keep your heart rate in your target zone when exercising.

to achieve and maintain total fitness. For most people, however, trying to fulfill such a big goal would be overwhelming. You need to break this goal down into smaller, more manageable goals.

Begin by identifying which component of fitness you want to improve first. Then think about activities that can help you improve in that area. Review the choices of activities presented in 15-13. Then select those activities that are of interest to you. Make a specific plan to include those activities in your weekly routine.

One way to stay focused in your exercise program is to write down your fitness goals. Start with one specific and attainable goal. Your goal might read "I will improve my cardiovascular fitness until my pulse drops to 100 beats per minute following a three-minute step test." Then list specific steps for achieving your goal. You might write "I will bicycle for 30 minutes after school on Monday and Thursday.

Building Health Components of Fitness

Health Component of Physical Fitness	Activities
Cardiorespiratory fitness	Aerobic dancing, bicycling, cross-country skiing, hiking, in-line skating, rope jumping, rowing, racquetball, soccer, swimming
Muscular endurance	Backpacking, calisthenics, cross-country skiing, football, gymnastics, ice skating, in-line skating, mountain climbing, rowing, swimming, weight training
Strength	Backpacking, ballet, football, gymnastics, walking, weight training
Flexibility	Aerobic dancing, ballet, calisthenics, gymnastics, modern dance
Body composition	Aerobic dancing, bicycling, cross-country skiing, handball, hiking, in-line skating, mountain climbing, racquetball, rope jumping, rowing, soccer, swimming, walking

15-13 Choose activities you enjoy that will help you develop health components of fitness in which you are weak.

I will skate for 30 minutes after school on Tuesday and Friday." You might want to write your goal and the steps for achieving it as a personal exercise contract. Post a copy of the contract in a spot where you will see it several times a day. See 15-14.

Your chances for success are much better if you write down what you accomplish. Keep a record of when you exercise and for how long. You will be less likely to skip an exercise session if you know it will show up on your record. You will feel good about yourself when you see how faithfully you are following your exercise contract. Be sure to praise yourself for your success.

Fitness goals take time to achieve. However, you should see some signs of improvement within a few weeks. If you have been following your contract and do not see improvement, evaluate your exercise plan carefully. You may need to revise the steps you are using to reach your goal. You may

also want to consider seeing a fitness counselor. When you achieve your goal, congratulate yourself for a job well done. Then set a new goal and begin working toward it.

● Choose Activities You Enjoy

Physical activity should be fun, not a chore. If you choose activities you enjoy, you will be more likely to stick with your exercise program. You may enjoy outdoor activities like hiking and canoeing. Perhaps you like the competition of team sports. Maybe you prefer partner sports, such as tennis or handball, that you can play with a friend. No matter what activity you choose, the important point is to be active.

Variety can help keep an exercise program enjoyable. You may become bored following the same exercise routine day after day. Doing different types of activities can keep you from getting into a rut. Different

Personal Exercise Contract

Goal

I will improve my cardiovascular fitness until my pulse drops to 100 beats per minute following a three-minute step test.

Action Plan

I will do one of the following activities at least five days a week.

Progress - Week 1

Activity	Sunday	Monday	Tuesday	Wednesday	Thursday	Friday	Saturday
bicycle 30 minutes	✓						
skate 30 minutes							✓
swim 20 laps			✓		✓		
walk 30 minutes				✓			

Progress - Week 2

Activity	Sunday	Monday	Tuesday	Wednesday	Thursday	Friday	Saturday
bicycle 30 minutes							✓
skate 30 minutes		✓				✓	
swim 20 laps			✓		✓		
walk 30 minutes	✓						

15-14 Using a personal exercise contract can motivate you to stick with an exercise program to meet your fitness goals.

activities also help develop different components of fitness. This will help you reach your long-term goal of achieving a good level of total fitness. If you enjoy anaerobic activities, try to include some aerobic activities in your exercise program, too. Also remember to choose activities that focus on different large muscle groups. For instance, you might try rowing to develop upper body strength and jogging to build leg muscles.

Although your exercise program should meet your personal fitness needs, you do not have to exercise alone. Working out with friends or family members can make a fitness program more fun. Doing activities with other people can also help you stay motivated. On a day when you are tempted to cancel your workout, a friend can encourage you to get going. See 15-15.

● Choose a Convenient Time

Scheduling physical activity at a convenient time will increase your likelihood of following through with your exercise program. You may want to work out first thing

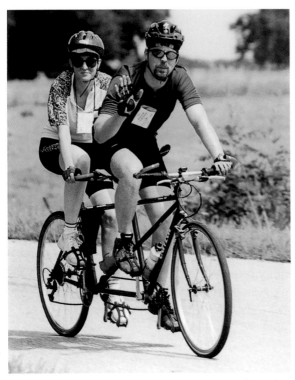

15-15 Exercising or playing sports with a friend can make physical activity more fun.

health components. Ask a fitness counselor or health or physical education teacher for information about self-assessment exercises. Also review the checklist in 15-16 to see if you need to seek medical advice before you start exercising. If you are in good health, you can begin a sensible exercise plan.

Gaining physical fitness is a building process. It involves three key factors: frequency, intensity, and duration. *Frequency* is how often you exercise. *Intensity* is how hard you exercise. *Duration* refers to how long an exercise session lasts.

Begin your exercise program with moderate frequency, low intensity, and short duration. You might start by exercising three times a week. Keep your pulse at about 60 percent of your maximum heart rate for 20 minutes. As you notice improvements in your state of fitness, gradually increase the frequency, intensity, and duration of your exercise. Compete with yourself to achieve

in the morning to get your day off to a good start. You might have some free time after school when you can enjoy activities with friends. Perhaps you would rather exercise at night before going to bed. It does not matter when you exercise as long as you do it.

Once you find an exercise time that is convenient for you, make it a set part of your daily schedule. This will help you form a habit that is easy to follow.

● Know Your Fitness Level

For your exercise program to be successful, you need to know your fitness level. In striving to meet your goal for total fitness, resist the temptation to begin working out too hard too soon. This increases your risk of fatigue and injury and, thereby, increases your likelihood of discontinuing your fitness program.

Before you begin an exercise program, measure your level of fitness in each of the

Proceed with Caution

_____ Your doctor said you have a heart condition, such as a heart murmur.

_____ Your doctor said you have high blood pressure.

_____ You have a medical condition, such as Type I diabetes, that might require special attention in an exercise program.

_____ You have pain in your joints, arms, or legs.

_____ You weigh 25 or more pounds above healthy weight.

_____ You often feel faint or have periods of dizziness.

_____ You experience pain or shortage of breath after moderate physical activity.

15-16 If any of these statements applies to you, see your doctor before starting an exercise program.

new, higher-level goals. Try increasing your frequency to five to seven days per week. Build your intensity up to 70 or 80 percent of your maximum heart rate. Extend the duration of your workouts up to 60 minutes.

Being aware of your fitness level can protect you from injuries caused by too much stress on your body. Exercise should not be painful. You need to learn to tune in to what your body tells you. Burning muscles and feeling as if you cannot catch your breath are signs you are working too hard. These symptoms may occur more rapidly as you increase your speed, exercise in heat or high humidity, or grow tired. If you experience these symptoms, you need to slow down your exercise pace.

Following basic safety precautions can help you avoid other types of injuries when exercising. Know how to use equipment and use it correctly. Wear protective gear, such as helmets and body pads, when appropriate. If you will be exercising outdoors, be prepared for the environmental conditions. If you are injured, follow first aid practices and seek prompt medical attention if necessary. See 15-17.

Planning an Exercise Program

Your exercise program should include three phases for each workout session. You need a warm-up period, workout period, and cool-down period.

Warm-Up Period

On a cold morning, a car engine needs to warm up before you start driving. In a similar way, your muscles need to warm up before you start exercising. Warming up prepares your heart and other muscles for work. Many people ignore this important phase of an exercise program. If you do not warm up, you may be more likely to end up with sore muscles or an injury.

The warm-up period should last about 5 to 10 minutes. Begin by gradually increasing your heart rate. Some people choose a slow jog for this purpose. If you will be swimming or bicycling, you can simply start the activity at a slow pace. Gradually increase to a moderate pace to bring your heart rate near your target zone.

Preparing for Environmental Conditions

- Use caution when exercising in hot, humid weather. High temperatures combined with high humidity increase the risk of heat exhaustion and heatstroke. Wait until temperatures have cooled or choose to exercise in an air-conditioned facility. Be sure to drink plenty of water before, during, and after exercise.
- Use caution when exercising in extremely cold weather. Cold temperatures can cause frostbite and a drop in body temperature. If you feel cold, stop the activity and get to a warmer place. Warm showers are helpful after feeling cold.
- Use caution when exercising on wet, icy, and snow-covered surfaces.
- In stormy weather, head indoors at the first sight of lightning.
- Allow the body time to adjust to the lower air pressure before exercising vigorously in high altitudes (over 5,000 feet).
- Avoid exercising in areas that have high levels of fume exhaust from cars and industry. Polluted air can cause headaches, painful breathing, and watery eyes.

15-17 Following these recommendations can make your exercise activities safe and rewarding.

Following your heart warm-up, warm up the muscles you will be using in your workout. Do a series of gentle stretches, but avoid bouncing motions. Your movements should resemble those you will use in your exercise activity. If you will be playing tennis, slowly move your arms as though you are making broad forehand and backhand strokes. Make these motions several times with empty hands. Then pick up a tennis racquet and repeat them several more times. After a brief warm-up session such as this, you will be ready for a more vigorous workout. See 15-18.

Workout Period

The workout period is the main part of your exercise program. It should last at least 20 minutes. During this time, do activities that will help you develop the health components of fitness. When choosing activities for your workout period, remember the keys for success you read about earlier in the chapter.

Cool-Down Period

Never sit down or enter a hot shower immediately after exercise without a cool-down period. The body needs to slowly return to its pre-exercise state.

During exercise, your heart pumps extra blood to your muscles to meet their increased demand for oxygen and energy. The action of your muscles keeps blood circulating back to the heart. If you stop muscle action too quickly, the extra blood temporarily collects in your muscles. This reduces the amount of oxygen-rich blood available for the heart to pump to the brain, and dizziness results.

The cool-down period should last about 10 minutes. You can use the same activities for your cooldown as you used for your warm-up. A slow jog will help reduce your heart rate and allow the muscles to push more blood toward the heart. Some stretching exercises will help prevent muscle cramps and soreness by loosening muscles that have become tight from exercise. See 15-19.

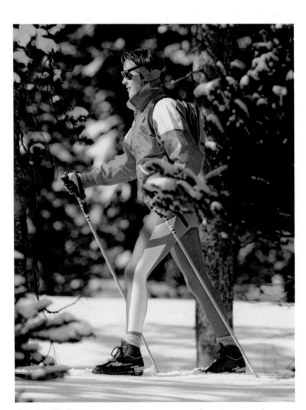

15-19 Following a strenuous workout, a cool-down period is needed to prevent dizziness and muscle cramps.

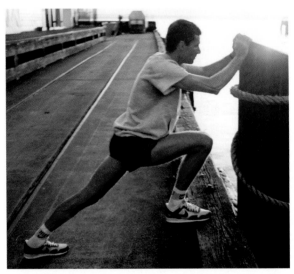

15-18 Stretching before a workout helps warm up muscles and prepare them for activity.

Chapter 15 Review

Summary

Physical activity is needed for physical fitness. The kinds of activities you do and the way you do them will help you reach different fitness goals. To achieve good health, you need to accumulate at least 60 minutes of moderate activity nearly every day. Physical activity can also help you achieve the goals of total fitness or peak athletic performance.

Physical activity has several key benefits. It improves your appearance by helping you develop good posture, graceful movements, and healthy weight. It reduces the risk of several diseases, including coronary heart disease. Physical activity can also help improve your mental outlook.

Through physical activity, you develop the five health components of physical fitness. They are cardiorespiratory fitness, muscular endurance, strength, flexibility, and healthy body composition. Physical activity can also help you build six skill components that will improve your sports performance. The skill components of physical fitness are power, agility, balance, coordination, speed, and reaction time. You can measure your fitness level for all eleven of these components through simple self-assessment tests.

Exercise benefits heart health in several ways. It helps strengthen the heart muscle, improves blood lipid levels, and lowers blood pressure. Measuring your heart rate can help you see how exercise is affecting your heart. To give your heart the best workout, try to stay within your target heart rate zone when exercising.

There are several keys to a successful exercise program. Put your fitness goals in writing. Choose activities you enjoy and do them at a convenient time. Also, be sure to keep your workouts in line with your fitness level.

Each exercise session should have a warm-up, workout, and cool-down period. Try following this format to do at least 20 minutes of moderate-intensity activity nearly every day. You will find physical activity is a lifestyle choice with lifetime benefits.

Check Your Knowledge

1. What is the guideline for teens for achieving good health through lifestyle physical activities?

2. What are three ways physical activity can improve appearance?

3. What types of activities are good for building cardiorespiratory fitness?

4. Which health component of physical fitness is demonstrated by an ability to repeatedly use muscles without tiring?

5. List four skill components of physical fitness and give an example of an activity that would help develop each component.

6. Why does someone with a high level of cardiorespiratory fitness have a slower heartbeat than someone who is less fit?

7. Where is heart rate usually measured?

8. What is the maximum heart rate for a 30-year-old man?

9. What percentage of the maximum heart rate is the target heart rate zone?

10. Why is an exercise program more likely to be successful if a written record of exercise sessions is kept?

11. What are two advantages of varying the activities in an exercise program?

12. What are the three key factors involved in gaining physical fitness?

13. True or false. Burning muscles are a sign of a good workout.

14. What is the purpose of the warm-up period of an exercise session?

15. Why might skipping the cool-down period at the end of an exercise session result in dizziness?

Put Learning into Action

1. Interview a physically active person about his or her goal for physical activity. Find out how long the person has been working toward the goal and what progress he or she has made. Also find out what kind of exercise program the person is following to try to reach his or her goal. Share your findings in class.

2. List five excuses people commonly give for not being physically active. Write a counterpoint you could give someone using each excuse to encourage him or her to be more active.

3. Make a bulletin board or poster illustrating activities that help develop the five health components of physical fitness.

4. Make a list of 10 sports. Rank the importance of each skill component of physical fitness for each sport. Discuss your list with a small group of your classmates to see if they agree with your rankings.

5. Measure your resting heart rate. Compute your maximum heart rate and your target heart rate zone.

6. Write a personal exercise contract. Identify a specific, attainable fitness goal and list the steps you intend to follow to achieve it. Follow the contract for three weeks. Then evaluate the strengths and weaknesses of your plan.

Explore Further

1. Write a research report about the effects physical activity has on the risks of developing a specific disease. Explain how and why activity seems to have an effect.

2. Prepare an oral report on the causes and treatment of a common sports injury.

3. Compare costs and services of three local health clubs, community fitness centers, and/or group exercise programs. Talk to several people who have used each fitness resource to find out what they like and dislike about it. Develop a checklist of features to look for when choosing a fitness facility or program.

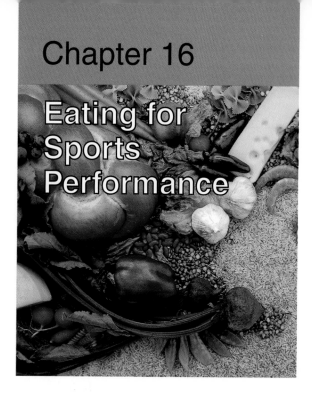

Chapter 16

Eating for Sports Performance

● Learn the Language

lactic acid
endurance athlete

carbohydrate
loading

● Objectives

After studying this chapter you will be able to

- explain an athlete's dietary and fluid needs.
- plan a performance day or pregame meal for an athlete.
- describe techniques athletes can use to safely lose or gain weight for competition.
- state consumer cautions related to performance aids marketed to athletes.

Sports activities have been an important part of everyday life from the beginning of recorded time. Sports are relaxing, fun, and available for people of all ages and both sexes. These activities provide health and wellness benefits for all who take part. They promote self-esteem, and they help people build physical skills. Through teamwork, sports also help people grow socially and emotionally.

Athletes often have an intense desire to excel. Team and partner sports are competitive. The focus is on beating an opponent. Individual sports present athletes with a challenge to surpass their previous best performance. See 16-1.

The drive for peak performance has led some athletes to seek a winning edge through their diet. Their search has fostered the spread of nutrition myths and misinformation. This chapter will help you sort the facts from the fallacies. You will learn which diet choices can make a difference in how well you perform.

● The Nutrient Needs of an Athlete

What should an athlete eat? What foods will improve his or her performance? Which foods should be avoided before and during athletic participation?

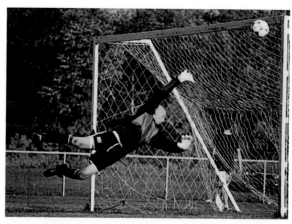

16-1 In team sports, athletes compete against other players.

The typical athlete burns many calories through exercise. The number of calories athletes use is determined by their body weight and the types of activities they are doing. The length of the exercise period will also affect the number of calories used. People who weigh more burn more calories through a given activity. This is because more energy is required to move their heavier body mass. More vigorous activities require more energy than less active sports. For instance, running requires more energy than jogging. The longer the workout lasts, the more calories will be burned. See 16-2.

An athlete who burns more calories through exercise than he or she takes in

How Many Calories Do Athletes Burn?					
Activity	**Calories Burned per Minute**				
	100 lbs. *(45 kg)*	*125 lbs.* *(57 kg)*	*150 lbs.* *(68 kg)*	*175 lbs.* *(80 kg)*	*200 lbs.* *(91 kg)*
Aerobic dance	6.0	7.6	9.1	10.6	12.1
Baseball	3.1	4.0	4.7	5.5	6.3
Basketball, recreational	4.9	6.2	7.5	8.7	10.0
Bicycling, 10 mph	4.2	5.3	6.4	7.4	8.5
Canoeing, 4 mph	4.4	5.5	6.7	7.8	8.9
Dancing, active	4.5	5.6	6.8	7.9	9.1
Football, vigorous touch	5.5	6.9	8.3	9.7	11.1
Golf, carrying clubs	3.6	4.6	5.4	6.4	7.3
Hockey	6.6	8.3	10.0	11.7	13.4
Horseback riding	2.7	3.4	4.1	4.8	5.4
Ice skating	4.2	5.2	6.4	7.4	8.5
Jogging, 5.5 mph	6.7	8.4	10.0	11.7	13.4
Racquetball	6.5	8.1	9.8	11.4	13.0
Roller skating	4.2	5.3	6.4	7.4	8.5
Running, 8 mph	9.7	12.1	14.6	17.1	19.5
Skiing, cross-country, 4 mph	6.5	8.2	9.9	11.5	13.2
Skiing, downhill	6.5	8.2	9.9	11.5	13.2
Soccer	5.9	7.5	9.0	10.5	12.0
Swimming, crawl, 35 yd./min.	4.8	6.1	7.3	8.5	9.7
Table tennis	3.4	4.3	5.2	6.1	7.0
Tennis, recreational singles	5.0	6.2	7.5	8.8	10.0
Volleyball, recreational	2.9	3.6	4.4	5.1	5.9
Walking, 4 mph	4.2	5.3	6.4	7.4	8.5
Wrestling	8.5	10.6	12.8	14.9	17.1

Note: The energy costs in calories will vary. Values are approximate. Factors that influence calorie needs include wind resistance, ground levels, weight of clothes, and other conditions.

16-2 Locate the column closest to your weight for an activity you enjoy. Multiply the calories burned per minute by the number of minutes spent in the activity to figure total energy expenditure.

through food will lose weight. (Refer to Chapter 12, "The Energy Balancing Act" for more information on energy imbalance.) An athlete burns more calories than a nonathlete. Therefore, he or she needs to consume more calories to maintain body size.

Most athletes can meet their energy needs by eating extra calories from a wide selection of nutritious foods. About 50 to 60 percent of the calories in an athlete's diet should come from carbohydrates. No more than 30 percent of the calories should come from fat. The remaining 10 to 15 percent of the calories an athlete consumes should come from protein.

● Sources of Muscle Energy

What type of fuel do muscles use to supply the energy needed for activity? As you know, carbohydrates, fats, and proteins all supply energy. The percentage of total fuel supplied by each of these nutrients depends on the duration and intensity of the activity.

Glucose is the body's chief source of energy. It is one of the simple sugars found in some of the foods you eat. Your liver also makes glucose from other sugars and starches in your diet. Glucose is stored in the liver and muscle tissues as *glycogen.* When muscular activity begins, glycogen stored in the muscles begins to be used as a source of energy.

The body breaks down glucose into carbon dioxide, water, and energy. Oxygen is needed for this chemical process to continue. Oxygen comes into the body through the lungs and the blood carries it to the muscles. Muscles then release energy so you can perform your sport. Muscles can continue to work as long as the breakdown of glucose occurs efficiently.

After about 20 minutes of aerobic activity, fats from body stores also begin to be metabolized for energy. The body can stockpile much more fat than carbohydrate. Therefore, fats serve as an almost unlimited energy

source. However, fat cannot be converted to energy without the presence of oxygen. This means fat is not burned for energy during anaerobic activity.

● Anaerobic Activity

When you are intensely active, more and more glucose must be metabolized to meet the increasing energy demands. This requires more oxygen. However, your heart and lungs cannot always supply enough oxygen to the muscles to completely oxidize glucose. (This describes anaerobic activity, as discussed in Chapter 15, "Staying Physically Active: A Way of Life.")

The incomplete breakdown of glucose results in a buildup of a product called *lactic acid* in the muscles. You experience a burning sensation and fatigue in the muscles. When this occurs, you may have to slow down and catch your breath. The muscles need to rest until they receive enough oxygen to move out some of the lactic acid. When they have enough oxygen and the cramping stops, energy can be produced more efficiently again.

As you know, some sports require athletes to use their muscles for long periods. These *endurance athletes* may be involved in sports such as marathon bicycle and foot races or distance swimming. Endurance athletes may require sustained muscle efforts for several hours at a time. You might wonder how they can extend their muscle performance to avoid exhausting their glycogen stores and "hitting the wall." Training helps improve the muscles' use of glucose. Trained muscles use more fat for fuel and conserve their glycogen. Trained muscles also become more tolerant of lactic acid. Thus, soreness and fatigue will not occur as quickly. As training proceeds, the lungs' capacity to carry oxygen also becomes more efficient. See 16-3.

Endurance athletes also learn to pace their activity so they can maintain the flow of oxygen for steady glucose metabolism. They relax their muscles at every opportunity so

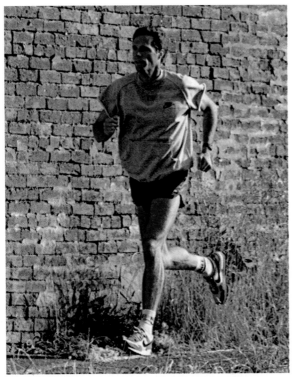

16-3 Marathon runners, who compete in 26-mile races, must train intensively. This improves their muscles' use of glucose and tolerance of lactic acid.

their blood can carry the lactic acid away and supply more oxygen.

● The Athlete's Dietary Needs

Good daily nutrition provides athletes (and nonathletes) with the ongoing foundation for peak performance. Athletes need to choose foods high in carbohydrate, moderate in protein, and low in fat. Carbohydrate is the preferred source of energy.

Athletes may need slightly more protein than nonathletes to build and maintain muscle tissue. Athletes also use some protein to meet energy needs. However, most athletes can meet their protein needs without making major diet modifications.

Many foods provide protein. A slice of bread and ½ cup (125 mL) of cooked vegetables each provides about 2 grams of protein. A cup (250 mL) of milk provides 8 grams.

A 3-ounce (84 g) cooked portion of meat or poultry provides about 26 grams.

Teen females who follow the Food Guide Pyramid consume about 107 grams of protein per day. Teen males who follow the Pyramid consume about 124 grams of protein daily. These amounts of protein are more than enough even for teens who are most involved in active sports. Protein supplements are not necessary. In fact, they may interfere with peak performance.

Athletes need to plan their diets around a variety of foods rich in vitamins and minerals. These nutrients are important for the conversion of carbohydrates, fats, and protein to energy. Vitamin and mineral supplements are an added expense and are usually not necessary.

In special situations, an athlete may need a supplement. For example, a vegetarian athlete who avoids all dairy foods would need a calcium supplement. When a supplement is advised, athletes do not benefit from those that provide more than 100 percent of the RDAs or AIs. A multiple vitamin and mineral formula will meet most athletes' nutrient needs.

Some athletes need more energy than they can comfortably take in through food. These athletes may find it helpful to consume energy in concentrated forms, such as dried fruits. Drinking high-energy liquids, like yogurt shakes, may also be easier than eating solid foods. Supplements and special "power" foods are generally not needed and have not been shown to improve performance. See 16-4.

● Carbohydrate Loading

Carbohydrate loading is a technique used to trick the muscles into storing more glycogen for extra energy. Its use was intended to improve the performance only of endurance athletes. Carbohydrate loading involves eating a diet moderate in carbohydrates for a few days. Then during the three days before a sports event, an athlete consumes a high-carbohydrate diet. The

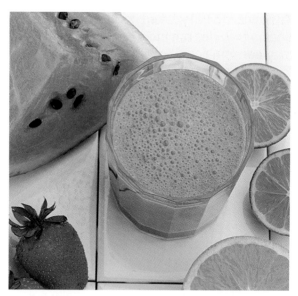

16-4 A high-energy fruit shake can provide an athlete with needed calories in a form that is easy to consume.

increase in carbohydrates is coupled with a decrease in training intensity.

Some problems have occurred for athletes practicing carbohydrate loading. These problems have included water retention, digestion distress, muscle stiffness, and sluggishness. Athletes with chronic diseases like diabetes are especially likely to have problems.

For most athletes, attempts to increase glycogen stores are not needed. If you are in a daily vigorous exercise program, eat a carbohydrate-rich diet. Include a rest day in your schedule now and then, too. Such rest days will help build up the glycogen stores you need.

● The Athlete's Need for Fluids

Drinking enough fluids may be the most critical aspect of sports nutrition. If fluid levels drop too low, dehydration results. Symptoms of dehydration include headache, dizziness, nausea, dry skin, shivering, and confusion. Dehydration also causes increases in body temperature and heart rate. Clearly, dehydration can impair performance.

Performing athletes may not feel thirsty because exercise masks the sense of thirst. Sweating during moderate exercise causes you to lose about 1 quart (1 L) of water per hour. If the workout is vigorous, a loss of 2 to 3 quarts (2 to 3 L) of water per hour may result. Therefore, athletes need to drink regardless of whether they feel thirsty.

Athletes can lose four to six pounds of water weight during a sports event. To determine how much water you lose, weigh yourself before and after an event. If you lose more than 3 percent of your body weight, your performance will deteriorate. For example, a 150-pound (67.5 kg) person should not lose more than 4½ pounds (2 kg) during an athletic activity ($150 \times .03 = 4.5$).

To avoid dehydration, athletes should drink water before, during, and after an event. The American Dietetics Association suggests the following plan for fluid intake:

- 2 hours before event: 3 cups (750 mL) water
- 10-15 minutes before event: 1-2 cups (250-500 mL) water
- 10-15 minute intervals during event: ½-1 cup (125-250 mL) water
- After event: 2 cups (500 mL) water for every pound of body weight lost

Athletes lose water during exercise even when the air temperature is comfortable. Water losses are greater when exercising in hot, humid weather. This makes heat cramps and heat exhaustion more likely. When exercising in these conditions, watching fluid replacement is even more critical.

Water is the preferred liquid for fluid replacement during a sporting event. Cold water (40°F) helps lower body temperature and empties from the stomach more quickly than any other fluid. The carbohydrates in some sweetened drinks can pull water from the body into the digestive tract, causing cramps. The carbohydrates in most sports drinks are designed to be easily absorbed to prevent such cramping. Even so, if you choose a sports drink, you may want to dilute it with water or ice. Caffeine and alcohol increase body water loss. They should be avoided during physical activity. See 16-5.

Besides water, athletes lose sodium when they sweat. Most athletes get enough sodium from the foods they eat. However, endurance athletes who compete in events lasting four or more hours may lose excessive amounts of water and sodium. These athletes may benefit from a sports drink that contains sodium, chloride, and potassium. Salting food a bit more liberally will also help them meet sodium needs.

Salt tablets are not recommended to replace sodium lost during physical activity.

They worsen dehydration and impair performance. They can also irritate the stomach and may cause severe vomiting. This is especially true when fluid intake is not adequate.

● Performance Day and Pregame Meal

Without a doubt, good nutrition is critical to top level performance. Special sports nutrition products and supplements do not have special benefits beyond a well-planned diet. Several guidelines for diet planning involve thinking about how food intake affects digestion and use of energy for top performance.

	Beverage Choices for Athletes			
Beverage	**15 to 30 Minutes Before Event**	**During Event**	**After Event**	**Reason**
Water (cool to cold)	Yes	Yes	Yes	Best fluid for your system; regulates body temperature
Special sports drinks	Maybe	Maybe	Yes	Depends on content; may be high in sugar, which slows fluids in emptying from the stomach; salt content may be too high
Carbonated soft drinks	No	No	Yes	Carbonation may cause problems during an event and sugar may prevent fluids from quickly emptying the stomach
Fruit juices	No	No	Yes	Sugar content is high; can be used to replace carbohydrates after an event
Coffee/tea	No	No	No	Caffeine pulls water from the body through increased urination; makes the heart work harder
Milk	No	No	No; Fat free—Yes	Too difficult to digest for fluid use
Alcohol	No	No	No	Undesirable, does not help performance, dehydrates cells and decreases muscle efficiency

16-5 What is the best drink before, during, and after an athletic event?

The goals of the pregame meal should be to provide appropriate amounts of energy and fluid. The meal should also help the athlete avoid feelings of fullness and digestive disturbances.

Very large meals before competition should be avoided. They require too much energy to digest. This does not mean you should go hungry. Hunger makes you feel tired and sluggish. For most sports events, the best diet plan includes a high-carbohydrate meal within 3 to 4 hours before competition.

Avoid the high-protein, high-fat steak dinners that were once training table standards.

Diets containing little or no carbohydrates have been found to have negative effects on performance. However, very sweet carbohydrates like syrups and candy bars can cause water to pool in the gastrointestinal tract. Discomfort and diarrhea may result.

Athletes should avoid bulky and fatty foods on the day of competition. High-fiber foods like whole grain breads and large portions of fresh fruits and vegetables should be limited. Also, avoid French fries, bacon, sausage, and other foods high in fat. Instead, choose foods like bread, rice cakes, potatoes, juices, or other high-carbohydrate, low-fat foods. See 16-6.

Pregame Meals		
Foods	**Calories**	**Carbohydrate (Grams)**
Pregame Breakfast		
Orange juice	112	27
Cornflakes with milk	152	30
Banana	104	27
Toast with jelly	103	22
Hard-cooked egg	78	1
Total	**549**	**107 (78% of calories)**
Pregame Lunch		
Pasta with meatless sauce	404	73
Roll	85	14
Applesauce	52	14
Fat free milk	86	12
Total	**627**	**113 (72% of calories)**
Pregame Snack Ideas		
Bagel		Frozen yogurt
Crackers		Dried fruit
Popcorn (unsalted, unbuttered)		Oatmeal, fig, or raisin cookies
Pretzels		Granola
Pudding		

16-6 A pregame meal, eaten 3 to 4 hours before a competition, should be rich in carbohydrates and moderate in calories.

Foods you have never eaten before are not recommended at pregame time. You cannot be sure how they will make you feel.

For some athletes, mental attitude can be just as important as the foods eaten. Suppose an athlete always eats pizza before a competition. For this athlete, it may be psychologically important to eat pizza to be ready to win. Follow the pattern that works best for you.

● Weight Concerns of Athletes

Achieving optimum weight can positively affect your athletic performance. What is optimum weight? The answer depends on your percentage of body fat, or your body composition.

Chapter 12, "The Energy Balancing Act," described the various methods for analyzing body composition. Knowing your percentage of body fat suggests whether you need to lose extra fat and/or build more muscle mass. Too much body fat increases energy needs. Energy needed for performance ends up being used to move excess body weight. Too little body fat makes you lose body heat too fast. Energy needed for competition ends up being used to maintain body warmth.

Lean body mass is especially valued by some athletes, such as gymnasts, distance runners, and body builders. For other athletes, like discus throwers and baseball players, body composition may not matter as much. Most male athletes do well with 10 to 15 percent body fat. An acceptable level for most female athletes is 18 to 24 percent body fat. Most females stop menstruating when body fat drops below 17 percent. This creates a hormonal imbalance that promotes mineral losses from bone tissue and increases the risk of developing osteoporosis. See 16-7.

● Losing Weight for Competition

Athletes in some sports, such as wrestling, boxing, and weight lifting, compete in specific weight classes, 16-8. Some of these athletes use harmful methods to try to reduce their body weight quickly to compete in lower weight classes. They may try to skip meals or refuse to drink fluids one or two days before competition. Some use laxatives, diuretics, and emetics (substances that induce vomiting) to rid their bodies of food and fluids. Such practices can weaken an athlete's endurance.

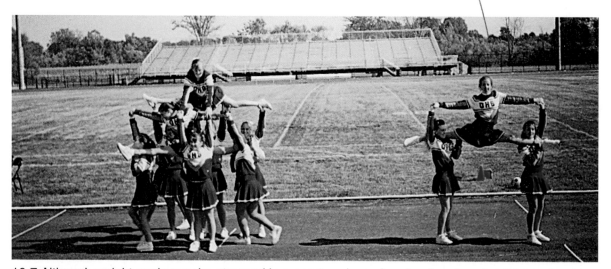

16-7 Although weight goals may be stressed in a sport such as cheerleading, female athletes should maintain 18 to 24 percent body fat.

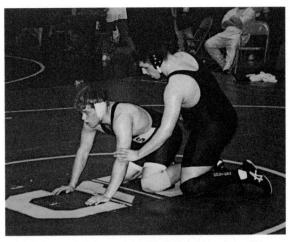

16-8 Athletes who want to compete in specific weight classes should adjust weight gradually *before* the start of their sport season.

Crash dieting can also harm an athlete's health. Severely restricting calorie intake while vigorously training can interfere with normal growth. The body will use energy to fuel activity rather than to support growth.

For females, severe dieting coupled with strenuous exercising may change hormone production. Females can experience irregular or absent menstrual periods. Hormonal changes can also trigger a decrease in bone density. This can delay healing if a bone injury occurs.

The best time to diet is before the official training season begins. Athletes need to weigh themselves well before the start of their sports season. Then they will have ample time to reduce body fat and reach weight goals before they begin competing.

Gradual weight loss is the best way to reduce pounds. Athletes need to set realistic goals for weight loss at a maximum of two pounds per week. Athletes who lose weight faster than this are probably losing more than fat. They will be losing body fluids and muscle mass, too.

To lose one pound of body fat, an athlete needs to consume 3,500 fewer calories than he or she expends. However, the athlete needs an adequate supply of nutrients to maintain strength and stamina while trying to lose weight. Most teen male athletes need at least 3,000 calories per day. Teen female athletes need a minimum of 2,200 calories daily. These amounts need to come from nutritious foods that provide the full range of vitamins and minerals. Eating more complex carbohydrates while reducing fats in the diet can help athletes limit calorie intake. Increasing energy expenditure by moderately extending workouts will help athletes gradually reach their weight goals.

Athletes should work with a registered dietitian while going through a weight loss program. (Many coaches do not have adequate nutrition training to supervise an athlete's weight loss.) A dietitian can make sure athletes are meeting their daily calorie and nutrient needs for growth and training. (More advice on weight loss is provided in Chapter 13, "Healthy Weight Management.")

● Gaining Weight for Competition

Some athletes, such as football and hockey players, want to gain weight or "bulk up." Their goal is to gain size as well as strength. A large body mass will make them seem more formidable to their opponents. See 16-9.

For many athletes, gaining weight is difficult because they burn so many calories through long, hard workout sessions. Experts recommend athletes choose nutritious foods to add an extra 2,500 calories to their weekly intake. Some athletes may need to consume 5,000 or more calories per day to meet this recommendation.

High-fiber foods like salads and whole grain breads and cereals are not emphasized in a weight-gain plan. These foods will cause an athlete to feel full too quickly. Athletes should include moderate amounts of monounsaturated and polyunsaturated oils because of their high calorie density. However, they should avoid saturated fats because of their link to heart disease.

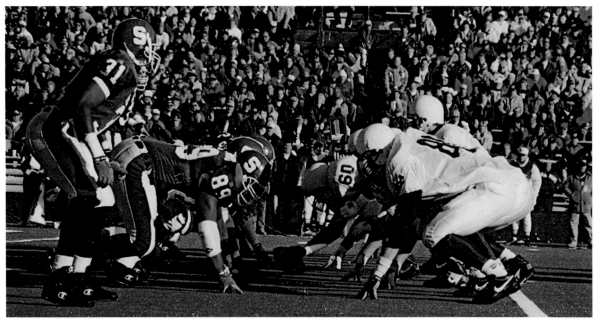

David West

16-9 Football players require strength, power, and body mass to be effective in their sport.

Athletes who are trying to gain weight may wish to reduce the length and intensity of their regular workout sessions. They may also want to increase their rest and sleep time. These efforts will decrease the number of calories athletes burn for energy. However, an athlete's weight-gain program must include exercise, particularly weight training. An athlete's weight-gain goal is to add muscle, not fat. Muscle size cannot be increased by consuming more calories. Weight gain without training will be fat gain, not muscle gain.

Athletes who consume coffee, tea, and colas should decrease their use of these products when trying to gain weight. The caffeine in these products tends to increase metabolic rates. Reducing caffeine consumption will help athletes burn fewer calories.

Modifying eating and exercise patterns will help athletes gain about 1 to 2 pounds (.5 to 1 kg) per week. Like those who are trying to lose weight, athletes trying to gain weight should work with a registered dietitian. (More advice on weight gain is provided in Chapter 13, "Healthy Weight Management.")

● Harmful Performance Aids

Perhaps you have wished there were a special drink or pill that would make you stronger or faster. If only you could find some magic key to success, you would be sure to win, right?

Unfortunately, there is no special food, drink, or pill that will safely make an athlete stronger or faster. Likewise, no safe methods exist to add muscle weight quickly. Schemes promoted to build muscle mass fast are often frauds. Some can negatively affect performance and health. They can even interfere with normal growth and development. The health effects of drugs and other substances can produce a range of symptoms. Mild symptoms include headache and nausea. Severe symptoms include liver disease, stroke, and death. See 16-10.

New "performance enhancers" appear on the shelves of health food stores every day. The sales pitches are creative, and the claims often sound miraculous. However, as a careful consumer and serious competitor, you must evaluate claims carefully. Keep in mind that if a claim sounds too good to be true, it probably is.

A planned program of supervised training and nutritious eating is the safest, most effective key to peak performance.

Harmful Effects of Performance Aids		
Performance Aid	**Reasons Used**	**Harmful Effects**
Anabolic steroids	A male sex hormone used to build strength and add muscle mass	Liver disorders, kidney disease, growth disorders, decreased level of HDLs (good cholesterol) and increased level of LDLs (bad cholesterol), high blood pressure, sexual problems, reproductive disorders (men—affects the production and functions of testosterone; women—growth of facial hair, baldness, menstrual irregularities, aggressiveness), unusual weight gain or loss, rashes or hives
Bee pollen	Used to improve overall athletic performance	Has no proven beneficial effects on performance, serious harm to those with certain kinds of allergies
Caffeine	A stimulant to the central nervous system used to increase endurance during strenuous exercise	Increases fluid losses; increases heart rate; can cause headaches, insomnia, and nervous irritability
Carnitine	An amino acid supplement used to strengthen endurance	Can cause muscle cramps, muscle weakness, and loss of iron-containing muscle protein
Human growth hormones	Used to build muscle and shorten recovery time	Thickening of bones, overgrowth of soft body tissues, possibility of grotesque body features
Pangamic acid (sometimes called vitamin B$_{15}$)	Used to improve efficient use of oxygen in aerobic exercises	Ruled illegal by the Food and Drug Administration, unsafe for humans
Bicarbonate of soda or soft drinks (soda loading)	Used to avoid muscle fatigue	A form of doping, no confirmed benefits for game performance
Vitamin supplements	Used to feel better and provide a competitive edge	False promises, promotes "pill popping," costs more than food sources, individual becomes less concerned about eating a variety of foods because the pill will cover his or her needs

16-10 These performance aids may appear to be quick fixes, but they may actually be harmful to your health.

Chapter 16 Review

Summary

Athletes have greater needs for energy and some nutrients than nonathletes. However, they meet their calorie and nutrient needs in the same way as everyone else—through diet.

The body breaks down sugars and starches in an athlete's diet and converts them to glucose. The athlete's muscles use oxygen to burn glucose for energy. During anaerobic activity, the heart and lungs cannot supply enough oxygen to keep up with the muscles' needs. This results in a burning sensation in the muscles due to a buildup of lactic acid.

Athletes have high energy needs to fuel their activity in training and competition. Most of this energy should come from carbohydrates in the diet. The diet should also provide moderate amounts of protein and fat. Athletes need vitamins and minerals to help metabolize the energy nutrients. Athletes need plenty of fluids before, during, and after sports events to avoid dehydration. Water is the preferred body fluid during vigorous exercise. Eating a high-carbohydrate diet a few days before an endurance event increases glycogen stores in the muscles. Athletes should avoid foods high in fat and fiber at pregame meals.

Reducing excess body fat and increasing lean body mass improves performance in many sports. However, weight adjustments should be gradual. They should occur before the start of an athlete's training season. Body fat should stay within recommended limits.

Check Your Knowledge

1. What are three factors that affect the number of calories an athlete burns through activity?

2. What is the storage form of glucose in the body?

3. Why does the body not use fat for energy during anaerobic activity?

4. True or false. Most athletes need to take protein supplements to build muscle tissue and fuel activity.

5. Describe the type of athletic activity that is most likely to benefit from carbohydrate loading.

6. How much liquid should an athlete consume after an event to replace fluid losses from the body?

7. Explain two tips for planning a pregame meal for an athlete.

8. What percentage of an athlete's body should be fat?

9. Why is exercise an important part of a weight-gain program for an athlete?

10. Why should athletes who are trying to lose or gain weight for competition work with a registered dietitian?

Put Learning into Action

1. Interview an athlete in your school about what foods he or she eats before a sports event. Find out the reasons behind the food choices. Write a report comparing the athlete's practices with the recommendations for pregame meals made in this chapter. In your report, identify the athlete's gender and sport, but do not use his or her name.

2. Prepare a brochure discussing the relationship between a nutritious diet and athletic performance. Give copies of your brochure to the coach of one of your school's athletic teams. Invite the coach to share the brochure with the athletes he or she directs.

Explore Further

1. Review the ingredients lists and Nutrition Facts panels on two commercial sports drinks. Note the cost per 8-ounce serving

of each product. Use the Internet to visit the Web sites of the manufacturers of the drinks. See what types of information they make available about the effects of their products on athletic performance. Detail your findings in a report comparing the two products.

2. Contact a national association for youth sports. Find out the association's official position on weight requirements for competition among adolescent athletes. Write an opinion paper agreeing or disagreeing with the association's position. Cite at least two references to support your opinion.

Chapter 17

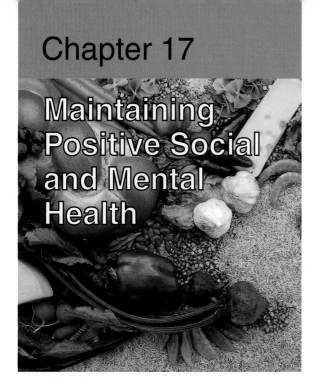

Maintaining Positive Social and Mental Health

● Learn the Language

self-actualization
relationship
social development
communication
verbal
  communication
nonverbal
  communication
conflict

compromise
assertiveness
teamwork
self-concept
self-esteem
personality
balance
burnout

● Objectives

After studying this chapter, you will be able to

- determine the order in which a person will typically strive to meet specific human needs.
- list characteristics of a socially healthy person.
- explain techniques for promoting positive social health.
- summarize how self-concept and personality are related to mental health.
- identify strategies for promoting positive mental health.
- propose a self-management plan to make a positive life change.
- describe a situation that might require the help of a mental or social health care professional.

Have you ever felt torn when you and your friends were on opposite sides of an issue? Has there ever been a time when you felt overwhelmed by more school assignments than you had time to complete? Have these kinds of situations ever caused you to lose sleep, lose your appetite, or feel ill? If so, you may not be surprised to learn that your social and mental health can affect your physical health. See 17-1.

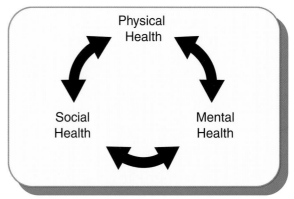

17-1 Physical, social, and mental health affect one another. When positive gains are made in one area, an individual often senses positive outcomes in the other two areas.

In this chapter, you will learn that your interactions with others and your mental state are important aspects of wellness. You will find out how communication skills can help you relate to others. You will also study strategies that will help you develop a healthy mental outlook.

Basic Human Needs

As a human being, you have basic needs. The degree to which these needs are met affects your state of physical, social, and mental health. When your human needs are met, your potential for achieving a high level of wellness greatly improves.

Abraham Maslow, a psychologist, proposed a theory that human needs form a *hierarchy,* or a ranked series. He grouped needs into five basic levels. He believed people must meet their needs at the lowest level first, at least in part. Until they address these needs, people cannot focus on needs at the next level. Maslow's theory can be represented as a triangle, which has a base broader than the peak. This suggests needs shown at the base of the triangle provide a foundation for healthy growth and development. See 17-2.

Physical Needs

The first level of needs in Maslow's hierarchy is made up of physical needs that are basic to survival. These include needs for oxygen, water, food, shelter, clothing, and sleep. You are likely to have trouble thinking about much else until these needs are met to some degree. For instance, think about sitting in a football stadium when a terrible storm suddenly begins. Watching the game is likely to become less important than finding some way to meet your basic need for shelter.

Safety and security needs, which form the second level in the hierarchy, also affect physical health. You need to feel protected from physical harm. You also need to feel

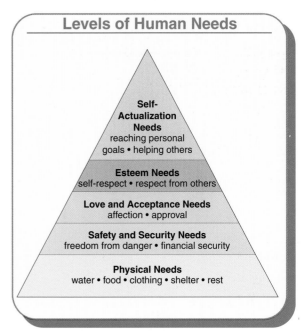

17-2 The needs at the base of Maslow's hierarchy must be at least partially met before addressing needs at the next level.

financially secure. When these needs are threatened or not met, your state of total health is jeopardized. For instance, safety needs are not being met if you are being driven by someone who has been drinking alcohol. Until you get out of this situation, your life is at risk.

Social Needs

If basic physical and security needs are adequately met, it will be possible to fulfill needs for love and acceptance. This third level of the hierarchy affects social health. These needs stem from a human desire to experience positive connections with people. All people need to know others care about them. Everyone needs to feel wanted as a member of a group. You may feel loved when a parent expresses concern about you. Perhaps you feel acceptance when a friend invites you to join in an activity. This group of needs also includes your need to be able to show love and acceptance for others. Loving others helps you feel good about yourself.

Another set of social needs falls at Maslow's fourth level in the hierarchy. This level includes needs for esteem. You need to feel others value you as a person. You must also value yourself. When others recognize your achievements or ask for your opinion, they are helping to address this need. When you congratulate yourself on a job well done, you are showing self-esteem.

Mental Needs

The peak of Maslow's hierarchy relates to mental needs. These are needs for people to believe they are doing their best to reach their full human potential. Maslow referred to this as *self-actualization*. Meeting needs at this level involves more than facing and managing daily tasks. It requires you to work at the peak of your abilities. People who do volunteer work are often addressing their need for self-actualization. They find the experience rewarding, and they feel they are helping others.

The need for self-actualization expands as you pursue it. Meeting this need is a lifelong process. After achieving one goal toward self-actualization, you need to set new goals. Few people reach a point where they feel they have reached the highest level of achievement in every area.

What Is Social Health?

The degree to which your social needs for love, acceptance, and esteem are met affects your social health. Social health is reflected in your ability to get along with the people around you. It is measured by the quality of your relationships. *Relationships* are the connections you form with family members, friends, and other people.

People enrich their lives as they build relationships with others. They learn what types of interactions meet their social needs. Learning more about themselves enables people to form stronger relationships.

Socially healthy people enjoy making new friends and keeping old ones. People who have good social health generally have certain traits that help them relate to others. Such traits include patience, empathy, courtesy, and selflessness. Socially healthy people exhibit these traits through their daily words and actions when they are around others. They can share thoughts and ideas while showing respect for other's needs.

Social Development

One sign of social health is positive social development during childhood and adolescence. *Social development* is learning how to get along with others. It involves more than forming close personal relationships. It involves being able to act appropriately in all kinds of situations that involve people. Not talking in a movie theater, thanking a clerk for help, and raising your hand in class are social skills. Having such skills may not be enough to help you form close friendships. However, these skills should help you feel more at ease in social settings. See 17-3.

How does social development take place in your childhood years? In a physically safe and secure environment, children learn positive social skills by watching others. They identify with and imitate the people who are

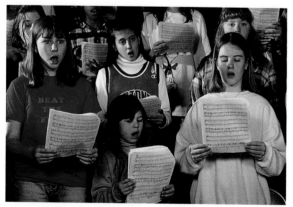

Photo courtesy of University Relations, MSU, Bruce A. Fox, photographer

17-3 Sharing activities, such as choral singing, is one way to build relationships with people.

closest to them. The people children first model are most often parents, family members, and caregivers. Boys tend to copy the social behaviors of males. Girls usually mimic the social behaviors of females.

As children grow, they generally begin spending more time with people away from home. Friends and classmates become new models for children to follow. If children observe people who use socially appropriate behaviors, the children will learn positive social skills.

Social development continues during adolescence. Most adolescents want to form more adult social relationships with their peers. Masculine and feminine social roles become more defined. Many teens begin forming dating relationships. As teens form and end relationships with friends and dating partners, they gain understanding of their social needs. They also learn new social skills that will help them build more lasting relationships as adults. See 17-4.

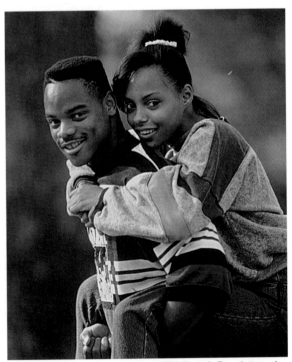

Photo courtesy of University Relations, MSU, Bruce A. Fox, photographer

17-4 A socially healthy person enjoys the companionship of others.

Like children, teens tend to model the conduct of their peers. Peers who model inappropriate social actions can have a negative effect on social development. Teens who learn to recognize and reject inappropriate behavior can protect their social health status.

Adult relationships involve getting along with coworkers as well as friends and family members. Job success depends on achieving social competence. Skills developed early in life can help people reach career advancement goals as adults.

● People in Your Social Circle

For most people, the closest and most continuous relationships occur within families. These relationships begin at birth as family members respond to a baby's needs. A family that demonstrates care and respect for each of its members displays signs of positive social health. See 17-5.

Sharing friendships is an important way to achieve social health. Friends provide people with a source of shared fun and companionship. You feel free to exchange joys and sorrows with a friend. Most importantly, friends can help you work through problems and give you feedback on ideas. As your friends provide this type of support for you, you can provide it for them. This two-way interaction makes friends a valuable source of self-discovery.

Beyond family members and friends, your social connections can expand through Internet communications, travel, media, and group activities. You face new social challenges as you include people from other cultures in your social network. As you interact with others, they influence your thoughts and feelings and you influence theirs.

● Promoting Positive Social Health

You can take steps to build positive relationships that will meet your social needs. Many experts would agree that an ability to

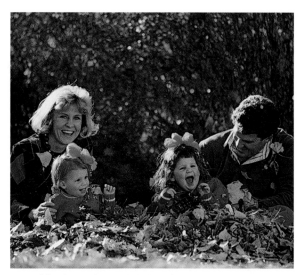

17-5 Much early social development occurs within the family unit.

share ideas with others is the most important social skill. With this skill, you can solve problems with others and make your needs known to them. You can also express care for others and work with them to achieve goals.

● Develop Communication Skills

Communication is the sending of a message from one source to another. Two basic types of communication are used to convey messages. *Verbal communication* uses words. It may be spoken or unspoken. Speaking to someone and writing a letter are both examples of verbal communication. *Nonverbal communication* transmits messages without the use of words. Posture, facial expressions, tone of voice, and symbols are nonverbal ways of communicating. When verbal and nonverbal communication both send the same message, communication is clear.

Communication can take place between two people, such as when you call a friend on the telephone. Communication can also occur among millions of people. When a news anchor reports a national event, he or she is engaging in this type of mass communication.

You need effective communication skills to be able to clearly exchange ideas with others. These skills can greatly affect your relationships and, thus, your social health. The following guidelines will help you plainly and openly communicate your ideas with others:

- Know what you want to say.
- Speak clearly and loudly enough to be understood.
- Avoid using slang terms that may not be familiar to your listener.
- Avoid sending nonverbal signals that contradict your spoken message, such as rolling your eyes when giving a compliment.
- Use specific words to convey your exact meaning.
- Maintain eye contact when you are communicating with someone in person.
- Be honest.

Communication involves listening as well as speaking. You need to listen carefully to be sure you understand the message someone else is sending. Try restating information that has been shared. Ask questions about any points that are not clear. These steps will allow you to confirm that you have correctly understood what the speaker was saying. See 17-6.

With the increasing use of e-mail and Web sites, electronic communication is being used more than ever. This makes good writing skills more important than ever. A message that contains errors could end up making a bad impression on people all over the world in a matter of seconds.

You need to learn how to write effectively. You must select the right words and construct clear sentences. You also need to use a writing style that conveys your intended tone. You must be sure the message you send cannot be interpreted as offensive to another person or group of people. For informative writing, keep sentences short and limit your use of technical words. Sentences that are long and contain many complex terms are harder for people to read and understand. Following these suggestions will help you represent yourself well as you use written communication to build personal relationships.

● Resolve Conflicts

A **conflict** is a disagreement. Conflicts tend to arise between people in social situations. Perhaps someone has blamed you for something you did not do. You may have gotten into an argument with a good friend. These are examples of conflict.

If you do not handle conflicts carefully, they can grow. A conflict that gets out of hand can eventually destroy a relationship. This is why an ability to *resolve,* or settle, conflicts is important for maintaining good social health. You can use your communication skills to help you resolve conflicts.

Handling conflicts as soon as possible helps keep them under control. However, you should wait until you have a chance to talk about the problem privately. Airing your disagreement publicly is likely to make the other person uncomfortable and defensive.

Stay focused on the facts related to the problem. Try not to bring emotions into your discussion. Also avoid becoming sidetracked by other issues. Explain why you are unhappy with the person's *actions,* not why you are unhappy with the *person.*

Use "I" messages to state how you feel and why you feel that way. This allows you to take ownership of your feelings. In contrast, a "you" message blames your feelings on someone else. Compare the following examples:

- "I feel uncomfortable when we arrive late for our exercise class. I would appreciate your help in getting there on time."
- "You embarrass me by making us late for our exercise class. You better start getting us there on time."

The "I" statements in the first example are likely to evoke a more positive response from the other person.

Try to monitor your voice. Tone of voice greatly influences the quality of a conversation. A loud, angry voice will cause the other person to feel as though he or she is being attacked.

Do not simply criticize what is wrong with a situation. Explain what could be done differently. Suggest a plan that might work better. Describe why you think this solution would work. Stay flexible as you discuss various solutions to the problem. The other person may also have some good ideas. Together you may be able to reach a **compromise.** This is a solution that blends ideas from two differing parties.

● Practice Assertiveness

Learning to be assertive will help you develop positive social health. **Assertiveness** is a personality trait. It is the boldness to express what you think and feel in a way that does not offend others. It is different from aggressiveness and goes beyond passiveness. To be *aggressive* is to express your feelings in a way that is pushy and offensive. To be *passive* may mean failing to express your feelings at all. See 17-7.

Assertiveness allows you to take steps to reach desired outcomes. It allows you to feel

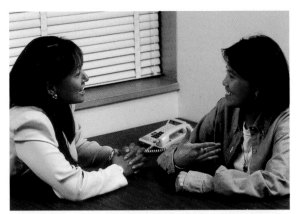

Photo courtesy of University Relations, MSU, Bruce A. Fox, photographer

17-6 Eye contact and body language can help people communicate clearly with each other.

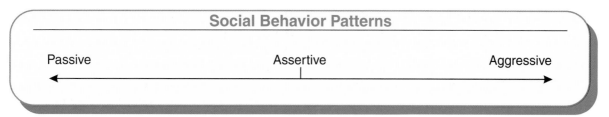

Social Behavior Patterns

Passive   Assertive   Aggressive

17-7 Assertiveness is the ability to express a personal point of view without offending others. You are neither passive nor aggressive in your words and actions.

actively involved in the decisions that must be made. It gives you the courage to ask important questions and locate necessary resources to achieve your needs and interests.

Assertiveness can help you feel more confident in socially challenging situations. You will be able to say no when an activity does not agree with your personal values and beliefs. You will be able to turn down offers to join in activities that do not fit into your schedule. You will be able to pursue opportunities that are important to you.

You can practice assertiveness if it does not come naturally to you. Make a point of expressing your opinions to others. Be firm when asking for what you want. However, if the answer is no, let go of the issue. Avoid becoming angry, demanding, and argumentative. (This would be aggressive behavior.) Do not be afraid of your position or feel you have to defend it. (This would be passive behavior.) Just state your feelings calmly and openly. In most cases, people will respect your honesty.

When you encounter someone who is aggressive, your most assertive response is to simply get away. You will not be able to reason with someone who is out of control. To protect yourself from potential violence, you need to remove yourself from the situation.

● Develop Qualities of a Friend

You read earlier that social health is measured by the nature of your relationships. Friendships are among your most important relationships. Developing the qualities of a friend will improve your social health

by helping you form strong friendships. See 17-8.

You need to offer others the same qualities you desire in a friend. People list a number of characteristics they seek in a good friend. These characteristics include loyalty, or being there when someone needs you. Good friends are also reliable. You can count on them to do what they say they will do. Friends need to be understanding and sensitive to how you feel at any given time. Friends must be caring, too. They must show you they value your feelings

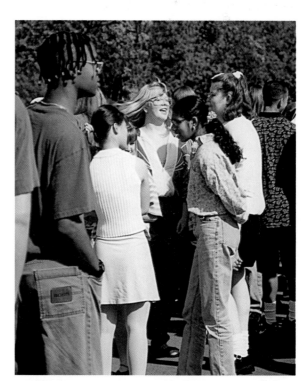

17-8 Friends will support your ideas and listen to your thoughts without criticism.

as much as their own. What other words would you use to describe your best friend?

● Be a Team Member

To be a socially healthy person, you must be able to be an effective member of a group. You must be willing to participate in teamwork. *Teamwork* is effort of two or more people toward a common goal. Teamwork is often required to solve complex problems or complete involved tasks. For instance, making a parade float for a school club would require teamwork among club members.

Each person can contribute unique talents, giving the project balance and completeness. A club member with artistic skill could design the float. Someone with consumer skills could buy the supplies. A member who has construction skills could help build the float. Completing the project successfully would be much more difficult without the addition of each person's special

abilities. By helping and encouraging one another, team members can accomplish more as a group than they can individually. See 17-9.

What are the characteristics of an effective team or group member? Groups who work together effectively have members who

- focus on the team goals
- show willingness to compromise
- value the importance of each person's job to the team's success
- cooperate and offer help when needed
- treat each person as a valued member by seeking his or her ideas and opinions

Teamwork is often identified as an important job skill. Therefore, being a team member will do more than promote your positive social health. It will also help you achieve career success. You can develop teamwork skills by taking an active role in school and community group projects.

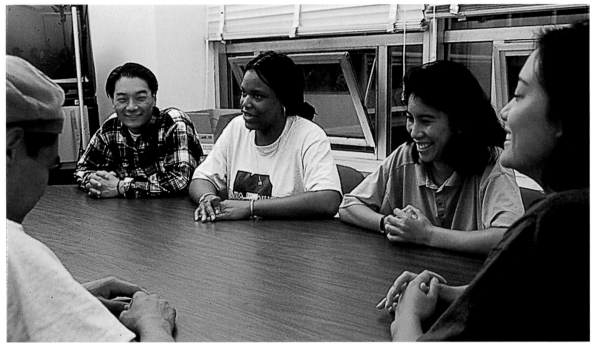

Photo courtesy of University Relations, MSU, Bruce A. Fox, photographer

17-9 To work together effectively, team members need listening skills and a willingness to cooperate.

Team members often develop into team leaders. You can recognize members who might become leaders. Such members are the ones who urge others to participate. Besides helping others get involved, leaders are willing to share ideas and knowledge. Leaders try to make others feel their roles in the group are important. They know how to give credit and praise to others as signs of recognition. Developing these leadership traits will help you to achieve success in the job market.

● What Is Mental Health?

Most health care professionals agree that people's mental health reflects the ways they see themselves. People with positive mental health feel comfortable with their work and family lives. They can usually adapt to the demands and challenges they must face each day. Mentally healthy people also seek positive ways to meet their physical and social needs. See 17-10.

Mentally healthy people are not always smiling and happy. They sometimes have periods of fear, insecurity, and loss of control. These are normal emotional events. However, people with good mental health have learned to deal effectively with their emotional ups and downs.

Mentally healthy people have also learned how to react positively to major life events. They may become distressed after an emotional crisis, such as losing a job or ending a relationship. They may feel uneasy about a lifestyle change, such as a move to a new community. However, they find ways to control and reshape the effects of these

---

Characteristics of Positive Mental and Social Health

Positive mental and social health may be reflected in someone who

- maintains a positive self-image
- respects self and takes good care of self
- finds pleasure in life; is happy and active most of the time
- shows awareness of personal thoughts and feelings and can express them in positive ways
- works to meet daily problems and challenges
- is not afraid to face problems and is willing to seek help when crises arise
- plans for achieving future goals
- enjoys humor and can laugh at self
- knows how to end personal relationships that are hurtful
- shows interest in learning and growing from mistakes; knows how to accept criticism
- tolerates frustration without undue anger
- works well in group situations
- continues to work with an individual or group even when his or her ideas are rejected
- develops talents and abilities to their fullest
- enjoys positive interpersonal relations with people of both sexes
- genuinely likes people and shows interest in meeting new people
- considers the needs and rights of others when expressing personal needs and rights
- respects differences in appearances, race, religion, interests, and abilities

17-10 People who display many of these characteristics tend to have positive views of themselves and strong relationships with others.

emotional upheavals. They focus on improving the conditions they can change.

Mentally healthy people are likely to view life's challenges as opportunities for growth. When an event occurs, they identify the issues involved. They think clearly about their goals. Then they search for solutions to resolve the problem. If a situation becomes too overwhelming, mentally healthy people are not afraid to ask others for help.

● Self-Concept and Mental Health

Your *self-concept* is the idea you have about yourself. It is how you see your behavior in relation to other people and tasks. Part of having good mental health is having a positive self-concept. You have a realistic view of yourself and the events in your life. You realize most situations have pluses and minuses.

Through your early social interactions with family and friends, you begin to develop a concept of who you are. Your self-concept is often a reflection of the way you believe other people see you. If other people focus only on your strengths, you may form a *negative self-concept.* This means you have an inaccurate picture of yourself. You fail to realize you have faults as well as gifts. You are also likely to form a negative self-concept if other people dwell on your failures. You may not recognize you have both positive and negative qualities. If other people acknowledge both your strengths and weaknesses, you are likely to form a *positive self-concept.* This means you have an accurate picture of yourself. You understand you have abilities as well as shortcomings.

As you grow and change, your self-concept can change. Feedback from family members, friends, teachers, and community leaders may reinforce your self-concept. It may also cause you to reevaluate and redefine your self-concept. This is part of human growth over the life cycle.

Good mental health is also linked with having a high level of self-esteem. ***Self-esteem*** is the worth or value you assign yourself.

Like your self-concept, your self-esteem is affected by the people around you. When people give you the impression you do not matter, they can decrease your level of self-esteem. For instance, picture your teachers never calling on you when you raise your hand. Imagine your family members ignoring your opinions. Think about your friends always interrupting you. Over time, these actions may cause you to feel worthless.

A person who has low self-esteem may feel helpless to make decisions. He or she may not feel deserving of good fortune. This person may be easily influenced by peer pressure.

When people express the opinion that you are worthwhile and important, they help build your self-esteem. For example, a teacher may say you did a good job on your science report. Your parents may show pride when you make a mature decision. Your friend may thank you for your loyalty. These types of positive feedback help you feel good about yourself.

With a high level of self-esteem, you will feel like a capable, secure, and creative person most of the time. You care about how situations will affect you. This helps you recognize negative peer pressure. It also empowers you to resist pressure urging you to take part in activities that could be harmful to you. A high level of self-esteem enables you to set goals and take actions to achieve them. Your self-esteem grows as you accomplish tasks that are important to you. See 17-11.

● Personality and Mental Health

Your personality can affect the impact events have on your mental health. Your ***personality*** includes all the characteristics that make you a unique person. It includes your thoughts, feelings, and behaviors as you interact with your surroundings.

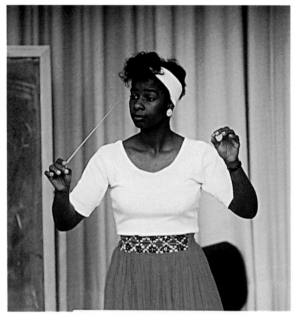

Photo courtesy of University Relations, MSU, Bruce A. Fox, photographer

17-11 Self-esteem can help you make a presentation confidently.

No two people are exactly the same. Personality characteristics take form early in life. They are shaped by your experiences, culture, and genetic makeup.

Some people have tense personalities. They tend to worry about unpleasant events before the events happen. Such people often express anger over situations they cannot control. This type of personality can have a negative effect on mental health. (It can affect physical and social health, too.) Needless worrying and unfounded anger can cloud a person's overall outlook.

Other people have relaxed personalities. They are not bothered by problems that *might* occur, only those that *do* occur. Such people tend to be resilient to the effects of negative events. Their resiliency allows them to draw on their personal strengths. This type of personality can help a person maintain good mental health. Avoiding needless worrying can help a person reserve mental energy for times when he or she needs it most.

● Promoting Positive Mental Health

You can take steps to promote good mental health. Having positive mental health can help you meet your mental needs. A realistic view of yourself can point you in the direction of activities that move you toward self-actualization.

● Surround Yourself with Supportive People

Having good social health can boost your mental health. You need to surround yourself with people who will fulfill your needs to feel loved, accepted, and valued. Such people will help you build a positive self-concept and a high level of self-esteem. Their love and support will help you develop the confidence you need to succeed.

Try to connect with encouraging friends and adult role models. These supportive people can help you build on your strengths and learn from your mistakes. Avoid people who always send negative messages to you. See 17-12.

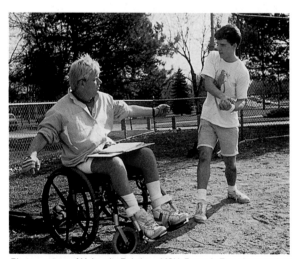

Photo courtesy of University Relations, MSU, Bruce A. Fox, photographer

17-12 Friends who model socially acceptable behaviors can be a source of support.

Keep in mind that healthy relationships involve giving as well as receiving. Just as you need support from others, others need support from you. When you encourage others, you are playing an important role in helping to fulfill their social and mental needs.

Remember that you need to be supportive of yourself. Encouragement from others will not go very far if you have a poor opinion of yourself. Try to avoid negative thoughts about yourself. Concentrate on using your strengths and improving your weaknesses.

The connection between social health and mental health goes both ways. When you have good mental health, you will find it easier to attract people who meet your social needs. Other people will be drawn to your positive outlook. They will appreciate your realistic view of yourself.

● Protect Your Physical Health

Your physical health can also affect your mental health. When you feel physically well, you have the energy you need to face your problems. You have the strength to look for positive ways to help yourself feel good. For instance, you may find exercise is a great way to beat negative emotions.

Here again, you will find a two-way link between health areas. Feeling mentally content may contribute in significant ways to good physical health. When someone feels down for a long period, he or she can lose interest in fitness. This person may have little desire to eat a nutritious diet. The body's immune system may become impaired. The person's physical health may deteriorate. By contrast, when people are in a good state of mental health, their bodies seem to fight disease more effectively.

Knowing there is a relationship between body and mind, you can see the importance of protecting your physical health. Make a point of eating healthful foods. Be sure to get enough rest and exercise. Avoid harmful substances, too. By following these guidelines,

you will be caring for your mental health as well as your physical health.

● Maintain Balance in Your Life

Have you ever been so busy going out with your friends that you barely have time to see your family? Have you ever been so involved with a school project that you forgot to eat a meal? From time to time, many people get excessively focused on one area of their lives. As a result, they lose touch with other areas. Their lives lack balance.

Balance refers to a sense of proportional distribution given to life's roles and responsibilities. A lack of balance can have a negative effect on mental health. People whose lives are out of balance may find themselves feeling emotionally exhausted. They are likely to experience ***burnout***. This is a lack of energy and motivation to work toward goals. Burnout causes a reduced sense of personal accomplishment.

Maintaining balance requires you to step away from yourself. Look at your life from an outsider's point of view. This will help you see how your daily actions affect the quality of your whole life. It will help you get a better perspective of what really matters to you in the long run.

Balance comes from devoting an appropriate amount of time and energy to each of your roles. These roles may include family, school or job, and community roles. Each demands your personal attention. See 17-13.

Family roles include your responsibilities as a son or daughter, brother or sister, niece or nephew. Fulfilling these roles can give you a strong sense of security and support during happy and sad times. You need to give yourself enough time and energy to help family members when they need you. You need to allow yourself to rely on them, too.

School and job roles are often fulfilled outside the home. These roles can provide intellectual challenges, which can be stimulating and rewarding. These roles also prepare you

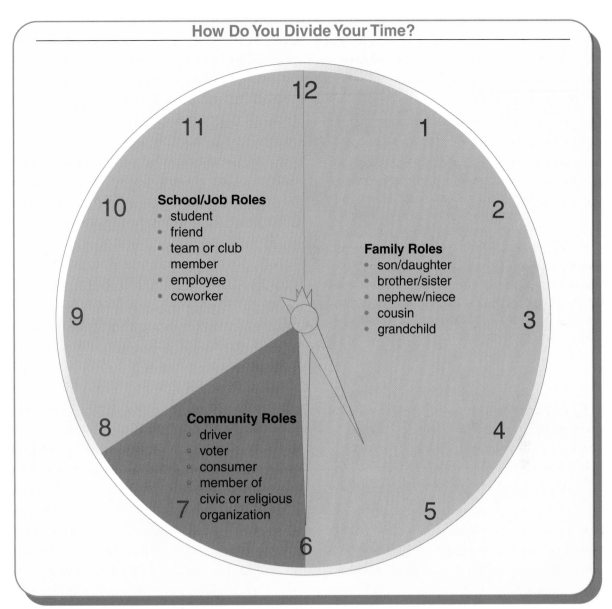

How Do You Divide Your Time?

School/Job Roles
- student
- friend
- team or club member
- employee
- coworker

Family Roles
- son/daughter
- brother/sister
- nephew/niece
- cousin
- grandchild

Community Roles
- driver
- voter
- consumer
- member of civic or religious organization

17-13 Promoting positive mental health involves allotting an appropriate amount of time to each of your roles.

for or provide you with a way to earn income. When career demands become great, other life roles may be ignored. Seeking a balance between work and family roles is a challenge for many people.

Community roles may take a variety of forms. They can include roles in clubs, civic groups, and religious organizations. For many people, community roles provide a way to offer services to others. Important values can be shared as you express commitment to selected community projects. Community roles offer the chance to meet and work with a diverse group of people.

While dividing your time among all your roles, do not forget to save some time for yourself. You need to take care of your physical, social, and mental needs. You need to allow yourself the time to select nutritious foods and get adequate amounts of rest and exercise. You need to take the time to relax and enjoy hobbies and friends, too. Taking this time for yourself makes you feel more prepared to face all your roles and responsibilities. See 17-14.

When one role in life overshadows other important roles, life often feels out of balance. This sometimes happens when roles on sports teams take teens away from family and school roles. Such a temporary imbalance may not be as harmful to health as a lifestyle of imbalance. Evaluate the amount of time and energy you spend on each of your roles. Make whatever adjustments you can to help you get through temporary imbalances and avoid long-term ones. Seeking a healthy sense of balance in your life is key to promoting positive mental health.

Making Positive Life Changes

Perhaps you have a desire to improve your social and/or mental health. You have read several suggestions for helping you reach this goal. However, following these suggestions may require you to adopt some new behaviors. Making such changes in your life can be difficult. It involves conscious and responsible efforts.

Using a self-management plan can make this change process easier. A *self-management plan* is a tool for making a positive behavior change. It involves carefully analyzing goals, priorities, and choices. It requires you to identify options before making and acting on decisions. A self-management plan involves the following steps:

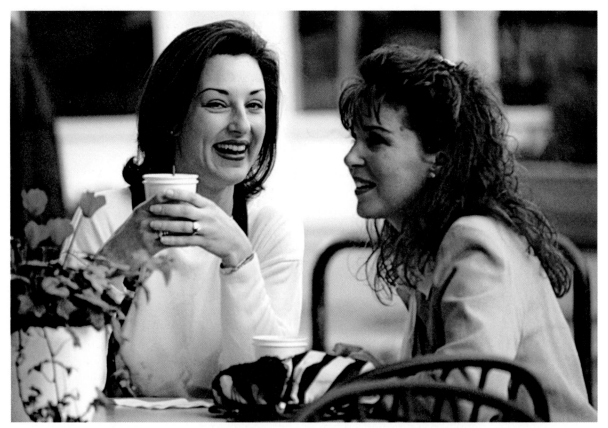

17-14 Relaxing with family and friends can help you feel refreshed and ready to face responsibilities.

1. List your strengths.
2. List your "needs improvement" behaviors.
3. Prioritize your "needs improvement" behaviors.
4. Clarify your goal.
5. List your alternatives for achieving your goal.
6. Evaluate the pros and cons of each alternative.
7. Make a choice and act on it.
8. Evaluate the outcomes of your choice.

As you read about each step in the self-management plan, begin to prepare a plan of your own. This will allow you to clearly see the step-by-step actions you intend to take. It will help you monitor your progress. It will also enable you to reward yourself when you achieve successes.

List Your Strengths

Most people have experienced many successes in life. No one has a life full of failures. Begin your self-management plan by examining your strengths in the health area you want to improve. For example, suppose you want to improve your social health. Your current social strengths may include your honesty as a friend and your cooperative attitude when working on a team. See 17-15.

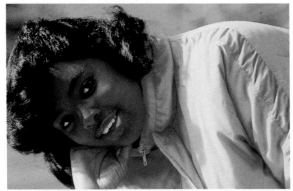

Photo courtesy of University Relations, MSU, Bruce A. Fox, photographer

17-15 Friendliness and a sense of humor may be strengths related to your social health.

List Your "Needs Improvement" Behaviors

Identify health-related behaviors you feel you need to improve. You might believe being assertive is one of your weaker social skills. Maybe you feel you often hesitate to express your needs to others. As a result, your wishes go unnoticed. You might also feel you have trouble resolving conflicts. Perhaps you do not tell other people when you disagree with them. Instead, you allow negative feelings to build up until you have an outburst of temper.

Prioritize Your "Needs Improvement" Behaviors

After you have identified the "needs improvement" behaviors, you must narrow your focus. You are less likely to be successful if you scatter your attention in too many directions. Look at the list of behaviors you identified in the second step. Rank your list, placing the behavior that concerns you most at the top. You may believe assertiveness will help you resolve conflicts. Therefore, you decide to put "being more assertive" at the top of your "needs improvement" list.

Clarify Your Goal

Now that you have identified your main area for self-improvement, shape it into a specific goal. This will give you a sense of direction. State your goal in writing, using concrete, measurable terms. When possible, include a time frame for meeting your goal. Be sure to be realistic about what you can achieve.

Try to break your goal down into manageable subgoals. For example, your main goal is "I want to be more assertive." This is a broad goal. A measurable subgoal might be "I will ask one question or state one opinion every day." Another subgoal might be "I will not apologize when I have to say no to an activity." You can easily see how well you are achieving these specific subgoals. This will give you motivation to continue working toward your main goal.

As you are clarifying your goal, decide how important it is to you. Ask yourself if you are willing to do what it will take to create a change. Also consider how the achievement of your goal will affect others. For example, how will your goal to be more assertive affect your family?

● List Your Alternatives

For each subgoal you have identified, list all the ways you can think of to achieve it. Usually there will be more than one choice available. For example, to learn how to boldly ask questions and state opinions, you could attend an assertiveness workshop. You might read a book about expressing yourself with confidence. You could ask advice from someone who has an ability to speak out. You could also ask a trusted friend to help you practice asking questions and stating opinions. All these choices have the possibility of helping you develop assertiveness skills.

You may want to do some research to become aware of different alternatives for reaching your goal. The more options you know about, the more likely you will be to find one that will work for you. Use the Internet or your community library to gather information. Seek the advice of a school counselor or someone else who may be knowledgeable on the subject.

● Evaluate the Pros and Cons

Identify as many advantages and disadvantages as you can for each alternative on your list. For example, an assertiveness workshop has the advantage of helping you gain new skills quickly. However, it may have the disadvantage of being costly. Weigh the pros against the cons for each alternative. Cross off any options on your list that have more drawbacks than benefits.

Think about how each alternative will affect your resources, including time, money,

and physical energy. Also consider the results of choosing one alternative over another. Choosing one option can often remove other options. If you spend your money to attend a workshop, you can no longer use that money to buy a book. See 17-16.

● Make a Choice and Act on It

After comparing your various alternatives, choose the one that seems to suit you best. Then act on your choice. Suppose you decide to read a book on expressing yourself with confidence. Go to a bookstore or library. Find a book on this topic that seems engaging. Buy or check out the book and read it. Then start following the worthwhile advice from the book in your daily interactions with others.

● Evaluate Outcomes

Evaluation is an ongoing process throughout a self-management plan. For example, in the first step, you evaluate your behaviors related to a particular type of health. This is

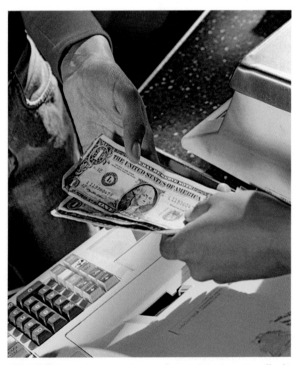

17-16 Some resources, such as money, may limit your alternatives.

an informal evaluation that occurs mainly in your head.

As a final step in a self-management plan, you need to do a more formal evaluation. Putting your evaluation in writing can help you think about how your chosen action helped you meet your main goal. You will be able to see whether following the advice from the book truly helped you become more assertive.

The following questions may help you evaluate the outcomes of your self-management plan:

- Am I satisfied with the results of my choices and actions?
- Do I feel better about myself than I did before?
- Is my health status better now than it was before?
- Do my friends and family show support of my newly developed behaviors and skills?
- Does my overall quality of life seem to be improved?

Answering no to any of these questions may indicate you did not choose the best way to improve your health. Try to view this situation as a chance to learn more about yourself. This will help you make better choices in the future.

If you can answer yes to each of these questions, your self-management plan worked for you. You took the necessary steps to make a change that helped you grow mentally and/or socially. Your physical health is also bound to improve as a result of your actions.

● Seeking Help for Social and Mental Health Problems

Positive social and mental health are key parts of your total state of wellness. Many people find the methods described earlier helpful for improving these two health areas. However, some people have social and mental

health problems that cannot be solved through self-help techniques. Such problems require the help of mental and social health care professionals. See 17-17.

Mental and social health problems can occur for many reasons. Some are the result of specific crisis events, such as divorce or the death of a loved one. Other problems arise out of long-term situations, such as emotional neglect or substance abuse. No matter what is causing the problem, the important point is to find needed help.

A physician can recommend professionals who can help people with social or mental problems. A professional will begin by helping a client define the problem. Treatment may involve individual, family, or group therapy. Therapy often focuses on helping clients develop the social and mental tools they need to help themselves. Treatment for some clients also involves medication.

Helpful therapists can convey interest, understanding, and respect to clients. They offer advice and support to help clients improve their mental and social health. However, the clients are responsible for making needed behavior changes.

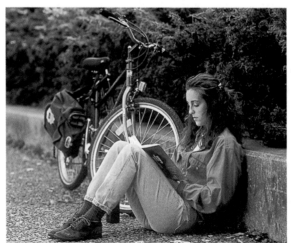

Photo courtesy of University Relations, MSU, Bruce A. Fox, photographer

17-17 If mental or social conflicts are too stressful, you may feel unable to solve problems alone. Professional counselors are available to help teens in conflict.

Chapter 17 Review

Summary

Your social and mental health play large roles in your wellness. These health areas are interrelated with your physical health.

All three health areas are affected by the degree to which your needs are met. You can group basic human needs into five levels. You have needs for physical survival, safety and security, love and acceptance, esteem, and self-actualization. Needs at each level must be at least partly met before you can focus on needs at the next level.

Your social health refers to your ability to form quality relationships with others. Your social health is influenced by your development of social skills as you grow up. It is also affected by the people in your social circle, especially family members and friends.

You can take steps to promote positive social health. One of the most important steps is to develop communication skills. Having these skills will help you resolve conflicts. You also need to practice assertiveness in social situations. Developing the qualities of a good friend and team member will help you build more positive relationships, too.

Your mental health is reflected in the way you see yourself and in the way you react to life events. Having good mental health involves having a positive self-concept and a high level of self-esteem. Having a resilient personality can reduce the negative effects life's problems can have on mental health.

As with social health, you can take steps to promote positive mental health. Surrounding yourself with supportive people can help you build a positive self-concept. Protecting your physical health will give you the strength to tackle problems that come your way. Maintaining balance among your various roles will help you avoid strain on your mental health.

A self-management plan can help you make positive life changes that will promote good social and mental health. However, some problems may seem too big for you to handle through self-management. In such cases, you may need to seek help from mental and social health care professionals.

Check Your Knowledge

1. Give examples of four physical needs that are basic to survival.
2. Explain why meeting the need for self-actualization is a lifelong process.
3. What are three traits that help people with good social health relate to others?
4. How does social development take place in the childhood years?
5. What are five guidelines for clear, open communication?
6. What are five tips for resolving conflict?
7. Which of the following would be an assertive way to express an opinion?
   A. Anyone who would buy that CD is an idiot. That music stinks.
   B. I would not buy that CD. I don't like that type of music.
   C. I'm not sure how I feel about that CD. What do you think?
   D. I would not buy that CD because I already have a lot of CDs. Besides, my mom says that music gives her a headache.
8. True or false. Having a negative self-concept means a person does not value himself or herself as a person.
9. How can a relaxed, resilient personality help a person maintain positive mental health?
10. Explain the two-way relationship between physical health and mental health.
11. Give three examples of each of the following types of roles: family, school or job, and community.

12. Why should a person prioritize "needs improvement" behaviors when preparing a self-management plan?

13. What are three resources a person should consider when evaluating alternatives for reaching a life-change goal?

14. What is the final step in a self-management plan?

15. What is often the focus of professional therapy for social and mental health problems?

Put Learning into Action

1. To practice your written and electronic communication skills, connect with an e-mail partner in a family and consumer sciences class from another school. Ask what projects your partner is engaged in for his or her classes. Share information about the projects you are doing for your classes.

2. Write a brief description of a situation that would require assertiveness skills. In a small group, role-play the situation to practice using assertiveness skills. Video-tape your role-play and invite your classmates to evaluate your use of the skills.

3. Make a self-esteem bulletin board. Cover the board with plain paper and invite classmates to write esteem-building phrases on it. Discuss how these phrases relate to human needs in Maslow's hierarchy.

4. Prepare a self-management plan for making a life change to promote positive social or mental health.

Explore Further

1. Imagine you are an elected official. Develop a proposal for a local or national program you would like to initiate to foster social or mental health. State the overall goal of the program. Give your rationale for why the program would be an effective way to achieve the goal. Provide details on how the program would operate, who would oversee it, and who would be served by it. Prepare a general budget estimating how much it would cost to start the program and keep it running for one year. Cite references to support your cost estimates.

2. As a class, develop a questionnaire about family, work, and community roles. Questions should identify what the respondents' roles are and how much time and energy they devote to each role. Questions should also focus on how satisfied respondents are with the balance in their lives. Finally, the questionnaire should invite respondents to share any tips they might have for maintaining balance in their lives. Each student should have two working parents complete the questionnaire. Compile your findings into an article for the school or local newspaper.

Chapter 18

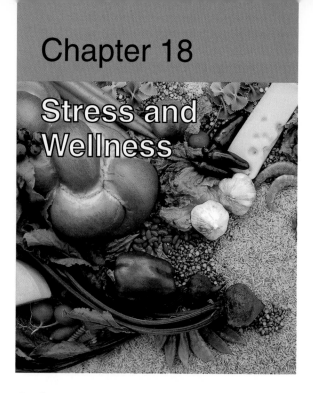

Stress and Wellness

● Learn the Language

stress	fight or flight
negative stress	response
distress	biofeedback
positive stress	support system
stressor	progressive muscle
life-change events	relaxation
daily hassles	self-talk

● Objectives

After reading this chapter, you will be able to
- recognize potential sources of stress in your life.
- describe the effects of stress on physical and mental health.
- explain how recognizing signs of stress, using support systems, relaxing, and using positive self-talk can help you manage stress.
- use strategies to prevent stress.

How would the following events affect you physically and emotionally?
- Your teacher announces there will be a unit test in two days, and you have not yet read the chapters.
- You and your dating partner had a major disagreement last night.
- Basketball tryouts are tomorrow afternoon, and you have been dreaming of making the team for six months.
- You won a contest, and suddenly people in your school and community are treating you like a minor celebrity.

Each situation described above can produce stress. **Stress** is the inner agitation you feel when you are exposed to change. Many people associate stress with the feeling of being tense. See 18-1.

All people experience daily stress throughout their lives. Some stress is good for you and some is bad. In this chapter you will learn to recognize when stress can be positive. You will also read about how to manage the stress that can harm your state of wellness.

● Stress Is Part of Life

To understand how stress can affect your life, you will need to examine the kinds of stress. You will also need to be aware of what causes stress and how your body reacts to it.

● Types of Stress

Most people are aware that some stress in their lives tends to motivate them to achieve and perform well. They also know stress can be negative. Both types of stress impact social, emotional, and physical performance.

● Negative Stress or Distress

When you see an event or situation as a threat to your well-being, you are likely to feel

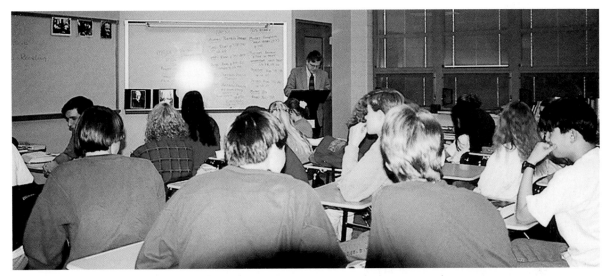

18-1 The announcement of an upcoming test may cause students to experience stress.

negative stress. **Negative stress***,* or ***distress****,* is harmful stress. Negative stress can reduce your effectiveness by causing you to be fearful and perform poorly. If a classmate threatens to tell a teacher you cheated on a test, you will probably feel negative stress. Fear over whether the teacher will confront you about cheating may keep you from focusing on class material. This, in turn, may keep you from doing well in the class.

Another time distress can occur is when you experience a number of minor changes within a short period. For instance, suppose you have a job and are regularly scheduled to work from six to nine on Thursday evenings. On Wednesday, your manager calls and asks you to work on Friday evening instead of Thursday. This change in your schedule might not seem like a problem. However, imagine it occurred on the same weekend your best friend from out of town was planning to visit you. Suppose you have no car available to get to work. Now, your work schedule, your visiting plans, and your travel arrangements are all being changed at the same time. This many changes can cause distress.

Distress can result when one change continues to affect you for a long time, too. In the previous work example, suppose your manager asked you to make Friday your regular night to work. The first week, the Friday schedule might not bother you. However, imagine you missed seeing a movie with your friends on the second Friday. On the third week, you had to turn down a party invitation because of your job. On the fourth week, you had to skip going to a basketball game. By this time, the negative stress caused by the change in your work schedule is probably starting to build.

● **Positive Stress**

Stress is not always bad. ***Positive stress*** motivates you to accomplish challenging goals. For example, athletes often feel positive stress when they are competing. The atmosphere during practice may not always prompt athletes to excel. At times, practice can feel like drudgery, and some athletes may have to push themselves to keep working. However, the atmosphere changes when opponents, fans, and officials are present. Athletes' response to this change in atmosphere is a form of positive stress. This stress of competition is the force that spurs athletes to give their best performance. They are inspired to achieve the goal of winning. See 18-2.

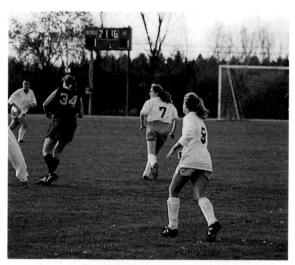

18-2 The positive stress of competition helps athletes work toward the reward of winning.

● Causes of Stress

A source of stress is called a **stressor**. It is a change in circumstances that produces feelings of agitation and discomfort. Stressors can be physical, such as a change in your daily routine. Stressors can also be emotional, such as an increase in the amount of pressure you feel at school. A stressor is what begins the stress response.

Some researchers refer to major stressors that occur to people as **life-change events**. These are situations that can greatly alter a person's lifestyle. Death, divorce, remarriage, legal problems, and sudden unemployment are examples of life-change events. The kind and number of life-change events a person experiences directly affect his or her stress level.

Not all the stress people experience comes from life-change events. Minor stressors that produce tension are often known as **daily hassles**. Long lines, heavy traffic, and misplaced belongings are common daily hassles. These types of persistent annoyances can strain a person's body, mind, and relationships. The result is negative stress. See 18-3.

Teens have many stressors in their lives. They face the physical changes associated with body growth and hormonal influences. Teens may also encounter emotional and

Common Stressors	
Life-Change Events	
Death of a family member	New baby in the household
Parents' divorce or separation	Pregnancy
Personal injury	Moving
Change in health of family member	Outstanding personal achievement
Loss of a job and financial resources	Parent loses or changes job
Death of a close friend	Change in schools, church, clubs, sports activities
Daily Hassles	
Misplacing or losing items	School/job responsibilities
Concern about physical appearance	Change in sleeping habits
Arguments in the household	Loneliness
Difficulties with friends	Peer pressure
Trouble with boyfriend/girlfriend	Uncertainty of the future
Decision making	Money concerns

18-3 What other stressors could you add to these lists?

social changes in relationships with family members and friends. Taking more challenging classes and making decisions that affect the future can create mental changes for teens, too.

Most people can manage one or two stressors at a time. However, life seems to present an overload of stressors to some people. For example, when a divorce occurs, family financial resources may become stretched to the limits. To help, a teen may get an after-school job. The job involves pressure to perform well. It also takes time away from schoolwork, which leads to stress over grades. Over time, the snowball effect of one stressor adding to another can damage a person's physical, social, and emotional well-being.

● The Body's Response to Stress

Your body goes through three stages when responding to a stressful event. These stages are alarm, resistance, and exhaustion.

To understand these three stages, imagine you just started a job in a fast-food restaurant. It is dinnertime and a long line of people is forming at your counter. Customers are reeling off orders, coworkers are bustling around, and children are crying in the background. You are trying to listen to orders, make change, package food, and keep the line moving. Suddenly one of your coworkers bumps into you. Your initial *alarm* response may include fear of spilling the food you are carrying. You may also feel mad at the coworker and discouraged about the delay in filling the customer's order.

These emotional responses during the alarm stage are coupled with physical responses. Inside your body, hormones are being released into your bloodstream. These hormones will cause your heart rate and blood pressure to increase. You will start breathing faster. Your face may flush, and you are likely to perspire. You may feel the muscles in your arms, legs, and stomach becoming tense. Your hearing will sharpen and your eyes will widen. All these reactions indicate your body is gathering its resources to conquer danger or escape to safety. This reaction to stress is often called the **fight or flight response**. See 18-4.

The next stage of the body's response to stress is *resistance.* As you serve customers and the line at your counter becomes shorter, your stress level will subside. Your body systems begin to return to their prestress state. You may stop perspiring and your arms, legs, and stomach may begin to relax.

If the rush of customers continues for several hours, your body may never have a chance to recover. In this case, you will progress to the third response stage of *exhaustion.* Physical and mental fatigue are a part of this stage. You may feel tired and have a hard time thinking clearly. Your inner resources to resist and adapt to stress are gone.

Suppose you experience this kind of stress every evening at work. Soon your body will automatically become tense each day as you begin your shift. After months of working under these stressful conditions, tensions may begin to spill over into other areas of your life. You may find you are becoming less and less able to handle minor daily stressors. Over time, your body will begin to show signs of weakness. If lifestyle changes and stress reduction methods do not occur, physical illness may follow.

● Effects of Stress on Health

Stress can affect your health. A continuous high level of negative stress can weaken body systems and increase your risks for certain diseases. Stress can also tax your emotional well-being. The type of personality you have can affect the degree to which stress impacts your health.

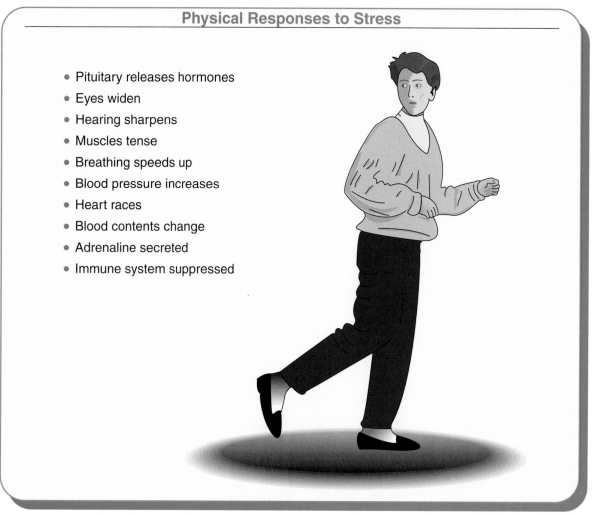

Physical Responses to Stress

- Pituitary releases hormones
- Eyes widen
- Hearing sharpens
- Muscles tense
- Breathing speeds up
- Blood pressure increases
- Heart races
- Blood contents change
- Adrenaline secreted
- Immune system suppressed

18-4 The fight or flight response will trigger certain physical reactions.

● Effects on Physical Health

Over time and without your awareness, too much stress can damage your physical health. Some researchers believe stress may be the greatest contributor to illness in the modern, industrialized world.

You read earlier about physical reactions triggered by the release of stress hormones into your bloodstream. You breathe harder and faster to bring more oxygen into your body. Your heart beats more rapidly to quickly pump that oxygen out to the muscles. Your liver releases glucose and fat cells release fat into the bloodstream. Your blood pressure increases to speed the glucose and fat to the muscles for use as energy. All these reactions are intended to prepare your body to take action. Your muscles are getting ready to either defend you against the source of stress or run from it.

Many sources of stress in today's society do not require a physical battle or escape to safety. For instance, you may feel stress about auditioning for a part in the school play. However, dealing with this stress will not involve fighting or running from the director of the play. Therefore, the increase in your heart rate and blood pressure serve only to strain your heart and blood vessels.

The extra fat released into your bloodstream may accumulate in your arteries. You can see how these results of stress can increase your risk for coronary heart disease, hypertension, and stroke.

● Effects on the Immune System

Your body's immune system helps protect you from getting diseases. During periods of stress, your immune system defenses can become lowered. This may explain why you feel run-down after a long siege of stress. During these times, you may find you have decreased resistance to infections, such as colds and flu. For example, during midterms or finals, you may be very worried about passing the tests. When the tests are over, your immune system may be so depressed you develop a cold.

● Effects on Sleep Patterns

When stress hormones are released into your bloodstream, you are likely to experience heightened awareness. Your senses of sight and hearing become keener. Your mind may be racing with thoughts of the stressor and how to address it. You may have reached the exhaustion stage of the stress response. However, your increased level of mental activity can keep you from falling asleep quickly. It can also prevent you from enjoying a sound, peaceful sleep that will refresh you. This lack of rest can add to your stress and further depress your immune system. See 18-5.

● Effects on Eating Habits

When stress hormones are circulating in the bloodstream, the body treats digesting food as a low priority. The body focuses its resources on the needs of the muscles and nerves rather than the digestive system.

Stress often affects people's eating habits and emotional responses to food. This is why stress is sometimes a factor in body weight problems. During emotional stress, some people nibble foods nervously. Others

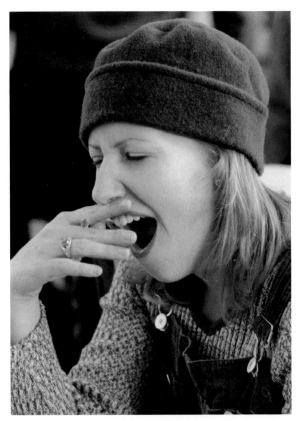

18-5 If stress causes you to lose sleep, you may be too tired during the day to fulfill school responsibilities. This, in turn, may cause you to feel more stressed.

binge, which involves eating excessive amounts of food in a short time. Eating may seem to relieve their feelings of frustration. Some people cannot eat when under stress. They do not feel hungry because they are so focused on the source of stress. Others may experience upset stomach. Stress can also contribute to the development of anorexia nervosa and bulimia nervosa. (These disorders were described in Chapter 14, "Eating Disorders.")

Eating habits affected by stress may change your nutritional status. Eating out of boredom or tension may cause you to eat excess calories. Not eating because you are too excited or nervous may cause you to lose weight and feel tired and cranky. These outcomes can compound stress.

● Effects on Emotional Health

Too much stress can make you irritable, tense, and anxious. You may reach a point where you lack the strength to keep preventable sources of stress out of your life. When this happens, worry can overtake productive thinking. See 18-6.

Many social and emotional problems for teens can be related to undue amounts of stress in the family. Reports of substance abuse and suicide are often tied to an inability to cope with high stress levels. For adults, stress at work as well as in the family can take a toll on emotional health. Many cases of adults who abuse or abandon family members are linked to stress.

● Personality Factors and Stress

Research has found health outcomes may be more related to your reaction to stress than to its cause. Many factors determine how you respond to the stressors in your life. These include heredity, experiences, and outlook. See 18-7.

Each person has different attitudes toward a given stressor. What may be stressful to one person may not be stressful to another. For instance, one student may agonize over getting a C on a test. Another student might be pleased to do that well. Also, events that cause stress may vary from one time in your life to another. Getting bitten by a mosquito can seem fairly stressful to some children. However, many adults would scarcely notice a mosquito bite.

Your reactions to stress depend partly on your personality type. Personality type refers to your general way of looking at life. You may have heard people refer to type A and type B personalities. People with *type A personalities* can be divided into two groups—hostile and nonhostile. People in both groups tend to be driven to achieve goals. However, people in the hostile group tend to be impatient and

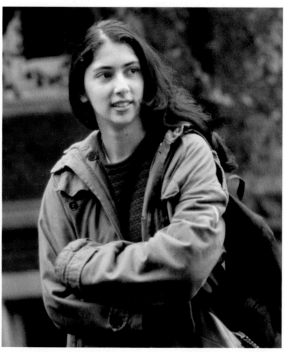

18-6 Stress at school may make you feel isolated and overwhelmed.

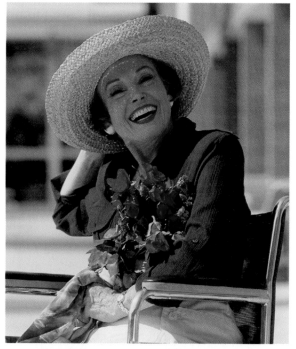

18-7 Positive attitudes can help people prevent stress from affecting their health.

pushy. They easily become irritated over stressful events. People in this group are at greatest risk for stress-related problems. People in the nonhostile type A group are less aggressive than hostile type A people. They are also less likely to become upset over stressful events. People with *type B personalities* are fairly relaxed and easy-going. Like nonhostile type A personalities, type B personalities are able to adapt to stress fairly well. See 18-8.

More important than your personality type is your attitude. If you approach problems as opportunities rather than threats, you are more likely to feel positive stress. Taking the following positive approaches toward life may help you have an easier time dealing with stressors:

- Look at new ideas and problems as exciting and challenging. Try not to feel threatened.

- Show a commitment to your work while showing a willingness to help others along the way.
- Take charge of your life, making decisions that will get you closer to your goals.
- Accept life's change with optimism rather than seeing it as a source of stress.
- Maintain positive health practices, taking good care of yourself.
- During times of personal crisis, talk openly with family members and friends.
- Be willing to seek the support of others. Do not wait for others to ask "What is wrong?"

Failing to react to life's events with these attitudes can create and promote excess personal stress. Excess stress can damage your mental and physical health. Stress can also hurt your relationships with family members and friends.

Managing Stress

You cannot avoid all stress. However, you can learn to manage it. Most healthy, productive people search for ways to manage the stress in their lives. Stress management provides them with opportunities for personal growth. Viewing stress as positive allows people the chance to be creative. Learning how to adapt to negative stress helps people rationally deal with the changes that occur throughout life.

You can use a number of techniques to help you manage stress. Begin by learning to recognize the signs of stress. Rely on available support systems. Learn how to relax and use positive self-talk.

The key is to choose the methods that most easily fit into your lifestyle. Combine a variety of methods for greatest effects on total health. Be sensitive to other techniques that seem to help you relax.

At the very least, learning how to lessen the negative effects of stress can help you enjoy life more. At best, you can reduce your

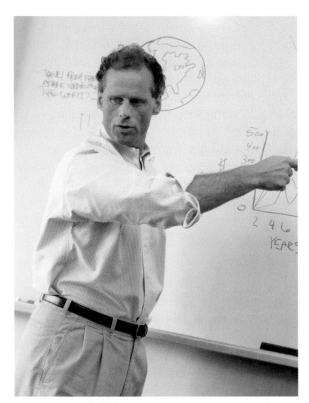

18-8 A person with a type B personality might find giving a presentation easier than a person with a type A personality would.

risks of disease and improve your state of wellness.

Recognize Signs of Stress

Identifying the warning signs of stress in your life is an important first step in stress management. Your emotions, behaviors, and physical health may all give you clues that negative stress is starting to take a toll. Frustration, irritability, and depression are common emotional signs of distress. Withdrawing from friends, grinding your teeth, and forgetting details are behaviors that may warn you of negative stress. Headaches, upset stomach, and fatigue are health indicators that you may have too much stress in your life.

You can learn to read your body's stress signals through biofeedback. **Biofeedback** is a technique of focusing on involuntary bodily processes in order to control them. Using biofeedback involves being aware of such conditions as your breath and pulse rates. Hard breathing or a rapid pulse rate may be a sign of distress. When you realize you are breathing hard or your pulse is racing, you will know you may be under stress. Then you can make a conscious effort to relax and bring your breathing and pulse back to normal levels. Through biofeedback, you may be able to avoid a headache or calm a nervous stomach caused by stress.

When you become aware that you are experiencing stress symptoms, try to determine what is causing them. Then you can take steps to either deal with or eliminate the source of the stressors.

If signs of stress occur on a regular basis, you may need to increase your stress management efforts. This will help you avoid the harmful effects of stress.

Use Support Systems

You need to identify people who can be part of your support system in times of stress or crisis. A **support system** is a person or group of people who can provide you with help and emotional comfort. Family members and friends can listen and offer insights to problems. School counselors, social workers, and psychologists can give their professional opinions about how to deal with stressful situations.

You must be willing to turn to these people when you are feeling overwhelmed. Your support system cannot help you if you do not access it. See 18-9.

Remember that you are part of other people's support systems. In this role, you can support people who are under stress by being a good listener. You may need to encourage others to talk about situations that are bothering them. If they are not ready to talk, do not pressure them. If they want to talk, however, be ready to listen attentively. Maintain eye contact and do not interrupt. Avoid offering advice unless someone asks you for it. Many times, people are not looking for advice. They simply want someone to listen to and understand their problems.

You may sometimes need to seek the help of an adult on your friend's behalf. Someone who mentions suicide is at great risk. Someone who talks about drinking or getting high to handle stress may also need professional help. Parents, teachers, guidance counselors, and members of the clergy can provide assistance when a friend is in potential danger.

Learn How to Relax

Learning how to play and see the joys of living will help relieve stress. Set aside time to enjoy leisure activities with your friends and family. Different people find different activities relaxing. For you, leisure may be listening to music, reading a book, or enjoying your favorite hobby. For someone else, playing sports or working out may be more relaxing. Learn to know when you need to take a break from work and other demands.

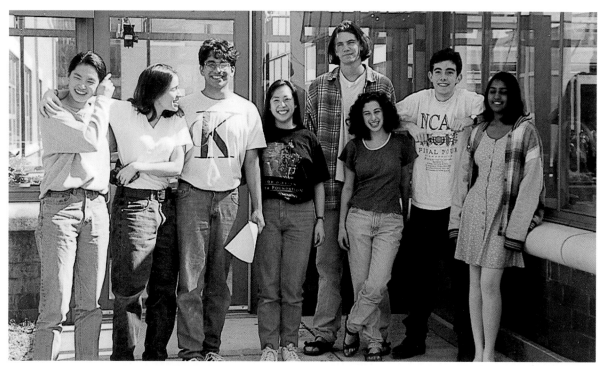

18-9 Friends can give support and comfort during times of stress.

● Relaxation Techniques

Besides enjoyable activities, you can use some techniques to help you relax when you begin to feel excess stress. One of these techniques is deep breathing. This involves pulling slow, regular breaths deep into the lungs. Then you release each breath in a long, controlled exhale. Deep breathing calms the whole body. It forces you to slow down and focus on something other than stressors. You can use this breathing technique almost anywhere. You might be driving in heavy traffic, standing in a long line, or sitting in class before a test. A few minutes of deep breathing in any of these situations can help you feel more relaxed.

Another technique sometimes used to reduce stress is *progressive muscle relaxation*. This method involves slowly tensing and then relaxing different groups of muscles. Begin with your feet. Then gradually work your way up the body to your legs, midsection, hands, arms, shoulders, neck, and face. Tense each muscle group, hold for five seconds, then release. Try to clear your mind of all thoughts, focusing only on your muscle groups. As you release the tension in your muscles, you will also be releasing stress. This technique will probably work best in a setting where you can be alone for a few minutes. You may find listening to quiet music while you perform this technique helps you relax further. Figure 18-10 describes other ways to practice relaxation before stressful events.

● Use Positive Self-Talk

Self-talk refers to your internal conversations about yourself and the situations you face. Unfortunately, self-talk for many people is filled with negative statements, such as "I'm stupid. I'll never be able to figure out how to solve this problem." This type of self-talk is harmful. It drains your emotional energy and produces stress. You begin to

Stress and Tension-Fighting Exercises

☺ Close your eyes and concentrate on breathing slowly. Imagine you are going down stairs in a 15-story building. Each time you exhale, you have reached a lower floor. When you reach ground level, resume normal activities by inhaling and counting to three.

☺ Close your eyes. Think of a beautiful scene and imagine you are there. Is it your last vacation spot or a favorite spot in your home? Spend a moment looking and enjoying every detail. Listen to the sounds. Can you smell the good smells?

☺ This exercise is intended to relax the muscles of your neck and back. Sit up straight. Let your chin fall to your neck as you exhale. Inhale and move your head back slowly. Pretend you are trying to touch the back of your neck with your head. Then pull your shoulders up and try to touch them with your ears. Release your muscles and relax.

☺ Take a deep breath. As you do, scan your body for tense muscles. Check out each group: face, neck, shoulders, arms, abdomen, legs, feet. Seek out the tense ones. As you exhale, relax all that are tense.

18-10 These relaxation exercises are easy to do, even in public places such as a classroom.

feel awful because you tell yourself how incompetent you are.

Positive self-talk, on the other hand, is beneficial and helps reduce stress. This type of self-talk is filled with statements such as "I'm as smart as the next person. If I take my time, I'm sure I'll be able to figure out how to solve this problem." As you substitute positive statements for negative ones in your self-talk, you will build your confidence. When you feel positive about your abilities, you can more effectively deal with life's stressors. See 18-11.

Preventing Stress

Perhaps the best stress management technique is to prevent stress from occurring in the first place. You cannot stop all sources of stress. However, addressing the root causes of stress can go a long way toward improving your overall well-being. Root causes include lack of time, physical illness, fatigue, and substance abuse. Using time wisely and staying physically fit can help you keep many situations from turning into stressors. Eating nutritiously and getting enough sleep will help you prevent stress, too.

Learn to Manage Your Time

One key cause of stress for many people is poor time management. Imagine you have three tests tomorrow, a paper to write, and an after-school job. Having too little time to handle all the tasks you need to do can produce stress.

The overwhelming feeling of facing a number of tasks can be paralyzing. You may not know where to begin. You might feel there is no point in starting work because you will never be able to complete everything. Overcoming your fear and taking action is the only way to eliminate this source of stress.

Using some time management strategies can help you avoid the stress of having too little time. You may want to study how you currently use your time by keeping a time-activity diary. Record how you spend the minutes of your day. Study your results.

As you review your time-activity diary, do you see periods when you could be using time more efficiently? Perhaps you could double up on some tasks, such as making a phone call while washing dishes. Maybe you could spend less time watching television or looking for misplaced items.

Positive Self-Talk

Instead of saying . . .	Try saying . . .
• everything I do must be perfect.	• I will do the best I can.
• if I want it done right, I have to do it myself.	• I can delegate tasks to others.
• my life is running me.	• I can take control of my life.
• I must not fail.	• I will try my best.
• I feel life is treating me unfairly.	• I will get through hard times— better days are ahead.

18-11 Try using positive self-talk to relieve stress.

Use what you learn from your time-activity diary to plan a time schedule. The best way to handle important tasks is to assign a priority to each one. Decide how many minutes and hours you will need to complete it. Write a schedule showing when you plan to do each task. Schedule the tasks with the highest priority first. This will give you some idea of what you can accomplish in one day. You may not have time to do everything, but using a schedule should help you do the most important tasks.

Do not forget to schedule time for leisure as well as work. Without taking time to relax, your efforts to complete tasks may become less efficient. For example, you may have trouble focusing on your studies if you become tense and tired from studying too long. Taking a short break can refresh you and help you work more effectively, 18-12.

Realize you do not need to do everything perfectly. Also keep in mind you do not need to do every task yourself. When possible, delegate responsibilities to other people.

When other people request your time, examine their requests. If you have a chance to learn or do something new, you may want to accept the opportunity. This may mean giving up an existing event in your schedule. For instance, going to a book signing of your favorite author may mean skipping a movie with your friends. You may have to turn down requests that interfere with achieving higher priority goals. Avoid adding to your level of stress by overloading your schedule.

Cross items off your schedule as you accomplish them. This will give you a feeling of success. The stress of your schedule should lessen with each task you complete.

● Eat a Nutritious Diet

Health problems can be a major source of stress. Therefore, steps you take to maintain good health are also steps for preventing stress. Eating a nutritious diet is one such step.

Eating right means following the recommendations of the Food Guide Pyramid on a day-to-day basis. Regularly choose the appropriate number of servings of healthful, nutrient-dense foods. Limit snacks that are high in fat, sugar, and sodium. Also drink plenty of liquids to replenish body fluids and keep kidneys functioning properly.

You may have seen stress formula nutrient supplements on store shelves. Stress causes the release of hormones that trigger nerve reactions. However, a high stress level does not increase your need for nutrients involved in hormone synthesis and nerve functioning. On the other hand, if stress is prolonged, it can negatively affect your diet, exercise, and sleeping. In this case, it can deplete your nutrient stores and increase your risk of disease. Unfortunately, taking vitamin and mineral supplements will not reduce your stress level. If you eat a healthful diet,

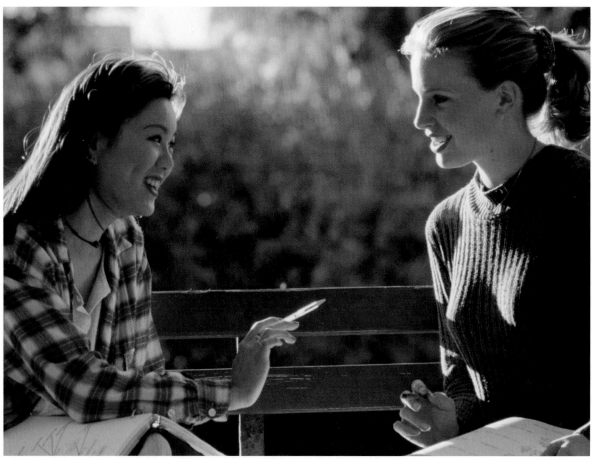

18-12 Taking short breaks during study time will help you feel more energized when you are working.

you will be getting the nutrients your body needs to respond to stressful situations.

Stay Physically Fit

Staying physically fit can help you prevent stress. Your body and mind must work together to solve problems. Regular physical activity helps you stay healthy. It gives your body the strength to respond more efficiently to stressful situations. Physical activity refreshes your mind, too. It gives you the renewed energy to think more clearly about solutions to problems.

Physical activity also helps relieve stress when it occurs. You can work out frustrations and release tensions through movement. When your body is giving you signs of stress, plan an activity break. Participate in a favorite sport. Walk, swim, jog, skate, bicycle, or do some other activity. While your body is moving, your mind is less likely to be focused on your problems. After your activity, you may find you are able to face troubles with a clear mind and new insights. See 18-13.

Get Adequate Rest

Like staying fit and eating well, getting enough rest will help you prevent stress by guarding your health. Most people need at least seven to eight hours of sleep each night. Getting enough sleep can make you more alert, less irritable, and better able to manage stressful situations. When you have had adequate sleep, you should awaken feeling refreshed and ready to start your daily tasks.

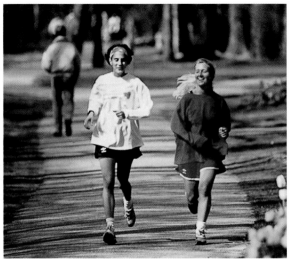

Photo courtesy of University Relations, MSU. Bruce A. Fox, Photographer

18-13 Physical activity is a positive alternative for managing stress.

● Avoid Substance Abuse

Avoiding substance abuse is a key way to prevent stress. People who think alcohol and other drugs relieve stress are mistaken. These substances only temporarily mask the symptoms of stress. At the same time, they create a huge new source of stress for people who abuse them.

The use of alcohol and other drugs can cause stress by creating physical and mental health problems. Substance abuse can be a tremendous source of tension in relationships with others. It can also add to stress by increasing the possibilities of fights, accidents, and arrests.

No technique exists for preventing all sources of stress. Likewise, no strategy will instantly eliminate any stressors that creep into your life. However, being aware of stressful situations will help you take action to manage stress before it gets out of hand. Being aware of how stress can affect your health will prompt you to try to manage stress before it builds. See 18-14.

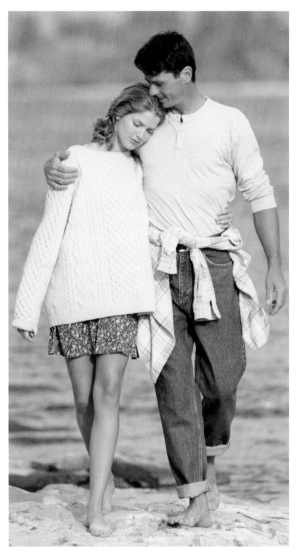

18-14 Vacation time helps people release stress that has built up from everyday responsibilities.

Chapter 18 Review

Summary

Everyone experiences stress in their lives. Some forms of stress are negative and can harm your physical and emotional health. Other forms of stress are positive. They can motivate you and make your life exciting. The causes of stress vary from person to person. They can range from daily hassles to life-change events. The body responds to stress in three stages that each involves a number of specific reactions.

Stress can affect health in a variety of ways. Physical health outcomes include effects on the immune system as well as effects on sleep patterns and eating habits. Effects of stress on emotional health are often exhibited as irritability and anxiety. Your reactions to stress, which are partly a factor of your personality, determine how stress will affect you.

You can take steps to manage stress. Learning to recognize your body's initial signs of stress can help you deal with stressors quickly. Using support systems, relaxation techniques, and positive self-talk can help you reduce the impact of stress.

You can prevent some sources of stress from creeping into your life. Learning to manage your time can help you avoid much stress. Staying physically fit, eating a nutritious diet, and getting adequate rest are also keys to keeping stress at bay. Avoiding substance abuse is an important stress prevention step, too.

Check Your Knowledge

1. Describe two types of situations that can cause negative stress.
2. List three life-change events and three daily hassles that are common sources of stress.
3. What are the three stages of the body's response to stress?
4. What are three internal physical reactions that occur when the body releases stress hormones?
5. How can stress affect the body's immune system?
6. How can the effects of stress on sleep patterns further add to stress?
7. What are three eating habits or emotional responses to food that can be triggered by stress?
8. What are four positive approaches toward life that may help people deal with stressors?
9. Give one example each of an emotional, behavioral, and physical sign of stress.
10. List three people who may be part of a person's support system.
11. Describe two relaxation techniques people can use when they begin to feel excess stress.
12. Which of the following is *not* a time management strategy that would help avoid stress?
    A. Delegate responsibilities.
    B. Double up on tasks.
    C. Prioritize tasks.
    D. Remove leisure activities from the schedule.
13. True or false. Physical activity can help a person both prevent and manage stress.
14. True or false. Taking stress formula nutrient supplements can help reduce a person's stress level.
15. Why are alcohol and drug use not effective stress-management strategies?

Put Learning into Action

1. Keep a "stress diary" for one day. Every time you feel stress, write down the source of the stress. At the end of the day, categorize your list of stressors into two groups. The groups are stressors you can change and stressors you

cannot change. For each stressor you can change, jot down steps you can take to reduce the source of stress. With a trusted, caring friend, talk about ways you can approach the root causes of your stressors.

2. Practice two of the relaxation techniques described in the chapter. Write a brief evaluation stating which technique you found more effective and explaining your choice.

3. Practice changing negative self-talk into positive self-talk. Working with a partner, list 10 common negative self-talk statements. Take turns suggesting how to turn each statement into positive self-talk.

4. Prepare a bulletin board showing ways to manage and prevent stress. A possible title might be "How to Safely Let the Steam Out of the Kettle." Use pictures to convey such concepts as relaxation, nutritious food, physical activity, hobbies, and time management.

Explore Further

1. Research the relationship between personality types and stress responses. Summarize your findings in a poster presentation.

2. Use the Internet or library resources to research statistics of work-related injuries and employee absences. See if you can find any research linking employee stress levels with injuries and absences. Illustrate your findings in a chart or graph format.

3. Investigate a prescription drug used to treat stress disorders. Write a report describing the drug's effectiveness and possible side effects.

Chapter 19

The Use and Abuse of Drugs

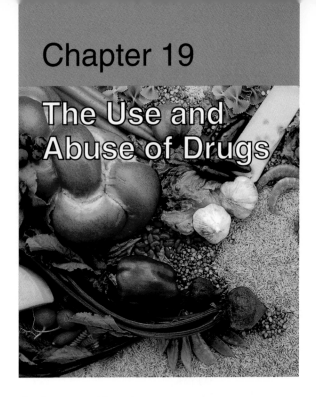

● Learn the Language

drug	amphetamine
medicine	tolerance
prescription drug	overdose
side effect	secondhand
over-the-counter	smoking
(OTC) drug	smokeless tobacco
generic drug	depressant
food-drug interaction	cirrhosis
drug misuse	alcoholism
drug abuse	inhalant
illegal drug	narcotic
addiction	opiate
withdrawal	hallucinogen
psychoactive drug	designer drug
stimulant	anabolic steroid

● Objectives

After studying this chapter, you will be able to

- describe appropriate uses of drugs as medicine.
- distinguish between drug misuse and drug abuse.
- identify health risks associated with the abuse of stimulants, depressants, hallucinogens, and anabolic steroids.
- suggest ways to offer help for someone with a substance abuse problem.

More drugs and medicines are available today than ever before. A **drug** is any substance other than food or water that changes the way the body or mind operates. A **medicine** is a drug used to treat an ailment or improve a disabling condition.

At least one out of five people takes medicine every day. Unfortunately, much of this medicine is unnecessary. Taking unnecessary drugs is a health risk, not a health benefit. Misuse of drugs can have serious health consequences.

This chapter will describe how various types of drugs can affect your health. It will also discuss the physical, emotional, and social effects of the misuse and abuse of drugs.

● Drugs as Medicine

Drugs used for medical reasons may be grouped according to their uses, as shown in 19-1. The list is not complete. New drugs are always being developed, and old ones are discontinued. Legal drugs are available to the consumer through prescription or as over-the-counter drugs.

● Prescription Drugs

A **prescription drug** is a medicine that can only be obtained from a pharmacy with a written or phoned order from a doctor. See 19-2. A physician has the training to decide

Medical Drug Classifications

Drug Group	Use
Analgesic	Relieve pain
Antacid	Reduce stomach acidity levels
Anticoagulant	Dissolve and prevent formation of blood clots
Anticonvulsant	Prevent seizures
Antidepressant	Reduce depression and anxiety
Antihistamine	Treat allergies
Antihypertensive	Reduce high blood pressure
Anti-infective	Fight infections; destroy disease-causing organisms
Anti-inflammatory	Reduce fever and inflammation
Antineoplastic (Chemotherapeutic)	Fight cancers
Diuretic	Reduce water retention

19-1 Each drug is usually classified according its primary effect on the body.

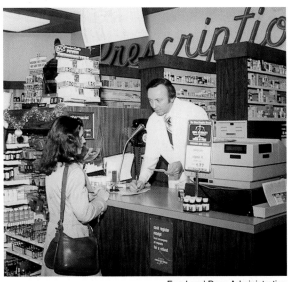

Food and Drug Administration

19-2 The sale of prescription drugs is carefully regulated by law to protect consumers.

which prescription drug best suits the needs of a patient.

When a doctor prescribes medicine for you, you need to be sure you know how to use it effectively. You should ask your physician and pharmacist the following questions about a prescription drug.

- What will it do and what results can be expected?
- How often should it be taken?
- If other medicines are currently being taken, how will it interact with them?
- Should the medicine be taken on a full or empty stomach?
- Should certain foods be avoided?
- What are its side effects?

A *side effect* is a reaction that differs from the desired effect. However, it occurs alongside the desired effect. For instance, many drugs that relieve the sneezing and runny nose associated with colds and allergies also cause drowsiness. Most drugs produce some side effects in some people. For most people, however, the side effects are not even noticeable.

With each prescription, pharmacists often provide an information sheet explaining what the medicine is and how it should be used. Possible side effects are explained, too, as well as other conditions to watch. Your health is at stake, so use prescription drugs according to directions. See 19-3.

● Over-the-Counter Drugs

Over-the-counter (OTC) drugs are the drugs sold legally that do not require a physician's prescription. OTC drugs are often called nonprescription drugs. They are generally purchased off the shelves of supermarkets, drugstores, and convenience stores. When used as directed, OTC drugs are not as strong as prescription drugs. They also pose less potential risk than prescription drugs, even when self-administered.

The Food and Drug Administration (FDA) regulates the manufacture and sale of all drugs, including OTC drugs. A drug manufacturer must provide conclusive evidence to the FDA that a drug is safe and effective for the intended use. Only then is it approved for sale.

As a consumer, you decide which OTC drug to buy to treat a health problem or ailment. Read package labels carefully when choosing these products. Avoid buying OTC products designed to relieve symptoms you do not have.

When you have questions, ask your doctor or pharmacist. After choosing a product, be sure to read all information that comes with the drug. Heed all cautions and do not take more than the recommended dosage. Using the medication incorrectly could be dangerous and may damage your health.

● Generic Versus Trade Name Drugs

Most drugs have three names: a chemical name, a generic name, and a trade or brand name. The *chemical drug name* describes the chemical composition of a drug. The *generic drug name* is the officially accepted name of the drug. A *brand name* or *trade name* is a name a manufacturer uses to promote a drug product.

When the FDA approves a new drug for sale, the manufacturer has exclusive

---

Using Prescription Drugs Safely

- Ask the physician or the pharmacist about the medicine if you are not sure what it is and how it will help you. Ask whether the prescription can be refilled without a doctor's appointment.
- Read all the instructions and follow them carefully. Do not take more or less of the drug than the physician recommends.
- Take the medicine for the prescribed period of time even if you begin to feel better.
- While taking the drug, be sure to tell your physician about any unusual symptoms you experience.
- Use only one medicine at a time unless the physician indicates otherwise. Make sure the physician knows about all other drugs you are taking, even headache remedies, cold medicine, laxatives, or other nonprescription drugs.
- Never drink alcoholic beverages when taking medicine. Find out what other foods or medicines should be avoided.
- Never take someone else's prescribed medicine.
- Safely dispose of old medicines.

19-3 Follow these guidelines to use prescription drugs safely.

marketing rights to it for 17 years. During this period, the drug is available only under the company's brand name. See 19-4. After 17 years, other manufacturers can sell the product under their own brand names and/or under the generic name. This is true for both prescription and OTC drugs.

A *generic drug* is a drug available under its generic name. For example, acetaminophen is the generic name for a common OTC drug. It relieves headache and pain in people sensitive to aspirin. You can buy it labeled *Tylenol, Anacin, Datril,* or any of the many other brand names currently used. You can also buy it labeled *acetaminophen,* which is the generic form of this product.

Many drug manufacturers produce a drug product in various forms, such as

powder, liquid, tablets, caplets, and capsules. They often sell a product under a brand name while providing it under its generic name to pharmacies. Generic drugs contain the same active ingredients as comparable trade name drugs. They are just as safe and effective as the brand name products.

A company usually spends money to advertise its brand name products. These costs are passed on to consumers. Therefore, brand name drugs usually cost 20 to 70 percent more than generic drugs.

● What the Body Does with Drugs

Like nutrients, drugs taken orally must be absorbed before they can have their intended effect on the body. Depending on the type of drug, absorption may take place in the mouth, stomach, or small intestine. As drugs are absorbed, they pass into the bloodstream. Then the blood carries them throughout the body.

The liver changes the structure of some drug chemicals to prepare them for use in the body. If the chemicals are toxic, the liver tries to convert them to less toxic substances. The liver also processes some chemicals for elimination, which usually occurs via the kidneys through the urine.

The body does not act on every chemical in the same way. Some chemicals may not be absorbed at all. Others may be absorbed, but not reduced to usable forms. The way the body uses the chemicals from drugs depends on many factors. These include the person's age, health status, use of other drugs, and diet. The timing and content of meals also affect the body's use of drugs. Genetics play a role in drug utilization, too.

● Food and Drug Interactions

Drugs and food can have physical and chemical effects on each other. These effects are called *food-drug interactions*. A food and a drug may affect the body differently

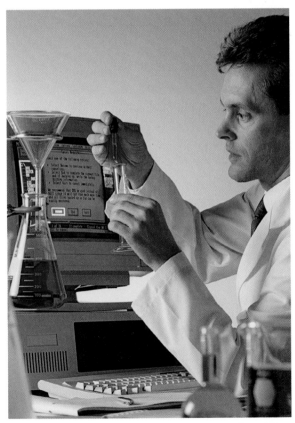

19-4 The exclusive right to a drug for its first 17 years helps to pay for the company's enormous research and development costs.

when consumed together than when consumed separately. Food-drug interactions may increase or decrease the effectiveness of the drug. They may also have an effect on nutrients.

Interference with Appetite

Long-term use of some drugs can alter a person's nutritional status. One way drugs can do this is by interfering with appetite. For instance, cancer treatment drugs often cause nausea, vomiting, diarrhea, and an altered sense of taste. Someone who is in a weakened state of health needs a full supply of nutrients to promote healing. This is why offering nutritious, appealing foods that will stimulate a patient's appetite is an important aspect of health care.

Interference with Absorption

The most common interaction between foods and drugs is an interference with absorption. Pills and capsules need to dissolve before they release chemicals into the rest of the body. The amount and type of liquid consumed with drugs can affect how fast they will dissolve and be absorbed.

Soft drinks and fruit juices, as in 19-5, can increase the acidity levels of the mouth and stomach. This can block the absorption of some drugs. The calcium and protein in milk can also interfere with the absorption of some drugs. Unless otherwise directed by a physician or pharmacist, you should drink plenty of water when taking medicine. Water allows most drugs to dissolve and be absorbed efficiently.

Food in the stomach slows the absorption of many drugs. For some drugs, this is desirable because it allows the chemicals to reach the body more gradually. For other drugs, slowed absorption is undesirable because it reduces their effectiveness. This is why it is important to read and follow information about taking drugs with food.

Just as food can interfere with drug absorption, drugs can interfere with nutrient

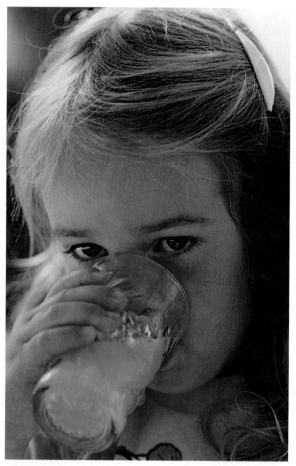

19-5 Juice and other beverages can prevent the absorption of some drugs. Drinking plenty of water is best.

absorption. For instance, laxatives can reduce the absorption of fat-soluble vitamins. Antacids can hinder the absorption of iron. Long-term use of antibiotics can decrease the absorption of fats, amino acids, and a number of vitamins and minerals. When the body does not absorb enough nutrients, deficiency symptoms may begin to appear.

Interference with Metabolism

Taking drugs for a long time may gradually reduce the amounts of some nutrients in the body. For instance, bacteria in the intestinal tract make vitamin K. Antibiotics taken to kill the bacteria causing an infection can kill these helpful bacteria, too. This will reduce the amount of vitamin K available in the body.

Some drugs have a diuretic effect. They cause the body to increase urine production. When the body loses fluids, it also loses some minerals. These losses can lead to nutritional problems.

The labels on medicine, provide warnings of potential food and drug interactions. You should consult your physician or pharmacist with any specific concerns you may have.

● Drug Misuse and Abuse

Drug misuse refers to using medicine in a way that was not intended. Drug misuse occurs among people, especially older adults, who take several medicines daily. Sometimes they confuse *what* to take *when.* See 19-6. Common examples of drug misuse include the following:

- taking more or less medicine than the recommended dose
- taking medicine more or less frequently per day or for longer or shorter periods than the directions state
- taking someone else's prescription medicine or sharing yours with others
- leaving medicine within children's reach, 19-7

Misusing drugs presents a serious health risk because it may result in adverse drug reactions. Dangerous interactions can occur when various drugs are combined. One medication may increase or decrease the effectiveness of other medications. Therefore, drugs should not be taken in combination unless directed by a doctor.

Drugs should never be taken with alcohol because it alters the effects of drugs. Depending on the quantity consumed and the frequency of use, alcohol can dull or magnify a drug's effects. Also, too much alcohol can

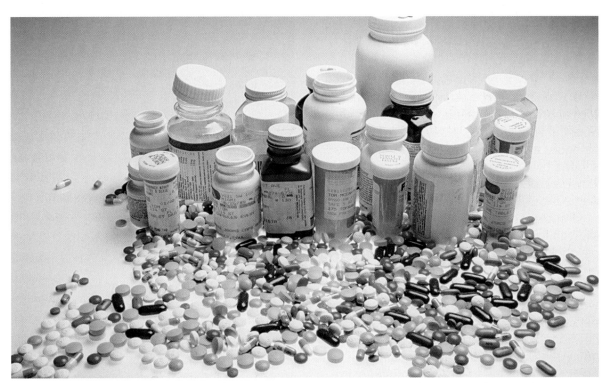

19-6 Even though pills and capsules have different sizes and colors, it is common for people to confuse them.

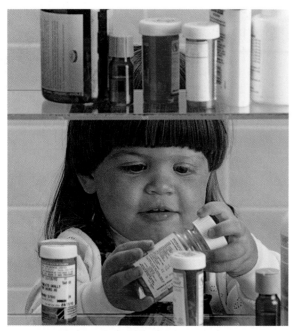

19-7 Special care must be taken to keep medicine away from children.

damage the liver, making it less able to process certain drugs.

Drug abuse is the use of a drug for other than medical reasons. Experimenting with drugs and their effects is one example of drug abuse. Any type of drug can be abused, but most drug abuse occurs with illegal drugs. *Illegal drugs*, also called "street drugs," are unlawful to buy or use. Many drugs fall in this category, some of which are legal when prescribed by a physician for treating patients. However, obtaining legal drugs through illegal means is against the law.

People who misuse or abuse drugs are likely to form addictions. An *addiction* is a psychological and/or physical dependence on a drug. When people stop taking an addictive drug, they are likely to go through *withdrawal*. Withdrawal symptoms vary from person to person. Symptoms also depend on how long and how much of the drug has been consumed. Withdrawal usually includes one or more of the following symptoms: irritability, nervousness, sleeplessness, nausea, vomiting, trembling, and cramps. To avoid

forming dependencies, patients must carefully follow their doctors' directions when taking drugs that can be addictive.

The most commonly misused and abused drugs are psychoactive drugs. *Psychoactive drugs* affect the central nervous system. They interfere with normal brain activity and can affect moods and feelings. Psychoactive drugs can serve beneficial purposes when administered according to accepted medical use. However, a few psychoactive drugs have no known medical benefits or are too unsafe to use. Psychoactive drugs include stimulants, depressants, and hallucinogens. See 19-8.

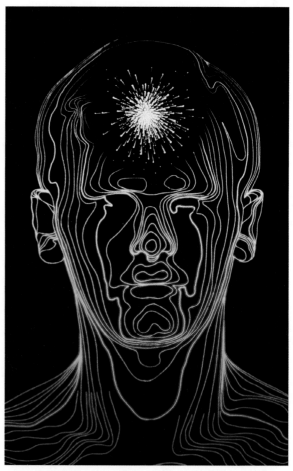

19-8 Psychoactive drugs affect the brain, influencing a person's mood, reasoning ability, and behavior.

Stimulants

Stimulants are a kind of psychoactive drug that speeds up the nervous system. They produce feelings of keen alertness and boundless energy. Stimulants have a number of effects on the body. They increase heart rate, blood pressure, and breathing rate. They can also affect appetite and cause headaches, dizziness, and insomnia. Many coffees, colas, and teas contain caffeine, a mild stimulant. Other well-known stimulants include amphetamines, cocaine, and nicotine.

Caffeine

Caffeine is a mild stimulant drug that occurs naturally in the leaves, seeds, or fruits of more than 60 plants. It is found in coffee, tea, cola drinks, and cocoa products. Caffeine is often used in OTC and prescription drugs.

Many people in the United States consume caffeine on a daily basis. A morning mug of coffee may have 200 to 300 milligrams of caffeine. An after-school cola may contain approximately 50 milligrams. A cup of tea at bedtime contributes about 40 milligrams, whereas cocoa provides under 20. See 19-9.

Caffeine affects the body in a number of ways. As with all stimulants, it increases breathing rate, heart rate, blood pressure, and the secretion of stress hormones. Too much caffeine may lead to irritability, lack of sleep, and an upset stomach. Caffeine causes diarrhea in some people.

Caffeine also acts as a diuretic. It stimulates the kidneys to increase urine output. Therefore, a drink containing caffeine is not the best choice when you have been perspiring. Water is the preferred liquid for replacing body fluids.

Caffeine has been the subject of much research. However, there is little proof linking caffeine to any specific diseases or health problems. As with other foods and drinks, it is wise to practice moderation with products

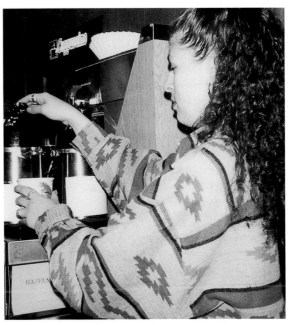

19-9 Coffee contains caffeine, a stimulant drug.

containing caffeine. Many experts recommend limiting intake to the equivalent of two cups of coffee per day.

To avoid the physical effects of caffeine, many people prefer to use caffeine-free products. Today, more choices of decaffeinated soft drinks, coffees, and teas are available than ever before. These products contain very little or no caffeine.

Caffeine is not an addictive drug, but it can be habit forming. People who suddenly stop drinking three or four cups of cola or coffee a day may experience withdrawal-like symptoms. These symptoms may include headaches, nausea, drowsiness, and irritability. A gradual withdrawal of caffeine will reduce these symptoms. To avoid feelings of fatigue from caffeine withdrawal, add daily exercise to your lifestyle.

Amphetamines

Amphetamines are commonly abused stimulant drugs. They are found in medicines used to treat certain sleep and attention disorders. They are also in some prescription medicines used to curb appetite for weight control.

Use of amphetamines to control weight is usually unsuccessful. The drugs only reduce appetite. They do not help dieters learn new eating behaviors. Once dieters stop using amphetamines, they usually regain weight rapidly. Also, dieters tend to build tolerance quickly to these drugs.

Amphetamines cause the same physical effects as other stimulants. In addition, long-term use can result in malnutrition and various nutrient deficiency diseases. Amphetamine abusers sometimes report having strange visions and thoughts. Continued use can result in the development of **tolerance**. This is the ability of the body and mind to become less responsive to a drug.

When a user develops a drug tolerance, he or she must take ever larger doses to feel a drug's effects. Taking larger and more dangerous doses of a drug can lead to a drug **overdose**. This means taking an unsafe quantity of a drug. It can cause a slowdown in brain activity, coma, or even death.

Cocaine

Cocaine is a white powder made from the coca plant. The powder, often called "coke," is usually inhaled through the nose. When consumed, cocaine causes impulses that flood the brain within seconds. These chemical reactions affect appetite, sleep, and emotions. A feeling of high energy is often followed by an emotional letdown, anger, and irritability. Cocaine is highly addictive.

Crack cocaine is a newer, less expensive form of cocaine. Because crack cocaine is smoked, its effects are felt quickly, usually within seconds.

Cocaine can cause a number of nutritional and health problems related to weight loss and poor sleep patterns. Just one use can cause a heart attack or lung failure, resulting in death.

Nicotine

Nicotine is a drug that occurs naturally in tobacco leaves, 19-10. This highly addictive

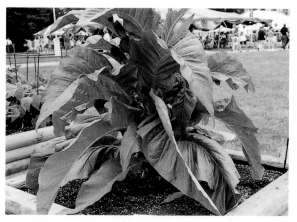

19-10 Tobacco leaves are harvested and dried before being processed into tobacco products that are smoked or chewed.

drug is found in cigarettes and all other tobacco products. It kills more people than all other drugs. According to the Surgeon General, about 1,000 people in the United States die each day from smoking-related causes. See 19-11.

The Effects of Nicotine

What happens when smoke is inhaled? Nicotine first goes to the lungs and bloodstream. Within seconds, much of the nicotine has traveled through the bloodstream to the

Percent of Deaths Linked to Smoking	
Lung cancer	75–90%
Bronchitis and emphysema	85%
Larynx cancer	40–75%
Mouth cancers	40–75%
Pharynx cancer	40–75%
Esophageal cancer	30–75%
Bladder cancer	30–50%
Pancreatic cancer	25–40%
Heart disease	15%

U.S. Department of Health and Human Services

19-11 Smoking is directly related to many fatal diseases.

brain. Nicotine then begins to affect mood and alertness.

Health Risks of Smoking

According to estimates, each cigarette a person smokes shortens his or her life by about seven minutes. This means a person loses one day of the future for every ten packs of cigarettes he or she smokes. The main reasons for a smoker's reduced life expectancy are the effects of tobacco on the heart and lungs.

Smoking is a major contributor to heart disease. Nicotine increases the heart rate. Carbon monoxide, a poisonous gas in cigarette smoke, decreases the amount of oxygen available in the blood. These two factors make the heart work harder. Smoking also causes blood clots to form more easily. This increases the risk of heart attack and stroke.

Tobacco smoke is the major cause of lung diseases, including lung cancer. When someone inhales smoke, irritating gases and particles slow the functioning of the lung's defense systems. Cigarette smoke can cause air passages to close up and make breathing more difficult. Cigarette smoke causes a sticky substance called *tar* to collect in the lungs. It can cause chronic swelling in the lungs, leading to coughs and bronchial infections. Lung tissue can be destroyed.

Smoking seems to increase the rate at which the body breaks down vitamin C. Nutrition researchers have found cigarette smokers need 35 milligrams more vitamin C each day than nonsmokers. Smokers must include extra sources of vitamin C in their diets to prevent deficiency.

A smoker is not the only one affected by his or her smoke. Other people inhale the smoke released into the air during smoking. This is called *secondhand smoking*. According to the American Lung Association, secondhand smoke can contain more cancer-causing compounds than the smoke inhaled by the smoker. The presence of smoke is especially harmful to infants and children.

According to studies, babies of parents who smoke have a higher rate of respiratory problems than babies of nonsmokers.

Tobacco products that are not intended to be smoked, such as chewing tobacco or snuff, are called *smokeless tobacco*. These products also contain nicotine, making them addictive and harmful to health. Chewing tobacco is associated with cancer of the cheeks, gums, and throat. Some people's mouths begin to be affected within a few weeks after starting to use smokeless tobacco. Gums and lips can sting, crack, bleed, wrinkle, and develop sores and white patches.

Say No to Smoking

Fortunately, information about the dangers of smoking has prompted many people to quit. The reasons to say no to smoking are many. Some of them are summarized in 19-12.

Anyone who smokes or uses other forms of tobacco knows that breaking the habit is not easy. Part of the dependence on nicotine is psychological. Some smokers associate smoking with relaxation, good food, and

---

Reasons to Avoid Smoking

- Obedience to the law (regarding underage purchasers)
- Healthier lungs, fewer colds, and less coughing and shortness of breath
- Decreased risk of blood clot formation
- Reduced cancer risk
- No nicotine addiction
- No risk of the shortened life span or premature aging of skin (especially the face) associated with smoking
- Fresher breath and whiter teeth
- Less debt (more spending money)
- No release of secondhand smoke

19-12 Can you name other reasons for not smoking?

friends. Quitting smoking can be especially hard in a social network of friends who smoke.

Nicotine addiction is also physical. Common withdrawal symptoms include shakiness, anxiety, and grouchiness. Dizziness, headaches, difficulty sleeping, and changes in appetite are symptoms, too.

Some people claim they gain weight when they stop smoking. This may be partly because smoking elevates the body's basal metabolism about 10 percent. When a person quits smoking, his or her basal metabolism will drop back to normal. This accounts for a reduced energy need of about 100 calories a day. When a person is adjusting to not smoking, an extra walk or other physical activity will help control weight. Added activity will also help a smoker take his or her mind off smoking.

Making wellness a lifestyle means never starting to smoke. See 19-13. People who do smoke should quit. Programs are available to help people quit smoking. Doctors can prescribe medical aids to help the body adjust to nicotine withdrawal. Family members and friends can provide emotional support.

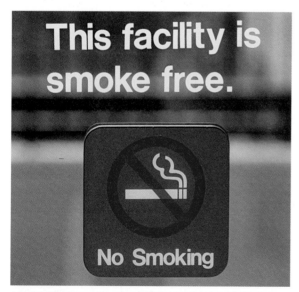

19-13 More and more public and private facilities are banning tobacco smoke.

Former smokers must be patient and stay firm in their commitment to end the smoking habit. Withdrawal symptoms may last several months. In time, a former smoker will realize the benefits of not smoking far outweigh any pleasures received from smoking. In addition, the financial rewards of not buying cigarettes can add up quickly.

● Depressants

Depressants are drugs that decrease the activity of the central nervous system. They slow down certain body functions and reactions. Many drugs fall in this category. They can be grouped as barbiturates, tranquilizers, inhalants, and narcotics. Among the list of depressants, alcohol is the most often abused.

● Alcohol

Alcohol, which is chemically called *ethanol,* is a drug. It is not a nutrient, although it supplies seven calories of energy per gram. Carbohydrates, fats, and proteins must be digested before they are absorbed through the walls of the small intestine. Alcohol, by contrast, requires no digestion and can be absorbed through cells in the mouth and the walls of the stomach. This is what causes a person to feel the effects of alcohol so quickly. Food in the stomach helps slow the absorption of alcohol.

● Alcohol in the Body

Once alcohol is absorbed, the bloodstream carries it to the liver. The liver is where alcohol metabolism occurs. The rate at which the liver can break down alcohol varies from person to person. Until alcohol is metabolized, it flows through the bloodstream, allowing it to reach and affect the brain.

In the brain, alcohol first suppresses the action of the area that controls judgment. Increased alcohol consumption affects the part of the brain that controls large muscle movements. This is why people who have consumed much alcohol begin to stagger when they walk. Loss of inhibitions, confusion, drowsiness, nausea, and vomiting are other symptoms. Further consumption affects the part of the brain that controls breathing and heartbeat.

The higher the level of blood alcohol, the greater are the risks to health and life. As blood alcohol content rises, more centers of the brain shut down. Many states declare a driver "drunk" when the blood alcohol level reaches 0.08 percent. However, a driver's judgment starts becoming impaired at a blood alcohol level of 0.05 percent. Even death can result at this blood alcohol level. See 19-14.

If a person passes out, it means the entire consciousness section of the brain has closed off. Meanwhile, the body continues to absorb the alcohol still in the stomach. This causes the blood alcohol levels to rise even though the person has stopped drinking.

The liver can metabolize alcohol only so fast. The higher the blood alcohol concentration, the longer it will take the liver to clear the body of the drug. The liver takes about six hours to break down the alcohol contained in four drinks. Drinking coffee, exercising, and using other techniques cannot speed up this process.

A person can feel sick the day after drinking large amounts of alcohol. This condition is called a *hangover*. A person with a hangover may experience headache, nausea, vomiting, fatigue, thirst, and irritability. Alcohol consumption can also lower blood sugar levels and increase the heart rate.

Smoking seems to intensify the symptoms of a hangover. Drinking plenty of water will help prevent dehydration. Bland foods such as gelatin, puddings, and yogurt can help relieve stomach irritation. Complex carbohydrates like whole grain breads and cereals can counteract the low blood sugar. However, no remedy exists for curing a hangover. A person simply has to wait until his or her body has time to recuperate.

● **Health Risks of Alcohol Abuse**

One effect of long-term alcohol abuse is vitamin deficiencies. Many vitamins are affected, including vitamins A, C, D, K, and several B vitamins. Deficiencies may occur due to a couple of factors. If many calories in the diet come from alcohol, the diet may be poor in nutrients. Alcohol in the system also reduces the body's ability to absorb and use nutrients.

Alcohol abuse over time causes a fat buildup in the liver. Fat accumulation in the liver eventually chokes off the supply of

Effects of Alcohol on Behavior

Percent of Blood Alcohol Concentration	Behavioral Effect
.00–.05%	Slight change in feeling; decreased alertness
.05–.10%	Reduced social inhibitions and motor coordination; slowed reaction time; legally drunk in many states
.10–.15%	Unsteadiness in standing and walking; loss of peripheral (side) vision
.15–.30%	Staggered walk and slurred speech; impaired pain receptors
.30 and greater	Possible shutdown of heart and lungs; complete unconsciousness; death possible

19-14 As alcohol becomes more concentrated in the blood, health risks increase.

blood to liver cells. Scar tissue forms. Eventually, liver cells begin to die. This is characteristic of a liver disease called **cirrhosis**. As cells die, the liver loses its ability to work. Without the function of this vital organ, a person will die. Seventy percent of deaths from cirrhosis are related to alcohol abuse.

Other health risks of alcohol abuse include stomach problems, heart disease, and brain damage. Alcohol affects the immune system and the reproductive system, too. Great health risks also result from impaired judgment and slowed motor responses. These effects can lead to serious accidents. See 19-15.

● **Alcoholism**
Alcoholism is an addiction to alcohol. It is fatal if left untreated. People who have this disease are called *alcoholics*. They cannot control the amount of alcohol they consume. Alcoholics do not always realize they have a disease. See 19-16. Many alcoholics find it hard to seek help. Close friends or family members can sometimes encourage an alcoholic to recognize he or she needs help to

recover. However, few alcohol abusers seek help without facing a crisis.

One of the most successful resources for helping alcoholics recover is *Alcoholics Anonymous (AA)*. AA is a community-based program. It uses a self-help group format. This approach helps alcoholics learn to deal with its consequences and accept the fact they have a disease. Al-Anon and Alateen are support groups that help people who have alcoholic family members. Addresses and phone numbers for these groups can easily be found in the Yellow Pages.

● **Say No to Alcohol**
Information about the dangers linked with alcohol has prompted many adults to use alcohol more responsibly. People who host parties make a point of offering nonalcoholic drinks. More people are avoiding driving if they have been drinking. Many people who drink alcohol limit their intake so they do not become drunk. They may alternate between alcohol and soft drinks. They also consume food along with alcohol to help slow alcohol's absorption.

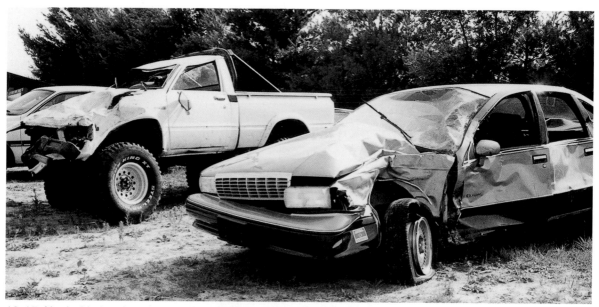

19-15 Alcohol is involved in nearly half of all vehicle accidents.

From a wellness standpoint, the health hazards of consuming alcohol are greatest for someone who is still growing. Therefore, drinking alcohol is very hazardous for teens. In addition, drinking alcohol is illegal for teens. The many reasons that teens say no to alcohol are summarized in 19-17.

Barbiturates and Tranquilizers

Two groups of depressants are barbiturates and tranquilizers. *Barbiturates* create a feeling of drowsiness. Doctors may prescribe them for people who have trouble sleeping. *Tranquilizers* can calm emotions and relax muscles. Doctors may prescribe them for people who are feeling overly anxious or having muscle pain. Both of these groups of drugs can be addictive.

People who are taking barbiturates or tranquilizers must avoid drinking alcohol. The chemicals in the drugs and alcohol each intensify the effects of the other. The mixture can be deadly.

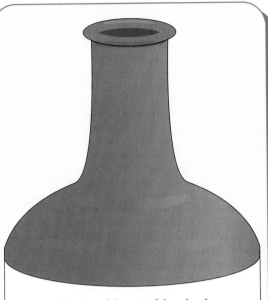

Facts About Alcohol and Alcoholism

- Alcoholism is a disease, not a moral weakness. Alcoholism is treatable.
- More than two drinks a day doubles the chances of developing high blood pressure.
- Fifteen million Americans are allergic to the ingredients in alcoholic beverages.
- Teens and preteens are more vulnerable than adults to the toxic effects of alcohol.
- Many teenage suicides are directly related to alcohol and drug use.
- Approximately 45–60% of all fatal auto accidents are alcohol related.
- Over 50% of fire, drowning, and falling accidents are related to alcohol.

19-16 Alcohol abuse and addiction are linked to a number of health and safety risks.

Reasons to Avoid Alcohol

- Less likely to have accidents
- Stay mentally alert
- Avoid dependency on alcohol to solve problems
- Reduce the risks of cancer
- Reduce the risk of nutritional and immune deficiencies
- Remain dependable for family and friends
- Avoid trouble with the law
- Maintain a healthy appearance
- Helps avoid liver disease
- Avoid dealing with hangovers
- Saves money

19-17 There are many reasons for saying no to alcohol. Can you think of others?

Inhalants

Inhalants are substances that are inhaled for their mind-numbing effects. Products used as inhalants include glue, spray paints, aerosols, and some petroleum products. People who abuse inhalants deeply breathe in their fumes. Inhalants can produce dizziness, confusion, and unconsciousness. See 19-18.

Abusing inhalants is very dangerous to health. Risks include a rapid increase in heart rate. Deeply breathing some substances can cause irreversible damage to lungs. Some inhalant abusers have also seen frightening visions and suffered permanent brain damage. Death from heart failure or suffocation is possible even with first-time inhalant use.

Narcotics

Narcotics are drugs that bring on sleep, relieve pain, and dull the senses. Some narcotics are made in a laboratory.

Most, however, are made from the opium poppy and are called **opiates**. The opiates include codeine, morphine, opium, and heroin.

Some opiates are used medically to help people who are suffering from pain and discomfort. For example, codeine is used to control coughing. OTC cough medications are allowed to contain small amounts of this drug. Morphine, used to ease pain, is available only with a doctor's prescription. Doctors and pharmacists carefully monitor the availability and use of these drugs because they can cause addictions quickly.

Heroin is the most addictive and dangerous narcotic known today. It is illegal in the United States, even for medical use. Heroin is illegal in most other countries, too.

Hallucinogens

Drugs that cause the mind to create images that do not really exist are called **hallucinogens**. The images the mind

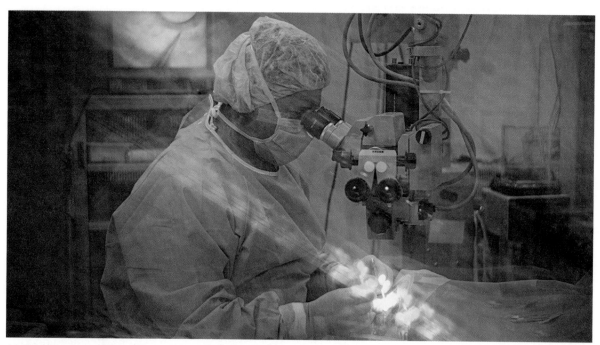

19-18 The powerful inhalant given to patients before surgery numbs all sense of pain. It is an example of a beneficial inhalant.

creates are called *hallucinations.* They may involve sounds and smells as well as visual images. See 19-19.

Users of hallucinogens cannot predict what effects the drugs will have from one time to the next. Some effects can be terrifying; some can be long lasting. Hallucinogens include marijuana, LSD, PCP, and designer drugs.

● Marijuana

Large doses of marijuana can produce hallucinations. *Marijuana* is an illegal drug that comes from the cannabis plant. It is usually smoked and often referred to as "pot" or "grass." Marijuana contains over 400 chemicals. The effects of all these chemicals on the body are not fully known.

THC is the chief mood-altering ingredient in marijuana. It passes rapidly from the bloodstream into the brain. THC is fat-soluble and is attracted to the body's fatty tissues, where it can be stored for long periods. It takes about four weeks to rid the body of the THC from one marijuana cigarette.

● Effects of Marijuana

Marijuana users cannot predict what the drug's effects will be. Purity levels of the drug may vary. Other substances may also be added to marijuana. These substances can alter the drug's effects.

Short-term effects of marijuana include apathy, mood swings, and a loss of concentration. Memory and coordination can also be affected. Someone who has used marijuana may feel its effects for only an hour or two. However, his or her judgment may be impaired for four or more hours.

Marijuana cigarettes release five times as much carbon monoxide into the lungs as tobacco cigarettes. They also release three times as much tar. These agents can damage the heart and lungs. Marijuana adversely affects the body's nervous and immune systems, too.

People who use marijuana can become psychologically dependent on it. It is common for marijuana users to experiment with more powerful drugs.

● LSD and PCP

LSD (lysergic acid diethylamide) and *PCP* (phencyclidine) are two very powerful, illegal, and dangerous hallucinogens. They are made in illegal laboratories. LSD can cause *flashbacks.* These are hallucinations that occur long after the drug has been used. PCP has been known to produce confusion and violent behavior.

Users of both of these drugs can quickly develop tolerance. Even a single use of either drug can cause mental illness. While under the effects of these drugs, many people engage in bizarre or dangerous behaviors. A number of users have died as a result of these behaviors. See 19-20.

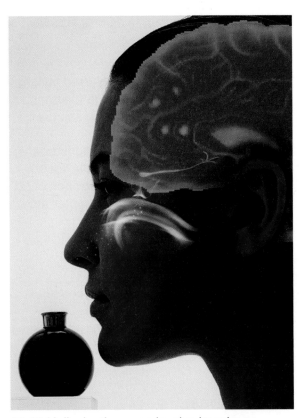

19-19 Hallucinations can involve imaginary smells, with or without imaginary images.

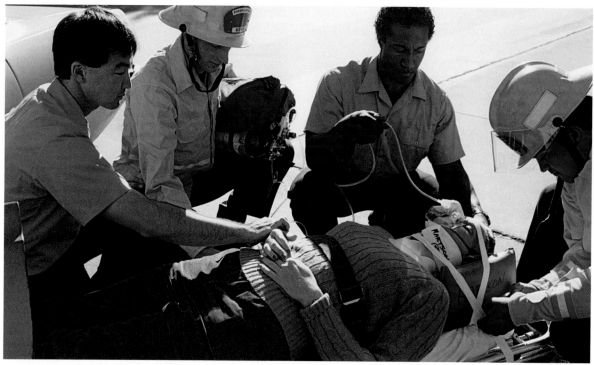

19-20 Believing that one can fly is a sensation associated with LSD use. Some users have walked off roofs and balconies under its influence.

Designer Drugs

Designer drugs are lab-created imitations of other street drugs. Most are much stronger than the drugs they are designed to imitate. When the drugs are being made in illegal laboratories, there is little concern for purity. They are never tested for contamination. These factors increase the already high risks of drug use.

Depending on the drug, effects may include confusion, depression, blurred vision, and nausea. Health risks include elevated blood pressure, rapid heart beat, seizures, and permanent brain damage.

Some designer drugs are hallucinogens. Others are classified as stimulants. Yet others are narcotics. The three categories of addictive drugs discussed in this chapter are summarized in 19-21.

Psychoactive Drugs		
Stimulants	**Depressants**	**Hallucinogens**
caffeine	alcohol	marijuana
amphetamines	barbiturates	LSD
cocaine	tranquilizers	PCP
nicotine	inhalants	designer drugs
designer drugs	narcotics	
	designer drugs	

19-21 This chart lists the type of drugs that fall in the three main categories of psychoactive drugs.

● Drugs and Athletes

Drug testing of athletes is occurring at all levels of sports. Of course illegal drug use is prohibited. However, most prescription stimulants and narcotics are banned from use, too. Also banned are diuretics and certain steroids. Most people agree sports should be a display of natural rather than chemically altered physical ability.

● Anabolic Steroids

Anabolic steroids are artificial hormones used to build a more muscular body. *Anabolic* means tissue-building. These steroids are a synthetic version of the male sex hormone *testosterone.* Both males and females have been known to use anabolic steroids to help build muscles, 19-22. Some people use them simply to look better. Others are motivated to use the steroids because they believe the drugs will help them excel in sports.

Some anabolic steroids are prescribed by doctors for medical reasons. However, many of these steroids are made and sold illegally. Like designer drugs, steroids may be produced under unsafe conditions and contamination may occur. Some products sold as muscle-building steroids are bogus. They contain no ingredients that promote muscle growth.

As long as people want to look bigger, run faster, and be stronger, the temptation to use these steroids will exist. Before giving in to this temptation, athletes need to know the facts about the dangers of anabolic steroid use. Even brief use of the steroids can have harmful effects on a growing body. Women have experienced baldness, increased body hair, voice deepening, and decreased breast size. In people of both sexes, anabolic steroids have caused acne, stunted growth, and sterility. Use of these steroids has also led to coronary artery disease, liver tumors, and death. With these dangers, it is easy to understand why so many professional athletes

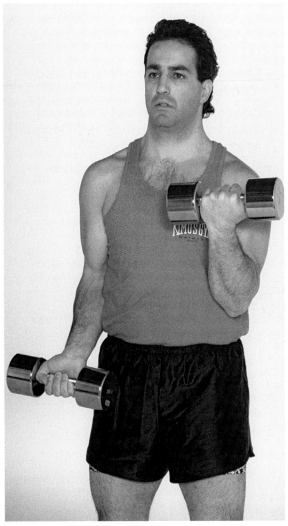

19-22 Exercise is a much better choice than anabolic steroids for building muscle.

have spoken out strongly against anabolic steroid use.

● Getting Help for a Substance Abuse Problem

Someone with a substance abuse problem needs to recognize a problem exists. A giant step toward recovery is the desire to seek help. The questions in 19-23 may help a person determine whether he or she has a problem.

Is There a Drug Problem?

- Do you miss school or work because of drinking or drugs?
- Does a drink or drugs help you build confidence?
- Do your friends comment about how much you drink or use drugs? Do you secretly feel angry at them?
- Do you drink or use drugs to break away from social, family, work, or school worries?
- Does a drink or other drug help you prepare for a date?
- Is finding enough money to buy alcohol or drugs a problem you are frequently facing?
- Do you choose to be friends with people who can get liquor or drugs easily?
- Do you eat very little or irregularly when you are drinking or getting high?
- Do you require more and more of the drug to get drunk or high?
- Have you ever been arrested for drunk driving or the illegal use of drugs?
- Do you get annoyed when friends or class discussions focus on the dangers of alcohol or drugs?
- Do you often think about alcohol or drugs?

19-23 Asking these questions might help a person determine if a drug problem exists.

Many forms of treatment are available for someone who has identified a substance abuse problem. Treatments range from inpatient therapy to self-help groups. No one approach is right for everyone.

Therapy programs are offered through hospitals and clinics. If needed, clients receive medical treatment for the physical effects of substance abuse. Trained counselors help them understand the effects of substance abuse at a personal level. For example, a drug problem for one family member creates stress for all other members. Therapy programs help clients develop the emotional tools they need to stay drug-free. Physicians and school counselors can refer people to therapy programs in their area.

Learning to control substance dependency can be a life-long process. Participation in self-help groups often follows other forms of treatment. These groups help people maintain drug-free lifestyles by attending regular meetings with supportive friends. Many self-help groups can be located by referring to the Yellow Pages.

Practicing wellness means taking drugs only when needed, as directed, and for their intended purposes. To protect your health, guard against the misuse of drugs.

Chapter 19 Review

Summary

Drug use has the potential for both positive and negative effects on wellness. When used appropriately, drugs can cure illness and save lives. However, drugs also have the potential to destroy health and even cause death. Drugs taken as medicine must be used as prescribed by a physician or as directed on the label. They contain chemicals that interact with the body in specific ways. As a consumer, you have a right to ask questions of the physician and the pharmacist about the medicines you are taking.

Drugs should never be misused or abused. Misuse means using drugs in ways not intended. Drug abuse refers to using drugs for reasons that are not medical. The most commonly misused and abused drugs are the psychoactive drugs. These include stimulants, depressants, and hallucinogens. The use of anabolic steroids by athletes is another example of drug abuse.

Body functioning and brain activity are affected in many ways by drugs. Mixing different drugs can compound the reactions. Prolonged drug use can lead to dependency and addiction. Illegal drugs present added dangers from impurities and contaminants. Some drugs are powerful enough to instantly cause brain damage, heart attack, coma, or death.

Saying no to substances that may harm your health is a lifelong wellness choice. The risks to an individual's health and personal life from using these substances are enormous. People who decide to quit using them can turn to their physician or school counselor for help. The Yellow Pages is another source of information on drug treatment services.

Check Your Knowledge

1. Describe the difference between a drug and a medicine.

2. True or false. Trade or brand name drugs are much stronger than generic drugs.

3. Which internal organ breaks down most of the toxins and chemicals in the body?

4. List the three basic ways in which food-drug interactions may interfere with a person's nutritional status.

5. State three examples of drug misuse.

6. True or false. Coffee and tobacco both contain stimulants.

7. Name the most common depressant.

8. Which is the most addictive and dangerous narcotic?

9. What are three possible reasons for drug abuse problems among teens?

10. To what sources of help may a person with a drug problem turn?

Put Learning into Action

1. Conduct a debate with your fellow classmates. Possible topics include: (A) Are we a drug-dependent society? (B) A drug problem exists in our society because medicine and other drugs are too available and affordable.

2. Invite a pharmacist or a representative from a pharmaceutical company to speak to the class. Ask the person to discuss how drugs are developed, approved, and marketed to the public.

3. Examine the labels on containers of muscle enhancers available in the health foods section of a store. What factors would help you decide if the claims are accurate?

4. Develop campaign messages to inform teens about the effects of drugs on wellness. Post them throughout your school.

5. Develop a newsletter for the athletic department in your school. Inform readers about the dangers of using anabolic steroids to build muscles. Provide

scientifically sound ideas for building body strength and endurance.

Explore Further

1. Research the drug treatment services available in your community. Interview three groups or agencies to determine the following: treatment policy, procedure, and cost. Also ask about the admissions policy and the recovery rate.

2. Find a reference that lists the caffeine content of foods. Determine how many milligrams of caffeine you consume in an average day.

3. Identify the drug prevention programs in your community. What is the prevention message delivered in each? Who receives the information? Find out how each program sponsor determines whether its program is effective.

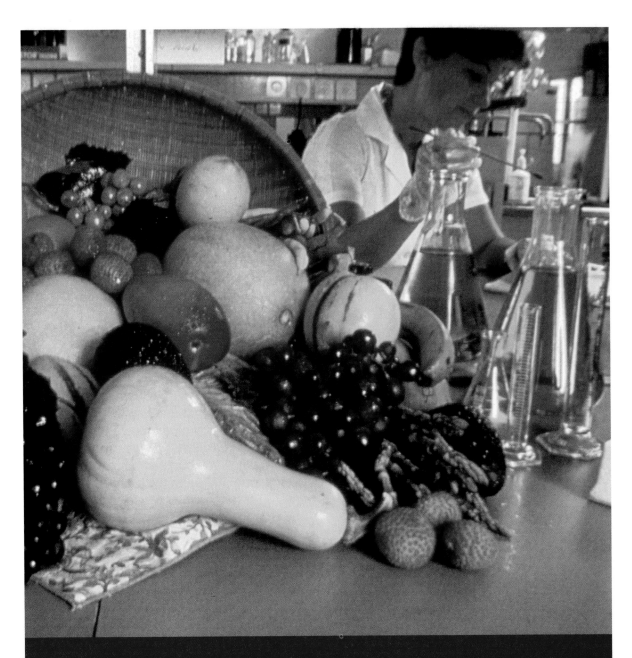

Part Six
Making Informed Choices

Chapter 20

Keeping Food Safe

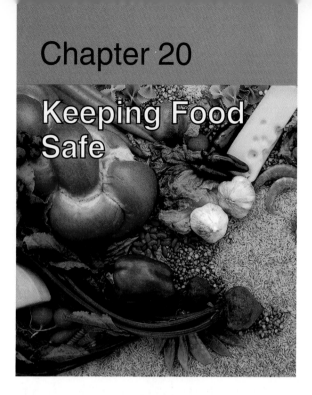

Objectives

After studying this chapter, you will be able to
- list common food contaminants.
- practice preventive measures when shopping for, storing, and preparing food to avoid foodborne illness.
- identify population groups that are most at risk for foodborne illness.
- recognize symptoms of foodborne illnesses.
- discuss the roles of food producers, food processors, government agencies, and consumers in protecting the safety of the food supply.

Foodborne illness, also called *food poisoning,* is a disease transmitted by food. It can strike anyone. In fact, millions of people in the United States get some type of foodborne illness each year. However, many of these cases go unreported because people mistake their symptoms for "stomach flu."

Foodborne illness can be avoided. This chapter will help you learn how organisms that cause foodborne illness get into food. It will also help you apply guidelines to prevent the spread of these organisms. You will read about steps to take if foodborne illness occurs. You will study about agencies that are responsible for protecting the food supply, too.

Common Food Contaminants

Foodborne illness occurs when food is contaminated. A **contaminant** is an undesirable substance that unintentionally gets into food. The most common food contaminants are **microorganisms**. These are living beings so small you can see them only under a microscope. Although microorganisms are tiny, the diseases they cause can have big impacts on people.

Harmful Bacteria

By far, the most common cause of foodborne illness in the United States is harmful **bacteria**. These are single-celled microorganisms that live in soil, water, and the bodies of plants and animals. Knowing how bacteria grow and multiply can help you prevent foodborne illnesses. See 20-1.

All foods contain bacteria, but not all bacteria are harmful. Certain types of bacteria are intentionally added to foods to produce desired effects. For instance, bacteria are used to make cultured milk products, such as buttermilk and yogurt.

Bacteria is one of the factors that cause foods to spoil. However, foods that contain illness-causing bacteria often look, smell, and

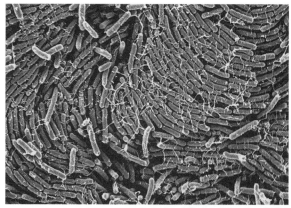

Agricultural Research Service, USDA

20-1 This picture of bacteria, magnified about 10,000 times, shows the filaments bacteria use to attach themselves to a surface. These same filaments are used to attach to other bacteria and microorganisms.

taste wholesome. Spoilage and contamination are not the same. *Spoiled* food has lost nutritional value and quality characteristics, such as flavor and texture, due to decay. *Contaminated* food has become unfit to eat due to the introduction of undesirable substances.

A number of bacteria are known to cause foodborne illness. Health experts are most concerned about controlling the five types that cause the most common and/or serious illnesses. These types are *E. coli* 0157:H7, *Salmonella, Listeria monocytogenes, Campylobacter jejuni,* and *Staphylococcus aureus.* Some bacteria cause sickness by irritating the lining of the intestines. Others produce **toxins**, or poisons, that cause illness. Several types of harmful bacteria and the illnesses they cause are summarized in Chart 20-2.

● Other Microorganisms

Other foodborne microorganisms that can cause illness include parasites, viruses, and molds. A **parasite** is an organism that lives off another organism, called a *host. Trichinella* is a food parasite sometimes found in raw or undercooked pork. It can cause a disease called *trichinosis.* Improved feeding conditions

of hogs have made trichinosis rare in the United States today. Trichinosis can be prevented by cooking pork to an internal temperature of at least 160°F (71°C).

Protozoa are single-celled animals. Some types of protozoa are parasites that can cause foodborne illness. *Entamoeba histolytica* and *Giardia lamblia* are two such protozoa. They are both found in water polluted with animal or human feces. Safe drinking water is tested and treated to destroy these and other harmful microorganisms.

A **virus** is a disease-causing agent that is the smallest type of life-form. A few viruses, such as *hepatitis A* and *Norwalk virus,* can be transmitted by foods. People are most likely to contract these viruses by eating raw or undercooked shellfish, such as oysters, clams, and mussels. Although most shellfish are safe, those taken from polluted waters or handled by infected workers may be contaminated.

Molds are mainly associated with food spoilage. Molds often form on foods that have been stored for extended periods after opening. Some molds produce toxins. When mold forms on liquids or soft foods, such as jelly, you should discard the whole food. When mold forms on solid foods, such as breads and hard cheeses, you can cut it off. Cut into the food one-half inch deeper than the mold and discard the moldy portion.

● Natural Toxins

Many plants produce substances to defend themselves against insects, birds, and animals. These substances are called *natural toxins.* Although many of these substances are not toxic to humans, others are. For instance, eating some varieties of wild berries and mushrooms can cause illness. Avoid foods that do not come from reputable food sellers.

Some types of fish, such as tuna and blue marlin, also produce a natural toxin when they begin to spoil. This toxin, *scombroid toxin,* is not destroyed by cooking. People who eat fish

Bacterial Foodborne Illnesses

Bacteria	Food Sources	Symptoms
Campylobacter jejuni	Raw poultry, meat, and unpasteurized milk	Diarrhea, abdominal cramping, fever Appear: 2–5 days after eating Last: 7–10 days
Clostridium botulinum	Canned goods, improperly processed home-canned foods, luncheon meats	Double vision, inability to swallow, speech difficulty, progressive paralysis of the respiratory system that can lead to death Appear: 12–36 hours after toxin enters the body
Clostridium perfringens	Meats and meat products, such as gravies and stuffing; frequently occurs in hot foods that cool down	Abdominal pain and diarrhea, sometimes nausea and vomiting Appear: 8–12 hours after eating Last: 1 day or less
E. coli 0157:H7	Raw or undercooked ground beef, raw milk, produce	Bloody stools, stomachache, nausea, vomiting Appear: 12–72 hours after eating Last: 4–10 days
Listeria monocytogenes	Soft cheese, unpasteurized milk, seafood products	Fever, headache, nausea, vomiting; can cause fetal and infant death Appear: 48–72 hours after eating
Salmonella	Raw meats, poultry, milk and dairy products, eggs	Severe headache, abdominal pain, diarrhea, fever Appear: 8–12 hours after eating Last: 2–3 days
Staphylococcus aureus	Meats; poultry; egg products; tuna, potato, and macaroni salads; cream-filled pastries	Diarrhea, vomiting, nausea, abdominal pain, cramps Appear: 30 minutes–8 hours after eating Last: 24–48 hours

20-2 These bacteria can cause illnesses with symptoms of varying degree.

containing this toxin may develop symptoms of foodborne illness immediately. These symptoms last less than 24 hours.

● Chemicals

Chemicals that come in contact with the food supply can be another source of foodborne illness. Some chemicals are purposely used to produce and process foods. Such chemicals include pesticides and food additives. A *pesticide* is a substance used to repel or destroy insects, weeds, or fungi on plant crops. Pesticides are also used to protect foods during transportation. *Food additives* are chemicals added to food during processing. (Additives will be discussed further in Chapter 22, "Making Wise Consumer Choices.")

Pesticide residues are chemical pesticide particles left on food after it is prepared for consumption. Some consumers are concerned about the effects long-term exposure to these residues may have. Farmers must follow strict guidelines when applying pesticides.

They must keep residues within legal limits. These limits are set by state and federal agencies to protect public health. Government agencies also check the food supply to be sure foods are safe. Washing and drying produce and removing outer leaves of leafy vegetables will help limit your intake of residues. See 20-3.

Some chemicals unintentionally come in contact with the food supply. ***Environmental contaminants*** are substances released into the air or water by industrial plants. These substances eventually make their way into foods. They can build up in the body over time until they reach toxic levels.

Environmental contaminants can accumulate in fish that live in waters polluted by industrial wastes. The larger the fish, the more time it had to store toxins. Eating lean fish may help you avoid chemical toxins, which tend to be stored in fishes' fatty tissues. Some health experts caution people to eat freshwater fish no more than once a week. This helps you avoid the potential buildup of toxins, just in case contamination exists.

● Helpful Microorganisms

Some microorganisms are used to change foods to create positive effects on food taste and texture. For instance, special molds are used to age some cheeses. Lactic acid bacteria are used to give yogurt its tangy taste and thick, creamy texture. Yeasts are another type of microorganism. One type of yeast is used as a *leavening agent.* This is a substance used to produce a gas that causes batter or dough to rise. See 20-4.

● Outwitting the Food Contaminators

Most foodborne illness is due to improper food handling. You need to use care when buying, storing, and preparing food. You must correct conditions that allow bacte-

Removing Pesticide Residues

- Thoroughly wash and dry fresh fruits and vegetables. Do not use soap or detergents to wash food; these products also leave residues.

- Remove outer leaves of vegetables such as lettuce and cabbage.

- Trim fat from meat and poultry. Discard fats and oils from broth and pan drippings. Some residue particles from animal feed concentrate in the fatty tissue.

- Eat kidneys, liver, and other organ meats sparingly. Feed chemical residues may also be stored in these organs.

- Eat a moderate, nutritious diet with plenty of variety to reduce the risk of toxicity from any one food source.

20-3 You may want to take added precautions to remove pesticide residues.

ria to spread and multiply. This will help you protect yourself and your family from foodborne illnesses.

● Shopping with Safety in Mind

Fortunately, the food supply in the United States is one of the safest in the world. However, you still need to be on guard for possible sources of contamination.

Bringing safe foods into your home is your first step toward outwitting the food contaminators. Begin by shopping at stores known for food safety and sanitation. ***Sanitation*** involves keeping everything that comes in contact with food clean to help prevent disease. Check to see if store refrigerators, shelves, and floors are clean. Poor sanitation in these areas may indicate low standards for food handling overall. See 20-5.

Select foods that appear fresh and wholesome. Look for freshness dates on food labels to help you know how long you

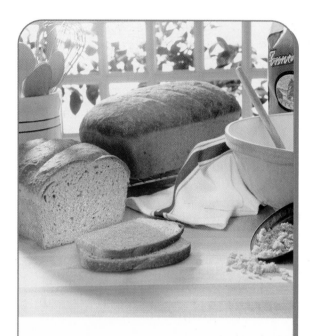

How Does Yeast Make Bread Rise?

1. Liquid ingredients used to make bread dough are heated to a temperature that helps activate the yeast.
2. Bread is kneaded, or folded and pushed with the hands. This action helps develop an elastic protein in the dough called gluten.
3. After kneading, the dough is allowed to rise in a warm environment, which promotes a process called fermentation. During this process, the yeast causes a chemical reaction that produces carbon dioxide gas.
4. After time, the carbon dioxide causes the dough to rise.
5. Physical changes to the size and shape of the dough result in a high-quality bread product that is flavorful and light in texture.

20-4 Yeast is a helpful microorganism that is used as a leavening agent to make bread rise.

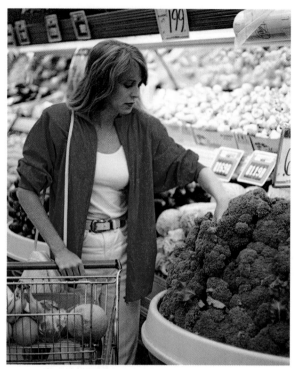

20-5 The clean appearance of a grocery store may indicate food has been kept in sanitary conditions.

can safely store foods at home. Do not buy food in cans that are swollen, rusted, or deeply dented. Bacteria may enter a can that is not sealed properly.

Shop for refrigerated and frozen foods last to help them stay cold. Put each package of raw meat, poultry, or fish in a separate plastic bag. This will keep their juices from dripping onto other food items. Avoid buying frozen foods that are leaky, misshapen, or covered with a heavy layer of frost. Also avoid frozen products that have watermarks on the packaging indicating the food has thawed and was refrozen. These are indications the food may not have been stored at safe freezer temperatures.

After shopping, get foods home quickly. Keep refrigerated and frozen items together so they help keep each other cold. Keep them well separated from hot foods from the deli.

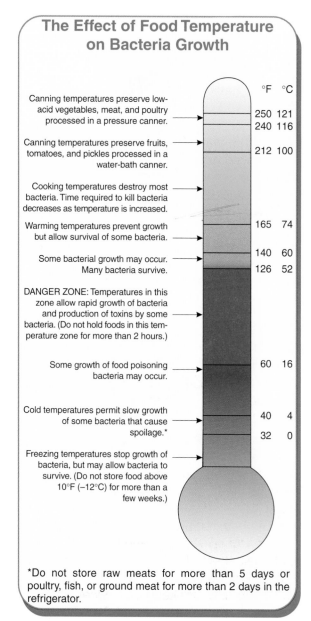

The Effect of Food Temperature on Bacteria Growth

	°F	°C
Canning temperatures preserve low-acid vegetables, meat, and poultry processed in a pressure canner.	250	121
	240	116
Canning temperatures preserve fruits, tomatoes, and pickles processed in a water-bath canner.	212	100
Cooking temperatures destroy most bacteria. Time required to kill bacteria decreases as temperature is increased.		
Warming temperatures prevent growth but allow survival of some bacteria.	165	74
	140	60
Some bacterial growth may occur. Many bacteria survive.	126	52
DANGER ZONE: Temperatures in this zone allow rapid growth of bacteria and production of toxins by some bacteria. (Do not hold foods in this temperature zone for more than 2 hours.)		
Some growth of food poisoning bacteria may occur.	60	16
Cold temperatures permit slow growth of some bacteria that cause spoilage.*	40	4
	32	0
Freezing temperatures stop growth of bacteria, but may allow bacteria to survive. (Do not store food above 10°F (−12°C) for more than a few weeks.)		

*Do not store raw meats for more than 5 days or poultry, fish, or ground meat for more than 2 days in the refrigerator.

20-6 Temperature can have an effect on the growth of bacteria.

The warmer the weather, the sooner you need to get foods home and store them properly.

● Storing Foods Safely

When you come home from the grocery store, put away your perishable foods first. The temperature in the refrigerator should be 40°F (4°C) or below. The freezer should be 0°F (−18°C) or lower. These cold temperatures do not kill bacteria. However, they do slow bacterial growth, 20-6. Consider keeping refrigerator/freezer thermometers in your refrigerator and freezer. This can help you make sure your appliances are maintaining the correct temperatures.

Store eggs in the cartons in which you purchased them. These cartons help reduce the evaporation of moisture from the egg through the porous eggshell. Place eggs on an interior shelf of the refrigerator. The refrigerator door is not as cold as the interior.

Wrap or cover all foods for refrigerator or freezer storage. This keeps bacteria from settling on foods. It also keeps foods from dripping onto one another. Plastic or glass lids are good covers because they can be reused. However, plastic wrap and aluminum foil make fine food covers, too. They cannot be reused because they cannot easily be sanitized.

The sooner foods are chilled, the less chance there will be for bacteria to grow to unsafe numbers. Store foods in shallow containers to promote quick cooling. Arrange foods in the refrigerator in a manner that allows air to circulate freely around the containers.

Put dates on leftovers. This will help you remember how soon you must use the food. Most leftovers can safely stay in the refrigerator for only three to four days. A cold storage chart for foods is listed in 20-7.

Store foods that do not need refrigeration, such as dry beans, pasta, and canned goods, in a cool, dry place. Store foods away from cleaning supplies, which are likely to be toxic. Also avoid storing foods in damp areas, such as under the sink. Dampness encourages bacterial growth. Check to be sure boxes and bottles are tightly closed and plastic bags are completely sealed.

● Keeping Clean in the Kitchen

Many people are unaware of basic safe food handling techniques. When working with food, one of the most important points to remember is to use good personal hygiene. **Hygiene** refers to practices that promote good health. It involves making a conscientious effort to keep dirt and germs from getting into food.

Always wash your hands with soap and warm running water for 20 seconds before beginning to work with food. Try singing "Happy Birthday" twice while you wash your hands to be sure you are spending a full 20 seconds. You need this much time to get hands thoroughly clean. Be sure to clean under your nails and around cuticles, too. Use paper towels or clean cloth towels to dry hands. Do not use the same towel you use to dry dishes. This will keep bacteria that multiply on a damp hand towel from getting on clean dishes.

If you have any kind of cut or infection on your hand, wear gloves when preparing foods. Bacteria grow in open wounds and may contaminate the food you are preparing. Treat gloved hands just like bare hands, washing them whenever they come in contact with unclean surfaces.

Rewash your hands every time you touch dirty objects, including pets, money, and unwashed utensils. Wash hands after coughing, sneezing, combing your hair, and using the bathroom, too.

Cold Storage Chart

Product	Refrigerator (40°F, 4°C)	Freezer (0°F, −18°C)
Bacon	7 days	1 month
Beef, fresh	3–5 days	6–12 months
Chicken, cooked	3–4 days	4 months
Chicken or turkey, whole	1–2 days	1 year
Eggs, fresh in shell	3 weeks	do not freeze
Eggs, hard-cooked	1 week	do not freeze well
Hamburger, ground turkey, veal, pork, and lamb	1–2 days	3–4 months
Ham, fully cooked	3–4 days slices, 7 days whole	1–2 months
Hot dogs	2 weeks unopened package, 1 week opened package	1–2 months
Lamb, fresh	3–5 days	6–9 months
Lunch meats	2 weeks unopened package, 3–5 days opened package	1–2 months
Mayonnaise	2 months	do not freeze
Meat and meat dishes, cooked	3–4 days	2–3 months
Pork, fresh	3–5 days	4–6 months
Sausage links, patties	7 days	1–2 months
Soups and stews	3–4 days	2–3 months

20-7 These guidelines will help you refrigerate or freeze perishable foods safely.

Wear clean clothes or a clean apron when working with food. If you have long hair, pull it back to keep loose strands from falling into food.

You need to keep your work area clean when preparing foods. ***Cross-contamination*** occurs when harmful bacteria from one food are transferred to another food. This can happen when one food drips on or touches another. Cross-contamination can also happen when an object that touches a contaminated food later touches another food. For instance, suppose a knife used to cut raw poultry is then used to cut fresh vegetables. Bacteria from the poultry can get on the knife and then be transferred to the vegetables.

To prevent cross-contamination, be sure to wash all utensils and surfaces thoroughly after each use. Using a bleach solution of two teaspoons bleach to a quart of water will help eliminate bacteria. Choose tools and cutting boards that are easy to clean. Plastic materials are good choices. Wooden surfaces are porous and more difficult to keep clean. Allow cutting boards to air dry rather than drying them with cloth towels, which can transmit bacteria.

Keep shelves and drawers clean. Bacteria from these surfaces can be transferred to foods by utensils and dishes. Carefully cleaning appliances is another way to avoid contamination. For example, cleaning the cutting edge of a can opener keeps it from transferring bacteria when it touches food.

Allow dish cloths and sponges to dry thoroughly. Damp cloths and sponges are breeding grounds for bacteria. Each day, replace dishcloths and wash sponges in a bleach solution.

● Preparing Foods Safely

Following safety guidelines when preparing and serving food is another major part of the food safety picture. Cooking temperatures kill most bacteria. Temperatures of 60°F to 125°F (16°C to 52°C) allow bacteria to grow rapidly. This is why you should never allow cooked foods to stay at room temperature for more than two hours. Keep cold foods at or below 40°F (4°C). Keep hot foods above 140°F (60°C). Refrigerate leftover foods as soon as possible. See 20-8.

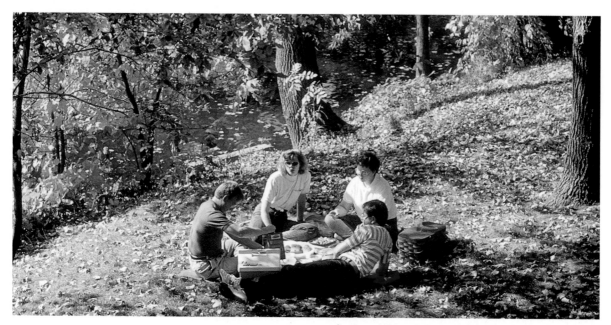

Courtesy of University Relations MSU, Bruce A. Fox, photographer

20-8 Foods at a picnic should not be left out for more than two hours.

Never thaw frozen meat on a countertop. Bacteria in the portions of the meat that reach room temperature will reproduce rapidly. The safest way to thaw all foods is to defrost them in the refrigerator. Another acceptable thawing technique is to place foods under cold running water. You can also use a microwave oven for quick, safe defrosting just before cooking. Follow the directions of the microwave manufacturer.

Do not eat or taste raw or partially cooked meat or poultry. Cook ground meat and all pork to an internal temperature of at least 160°F (71°C). Cook beef, veal, and lamb cuts to an internal temperature of at least 145°F (63°C). Cook whole poultry to an internal temperature of 180°F (82°C) and ground poultry to 165°F (74°C). Reheat leftovers to a temperature of 165°F (74°C). Use a meat thermometer to check the internal temperature. Insert the tip of the thermometer into the thickest part of the meat, avoiding fat and bone. See 20-9.

Do not put cooked meat on the same plate that held uncooked meat. Bacteria from the uncooked meat can remain on the plate and contaminate the cooked meat. Brush sauces only on cooked surfaces of meat and poultry. This prevents bacteria on raw meat and poultry surfaces from getting on the basting brush and contaminating the sauce. If you want to use a marinade as a sauce for cooked meat, reserve a portion before adding raw meat. Otherwise, you must boil the marinade for two minutes after removing raw meat to make it safe to use.

Eggs may be contaminated with salmonella bacteria. Therefore, avoid eating raw or undercooked eggs. Cooking eggs until whites are completely set and yolks are thickened helps destroy salmonella bacteria.

When cooking foods in a microwave oven, be sure to follow instructions on product labels. Keep in mind microwave ovens vary in power and operating efficiency. Also remember microwave ovens often do not cook foods evenly. Some parts of a food may not reach a high enough temperature to

Cooking Temperatures	
Food	**Temperature**
Eggs	
egg dishes	160°F, 71°C
fresh eggs	cook until whites are completely set and yolks are thickened
Beef and Lamb	
ground	160°F, 71°C
medium rare	145°F, 63°C
medium	160°F, 71°C
well done	170°F, 77°C
Pork	
fresh, medium	160°F, 71°C
fresh, well done	170°F, 77°C
ground	160°F, 71°C
ham, fresh	160°F, 71°C
ham, precooked	140°F, 60°C
Poultry	
chicken	180°F, 82°C
ground poultry	165°F, 74°C
turkey	180°F, 82°C

20-9 Cooking foods to an appropriate temperature will help kill any bacteria in the food.

destroy harmful microorganisms. To promote uniform cooking, arrange foods evenly in covered containers. Stir or rotate foods several times during the cooking period. (Many microwave ovens come with turntables for this purpose.) Use a temperature probe or meat thermometer to make sure food has reached a safe internal temperature.

Packing Food to Go

Some members of your family may pack lunches to take to work or school. You might need to transport a casserole to a relative's home for a holiday celebration. Perhaps you are going on a picnic with some friends. Whatever the situation, you need to take special steps to keep food safe when carrying it away from home.

When packing food to go, place all perishable items in an insulated bag or cooler. Be sure cold foods are frozen or well chilled before packing. For instance, you might freeze sandwiches for lunches the night before. The next day they will stay cold longer. (Freezing sandwiches with mayonnaise or fresh lettuce on them is not a good idea. Mayonnaise tends to separate and lettuce wilts during freezer storage.) Use ice packs to keep cold foods cold and safe for several hours. Try to keep foods out of the direct sun and avoid storage in a hot car. If possible, refrigerate packed food until you are ready to eat it.

You can store hot foods in a wide-mouth thermos to keep them at safe, high temperatures for several hours. Rinse the thermos with hot water before adding the food. Food should be hot to the touch at serving time. See 20-10.

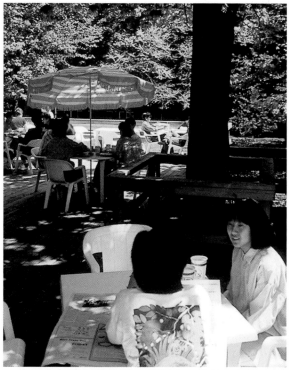

Courtesy of University Relations MSU, Bruce A. Fox, photographer

20-10 Picnics can be fun and safe if cold foods are kept cold and hot foods are kept hot.

When Foodborne Illness Happens

Foodborne illnesses can affect people differently. A contaminated food eaten by two people may cause different symptoms to appear in each person. One person may become sick and the other may not. Genetic makeup may play a role in the way your body reacts to certain contaminants. Your age and state of health may also affect how you will react to foodborne contaminants.

Who Is Most at Risk?

Foodborne illness can be more serious for some groups of people than others. Infants, children, pregnant women, older adults, substance abusers, and people with immune disorders are at the greatest risk. Infants' and children's immune systems are not mature enough to easily fight a virus or buildup of harmful bacteria. A given amount of toxin poses more danger to their small bodies than to the larger bodies of adults. Pregnant women need to avoid any type of illness due to potential danger to their fetuses. Contaminants from foods place added stress on the bodies of people who are already in poor health. People who are HIV positive or have AIDS are at a greater risk of problems from foodborne illness. People who have cancer, diabetes mellitus, or liver disease are also in more danger when foodborne illness occurs.

Recognizing the Symptoms

Foodborne illnesses produce an array of symptoms that range in severity. The most common symptoms are vomiting, stomach cramps, and diarrhea. The type and amount of bacteria in a food affects how sick a person becomes. The symptoms of most foodborne illnesses appear within a day or two after eating tainted food. However, some illnesses take up to 30 days to develop.

The symptoms of most foodborne illnesses last only a few days. A small percentage of cases lead to other illnesses. Spontaneous abortions (miscarriages), kidney failure, and arthritis have all been linked to foodborne illness. Complications caused by foodborne illnesses result in thousands of deaths each year.

Treating the Symptoms

Prevention is the best approach to foodborne illness. Do not eat any food you suspect might be contaminated. If in doubt about a food, throw it out! Dispose of it safely away from other humans and animals.

If foodborne illness does occur, you may be able to provide treatment at home. Self-treatment is appropriate when symptoms are mild and the person affected is not in a high-risk group. Replace the fluids lost through diarrhea and vomiting by drinking plenty of water. This will help prevent dehydration. Get a lot of rest. If symptoms continue for more than two or three days, call a physician.

If symptoms are severe, you should not wait to call a doctor. Severe symptoms include a high fever (102°F), blood in your stools, and dehydration (noticed by dizziness while standing). Diarrhea or vomiting lasting more than a few hours should be viewed as a severe symptom, too. You should also seek immediate medical advice when someone in a high-risk group presents symptoms of foodborne illness. Young children, pregnant women, older adults, and chronically ill people need prompt medical care. If symptoms include double vision, inability to swallow, or difficulty speaking, you should go directly to a hospital. These symptoms suggest *botulism,* which is a type of foodborne illness that can be fatal without immediate treatment.

Reporting Foodborne Illness

Determining the source of foodborne illness can be hard. This is because symptoms may not appear until a day or two after eating contaminated food. However, if you suspect the contaminated food came from a public source, you should call your local health department. If you ate the food at a restaurant or large gathering, such as a party, you should file a report. You should also report commercial products suspected of causing illness, such as canned goods or store-bought salads or cooked meats. Information you will need to present to the local health department when you phone in your report is presented in 20-11.

If you still have some of the suspected food, wrap it in a plastic bag. Clearly mark the bag to warn people not to eat the food. Store the bag in the refrigerator. Health officials may want to examine the food to see

---

Information to Report When Foodborne Illness Is Suspected

Your name, address, and phone number

Description of what happened: where the food was purchased, how many people ate the food, when the food was eaten

If food is a commercial product, the manufacturer's name and address listed on the container

On meat and poultry products, the USDA inspection stamp number for the identification of the processing plant or establishment number

Lot or batch number, which will indicate on what day and factory shift the item was produced

---

20-11 If foodborne illness is suspected and a number of people may be affected, health officials may request the above information.

if a product *recall* is necessary. This means removing the product from stores and warehouses and announcing a consumer alert to the public.

People and Public Food Safety

The food chain includes food producers, food processors and distributors, government agencies, and consumers. A weak link at any point in the chain may mean the difference between safety and illness. Poorly maintained farms and unclean processing plants can introduce microorganisms into the food supply. A careless inspection or improper handling at home can also allow tainted food to reach the dining table. Everyone in the chain has a role to play in keeping food safe.

Food Producers

Farmers who raise plants and animals for food have a duty to use chemicals carefully. They must use pesticides according to label directions. They might also explore alternatives to chemical pesticides as part of a crop management system. Farmers need to follow regulations when treating animals with medications. They must also be sure medications have cleared the animal's system before selling the animal for meat, 20-12.

Food Processors and Distributors

From the farm to the grocery store, the responsibility for safe foods lies with food processors and distributors. Reputable companies know safe food is good business. To compete in the food industry, they must provide wholesome foods. Processors should not accept farm products they suspect of being tainted. They need to keep their facilities clean. Distributors must be sure food is kept at safe temperatures during shipping.

To ensure food safety, some processing companies set guidelines that exceed government standards for handling food. They may have their own inspectors in addition to

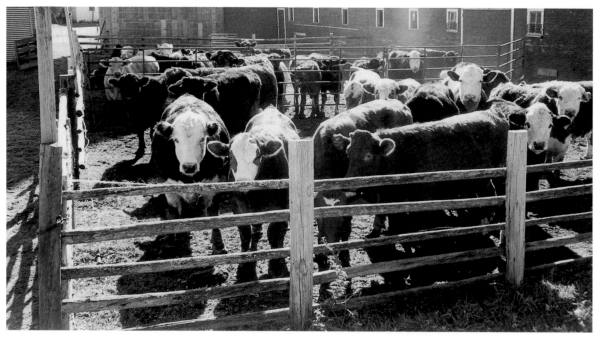

20-12 Animals bound for sale to meat producers must be free from medications.

government inspectors. These steps help guarantee the quality of products placed on grocery store shelves.

People who handle foods at supermarkets and restaurants also have a duty to protect public health. They must follow proper procedures to keep food wholesome.

Government Agencies

A number of federal and state agencies look after the food supply. Each agency plays a role in maintaining food safety.

U.S. Food and Drug Administration (FDA)

The FDA is in charge of ensuring the safety of all foods sold except meat, poultry, seafood, and eggs. The FDA monitors pesticide residues left on farm products. FDA inspectors check farms, food processing plants, and imported food products. They also oversee recalls of foods that have been found to be unsafe.

U.S. Department of Agriculture (USDA) and Food Safety and Inspection Service (FSIS)

The USDA and FSIS work together to monitor the safety and quality of poultry, egg, and meat products. USDA inspectors place a stamp of approval on food products that meet their standards for wholesomeness. They also check to be sure food handlers are practicing good sanitation.

Food processors may choose to have USDA inspectors judge the quality of products. A grade shield is placed on products to indicate their level of quality.

A large part of the USDA's and FSIS's efforts are geared to educating the public. They developed a safe food handling label to help consumers prepare and store foods with safety in mind, 20-13. The USDA also maintains the Meat and Poultry Hotline to answer consumers' food safety questions.

Safe Handling Instructions

This product was prepared from inspected and passed meat. Some animal products may contain bacteria that could cause illness if the product is mishandled or cooked improperly. For your protection, follow these safe handling instructions.

 Keep refrigerated or frozen. Thaw in refrigerator or microwave.

 Keep raw meats separate from other foods. Wash working surfaces (including cutting boards), utensils, and hands after touching raw meat.

 Cook thoroughly.

 Refrigerate leftovers within 2 hours.

20-13 This label, which is required on raw and partially cooked meat and poultry products, helps educate consumers about safe food handling.

National Marine Fisheries Service (NMFS)

The NMFS has a voluntary inspection program for fish products. Fish processors can choose to have their products inspected for quality. A quality seal can be placed on the labels of fish that meet quality standards.

U.S. Environmental Protection Agency (EPA)

The EPA plays a role in food safety by regulating pesticides. The EPA evaluates the safety of new pesticides and publishes directions for their safe use. It sets limits for pesticide residues and prosecutes growers who exceed these limits, too. The EPA also sets standards for water quality.

Federal Trade Commission (FTC)

The FTC's Bureau of Consumer Protection regulates food advertisements. Advertising claims must be truthful. They cannot mislead consumers about the contents or nutritional value of a product.

State and Local Agencies

Federal agencies cannot keep the food supply safe without support. State and local government agencies help ensure the safety of food produced in their regions. State departments of agriculture set standards and inspect farms. Local health departments check food handling in grocery stores. They also inspect food service operations, such as schools, nursing homes, and restaurants.

Food Consumers

As a consumer, you are the last link in the food chain. The responsibility for choosing wholesome food and handling it properly ultimately lies with you. You must select foods carefully to minimize food-related risks. You must practice safe food handling techniques to prevent foodborne illnesses. If illness occurs, you need to report it to the appropriate agencies. See 20-14.

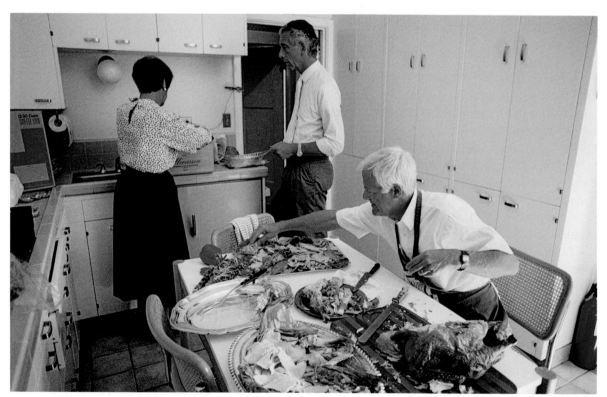

20-14 Consumers have a responsibility to prepare foods carefully and store leftovers promptly to help prevent foodborne illness.

Chapter 20 Review

Summary

Foodborne illness is common in the United States. Most foodborne illnesses are caused by harmful bacteria. Parasites, viruses, and molds in foods can cause illness, too. Natural toxins and chemicals can also contaminate foods.

You can take steps to help prevent foodborne illness. These steps begin with careful shopping to select only foods that appear wholesome. Then you need to store foods at safe temperatures. Prepare foods using safe food handling standards in a clean kitchen environment. When packing food to eat away from home, you need to take special precautions to keep it at safe temperatures.

Despite your best efforts, members of your family may still experience foodborne illness at some point. Knowing who is most at risk and recognizing the symptoms will help you know what steps to take. You can often treat mild symptoms at home. Severe symptoms and people in high-risk groups require treatment from a physician. If you suspect the cause of foodborne illness came from a public source, you should contact local health authorities.

Many people play a role in helping keep the food supply safe. Food producers, processors, and distributors each have a duty to maintain the wholesomeness of food before it reaches consumers. Government agencies set and enforce guidelines for food safety. The final burden for preventing foodborne illness lies with you, the consumer, through safe food handling practices.

Check Your Knowledge

1. What parasite is sometimes found in raw or undercooked pork and how can it be prevented from causing foodborne illness?

2. Disease-causing agents that are the smallest type of life-form are _____.
   A. bacteria
   B. contaminants
   C. protozoa
   D. viruses

3. What type of food produces scombroid toxin?

4. What are three steps a person can take to limit his or her intake of pesticide residues?

5. What are four signs that a frozen food may not have been stored at safe freezer temperatures?

6. How much time should a person spend washing his or her hands before handling food?

7. What are safe temperatures for serving hot and cold foods?

8. What six groups of people are most at risk when foodborne illness occurs?

9. What are the most common symptoms of foodborne illness?

10. Describe the treatment of mild symptoms of foodborne illness for someone who is not in a high-risk group.

11. What is the role of food distributors in keeping food safe?

12. Which government agency or agencies are responsible for monitoring the safety and quality of poultry, egg, and meat products?

Put Learning into Action

1. Look up Web sites related to food safety. Use the information you find to prepare food safety posters or a bulletin board.

2. Find out what a health inspector looks for when he or she is making an on-site inspection of a foodservice facility. Use these points to inspect your home kitchen or the kitchen in your school foods lab.

● Explore Further

1. Use a food science text or lab manual to research how to grow bacterial cultures. Follow the described procedure to transfer bacteria from at least three kitchen surfaces to a growth medium. Observe the bacterial growth over a three-day period. Record your observations and write a paper detailing your conclusions.

2. As a class, prepare a 10-question survey about basic food safety guidelines for selecting, storing, preparing, and transporting food. Each student should ask one adult and one student outside the class to complete the survey. Compile your survey findings. Then videotape a public service announcement to educate people about the food safety question that was most often answered incorrectly.

3. Research the functions and divisions of one of the governmental agencies involved in monitoring the safety of the food supply. Report your findings to the class.

Chapter 21

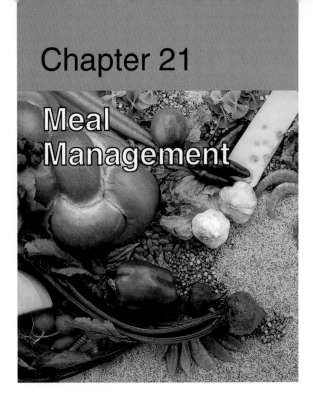

Meal Management

At mealtime, have you ever just opened the refrigerator and grabbed what was handy? Meals thrown together without planning often lack balanced nutrition and taste appeal. Meal management can help you avoid haphazard meals.

Meal management involves using resources to meet goals related to preparing and serving food. The resources a meal manager uses include knowledge of nutrition and food safety. Food preparation skills, time, and money are meal management resources, too. See 21-1.

In this chapter, you will learn how to plan meals that make wise use of these resources. By developing meal management skills, you will begin to focus on family food preferences and needs. You will also discover how to stay within a spending plan while preparing meals that suit your lifestyle. You will even pick up some pointers about managing your resources when eating

● Learn the Language

meal management   convenience food
budget

● Objectives

After studying this chapter, you will be able to
- plan menus that include a variety of food flavors, colors, textures, shapes, sizes, and temperatures.
- use the Food Guide Pyramid, the Dietary Guidelines for Americans, and meal patterns to plan nutritious menus for your family.
- describe techniques for controlling food spending to stay within the family food budget.
- identify methods for saving time when preparing foods.
- explain how to meet meal management goals when eating meals away from home.

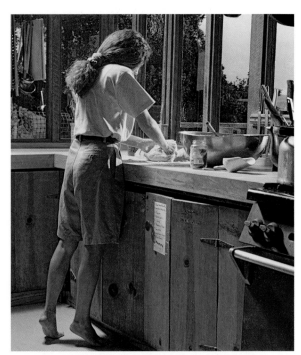

21-1 Today's lifestyles are hectic. The meal-planning process includes knowing how to prepare simple menus.

meals away from home. Applying this information will help everyone in your family enjoy daily meals.

● Planning for Appeal

Meal managers have found many advantages of planning meals. One advantage is being able to serve meals family members enjoy eating. A meal will not satisfy hunger if no one will eat it. Considering family members' likes and dislikes will help you plan a meal they will find appealing.

Besides family preferences, you can use variety to make meals more appealing. Variety adds interest to each meal served. It also adds interest to weekly menus because the same foods are not served repeatedly. You can add variety to meals with different flavors, colors, textures, shapes and sizes, and temperatures.

● Flavor

You may be tempted to always list favorite family foods in your meal plans. This assures you that your family members will find the meals appealing. For variety, however, consider introducing your family to new foods from time to time. Ethnic foods offer a broad range of interesting new flavors your family might enjoy. For example, you might want to try a quiche from France or refried beans from Mexico.

Keep in mind that eating habits change slowly. Family members may not like every new dish you try. Do not be discouraged. Continue to prepare tasty and attractive new foods now and then. Soon you will learn which flavor combinations generally meet with approval and which ones are usually disliked.

Using flavor variety in your meal planning means more than serving different dishes throughout the week. You need to include a variety of flavors in every meal. Think about a meal with tomato juice as an appetizer,

tomatoes on the salad, and tomato sauce on the pasta. So much tomato flavor would make the meal seem rather boring. Substituting apricot nectar for the appetizer and green pepper rings on the salad would introduce variety.

Make a point of balancing strongly flavored foods with those that are more subtle. For instance, you could complement a spicy burrito with some mild pinto beans. You might balance a dish of tart apple slices with a drizzle of sweet caramel topping.

● Color

Color appeals to the eye and stimulates appetite. Picture a meal of poached fish, scalloped potatoes, and steamed cabbage. These foods are all pale. Now envision how the plate would look if you sprinkled the fish with some bright red paprika. Change the scalloped potatoes to au gratin potatoes by adding some golden yellow cheese. Replace the cabbage with deep green broccoli. By making a few changes, a bland-looking meal has become quite colorful. See 21-2.

● Texture

Texture variety makes meals more enjoyable to eat. How appealing would you find a meal of creamed turkey, mashed sweet potatoes, and applesauce? These foods all have a smooth, creamy texture. A meal that includes crunchy and chewy textures as well as soft would be more appetizing. You could introduce some different textures by changing the menu to roast turkey with mashed sweet potatoes. Then replace the applesauce with a salad of crisp apple wedges on a bed of fresh spinach.

● Shape and Size

The shape of foods on your plate can affect how inviting they look. Think about a plate filled with strips of pepper steak, French fries, and carrot sticks. These foods are all in long, skinny pieces. The plate

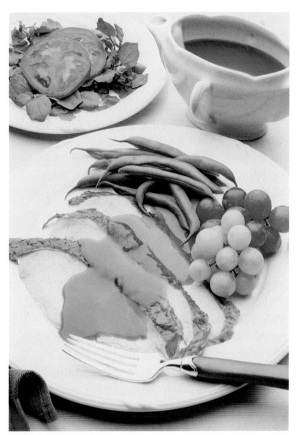

21-2 The variety of reds, greens, browns, and creams in this meal add interest and make the meal more attractive.

would be more appealing if you served a baked potato and sliced carrots with the pepper steak.

Also try to vary the size of food pieces. For instance, a tuna and rice casserole is made up of little pieces. Green peas and coleslaw might not be the best accompaniments for this casserole. They too are made up of little pieces. Snow peas and a salad of sliced tomatoes might complement the casserole better.

● Temperature

Most people enjoy a balance of hot and cold foods in their meals. Consider a breakfast of scrambled eggs, toast, warm fruit compote, and hot chocolate. These foods are all hot. Changing the fruit compote to a chilled

fruit salad and the hot chocolate to cold chocolate milk adds temperature variety.

Whatever foods are on your menu, be sure to serve them at the proper temperature. Few people enjoy lukewarm soup or milk that is barely cool. They prefer their soup to be piping hot and their milk to be icy cold. See 21-3. Besides being more appealing, foods are safer when they are served at the correct temperatures. Keep hot foods hot, above 140°F (60°C), and cold foods cold, below 40°F (5°C). This will help prevent growth of bacteria and other pathogens that can cause foodborne illness.

● Planning for Nutrition

A second advantage of meal planning is that it helps meal managers provide for their families' nutritional needs. Remember that no single food can provide all the needed nutrients. Serving a variety of foods is the best way to be sure family members are getting a variety of nutrients. Also keep in mind that each nutrient comes in many different foods. A family member who does not like one food

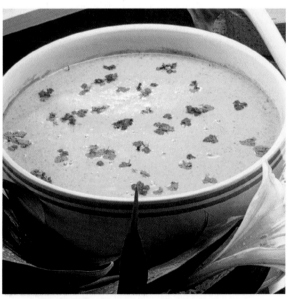

21-3 Soups such as this broccoli soup are more appealing when they are served hot.

source of a nutrient can get the nutrient from another source.

In some families, each member has different nutritional needs. Meal managers must consider each of these needs when planning menus. Special resources may be needed to help meal managers with this task.

Characteristics of Family Members

You have learned everyone needs the same set of nutrients. However, the amounts of nutrients each person needs may vary. For instance, children need smaller amounts of nutrients, but they have greater proportional needs than adults. The age, sex, body size, and activity level of each family member will affect his or her nutrient needs. Meal managers do not need to plan a separate menu to meet each person's needs. All family members can usually enjoy the same meal in different portion sizes.

Sometimes one or more members of a family follow a special diet. A family member with high blood pressure may follow a low-sodium diet. A vegetarian in the family does not include meat products in his or her diet. A registered dietitian can counsel a meal manager about meeting the special needs of family members when planning meals.

Nutrition Planning Resources

Meal managers can use a number of resources to help them meet their families' nutritional needs. These resources include the Food Guide Pyramid, the Dietary Guidelines for Americans, and basic meal patterns.

Following the Food Guide Pyramid can help you plan meals that provide recommended daily nutrients for your family. Each day's menus should provide family members with the suggested number of servings from the five major food groups. As you choose foods from each group, remember to keep the Dietary Guidelines for Americans in mind. Following the guidelines will help you

control the fat, saturated fat, cholesterol, sugar, sodium, and alcohol in your family's diet. At the same time, you will be selecting foods that are rich sources of vitamins, minerals, and fiber.

Meal patterns are outlines of what to serve at each meal. A meal pattern based on the Food Guide Pyramid includes the following servings at each meal:

- two to three servings from the bread, cereal, rice, and pasta group
- one to two servings from the vegetable group
- one to two servings from the fruit group
- one serving from the milk, yogurt, and cheese group
- one to three ounces from the meat, poultry, fish, dry beans, eggs, and nuts group (two to three servings per day)

This meal pattern works equally well for breakfast, lunch, and dinner. Following it will provide most people with the recommended daily servings from the Food Guide Pyramid. Snacks can be chosen to meet additional serving needs. See 21-4.

If you have too few or too many servings at one meal, you can make up for it at another meal. For instance, your dinner menu might not include any foods from the fruit group. You can simply choose an extra serving for breakfast, lunch, or snack. Keep serving sizes in mind. If you have a 6-ounce chicken breast for lunch, you have probably met your daily needs. You could skip the meat, poultry, fish, dry beans, eggs, and nuts group at breakfast and dinner.

Many meal managers plan for family members to meet nutrient needs by eating three meals a day. Breakfast generally supplies about one-fourth of the day's nutrient and calorie needs. Lunch and dinner each furnish one-third of the day's needs. Healthful snacks chosen from the five major food groups can provide the remaining needs. Some meal managers plan for family members to eat lighter meals and heartier

Menu Planning with a Meal Pattern

Menu	Bread, Cereal, Rice and Pasta Group 2-3 servings per meal	Vegetable Group 1-2 servings per meal	Fruit Group 1-2 servings per meal	Milk, Yogurt, and Cheese Group 1 serving per meal	Meat, Poultry, Fish, Dry Beans, Eggs, and Nuts Group 1-3 oz. per meal
Breakfast 2-egg omelet with mushrooms, onions, and peppers 2 slices wheat toast Sliced banana Milk	XX	X	X (orange juice)	X	XX
Snack Whole wheat crackers Grapes	X		X		(peanut butter)
Lunch Chicken breast, 1 oz., with Swiss cheese, lettuce, and tomato on a whole-wheat bun Apple	XX	X	X	X	X
Snack Popcorn, 1 cup (2 cups)	X (X)	(carrot sticks)			
Dinner Baked ham, 3 oz. Noodles, ½ cup (1 cup) Sweet potatoes Broccoli Dinner rolls, 2 Frozen yogurt	X (X) XX	X X		X	XXX
Total Daily Servings	9 (11)	4 (5)	3 (4)	3	6 (7)

21-4 These menus follow a meal pattern based on the Food Guide Pyramid. They meet the daily serving recommendations for most teenage females. Making the adjustments shown in parentheses allows them to meet the daily serving recommendations for most teenage males.

snacks. You can choose the meal schedule that is most convenient for members of your family. The important point is they receive their full allowance of nutrients throughout the day. See 21-5.

Selecting Equipment to Promote Nutrition

Your choice of kitchen equipment can affect the nutrients in foods. Choose cookware that provides even heat distribution. You want to avoid cookware that creates hotspots, which scorch foods, causing an unappealing taste and damage to some nutrients.

A microwave oven can be a wise choice in kitchen equipment that helps protect the nutrients in foods. High heat and long cooking periods can result in vitamin losses. A microwave oven cooks foods quickly, minimizing such losses. Microwave cooking also requires less water than conventional cooking methods. Therefore, fewer nutrients leach into the cooking liquid.

A deep fryer is a less healthful option in kitchen equipment. Frying adds fat and calories to foods. In addition, high frying temperatures can destroy heat-sensitive vitamins.

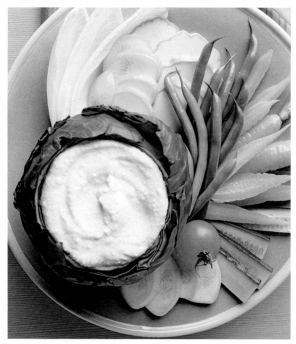

21-5 Choose nutritious snacks that will help you get the recommended number of servings from each food group.

Slow cookers can help you save time and energy as you prepare nutritious foods. You can put the ingredients for a one-dish dinner in a slow cooker in the morning. In the evening, your dinner will be ready with a minimal amount of preparation time. Slow cookers use low heat for long periods. Nutrients destroyed by high temperatures can be preserved. The cooking liquid is often eaten with one-dish meals prepared in slow cookers. Therefore, you will not lose the benefit of any nutrients that have escaped into the cooking liquid.

Choosing Preparation Methods to Promote Nutrition

The preparation methods you use as well as the equipment you choose can affect the nutrient content of your food. Whole, unpeeled fruits and vegetables generally retain more of their nutrients. Therefore, if you have the time to wash and trim produce yourself, avoid buying precut produce. When cooking fruits and vegetables, keep them in larger pieces to limit the amount of exposed surface area. This will help reduce the amount of nutrients that leach into the cooking liquid.

Use the smallest amount of cooking liquid possible to help preserve water-soluble nutrients. Protect heat-sensitive nutrients, such as folate and vitamin C, by cooking foods for the shortest time possible. Microwaving, steaming, and stir-frying are healthful choices for cooking foods quickly. Choose high-temperature cooking methods, such as grilling and deep frying, less often because they result in greater nutrient losses.

Controlling Food Costs

A third advantage of meal planning is being able to manage how much money your family spends on food. You can use a few techniques to help you control food costs without giving up appetite appeal or nutrients.

Use a Spending Plan

To plan meals that stay within your family's financial limits, you first need to decide what those limits are. Preparing a **budget**, or a spending plan, will help you make this decision. A budget helps you plan how to use your sources of income to meet your various expenses. Many expenses occur on a monthly basis. Therefore, many people find it convenient to set up a monthly budget.

It is not a good idea to spend more money than you receive. The amount of money you budget for food must fit in with all your other expenses. These include *fixed expenses,* such as rent and car payments, which are the same each month. You also have *flexible expenses,* such as clothing purchases and utility bills, which vary from month to month. The food category of a budget is generally considered a flexible expense.

As the meal manager, you are responsible for staying within the established food budget. Saving all your food receipts for a few weeks will help you see if you are meeting this goal. If you find you are spending too much, you will have to make some adjustments. Keep in mind that buying meats, gourmet foods, and convenience products adds to food expenses. Eating out and having frequent dinner guests increase food spending, too. You may have to cut back on these types of food purchases if you are not staying within your budget. See 21-6.

Cost-Cutting Menu Plans

Most people are concerned about food costs. When incomes are limited, food budgets must also be limited. One way to keep food spending under control is to build menus around low-cost foods in each food group. For instance, brown rice and fresh pasta are both in the bread, cereal, rice, and pasta group. You could use either as the basis of a tasty, nutritious casserole. However, fresh pasta costs about three times more than the brown rice.

When planning menus, plan to use the less costly foods from the other food groups in the same way. From the fruit and vegetable groups, choose fresh produce that is in season. Frozen and canned plain fruits and vegetables are usually good buys, too. Those that come with extras, like sauces, are more costly. See 21-7. In the milk, yogurt, and cheese group, you can save money by using nonfat dry milk in your menu plans. Dry legumes and peanut butter are the best buys in the meat, poultry, fish, dry beans, eggs, and nuts group. You can use them in high-fiber, lowfat meatless main dishes.

Plan menus that take advantage of advertised store specials. If broccoli is on sale, you might plan to serve it for several meals. You could use it in a salad one day and in a side dish another day.

Careful shopping can also help you save money when buying food. Smart shopping tips are listed in Chapter 22, "Making Wise Consumer Choices."

Saving Time

Saving time and effort is a fourth advantage of meal planning. Efficient use of time is important to people with busy schedules. Some people skip meals if they cannot prepare foods quickly and easily. For them, fast

Food Spending Plan		
Month: *January*		
Food Eaten at Home	**Money Planned**	**Money Spent**
Week one	*$150*	*$130*
Week two	*150*	*165*
Week three	*150*	*180*
Week four	*150*	*115*
Total	*$600*	*$590*
Restaurants/Takeout	**Money Planned**	**Money Spent**
Week one	*$30*	*$40*
Week two	*30*	*38*
Week three	*30*	*42*
Week four	*30*	*50*
Total	*$120*	*$170*
Total Food Expenses	*$720*	*$760*

21-6 If you are not meeting your monthly food budget, you may have to make adjustments in spending.

Cutting Fruit and Vegetable Costs

Form	Less Expensive Choices	More Expensive Choices
Fresh	In-season fruits and vegetables, apples, bananas, cabbage, carrots, greens, onions, oranges, potatoes	Out-of-season fruits and vegetables, asparagus, berries, Brussels sprouts, cauliflower, mangoes, mushrooms, pineapple, spinach, yams
Canned	Applesauce, beets, carrots, corn, fruit juices, green beans, greens, mixed vegetables, peas, tomatoes	Apricots, asparagus, berries, citrus sections, fruit nectars, individual juice boxes, mushrooms
Frozen	Concentrated citrus juices, corn, green beans, greens, peas, spinach, squash	Asparagus, corn on the cob, ethnic vegetable combinations, raspberries, vegetables in sauces
Dried	Dried beans, raisins	Apples, apricots, dates, mangoes, peaches

21-7 You can cut costs in food spending and still purchase foods you need for a nutritious diet.

and simple meal preparations are essential to good nutrition.

A number of tools can help you make the best use of your time in the kitchen. You can use organizational skills and timesaving appliances. You can also use recipes and food products designed to speed your food preparation tasks.

Organize Work Space and Equipment

A first step for saving time in food preparation is organizing your work space and equipment. Store kitchen utensils close to where you are likely to use them. For instance, you might store a pancake turner close to the range and a vegetable peeler close to the sink. Keeping cupboards and drawers neat makes it easier to find the items that are stored in them. Store appliances in handy locations. If appliances are difficult to get out and put away, you are less likely to use them.

Ingredients need to be on hand when you are ready to use them. Keeping a shopping list handy will help you remember to jot down items as you discover you need them. This will allow you to avoid running to the store at the last minute to pick up missing ingredients.

Use Timesaving Appliances

Many small appliances can save preparation and cooking time. Food processors can save time when chopping, grating, or mixing large portions of fruits, vegetables, or other ingredients. Pressure cookers reduce cooking time. Slow cookers and bread machines allow you to prepare foods in the morning and have them ready to eat at dinnertime. See 21-8.

Microwave ovens are useful for reducing time when cooking and reheating leftovers. Using a microwave oven can also save serving and cleanup time. This is because many foods can be cooked, served, and stored in the same container.

Select Quick and Easy Menu Items

With planning, you can prepare many meals in 30 minutes or less. These meals can be as tasty and healthful as those that take more time and trouble to prepare.

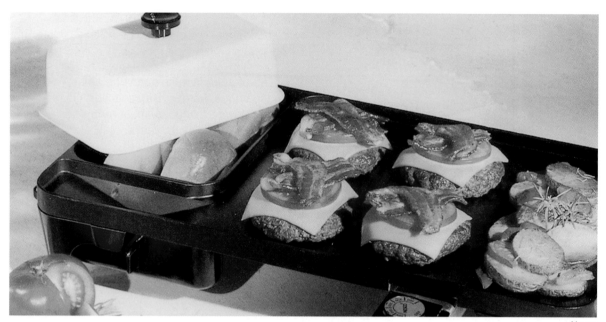

Nesco

21-8 The main dish and a side dish of a meal can be cooked on this electric skillet at the same time. This model also features a warming oven.

Quick and easy meals begin with quick and easy recipes. Most simple recipes require only a few ingredients. Ingredients are generally foods that most people have on hand. These recipes have a small number of preparation steps and require only a few utensils. They usually rely on fast cooking techniques, such as microwaving and stir-frying.

Keep a file of simple recipes your family enjoys. Organize them into categories, such as main dishes, salads, and desserts. You might also want to keep a file of quick menu ideas for various types of meals. This will make it easy for you to prepare complete meals when you are in a hurry.

Another way to prepare quick and easy meals is through the planned use of leftovers. When you have time to cook, double recipes and store half in the refrigerator or freezer. In the time it takes to cook or reheat the stored portion, you can prepare accompanying menu items. In a matter of minutes you will be able to serve a complete meal. Meat loaf, soups, and casseroles work especially well for this type of meal planning.

● Consider Convenience Foods

Nearly all meal managers use some convenience foods to help them save time in the kitchen. **Convenience foods** are food items that are purchased partially or completely prepared. Cake mixes, canned soups, and frozen entrees are typical convenience foods. See 21-9.

Convenience foods are popular for several reasons other than time savings. Meal managers who have limited cooking skills like convenience foods because the instructions are simple to follow. Many people enjoy the taste of convenience foods. Creative cooks appreciate recipes found on many convenience food packages calling for the convenience products as ingredients.

Convenience foods often cost more than foods made from scratch. You must decide whether the time savings, taste, and nutritional contributions of convenience products are worth the cost. Be sure to read nutrition labels when choosing convenience products. Many are higher in sodium and fat than foods you would prepare yourself.

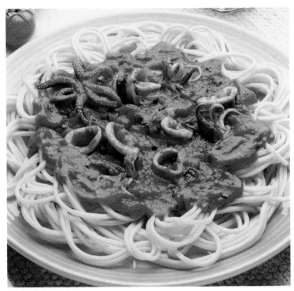

21-9 Heating ready-made spaghetti sauce and cooking the noodles for this dish could be done easily in a short time.

● Meals Away from Home

Meal managers are responsible for making sure family members' nutrient needs are met and the family food budget is maintained. This is true even when family members eat meals away from home. Managing nutrition and food costs is not difficult when meals are prepared at home and packed to go. These management tasks are more challenging when meals are prepared elsewhere.

● When You Pack a Lunch

Many students and working family members carry meals from home to eat at school or the workplace. These meals are most often lunches.

Carrying a lunch from home has many advantages over purchasing food from a restaurant or vending machine. When you pack a lunch, you can include your favorite foods. You can use ingredients that meet the Dietary Guidelines. You will save money, too.

Packing a lunch can also have a down side. Creatively choosing what to put into a lunch is not always easy. Finding the time to pack it requires planning.

Sandwiches are frequently the main course in a packed lunch. Look for new recipes if you like variety. You can add interest to sandwiches by using different kinds of breads and rolls and preparing various fillings.

When packing lunches, try to include a variety of foods from the five food groups. Limit snack foods, cookies, and cakes that are high in fats, sugars, and/or sodium. Choose some foods that are high in dietary fiber, such as whole grain breads and fresh fruits and vegetables.

Packing a lunch need not take much time. Many people pack lunches the night before and keep them in the refrigerator. When clearing the dinner table, store leftovers in serving-sized containers. Put them directly into lunch bags and refrigerate. Try setting up an assembly line to make sandwiches for the whole family. You can quickly complete each meal by adding a piece of fresh fruit. Packing a thermos of milk or a frozen box of juice will provide a cool drink with lunch.

Keep food safety in mind when packing lunches. Use food containers that will keep foods at the proper temperatures until they will be eaten. (Food safety is covered in detail in Chapter 20, "Keeping Food Safe.")

● When You Choose from a Menu

Eating out often serves as a solution to time problems for busy meal managers and their family members. In the United States, about 40¢ of every food dollar is spent on foods prepared away from home. This includes foods purchased from concession stands, vending machines, take-out counters, and all types of restaurants.

You have less control over the appeal, nutrient content, and cost of foods when eating out. However, your choice of restaurant will affect the type of foods available and how much you will spend.

Many restaurants offer a variety of choices for their health-conscious customers. Sometimes healthful options are marked by a special symbol on the menu. In addition, menu terms can help you identify foods that may be high in fat and sodium. See 21-10.

You may find healthful eating a bit more challenging when eating at fast-food restaurants. This is because many fast foods are high in sodium, fat, and calories. One large burger, French fries, and a milk shake can supply half a day's calorie needs for many teens. This meal is low in fiber and vitamins A and C. It contains approximately 1,400 milligrams of sodium, and over 50 percent of the calories come from fat. On the positive side, fast-food meals are usually excellent sources of protein and iron.

You do not have to avoid fast-food meals. Registered dietitians suggest selecting foods wisely and adjusting other meals throughout the day to balance calorie and nutrient intake.

The following tips can help you meet your goals for good nutrition when eating out:

- Resist the temptation to order double burgers, large fries, and super-sized drinks. Stick with regular-sized menu items.
- Order half-size, appetizer, or children's portions or consider sharing an entree with a friend.
- Limit high-fat creamy and oily salads, such as potato salad, tuna salad, and marinated pasta and vegetable salads.
- Go easy on toppings like cheese and bacon. Request that gravies, sauces, and salad dressings be served on the side. This will help you control fat intake.
- Use low-calorie condiments, such as reduced-fat dressings on salads and lemon juice on fish instead of tartar sauce.
- Avoid adding salt at the table.
- Trim fat from meat, skin from chicken, and breading from fish. Blot the oil on pizza with a napkin. See 21-11.
- Choose fruit or nonfat frozen yogurt for dessert.
- Order fruit juice instead of soda. Choose lowfat milk instead of a milk shake. Ask for water to drink with your meal along with or instead of other beverages.

Menu Clues

Higher Fat

Au gratin or in cheese sauce	Hollandaise
Breaded	In its own gravy, with gravy, pan gravy
Buttered or buttery	Pastry
Creamed, creamy, or in cream sauce	Rich
Fried, French-fried, deep-fried, batter-fried, panfried	Scalloped

Higher Sodium

Barbecued	Mustard sauce
Creole sauce	Parmesan
In a tomato base	Pickled
In broth	Smoked
In cocktail sauce	Soy sauce
Marinated	Teriyaki

21-10 Be aware of menu items described using these words. The food will be higher in fat and sodium.

Healthful Menu Choices

Chicken Menu Choices	Calories	Fat (g)	Sodium (mg)
3 oz. cooked skinless chicken breast	140	3	65
3 oz. cooked chicken breast (meat and skin)	165	7	60
3 oz. fried chicken breast (meat, skin, and breading)	220	11	235

21-11 When eating out, evaluate the choices available to you.

- Get some exercise after eating out. Walk home from the restaurant or plan other light activities to help burn a few calories.

Through planning, you can enjoy eating out. As people become more nutrition conscious, restaurants will increase their offerings of healthful menu items. This will allow meals eaten away from home to better meet all the goals of meal management.

Chapter 21 Review

Summary

Meal management involves using resources to plan and prepare meals. One of the goals of meal management is to make meals appealing. Planning meals that include foods with a variety of flavors, colors, textures, shapes, sizes, and temperatures will meet this goal.

A second goal of meal management is to plan meals that will meet nutritional needs. Different needs of each family member must be considered. The Dietary Guidelines for Americans and meal patterns based on the Food Guide Pyramid are resources for meeting this goal. Your choices of cooking equipment and food preparation methods can help you meet this goal, too.

A third meal management goal is to control food costs. A meal manager can prepare a budget. This will allow him or her to determine how much money is available to spend on food. A number of cost-cutting techniques can help a meal manager stay within his or her budget.

Saving time is a fourth goal for most meal managers. Keeping the kitchen and equipment organized and using timesaving appliances will help keep meal preparations moving. Choosing quick and easy recipes and taking advantage of convenience products will save time, too.

A meal manager must try to meet these four basic goals even when family members eat meals away from home. These goals are not difficult to achieve when packing meals to eat at school or the workplace. Meal management is more of a challenge when meals are purchased from sources such as restaurants. Meal managers can help family members learn to make nutritious choices that are within food spending limits.

Check Your Knowledge

1. What are two tips for adding flavor appeal to meals?
2. Which characteristic of an appealing meal is not met by a menu of cranberry juice, red cabbage slaw, and spaghetti with tomato sauce?
   A. Flavor.
   B. Color.
   C. Texture.
   D. Shape and size.
3. Besides making foods more appealing, why is it important to serve them at proper temperatures?
4. True or false. Meal managers usually need to plan separate menus to meet special dietary needs of individual family members.
5. Describe a meal pattern based on the Food Guide Pyramid.
6. What is the difference between fixed expenses and flexible expenses?
7. Give one example of a low-cost food in each of three food groups from the Food Guide Pyramid.
8. Give two examples of how appliances can help save time in the kitchen.
9. What are three characteristics of a quick and easy recipe?
10. What is one advantage and one disadvantage of using convenience foods?
11. What are two tips for saving time when packing lunches?
12. What are five tips for meeting the goal of good nutrition when eating out?

Put Learning into Action

1. Cut a picture of a plated meal from a magazine. Attach it to a written evaluation of the meal's flavors, colors, textures, shapes, sizes, and temperatures.

2. Write menus for your family for one day's meals. Be sure to follow the Dietary Guidelines for Americans and meal patterns based on the Food Guide Pyramid. Note how your choices of equipment and preparation methods can help promote good nutrition.

3. Collect menus from various local restaurants. Identify those that offer food choices in line within the Dietary Guidelines for Americans.

Explore Further

1. Plan and conduct a research project to evaluate the effect of flavor, color, texture, shape, size, or temperature on food choices. For instance, you might divide a batch of mashed potatoes in half. Color one half orange and leave the other half unaltered. Then ask people to try both samples and tell you which they prefer and why. Ask people to wear blindfolds when trying the potatoes to see if their responses are the same. Write a report describing your project in detail. Summarize your findings and draw a conclusion.

2. Prepare a food like spaghetti or chili from scratch. Use nutrient analysis software to evaluate your recipe. Then prepare two convenience forms of the food, such as a boxed mix and a canned product. Prepare a written evaluation comparing the three products for nutritional value and cost per serving. Also compare the taste and ease of preparation.

3. Survey three teens about what they ordered the last time they ate out. Be sure to note the age and gender of each teen. Compile your findings with those of your classmates to identify a "typical" food order. Analyze this order and make suggestions for improving the nutritional value of the food choices. Summarize your study and recommendations in an article for the school newspaper.

Chapter 22

Making Wise Consumer Choices

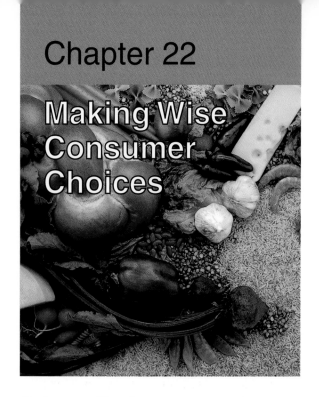

How do you decide which food and fitness items to buy? Are your decisions swayed by advertising? Do you base your food choices on the way products taste, their nutritional value, or their package appeal? Do you buy fitness equipment because it is the latest fad or because you are truly interested in an activity? How much does cost affect what you buy? Perhaps you buy certain products out of habit. These and many other factors influence your market decisions. See 22-1.

You are a **consumer**. That means you are someone who buys and uses products and services. You purchase food, sports equipment, clothing, movie tickets, and hundreds of other items. You pay people to serve you meals, lead your fitness classes, and dry-clean your clothes.

This chapter will help you develop skills as a consumer. You will consider your options for where to buy foods and fitness products and services. You will become aware of the impact advertising can have on you. You will determine what quality standards are

● Learn the Language

consumer
electronic shopping
food processing
food additive
GRAS (generally
  recognized as
  safe) list
organic food
comparison shopping
unit price
national brand
store brand
generic product
impulse buying

● Objectives

After studying this chapter, you will be able to
- describe at least six types of stores that sell food.
- explain how advertising, food processing, organic foods, and prices can affect consumer choices.
- use information on food labels to make healthful food choices.
- evaluate the quality of fitness products and services.
- identify your consumer rights and responsibilities.

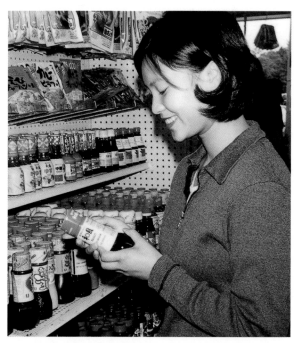

22-1 Your purchase decisions may be influenced by several factors.

important to you when choosing nutritious foods and quality fitness equipment. You will learn to read and interpret information on food and product labels. This chapter will also help you practice shopping skills to control spending. You will form a plan of action to take when you have problems in the marketplace, too.

● Where to Shop for Food

How do you decide where to buy the foods you need? If you are like most people, one of the factors that affects your choice of stores is food prices. However, you will probably not want price to be your only consideration. If you drive from store to store to get the lowest price, you may not end up saving money. This shopping strategy takes time and adds to your transportation costs.

You may find it more practical to do most of your shopping in one or two stores. Choose stores that give you the best overall price and quality. Look for stores that are conveniently located. You are likely to want stores that offer cleanliness, customer services, and variety, too. As you become familiar with favorite stores, you will learn where to quickly find the items on your shopping list.

● Types of Food Stores

Several types of stores sell food products. These include supermarkets, warehouse stores, convenience stores, cooperatives, outlet stores, specialty stores, and roadside stands and farmers' markets. Each alternative offers some advantages and disadvantages.

Supermarkets offer a wide range of products. Besides foods, they carry household items, health and beauty products, and pet supplies. Many stores have bakery, deli, and butcher departments. Some have pharmacies, bank branches, and cafeterias. Supermarkets offer consumers selection and convenience. However, some shoppers have trouble finding the products they need in such large stores.

Like supermarkets, most *warehouse stores* offer a variety of products other than foods. Selections may be limited, and the availability of given products may vary. Many items are sold in large containers and multi-unit packages. This can be a convenience for shoppers who like to stock up on food items. However, some consumers do not have enough storage space to accommodate large quantities. Prices at warehouse stores can be lower than supermarket prices. Some warehouses charge membership fees, and they may not accept coupons. These factors make warehouse prices less of a bargain.

Convenience stores usually have longer business hours than other food stores. Many stay open around the clock. They stock a limited variety of food items and household essentials. They often sell drinks and ready-to-eat foods, such as sandwiches and pizza. These stores are in locations that make it easy to quickly stop and pick up a few needed items. Prices at convenience stores are often higher than supermarket prices.

Most food *cooperatives,* or *co-ops,* are not open to the public. They are owned and run by a group of consumers. Only members of the group may take advantage of the discounted food prices. Food prices are low because the group buys foods in bulk and adds no charge for profit. Co-ops also save labor costs by requiring members to volunteer at the co-op for a few hours each month. Members may also have to pay an annual fee. See 22-2.

Outlet stores sell products made by one food manufacturer. Although these items are wholesome, some of them may not have met the manufacturer's standards for quality. For instance, bagels may be slightly misshapen or the frosting on a cake may be smudged. Products at outlet stores are usually sold at substantial discounts over retail prices. However, the consumer has no opportunity to compare and select competing brands.

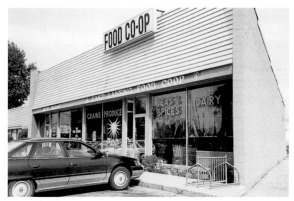

22-2 The low food prices at a co-op may make up for the annual fee members must pay.

Specialty stores include ethnic markets, dairies, bakeries, and butcher shops. These stores specialize in selling one type of product. Their products are usually high quality and very fresh. Most specialty stores charge premium prices.

Roadside stands and farmers' markets offer consumers the chance to buy fruits and vegetables fresh from the field. *Roadside stands* are operated by individual produce growers during the growing season. *Farmers' markets* sell produce from a number of farmers, often in a city location. Roadside stands and farmers' markets usually have limited hours. However, their produce is fresher and usually lower priced than supermarket produce. See 22-3.

● **Supermarket Trends**

Changes are taking place in supermarkets to meet emerging needs of consumers. Supermarkets are becoming larger and are focusing more on convenience. They are offering pharmacies, financial services, and ready-to-eat meals. They are adding more nonfood departments. New supermarket departments may include floral arranging, video rentals, and postal services. This trend allows consumers to do much of their shopping at one store. There may be separate entrances to specialty sections of the store, such as the deli and bakery departments.

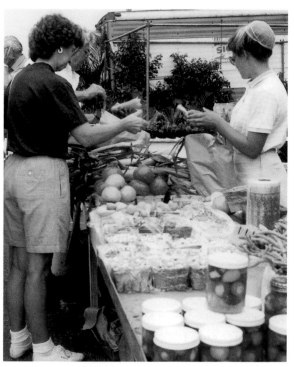

22-3 Freshly picked fruits and vegetables are offered at roadside stands and farmers' markets.

Some large supermarkets are adding educational centers. These are classrooms in which stores offer cooking and wellness classes for their customers.

Stores increasingly rely on *demographic data.* This is information about people in the communities in which the stores are located. This trend helps stores tailor the items they carry to the needs of their customers. For instance, a store might expand its ethnic food line to meet the needs of local consumers.

New marketing methods are being introduced in the supermarket. Look for food demonstrations or cooking contests as ways to advertise products. Video screens mounted on shopping carts may promote products as you walk up and down the store aisles. Monitors in specific store departments may show videotapes about how to prepare foods sold in those departments. Electronic coupons or automated discounts may be used to promote items. These forms of savings will be automatically deducted from your bill at the checkout.

Stores are introducing services that reduce the amount of time needed to shop. Self-service scanners are being used in some stores to speed checkout. Some supermarkets are allowing consumers to call in grocery orders for later pickup.

Online grocery shopping services eliminate the need for consumers to go to the store. These services provide people who sign up for the program with the software needed to do **electronic shopping**. This is a method of buying items over the Internet using a home computer. An electronic shopper can choose from a wide range of food and nonfood items. He or she can specify brands and sizes. The shopper can even see product labels on the computer screen. After a consumer completes a shopping list, he or she sends it electronically to the online service provider. Professional shoppers then fill the customer's order and deliver it to his or her home.

Many stores are also showing more concern for the environment. They may have facilities for recycling store bags and other materials. They may reduce the use of packaging by offering more foods in bulk, too.

● Factors That Affect Consumer Food Choices

A number of factors affect the choices you make when you are shopping for food. You may want to try products you learn about through advertising. You may think about how a food is processed and the types of additives it contains. You might evaluate the pros and cons of buying organic foods. You may be drawn to some products by their packaging. See 22-4.

● Food Advertising

Food advertising can influence your buying behavior. Manufacturers spend billions of dollars each year promoting products. Their

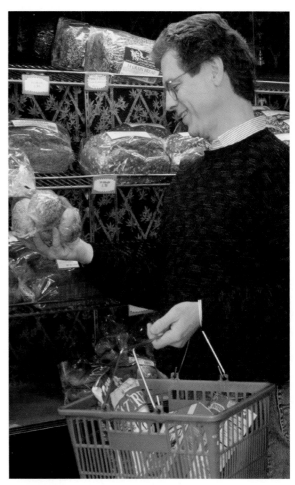

22-4 Evaluating the additives and price of a product will help you decide whether or not to purchase it.

intent is to sway how you spend your food dollars. They want to convince you one product is different from or better than a competing product.

Advertisers use a number of methods to encourage consumers to buy products. *Informational advertising* tends to focus on facts, such as ingredients, prices, and nutrients. This type of information can help you decide how products might fit into your meal planning. *Persuasive advertising* appeals to your human needs and desires for love, approval, fulfillment, and happiness. Often, food is advertised for its impact on your life rather than for its nutritional value. For instance, an advertisement may imply you will be more popular if you serve your friends a certain soft drink.

Be aware of how advertising is affecting your shopping decisions. Some ads are helpful, but others may cause you to overspend or buy items you do not need or want.

● Food Processing

The degree to which foods are processed may influence some of your consumer decisions. **Food processing** refers to any procedure performed on food to prepare it for consumers. Food processing offers consumers many advantages. Canning green beans preserves them for long-term storage. Pasteurizing milk kills harmful bacteria and makes the milk safer to drink. Washing, cutting, and boning chicken save consumers preparation time. Fortifying margarine makes it more nutritious. Table 22-5 describes some of the chemical and physical changes that occur during processing. As you may realize from these examples, preparing meals without some processed foods would be nearly impossible in today's society.

Food processing also has some disadvantages for consumers. Processing adds to the

Effects of Food Processing	
Processing Technique	**Chemical and Physical Effects on Foods**
Canning	Canning involves heating foods in sealed containers to destroy organisms that can cause disease or produce toxins. Heat causes changes in texture, color, and nutritive value of food products. Canned foods maintain quality for 1 to 2 years.
Aseptic canning	This processing method may use temperatures as high as 302°F (150°C) to sterilize food in as little as one second. This short time minimizes changes to the food product. Sterilized food is then placed in sterilized packages within a sterile environment.
Dehydration	Dehydration preserves food by lowering its water content. This stops microbe growth and inactivates enzymes. As food loses water, its weight and size are reduced. Its texture may become leathery or brittle. Flavors often become more concentrated. Treatments used to prevent enzymatic browning may destroy some vitamins in the food.
Fermentation	Microbes are added to cause specific enzymatic changes in some food products. As enzymes break down components in the food product, by-products such as carbon dioxide, acidic and lactic acids, and ethanol may be released. These by-products can change the texture, flavor, and keeping quality of foods such as bread, cheeses, and pickles.
Freezing	Freezing increases shelf life of food by slowing the growth of microbes and the chemical reaction rate of enzymes. Most frozen foods maintain their quality for three to nine months. Rapid freezing right after harvesting is best for preserving food texture and nutrients. Treatment of fruits and vegetables before freezing helps prevent darkening.
Pasteurization	Pasteurization involves heating a food product to reduce enzyme activity and destroy pathogens and some spoilage bacteria. This improves food safety and increases shelf life. Pasteurization can affect food flavors and destroy heat-sensitive nutrients, which may be replaced through fortification.

22-5 Food processing methods affect the chemical and physical characteristics of food products.

cost of foods. The more processed a food is, the higher its price tends to be. Some processing methods cause a loss of essential nutrients in foods. For instance, refining grains removes parts of the grain kernels that are rich in vitamins, minerals, protein, and fiber. Most refined grain products are enriched to add back some of the lost nutrients. However, enriched products still do not match the nutrient levels of whole grain products.

You must evaluate the convenience, cost, and nutritional value of processed foods. This will help you decide if you want to put them in your shopping cart.

Food Additives

Food additives are substances added to food products to cause desired changes in the products. Substances added to foods during processing may affect some of your consumer choices. The Food and Drug Administration (FDA) regulates the use of food additives. The FDA has placed food additives that have proved to be safe on the ***GRAS (generally recognized as safe) list***. The GRAS list includes sugar, salt, and about 700 other substances. GRAS list substances are also called *ingredients* of processed foods. The FDA has reviewed substances on the GRAS list and removed those whose safety is suspect. Manufacturers can freely use any of the substances on the GRAS list.

Manufacturers must seek FDA approval to use any food additives other than those on the GRAS list. The FDA will not approve the use of any substance found to cause cancer in humans or animals. Aspartame, nitrites, and synthetic food colorings are among the hundreds of additives used in foods.

Most packaged foods contain additives to perform one or more of the following functions:

- preserve food (For example, additives that control growth of bacteria, yeast, or molds improve keeping quality of foods. Additives that prevent damage due to oxidation keep fats from becoming rancid and fruits from turning brown.)
- enhance colors, flavors, or textures
- maintain or improve nutritional quality
- aid processing

Food manufacturers must limit additive use to the smallest amount needed to produce a desired effect. Even so, some people have adverse reactions to certain food additives. Others want to limit their intake of food additives. Reading ingredient labels will help people avoid food products that contain additives they want to avoid. As a wise consumer, you must weigh the costs and benefits of buying foods that contain additives.

Organic Foods

Like the chemicals used to process foods, the chemicals used to grow foods may concern you as a consumer. If so, you may want to shop for ***organic foods***. These are foods produced without the use of synthetic fertilizers, pesticides, or growth hormones. Organic farmers often use manure or compost to enrich the soil. They may hoe to control weeds and use natural pesticides to control insects. See 22-6.

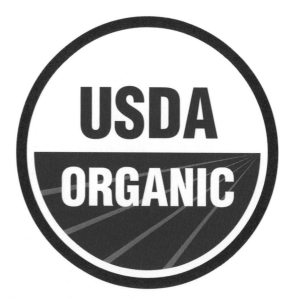

22-6 Look for this seal when buying organic foods to be sure thay have been produced according to USDA standards.

The average cost of organic foods is over 50 percent higher than nonorganic foods. Many organic farms are small. Therefore, organic farmers cannot produce and ship foods as economically as large farming operations.

Some health-conscious consumers choose organic produce. They may think it is more nutritious. However, research has not found this to be the case. Many consumers who choose organics are also concerned about the pesticide residues on nonorganic fruits and vegetables. However, many residues can be removed from nonorganics by washing them in running tap water and wiping them dry. Washing is an important step even when preparing organic produce to remove soil and insects.

Food Prices

Perhaps the price of products is one of the biggest factors that will affect your decisions when shopping for food. Most people have a certain amount of money available to spend on food. Comparison shopping will help you avoid overspending. *Comparison shopping* is assessing prices and quality of similar products. It enables you to choose those that best meet your needs and fit your price range.

Use Unit Prices

Unit pricing makes it easy to comparison shop. A *unit price* is a product's cost per standard unit of weight or volume. For instance, the unit price for breakfast cereal would tell you the cost in cents per ounce. The unit price for milk might be in cents per quart. Unit prices for products like eggs and paper napkins are based on count, such as cents per dozen.

Unit prices are usually on tags attached to the shelves on which products are sitting. You can use unit pricing to compare different forms, sizes, or brands of products to find the best buy. For example, you might compare frozen peas with canned peas. A 10-ounce box of frozen peas costs 69¢. A 15-ounce can of peas costs 79¢. Unit pricing tells you the frozen peas cost 6.9¢ per ounce whereas the canned peas cost 5.2¢ per ounce. Clearly, the canned peas are the better buy based on cost. See 22-7.

Compare Brands

You need to compare more than price when comparing brands. You also need to compare product quality. *National brand* products are distributed and advertised throughout the country by major food companies. These products are generally considered to be high quality. To cover the costs of nationwide advertising, the prices of these products are usually high.

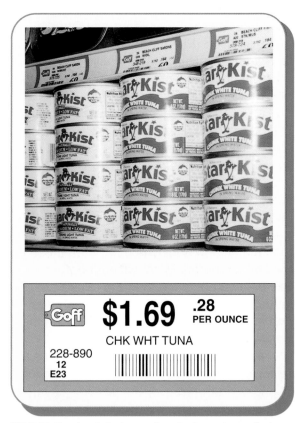

22-7 Unit price labels are located on store shelves beneath food items. Unit prices can help you determine which form, size, or brand of a product is the better buy.

Store brand products are sold only in specific chains of food stores. These products are often of similar quality to national brand products. However, because they are not widely advertised, their prices are usually lower than national brands.

Generic products are unbranded. You can identify them by their plain, simple packaging. You may find generic products to be of somewhat lower quality. For instance, the size of generic green beans may not be uniform. However, the nutritional value of generic products is comparable to other products. They are usually less expensive than national or store brands.

Consider how you intend to use a food when choosing among national brands, store brands, and generic products. For example, suppose you are going to cut up canned peaches for a salad. Irregular shapes and sizes will not be noticeable in this type of dish. Therefore, you do not need to pay a high price for the top-quality national brand. Consider buying store brand or generic peaches instead. The nutritional quality will remain the same, and you will save money.

● **Use a Shopping List**

One of the best ways to control food spending is to prepare a shopping list. A shopping list can help you avoid **impulse buying**, or making unplanned purchases. Impulse buying can cause you to spend money you had not planned to spend on items you do not need. A shopping list can also help you save the time required to return to the store for forgotten items.

To prepare your list, begin by reviewing the menus and recipes you plan to use. Write all the ingredients you do not have on hand on your shopping list. Keep the shopping list handy and add needed food items as supplies run low.

Organize your shopping list according to the way foods are grouped in the store. This will save you time and keep you from missing items you need. Your list might include such headings as *produce; canned foods; rice, beans, and pasta; baking needs; cereals;* and *breads.* Place the headings *meats, dairy products,* and *frozen foods* at the bottom of the list. You should pick up perishable foods in these categories last to reduce the chance of spoilage. See 22-8.

Shopping List

Fresh Produce
tomatoes
potatoes
celery
carrots
strawberries

Bakery and Deli
hamburger buns
whole wheat bread
potato salad

Canned Foods
tuna
mayonnaise
mushroom soup
noodle soup

Cereals and Packaged Foods
raisin bran
granola
pound cake mix

Household Items
dishwasher soap
60-watt lightbulbs

Meats/Fish/Poultry
chicken breasts (skinless)
hot dogs
ground round

Dairy and Refrigerated Products
milk
eggs
mozzarella cheese-shredded

Frozen Foods
whipped topping
sherbet

22-8 Food buyers can save time and money by using a shopping list set up according to store layout.

● Control Food Spending

The following shopping pointers may help you get more food value for your dollar:

- Plan meals around advertised specials.
- Try to avoid shopping when you are tired, hungry, or rushed. You are more likely to make unplanned purchases under these conditions.
- Buy foods in season. When foods are plentiful, they are usually a good buy. See 22-9.
- If you have the storage space, stock up on sale items that will stay fresh in your home.
- Avoid overbuying foods that will spoil if not eaten right away. Fresh produce spoils more quickly than canned, dried, or frozen fruits and vegetables.
- Avoid foods that are packaged in individual servings. Extra packaging usually adds to the costs of products. Packaging also places a strain on the environment.
- Compare prices of uncut and precut items, such as chunk and shredded cheeses or whole fruit and fruit salad. Precut items tend to cost more. They may also spoil more quickly.

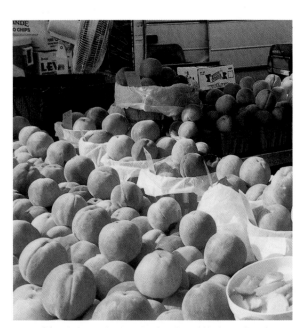

22-9 The best prices can be found when foods are in their growing season.

- Use coupons to buy items you need or use regularly. Before you use a coupon, however, compare quality and prices of similar products. Even with coupons, some foods are not cheaper than other brands.
- Be aware of methods stores use to entice you to make impulse purchases. Store displays may tempt you to buy items not on your shopping list. For example, a display of toppings with the frozen desserts may encourage you to make an unplanned purchase.

Preventing food spoilage helps you get the most from the money you spend. You can maintain wholesome quality of the foods you buy by storing them properly. Go directly home from the store. As soon as you get home, remember to refrigerate all perishable foods. Rewrap meats and other bulk items for the freezer in meal-sized portions. Place flour, mixes, and other dry foods in tightly covered containers to avoid insect problems. Store these items and canned foods in cool, dry places.

● Using Food Labels

As an informed consumer, you will want to use food labels to guide your buying decisions. Food labeling is regulated by the FDA. The United States Department of Agriculture (USDA) governs labels on meat and poultry products. Labels are your main source of information about food products.

Federal laws require certain information on the label of every processed, packaged food product. This information includes the name and form of the food, such as French cut green beans. The name and address of the manufacturer, packer, or distributor must appear, too. A list of ingredients and a Nutrition Facts panel are also required on almost all foods.

A few food products are exempt from labeling laws. Foods prepared by small businesses do not need complete label information. For example, the local baker does not need to label fresh baked goods. Restaurant and deli foods intended to be eaten right away do not need to supply label information. Custom processed fish and meats, donated foods, and individual foods from multiunit packages are exempt from labeling laws. Foods in small packages, such as chewing gum, do not need nutrition labeling. However, manufacturers must include a phone number or address for consumers to call or write if they have questions. Foods of limited nutritional value, such as tea and coffee, are not required to have nutrition labeling, either.

Ingredient Labeling

The law requires all the ingredients in a food product to be listed on the label. Manufacturers must list ingredients in descending order by weight. Flavorings, color additives, and some spices must be listed by their common names.

A complete list of ingredients helps consumers know what is in the foods they buy. People are interested in this information for various reasons. They may want to buy the canned beef stew that has more beef than any other ingredient. Some consumers want to avoid substances to which they may be allergic or sensitive. Others want to avoid certain ingredients for religious or cultural reasons. For instance, a vegetarian would want to know that a can of vegetable soup contains beef broth. See 22-10.

Health Claims

You may be swayed by words used on food packaging to make products sound healthful. For instance, lite whipped topping sounds more healthful than regular whipped topping. However, you need to know what the term *lite* means. Then you can decide if eating lite foods will improve the quality of your diet. Products must meet specific definitions for manufacturers to use terms such as *light, low sodium,* and *fat free* on labels. See 22-11.

Besides claims about nutrient content, manufacturers may put certain health claims on product labels. These claims are based on research showing solid evidence of links

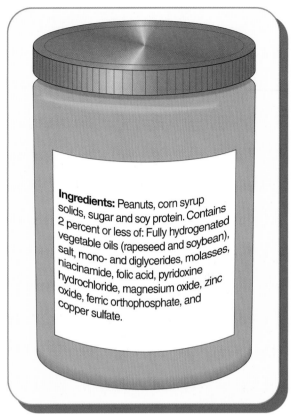

Ingredients: Peanuts, corn syrup solids, sugar and soy protein. Contains 2 percent or less of: Fully hydrogenated vegetable oils (rapeseed and soybean), salt, mono- and diglycerides, molasses, niacinamide, folic acid, pyridoxine hydrochloride, magnesium oxide, zinc oxide, ferric orthophosphate, and copper sulfate.

22-10 According to law, the ingredients on this label are listed in descending order by weight.

between foods or nutrients and diseases. For instance, a yogurt container might have a claim about the link between calcium and a reduced risk of osteoporosis. Statements cannot indicate that a certain food prevents or causes a disease. Only claims about the diet-health relationships listed in 22-12 are permitted on labels.

Nutrition Labeling

When purchasing a food item, take time to look at the Nutrition Facts panel on the product label. The information listed there can help you decide how the food will contribute to your day's total diet. It can help you meet special dietary needs, too. For instance, this information can help you select foods that are lower in fats or higher in fiber. The Nutrition Facts panel can also help you quickly compare the nutritional value of similar foods.

Nutrient Content Claims

Claim	Definition (per serving)
Calorie free	fewer than 5 calories
Low calorie	40 calories or fewer
Reduced or fewer calories	at least 25% fewer calories
Light or lite	one-third fewer calories or 50% less fat
Sugar free	fewer than 0.5 gram sugars
Reduced sugar or less sugar	at least 25% less sugars
No added sugar	no sugars added during processing or packing, including ingredients that contain sugars, such as juice or dry fruit
Fat free	fewer than 0.5 gram fat
Lowfat	3 grams or fewer of fat
Reduced or less fat	at least 25% less fat
Cholesterol free	fewer than 2 milligrams cholesterol and 2 grams or fewer of saturated fat
Low cholesterol	20 milligrams or fewer cholesterol and 2 grams or fewer of saturated fat
Reduced or less cholesterol	at least 25% less cholesterol and 2 grams or fewer saturated fat
Sodium free	fewer than 5 milligrams sodium
Very low sodium	35 milligrams or fewer sodium
Low sodium	140 milligrams or fewer sodium
Reduced or less sodium	at least 25% less sodium
Light in sodium	at least 50% less sodium

22-11 Foods labeled with a nutrient content claim must meet the appropriate criteria.

● Serving Sizes

On all labels, serving size of food products must be stated in common household terms and metric measures. For example, a serving of milk or yogurt is one cup (240 mL). Serving size is based on the amount of a food most people eat at one time.

Serving sizes are the same for all foods in the same general category. This allows you to compare the nutrient content of similar products. For example, you can easily compare vitamin C per serving of grape drink and grape juice. Both products will list nutrients based on the same serving size.

Compare the serving sizes listed on product labels with the sizes of portions you consume. Suppose a serving of cereal is one cup. However, you may pour one and a half cups into your bowl. This means you are consuming one and a half times the calories and nutrients listed on the cereal package. Knowing this will help you more accurately calculate your daily calorie and nutrient intakes. See 22-13.

Below the serving size on the Nutrition Facts panel is the number of servings per container. You can divide the total cost of the product by the number of servings to figure the cost per serving. This can help you compare food prices when shopping. For instance, suppose a 12-ounce can of frozen orange juice concentrate costs $1.29 and

Health Claims on Food Product Labels

Diet-Health Relationship	Possible Claim
Calcium and osteoporosis	A calcium-rich diet is linked to a reduced risk of osteoporosis, a condition in which bones become soft or brittle.
Fat and cancer	A diet low in total fat is linked to a reduced risk of some cancers.
Saturated fat and cholesterol and coronary heart disease	A diet low in saturated fat and cholesterol can help reduce the risk of heart disease.
Fiber-containing grain products, fruits, and vegetables and cancer	A diet rich in high-fiber grain products, fruits, and vegetables can reduce the risk of some cancers.
Fiber-rich fruits, vegetables, and grain products and heart disease	A diet rich in fruits, vegetables, and grain products that contain fiber can help reduce the risk for heart disease.
Sodium and hypertension (high blood pressure)	A low-sodium diet may help reduce the risk of high blood pressure, which is a risk factor for heart attacks and strokes.
Fruits and vegetables and some cancers	A lowfat diet rich in fruits and vegetables (foods that are low in fat and may contain dietary fiber, vitamin A, or vitamin C) is linked to a reduced risk of some cancers.
Folic acid and neural tube birth defects	Women who consume 0.4 mg folic acid daily reduce their risk of giving birth to a child affected with a neural tube defect.

22-12 Only health claims supported by scientific evidence are allowed on labels.

makes six servings. A 64-ounce carton of orange juice costs $1.69 and contains eight servings. (In this case, the unit price is not helpful. The concentrated weight of the frozen juice is not comparable to the fluid volume of the reconstituted juice.) You can figure the frozen juice costs $.22 per serving whereas juice from the carton costs $.21 per serving.

● Calories and Nutrients

The Nutrition Facts panel lists information about food products on a per serving basis. You will find the number of calories a serving of the product provides. The number of calories from fat is also stated. This information can help you limit your fat intake to no more than 30 percent of your total calories.

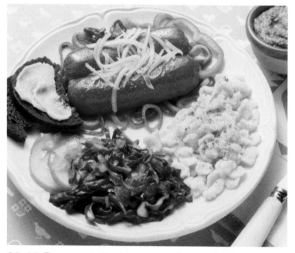

22-13 Be aware that your portions may be bigger than the serving sizes listed on product labels. This will help you accurately figure your nutrient and calorie intakes.

The next section of the Nutrition Facts panel contains the amounts of nutrients per serving. Amounts of total fat, saturated fat, cholesterol, sodium, total carbohydrates, dietary fiber, sugars, and protein are listed. The nutrient amounts are listed in grams or milligrams.

To the right of the nutrient amounts on the Nutrition Facts panel, you will see percent Daily Values (%DV). *Daily Values* are recommended nutrient intakes used as references on food labels. They are based on daily calorie needs. The percent Daily Values listed on food labels are based on a 2,000-calorie diet. If you need more or less than 2,000 calories daily, you will need to adjust your percent Daily Values accordingly. See 22-14.

Percent Daily Values for vitamins A and C, calcium, and iron are also required on the nutrition panel. Manufacturers may choose to list information about other nutrients, such as the B vitamins. They must provide information about all nutrients that are added to the food.

The percent Daily Values serve as general guidelines. They can help you know how a food serving fits into your daily nutrient needs. A high percent Daily Value for a given nutrient means a food provides a lot of that nutrient. A low percentage means the food provides a small amount of the nutrient.

The bottom of the Nutrition Facts panel provides some reference information. Daily Values are listed for several nutrients for a

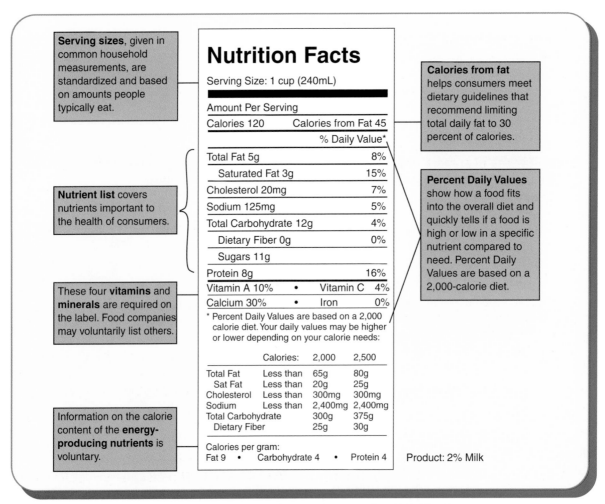

22-14 The nutrition label can help consumers choose the most healthful foods.

2,000- and a 2,500-calorie diet. You can use these numbers to estimate your daily limits for fat, saturated fat, cholesterol, and sodium. You can also estimate your recommended intakes of carbohydrate and dietary fiber. A conversion guide reminds you how many calories a gram of fat, carbohydrate, or protein provides.

● Modified Labels

You will find modified nutrition labels on some foods. For instance, no recommended fat intake levels are given on foods intended for children under two years of age. This is because restricting fat in the diets of young children may be harmful to health.

Another label modification you may notice is on boxed mixes for products like muffins and pudding. Two columns of nutrient amounts may appear on these products. Manufacturers must list nutrient amounts per serving of mix as packaged. However, manufacturers may also list nutrition information for the products as prepared.

You may find a simplified label on products like candy, which do not provide significant amounts of some nutrients. Also, smaller food items, such as canned tuna, may use simpler labels that fit more easily on their packages.

Fresh fruits, vegetables, meats, poultry, and fish may not have labels. However, most stores have posters, notebooks, or pamphlets with nutrition information about these foods. The produce department should offer information about the 20 most popular raw fruits and vegetables. The fish department should provide nutrition details about the 20 most common fish sold raw. The meat department has nutrient data on the 45 best-selling cuts of raw meat and poultry. See 22-15.

● Using Label Information to Meet Your Needs

Suppose you are reading the label on a can of baked beans. It tells you one serving provides 5 grams of total fat, or 8 percent of

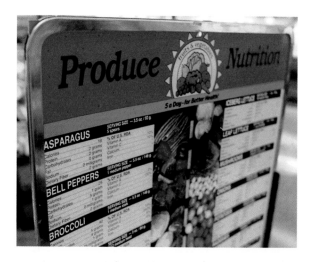

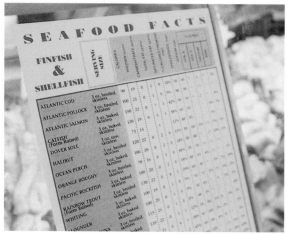

Courtesy of the U.S. Food and Drug Administration

22-15 Stores may use posters to present nutrition information for items such as vegetables and seafood.

the Daily Value. You know this percentage is based on a 2,000-calorie diet. How can you use this information if you need 2,800 calories per day?

Recommendations for daily total fat intake are based on 30 percent of daily calorie needs. If you need 2,800 calories per day, no more than 840 of those calories should come from fat (2,800 × .30 = 840). Fat provides 9 calories per gram. This means you should limit daily fat intake to no more than 93 grams (840 ÷ 9 = 93). Therefore, 5 grams of total fat from a serving of the baked beans equals 5 percent of *your* Daily Value (5 ÷ 93 = .05).

What if you need only 1,600 calories per day? The same series of calculations would tell you your daily limit for total fat is 53 grams. This means a serving of baked beans would provide 9 percent of your Daily Value for total fat.

Product Dating

Take note of dates on food product labels. The federal government does not require food products other than infant formula and some baby foods to be dated. Food manufacturers voluntarily use several types of dates. A *sell by* date shows how long the manufacturer recommends grocers keep the product on the shelf. A *use by* date is the last day the manufacturer recommends consumers use the product for peak quality. If foods have been stored properly, they should still be wholesome after the dates have expired. For maximum eating and keeping quality, however, avoid buying products with expired dates.

Being a Consumer of Fitness Products and Services

Unlike food, which is a basic physical need, fitness products and services are largely wants. They may be enjoyable, but they are not required for life. A significant portion of your family budget must be spent for food. Conversely, your consumer spending for fitness products and services may be minimal.

The only items required for taking part in physical activity are sturdy, comfortable shoes and nonbinding clothes. If you choose to buy more specialized fitness products and services, you need to know where to shop. You must also learn to use product information and evaluate quality. Taking these consumer steps will help you get the most value from your fitness dollars.

Shopping for Apparel

Some people prefer the comfort and appearance of fitness apparel that is tailored to specific activities. Sports clothing is designed to meet the needs of people who will be performing a certain set of motions. For instance, bicycle shorts are often made with padding in the seat to provide cushioning on a long ride. Tennis shorts are made with large pockets to hold spare tennis balls.

Fitness apparel is available at discount, department, and sporting goods stores. You can also buy it through catalogs and Internet shopping services. Some companies charge premium prices for their high-tech garments. You must decide if you want multipurpose clothing or items designed for specific activities. You will need to think about what garment features are most important to you. Then you can ask questions and compare prices to get the best value for your dollar.

One of the most important clothing items for fitness activities is shoes. You need to choose shoes that provide support for your feet. The shoes need to be flexible and lightweight to provide comfort as you move. They should not create any sore spots on your feet. The soles should be designed to give you an adequate amount of traction. You may also look for cushioning that absorbs shock and reduces jarring to the body. Absorbent socks will also help cushion and pull perspiration away from the feet. See 22-16.

Your choices of other fitness clothing will depend on the activities you plan to do. For some activities, you may prefer garments made from stretchy fabrics that hug the body. For other activities, loose-fitting clothes may be a better choice. Whatever the fit, you are likely to sweat when you exercise. Therefore, you will be more comfortable in garments made from fabrics that carry perspiration away from your body.

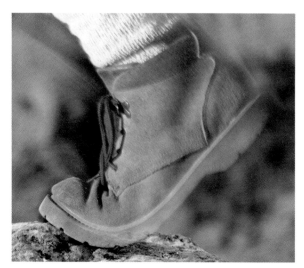

22-16 Shoes are specifically designed for different sports activities to provide the kind of support each activity requires.

● Shopping for Equipment

Many sports and exercise activities require special equipment. From golf clubs to free weights to treadmills, you need to know what to look for when shopping for fitness products.

Safety gear is one of the most important fitness purchases you can make. Even the most skilled athletes can have accidents when participating in physical activities. Equipment such as bicycle helmets and wrist guards for in-line skating can protect you from injury. Choose sturdy items that are designed to withstand the forces placed on them by a particular activity.

Having gym equipment at home may make it more convenient for you to exercise. Factors such as bad weather and lack of transportation will not hinder your ability to work out. For most people, less than $100 will set up a basic home gym. This includes a jump rope, a floor mat, and some hand weights. However, some people feel they can boost their motivation to exercise by working out on special gym equipment. Popular items include ski and rowing machines, exercise bikes, stair climbers, and all-in-one gyms.

Many brands and models of fitness equipment are available. To compare various pieces of equipment, you might begin by reading consumer articles. When you go to the store, study the features listed on product labels. You can also talk to salespeople. Sometimes talking to several salespeople is helpful because you can get more than one person's opinion about a product. Whenever possible, rent or borrow equipment to try it out before buying.

Ask yourself the following questions to help you evaluate a fitness equipment purchase:

● How often will I use this equipment? Choose equipment you will enjoy using regularly for months and years to come. The more you plan to use the equipment, the more important quality becomes. See 22-17.

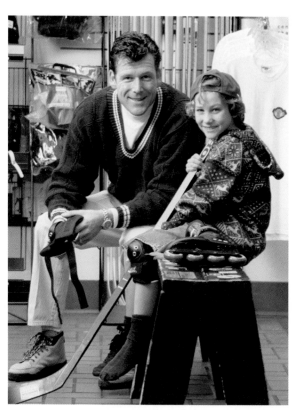

22-17 Someone planning to use sports equipment for many years may find it worthwhile to invest in better quality products.

- Can I afford this equipment? The more expensive the item, the more important it is to compare prices. Look at costs in retail stores, catalogs, and Internet shopping services.
- What safety features does this equipment have? The product should be designed to minimize the potential of common hazards, such as cuts and falls.
- Are clear instructions given for proper use? Detailed directions should explain how to use the equipment safely. Some companies provide videos to demonstrate proper use of fitness equipment.
- How good of a workout will I get from this equipment? Choose equipment that meets your personal training goals. Exercise should be challenging but not exhausting.
- Can I vary the intensity of exercise easily? The resistance levels should be adjustable, and the controls should be easy to reach.
- Will the equipment fit on the available floor space? Take measurements to be sure you have enough room. Consider the full range of motion of the equipment piece. Equipment that is easily folded for storage may help make the use of space more flexible.
- How sturdy is the equipment? Frames should not flex or scoot across the floor when in use. Springs should be heavy-duty.
- Will the equipment run smoothly? All moveable parts should glide easily.
- Will the machine fit my body size? If you are too short, tall, or heavy for the machine, you will not feel comfortable.
- Is the noise level acceptable? Consider how other members of your household will respond to any sounds the equipment makes.

Watch out for expensive gadgets that do not enhance fitness. Avoid passive devices driven by electric belts, shakers, or rollers. These machines cannot massage the inches away or reduce fat by jarring, squeezing, or rubbing it off.

Choosing Exercise Videos

Exercise videos let you work out at home. They provide some instruction and give you a sense of companionship. They are far less costly than hiring a trainer or joining a club.

Videos vary by the type and intensity of exercise they include. Some are aerobic for heart health; others are geared toward muscle conditioning for strength and toning. Stretching videos enhance flexibility. Some tapes combine all three types of exercise. Some video workouts are for beginners, whereas others are intended for advanced exercisers.

Before you buy a video, consider renting it or checking it out of a library. This will help you see if you like the music and the instructor. It will also allow you to evaluate whether the intensity of exercise is suited to your fitness level.

Watch out for videos involving dangerous techniques that can lead to injury. A safe workout should include a warm-up period and a cool-down period. The workout should encourage viewers to work at their own pace.

When doing a video workout, be sure to wear shoes that offer appropriate support. Work out on an exercise mat or carpet. Check your pulse to be sure you are staying within your safe target heart rate zone. (See Chapter 15, "Staying Physically Active: A Way of Life.") See 22-18.

Hiring a Personal Trainer

Personal trainers offer one-on-one coaching to help you reach your physical fitness goals. A good trainer should be able to design a safe program suited to your needs.

To find a trainer, call a fitness center, dance studio, or physical education department at a local college. Ask for the names of people who offer individualized fitness instruction.

When you interview a trainer, ask about his or her credentials. Certification and registration

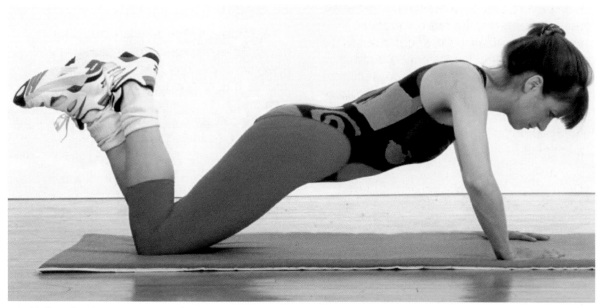

22-18 Sturdy shoes and an exercise mat will provide support and cushioning when working out with an exercise video.

programs are offered by a number of sports and fitness organizations. You might want to contact the organization through which a trainer received his or her credentials. Ask what qualifications this organization requires to bestow its credential. Decide whether these qualifications meet your standards for a personal trainer. Regardless of other credentials, a trainer should be certified in cardiopulmonary resuscitation (CPR). This will enable the trainer to offer help if a client has an exercise-related emergency.

Before hiring a trainer, ask for the names of people who have used his or her services. Call a few of these references to see if they were pleased with the trainer's work.

You may pay $25 to over $100 per hour for personalized fitness services. Ask about rates before signing a contract.

● Selecting a Health or Fitness Club

You may feel joining a health or fitness club will help you meet your exercise goals. Health facilities range from high-cost clubs with deluxe equipment and many services to inexpensive, no-frills gyms. When deciding what type of facility would meet your needs, examine all the options in your community. These may include spas, YMCAs, colleges, schools, and community centers. Weigh the costs and conveniences.

Choose a facility with a pleasant, non-threatening atmosphere. You should feel comfortable with the other people who go there. You should also feel comfortable with the instructors. Ask about their training and experience.

Evaluate the equipment and services a facility offers. You might be interested in a running track and a lap pool. Maybe you want basketball, tennis, and racquetball courts. Perhaps an aerobics class and a weight room are important to you. Look at the cleanliness of locker rooms, saunas, and hot tubs. You must decide if the features available will fit your needs.

The cost of membership will be part of your consumer decision. The costs should reflect the quality of the equipment and services offered by the facility. Many clubs have specials and package deals. Be sure to ask about any extra charges. Some clubs charge for court time and fitness classes in addition to basic membership fees. Comparison shop with other facilities. No matter what you pay, you must exercise regularly to get the full value of your membership dollar.

Choose a club that is conveniently located. Make sure the hours are convenient, too. You are more likely to go to a facility that is not out of your way. You will also be more inclined to use your membership if you can avoid waiting in line for equipment.

Work out at a facility several times before deciding to buy a membership. Choose a fitness center that is right for you and your budget. See 22-19.

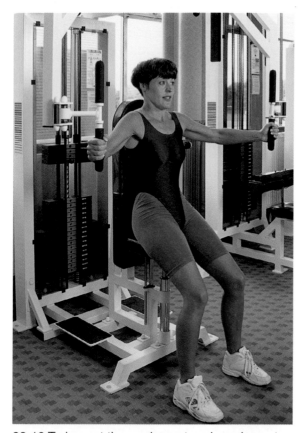

22-19 Trying out the equipment and services at a health club before joining will help you make a good consumer decision.

Your Consumer Rights

As a consumer, you have power. People who produce and sell goods and services want to keep you happy. They want you to keep spending your money on the items they offer.

You have specific rights as a consumer that are protected by federal laws. With these rights you also have responsibilities. You have to use your consumer power in appropriate ways when you have problems in the marketplace. The following points give some brief examples of your consumer rights and responsibilities when buying products:

- *You have the right to safety.* The foods you buy should be wholesome. Fitness products should list safety precautions. In turn, you have the responsibility to handle foods and fitness equipment correctly to avoid problems with use.

- *You have the right to be informed.* Labeling on food and other products should be complete and accurate. You have a responsibility to use package information to choose foods that do not contain ingredients you want to avoid. Read Nutrition Facts panels to select products that will meet your nutritional needs. You also have a responsibility to heed cautions on fitness equipment.

- *You have the right to choose.* You should be able to select from a variety of brands, forms, and sizes of products. You have a responsibility to choose carefully by comparing the cost, convenience, and value of items.

- *You have the right to be heard.* You should be able to expect a satisfactory response when you express your concern about a product. You have a responsibility to be truthful when making a complaint.

Making a Consumer Complaint

For one reason or another, you may find the need to make a consumer complaint. Perhaps you bought a package of cheese that was moldy when you opened it. Maybe a piece of fitness equipment did not operate as advertised. For these and other reasons, a complaint may be in order.

To receive a satisfactory response to your complaint, you need to complain to the right party. If the product you bought came from a local store, your first step is to return the item. If you have your receipt, take it along to help document when and where you bought the item. State your complaint to the manager. The manager may simply return your money or offer you a replacement product.

Sometimes it may be more appropriate to contact the manufacturer of a product. Look for a toll-free number, Web site, or e-mail address on the product package. You can use these resources to contact a consumer service representative. Clearly explain your problem. Be sure to have the product package handy. This will allow you to provide package code numbers and other information that helps the manufacturer identify the product. See 22-20.

If a store or manufacturer cannot resolve your problem, you may want to contact an appropriate government office. State, county, and city government consumer protection offices can settle complaints and conduct investigations. The FDA can help you with problems with food products. The U.S. Consumer Product Safety Commission (CPSC) can help solve problems related to other types of products. These agencies are listed under *government offices* in the telephone directory.

When you call, ask to speak to a consumer affairs officer. Again, clearly explain your problem. The officer may be able to take action on your behalf to find an acceptable solution. See 22-21.

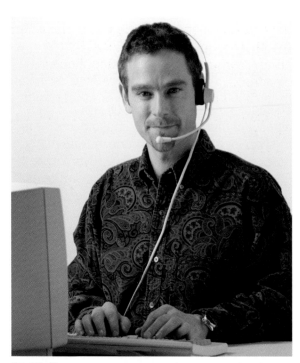

22-20 Consumer representatives are trained to answer calls and handle consumer complaints.

Making a Consumer Complaint

- First try to return the product. If you do not have your receipt, you may only be able to make an exchange instead of receiving a refund.

- If you do not get the desired response, call or write the manufacturer. State the problem clearly. Have any packaging nearby. Be able to give product code numbers or other identifying information.

- If the problem still is not resolved, contact a government office listed in the phone book.

22-21 Keeping these steps in mind can be helpful when making a consumer complaint.

Chapter 22 Review

Summary

Becoming familiar with some consumer skills and resources will help you make wise choices in the marketplace. One of the decisions you must make as a consumer is where to shop for food. You can choose from many types of food stores; each has advantages and disadvantages. The latest supermarket trends are geared toward making food shopping more convenient for consumers.

A number of factors affect your choices when shopping for food. You may be swayed by advertising. The degree to which foods are processed and the additives they contain may influence some of your food purchases. The availability of organic foods may attract your attention in the store. Food prices are likely to affect many of your choices, too. You can learn how to use unit prices, compare brands, and use a shopping list to control food spending.

Food labels provide much information that can help you as a consumer. Ingredient labeling allows you to identify what is in food products. Claims on packages may encourage you to choose some food products for health reasons. Nutrition labeling can help you analyze how a food will fit into your diet. Product dating can assist you in choosing foods that are fresh and wholesome.

You may be a consumer of fitness products and services as well as a consumer of foods. Look for apparel that meets your needs for comfort, appearance, and design features. Choose equipment that meets standards for safety and fits your budget and desired level of quality. When choosing an exercise video, look for one that is intended for your fitness level. When hiring a personal trainer or selecting a health club, find out all the details before signing any contracts.

As a consumer, you have a number of rights, which are protected by law. You must be aware these rights carry the weight of certain responsibilities. Going through proper channels to make a complaint can help you address problems in the marketplace.

Check Your Knowledge

1. List five types of food stores and give one advantage and one disadvantage of each.

2. Describe three supermarket trends that are intended to make shopping more convenient for consumers.

3. What is the difference between informational advertising and persuasive advertising?

4. What are the four main functions of food additives?

5. Why does organic food tend to cost more than nonorganic food?

6. Products sold only in specific chains of food stores are _____.
   A. generic products
   B. local brand products
   C. national brand products
   D. store brand products

7. Give five tips for controlling food spending.

8. In what order are ingredients listed on a food product label?

9. True or false. A product labeled "light in sodium" contains 35 milligrams or fewer sodium.

10. On what type of diet are the percent Daily Values on food labels based?

11. True or false. If foods have been stored properly, they should still be wholesome after the dates have expired.

12. What are three characteristics required in shoes for fitness activities?

13. What are five questions you might ask yourself when evaluating fitness equipment?

14. What are four factors you should consider when selecting a health or fitness club?

15. What are four consumer rights protected by law?

Put Learning into Action

1. Write the names, forms, and package sizes of five specific food products. Go to two types of food stores and record the prices of these products. Report your findings in class.

2. Watch television for one hour on a week-night and one hour on a weekend morning or afternoon. Record the specific days and times you watch. Also record the names of all the food products advertised during the times you watch. Note whether each ad is informational or persuasive. Compare your list with those of your classmates.

3. Analyze a food product label and write the following information from the label on a sheet of paper: nutrient or health claims; serving size; amounts per serving of fat, cholesterol, sodium, fiber, and sugars; percent Daily Values for vitamin A, vitamin C, calcium, and iron. Also list the most prevalent ingredient. Attach the label to your paper.

4. Visit a health or fitness club and write a one-page evaluation of the facilities.

Explore Further

1. Form teams to debate the pros and cons of additives in foods. Each team should conduct research to support its arguments.

2. Analyze the Nutrition Facts panels on fat free milk, whole milk, chocolate milk, and calcium-fortified orange juice. Prepare a poster comparing the products in terms of cost, calories, fat, cholesterol, sodium, fiber, sugars, protein, vitamin C, and calcium per serving.

3. Contact a sports and fitness organization that offers a credential program for personal fitness trainers. Ask what qualifications the organization requires to bestow its credential. Prepare a written evaluation of these qualifications.

4. Research the nature of the most frequent consumer complaints about a food or fitness product category. Share your findings in an oral report.

Chapter 23

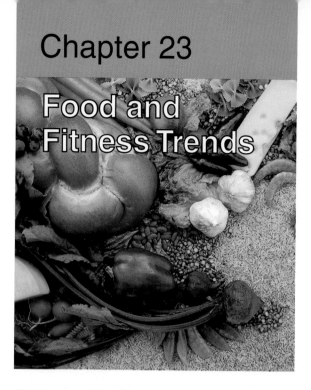

Food and Fitness Trends

Have you heard the expression "nothing stays the same forever"? It refers to the fact that life is constantly undergoing change. Generally, most of the changes in everyday life are too gradual to notice.

Changes that occur from one year to the next, however, are much more obvious. This is especially true when an entire nation is observed instead of a few individuals. By studying the actions and decisions of the general population, certain trends become obvious. A **trend** is a general pattern or direction. See 23-1. A trend reflects a new choice made by growing numbers of people. Trends indicate shifts away from the *norm,* or typical pattern.

In the areas of food and fitness, what do the trends show? This chapter answers that question by first examining food preferences. Then the possible effects of scientific advances on future food choices are discussed. Finally, the future of physical fitness is explored.

● Food Preferences

At any given moment, many food trends are obvious. Sometimes they conflict and point in different directions. The food industry addresses as many trends as possible by bringing hundreds of new products to market each year. This is a major reason for the wide variety of food choices in the United States.

The food trends that continually gain followers are most worth watching. One of these is the interest in international foods and new flavors. Another trend is the desire for food that is both fresh and convenient. A third key trend is the use of lowfat products to reduce dietary fat intake. A fourth important food trend is the growing popularity of supplements that do not provide nutrients.

● International Foods and Flavors

Common foods and mild flavors are boring to those desiring something new and different. Many people have a strong interest in

● Learn the Language

trend
mouth feel
olestra
nonnutrient
  supplement
botanical
megadose
bioengineering
herbicide

vaccine
immunity
functional food
competitive bacteria
DNA fingerprinting
product recall
active packaging
irradiation
service sector

● Objectives

After studying this chapter, you will be able to
- identify four food preferences that indicate trends.
- outline the pros and cons of nonnutrient supplements.
- list three ways that bioengineering may affect food and nutrition.
- explain the potential of functional foods.
- describe four technologies that will help keep food safe.
- identify five aspects of the growing fitness industry.

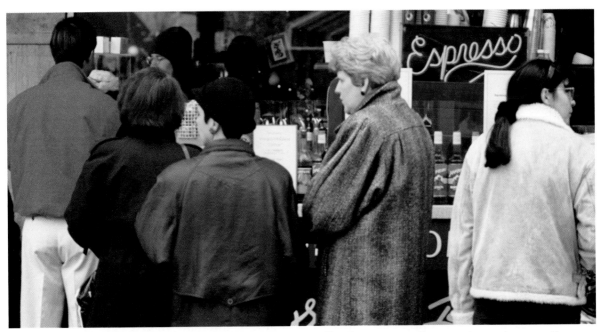

23-1 The trend to flavored coffee beverages inspired coffee bars across the country and new coffee blends in the supermarket.

food as an adventure. The rising popularity of ethnic restaurants and food festivals is evidence of this. A growing number of TV cooking shows is further proof. In addition, at least one cable channel is devoted solely to food.

Herbs, spices, and other flavorings help make each cuisine unique. Highly seasoned Szechwan (a region in China), Cajun, and Mexican dishes are among the favorites. Korean, Vietnamese, Thai, and Indian dishes are becoming new favorites. Consumers enjoy sampling ethnic dishes and preparing them at home. See 23-2.

The health benefits of various ethnic cuisines have been promoted by the media. Many cuisines feature dishes that are high in fiber and low in fat. This has given added incentive for people to try flavorful ethnic dishes. You might want to explore an unfamiliar culture and sample its foods.

● Freshness with Convenience

Not so long ago, food was either fresh or convenient, but rarely both. Using fresh ingredients meant spending much time cooking.

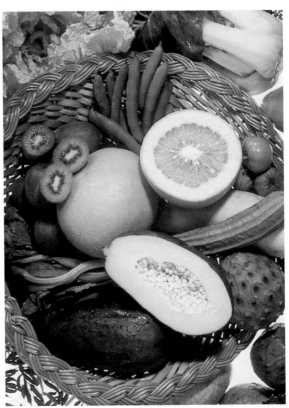

Agricultural Research Service, USDA

23-2 Foods like these from around the world are finding a place on American tables.

Using convenience foods meant making meals quickly, but sacrificing food appearance and texture somewhat to do so. Canning and freezing, the processes used to make convenience foods, tend to dull food colors and soften textures.

Today, however, consumers expect both freshness and convenience. They want food that takes little time and effort to prepare. They also want food that looks and tastes fresh. This means colorful ingredients and crisp textures, usually from fresh vegetables.

The demand for freshness with convenience is seen in the foods gaining popularity at the supermarket. They include ready-to-eat and ready-to-heat dishes. Chilled pasta with sauce from the refrigerated foods department is one example. A completely cooked meal from the deli section is another. Ready-to-eat salads, hot or cold side dishes, and hot entrées are available from many deli cases.

Freshness with convenience is also important in the produce department. Some fresh vegetables come ready to use. They have been cleaned, trimmed, cut, and packaged. Varieties include carrot sticks, mushroom slices, potato wedges, and tossed salad mixtures.

Outside the supermarket, some companies provide the ultimate convenience. They deliver meals to the home ready to eat. This service is a growing, multimillion-dollar business. It began with eat-in restaurants looking for new ways to expand. Other businesses that deliver ready-to-eat meals are nutrition consulting and diet planning services. See 23-3.

The major cause of the convenience trend is the need for satisfying meals at the end of business-filled days. Many adults need quick meal options on most days of the week. Foods in single servings are especially useful when family members eat at different times. Single servings also appeal to seniors living alone who have little desire or ability to cook.

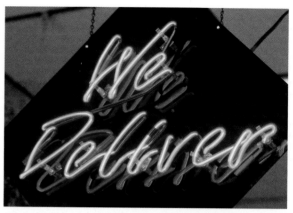

23-3 Delivery service makes food cost more, but some people feel it is worth the extra convenience.

● Foods with Less

Over one in three adults in the United States weigh more than is considered healthy. The answer to their weight problems involves both exercise and diet. However, many people focus on diet alone. To help lower their body weight and dietary fat intake, they seek lowfat and fat free foods. Fat replacers make it possible for food companies to develop these foods. (Fat replacers were discussed in Chapter 6, "Fats: A Concentrated Energy Source.")

Reducing a food's fat content is difficult because fat affects every aspect of food quality, including texture and color. Most importantly, fat affects flavor and provides a satisfying richness to food. It also affects *mouth feel*, which is a food industry term describing the sensation perceived by the tongue. Fat leaves a creamy mouth feel, such as you experience with ice cream and smooth peanut butter.

Finding reliable *fat replacers* involves continuous searching since each is effective only for certain foods. For example, Simplesse® is useful in ice cream, dips, and chilled spreads. It is made from egg whites and other food proteins. Oatrim, a flour made with oat bran, is useful in baked goods, cereals, frostings, and some candies. See 23-4.

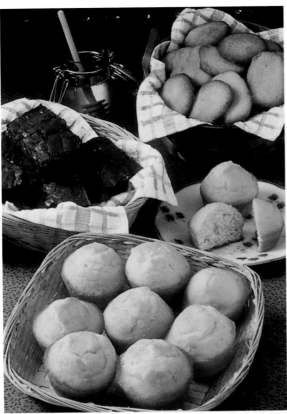

Agricultural Research Service, USDA

23-4 These breads are made with Oatrim, which reduces cholesterol and lowers the blood glucose linked to diabetes.

The first calorie-free fat replacer is *olestra,* currently marketed under the Olean® brand name. **Olestra** is made from soybean or cottonseed oil and sugar. It is approved for use as an ingredient in crackers and salted snacks. Some of the snacks on the market using this product include potato chips, corn chips, and tortilla chips. Olestra may be approved for other uses in the future.

The Census Bureau predicts the number of Americans over the age of 65 will nearly triple by 2030. Unfortunately, overweight older adults are likely to depend less on exercise and more on lowfat foods to manage weight. Reducing and eliminating fat from foods continues to be a priority for food scientists. See 23-5.

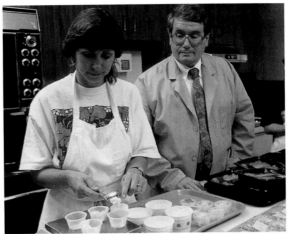

Agricultural Research Service, USDA

23-5 This USDA nutrition study is testing the effects of different table spreads on cholesterol levels.

The industry will also work to develop foods that help people prevent common diseases. These include heart disease, cancer, diabetes, and diseases associated with aging. Foods that address these goals will contain less sodium, less sugar, and fewer calories per serving.

Nonnutrient Supplements

A **nonnutrient supplement** is a pill, powder, or liquid that claims to promote health but has not been proven to do so. You often hear nonnutrient supplements called *dietary supplements.* They appear almost everywhere multivitamin tablets and other nutrient supplements are sold. You can buy them through health food stores, pharmacies, mail-order catalogs, and TV ads. These supplements should not be substituted for food, but their ads sometimes imply otherwise. See 23-6.

Nonnutrient supplements account for most of the rapidly expanding $12 billion supplement market. Nutrient supplements are also part of this market, but a very small part. (Nutrient supplements were discussed in Chapter 8, "Vitamins: Drivers of Cell Processes.")

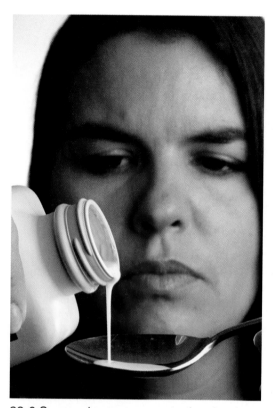
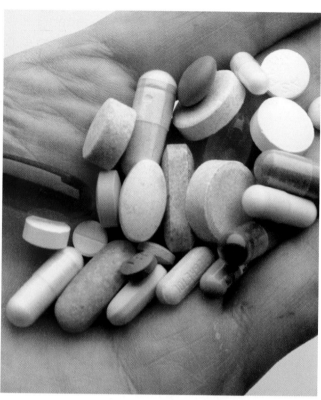

23-6 Some ads encourage starting the day with nonnutrient supplements in liquid form or powders that dissolve in liquids. Most nonnutrient supplements, however, are available in tablets and capsules.

The primary ingredients of nonnutrient supplements are plant sources, although animal extracts are sometimes used. Plant sources include herbals, botanicals, and phytochemicals. A **botanical** is plant material or part of a plant. *Phytochemicals* may have some disease-fighting properties, but their safety and effectiveness must still be determined. (Phytochemicals were discussed in Chapter 8.) None of these ingredients provide nutritional value, according to research conducted to date.

Plants thought to have healing or mystical powers are the main sources of ingredients for these supplements. Often the ingredients are present in megadoses. A **megadose** is a concentrated level many times higher than its natural occurrence in the diet.

● **Are Nonnutrient Supplements Safe?**

Heated controversy currently surrounds nonnutrient supplements for several reasons.

Advocates of these products believe they are nature's answer to staying healthy. They also believe the supplements are completely safe.

Opponents warn that some ingredients in these supplements can be harmful. They argue that supplements have not been tested to determine their real health effects, if any. A group of scientific organizations jointly issued a general caution to consumers about supplements. See 23-7.

Especially notice the first caution telling buyers to beware. The FDA also cautions consumers, especially when buying nonnutrient supplements. This is because no government authority checks these products before they enter the market. New foods and drugs, however, must be proven safe by the FDA before they can enter the market. See 23-8.

By law, the FDA safety checks that are required of new foods and drugs do not apply to nonnutrient supplements. Manufacturers are only required to give FDA a

Dietary Supplements—A Consumer Caution

The Food and Nutrition Science Alliance* urges consumers who purchase dietary supplements to consider the following:

- When buying dietary supplements, the buyer should beware.
- If it sounds too good to be true, it probably is not true.
- Dietary supplements include vitamins and minerals as well as herbals and botanicals.
- Multivitamins may help some people.
- Less is known about herbals and botanicals than about vitamins and minerals.
- High doses of some dietary supplements may be harmful.
- *Natural* is not the same as *safe*.
- For good health, eat a variety of foods.

The Food and Nutrition Science Alliance (FANSA) includes the Institute of Food Technologists, the American Dietetic Association, the American Society for Clinical Nutrition, and the American Society of Nutritional Sciences.

23-7 Use this guide to help clarify confusion about food and nutrition issues.

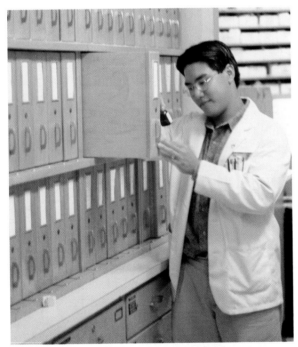

23-8 Medical professionals can refer to volumes of information that exist for FDA-approved drugs.

written explanation of why safety can reasonably be expected. Few scientific facts are known about these supplements, but many research projects are underway.

As a result of easy market-entry requirements, some harmful supplements have slipped through. Hazards have ranged from headaches, dizziness, and vomiting to strokes, seizures, and even death. Reports of these hazards have convinced government and industry leaders much more research is needed. Consequently, many changes are coming for this industry.

● **Are Nonnutrient Supplements Effective?**

Some people say nonnutrient supplements perform all the benefits claimed on their labels. Others insist they do not. What can a person believe? Here, again, research could provide an answer, but few scientific facts exist.

Usually ads for nonnutrient supplements include vague statements about making the user feel better. Some examples are "promotes relaxation" and "supports the immune system." See 23-9. Government action has stopped the use of claims that were judged false. Examples of false claims include "improves eyesight," "improves memory," and "slows the aging process."

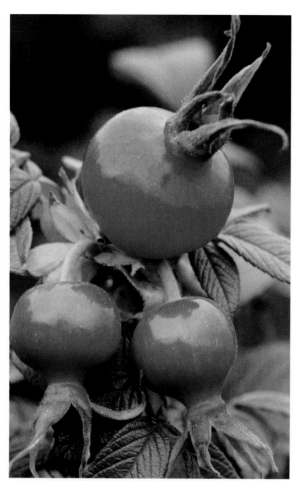

23-9 Ads for extracts from the bilberry plant claim to promote healthy blood vessels and good vision.

You will know that a supplement's claim is not scientifically proven when its ad or label includes the following: "This statement has not been evaluated by the Food and Drug Administration. This product is not intended to diagnose, treat, cure, or prevent any disease." These words are a sign that the product probably does not do what its literature may claim.

Some supplement claims, however, are true and reliable. These are the nutrition- or disease-related claims. An example of a nutrition claim is "excellent source of vitamin C." An example of a disease claim is "vitamin C prevents scurvy." FDA must review and approve these claims before they can be used. As a result, convincing facts exist to support them.

Food Science Trends

Food and nutrition in the future will benefit from the scientific discoveries in progress today. New technology at the cell level is opening many doors to improving and increasing the food supply. Food itself appears to contain disease fighters and health promoters besides nutrients. Finally, food safety advances are reducing food spoilage and foodborne illness.

Bioengineering

Bioengineering is the science of changing the genetic makeup of an organism. It involves altering DNA to change an organism's inherited traits. *DNA* is the molecular matter that makes up the genes in an organism. See 23-10. *Genes* are units in every cell that control an organism's inherited traits.

Taking a look back in time may help you better understand bioengineering. For years, farmers have worked to breed desirable qualities into plants and animals. They looked for plants that showed beneficial characteristics, such as resistance to disease. They crossbred those plants to produce young plants with the same characteristics. A new disease-resistant strain of the plant would gradually evolve. However, this required years of breeding the desired trait into one crop after another.

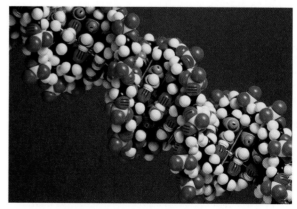

23-10 A gene, the longest living molecule, has a spiral form. It can form an exact replica of itself.

Sweet corn is an example of successful crossbreeding. Long ago, most corn was inedible. It was useful only for grinding into flour. After decades of plant breeding, farmers were able to grow the juicy sweet corn most people enjoy today.

Traditional crossbreeding has two main drawbacks. First, it is slow. It takes many years to achieve the desired results. Second, traditional crossbreeding methods pass on undesirable traits along with desirable ones.

Bioengineering is today's version of the crossbreeding techniques farmers have used for years. Researchers are learning to identify the exact genes that control certain traits in plants and animals. See 23-11. They are using this knowledge to transfer genes that govern useful traits from one species to another. Bioengineering is being used to produce hardier crops that resist pests and diseases.

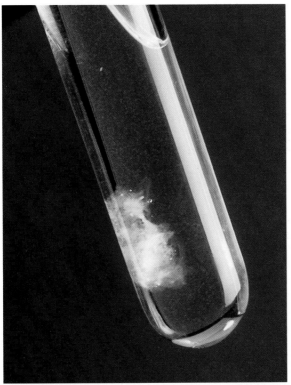

Agricultural Research Service, USDA

23-11 This test tube contains DNA strands from blueberry leaves, which helped scientists increase the hardiness of blueberry trees in cold weather.

Bioengineering overcomes both of the drawbacks of traditional crossbreeding. The time required to produce a plant with a desired trait through bioengineering is about five years. This technology provides certainty as well as speed. Scientists can isolate the gene for a specific desirable trait in an organism. Then they can introduce this gene to another organism. Bioengineering helps serve the needs of the world population. Food crops become more productive for farmers to grow and more nutritious and tasty for consumers to eat.

One common example of a food that uses bioengineering is cheese. More than half the cheese produced in the United States is now made with an enzyme prepared through bioengineering. Previously, a natural enzyme extracted from calf stomachs was used to make cheese. This enzyme caused slight variations in quality. The new enzyme is readily available. It also yields more consistent cheese quality.

Bioengineering is a fast-growing science. It has led to the use of new terms that you will hear more often in the future. Other names for bioengineering are *genetic engineering* and *biotechnology*. The process of recombining genes is called *recombinant DNA (rDNA) technology*. The term *gene-splicing* is also used.

Bioengineering can affect the future of nutrition and fitness in three ways. It can increase the quantity and quality of food. It can improve the nutrient content of food. It also has the potential to create foods that help prevent diseases in humans.

● **Increased Food Quantity and Quality**

Increasing food *quantity* is a very important goal of bioengineering. See 23-12. When food supplies are increased, the opportunity to eat a healthful and varied diet is available to more people. Also, more food is produced per acre of land. This is especially important in areas of the world where food is already scarce. Some examples of efforts currently in progress that will increase food quantity are

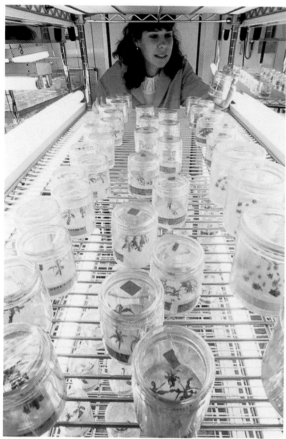

Agricultural Research Service, USDA

23-12 Each dish holds tiny experimental fruit trees grown from cells given new genes.

- insect-resistant apples, potatoes, and corn
- disease-resistant squash, potatoes, corn, papayas, and peaches
- freeze-resistant fruits and vegetables
- herbicide-resistant soybeans (An **herbicide** is a plant killer, used primarily to control weeds.)

Improving food *quality* is another important focus of bioengineering. It affects flavor, texture, appearance, and other important factors. Foods with improved quality are less likely to spoil or become damaged before use. Also, fresher and better-tasting produce is available throughout the year.

The first bioengineered whole product was a tomato, first marketed in 1994. This special tomato answered the public's desire for ripe tomatoes that did not rot quickly. Previously, only unripened tomatoes were available in supermarkets. These partially green tomatoes were firm enough to withstand the travel to distant markets. However, unripe tomatoes were flavorless.

Shoppers wanted ripe, flavorful tomatoes. Supermarket managers wanted tomatoes that did not arrive smashed. These two needs were satisfied by controlling the tomato gene that promoted fast rotting after ripening. The result was a ripe tomato that stayed fresh and relatively firm at room temperature for about 10 days. This is the average time needed to harvest, transport, sell, and use a tomato. See 23-13.

Enhanced Nutrient Content

Another benefit of bioengineering is the ability to make foods more nutritious. Nutrients can be added to or increased in grains, fruits, and vegetables. For example, USDA scientists recently developed new tomato strains with 10 to 25 times more beta-carotene. The human body converts beta-carotene into vitamin A. In the future, these specialty tomatoes will rival carrots as an excellent source of vitamin A.

Existing nutrient levels can also be reduced. Fat content, for example, can be

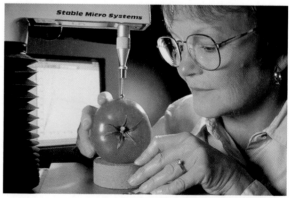

Agricultural Research Service, USDA

23-13 The search for the perfect tomato continues as USDA scientists examine properties that create ideal texture.

altered to lower total fat or saturated fat. See 23-14.

The potential of this technology is enormous. Imagine how protein-rich grain might reduce world hunger. Consider the impact of reducing fat in common foods. People following restricted or weight-control diets would benefit greatly. For example, people who avoid eggs because of the fat and cholesterol content could eat this ideal protein source again.

Possible Disease Prevention

Scientists are investigating ways to use biotechnology to attach disease fighters to common foods. The scientific principles involved in using a vaccine are at the heart of their work. A **vaccine** is a weakened strain of a disease-causing organism. It is usually grown in a laboratory. After a vaccination, your body responds by creating defenses. You then have **immunity**, or a high resistance to a disease. Each disease requires its unique vaccine.

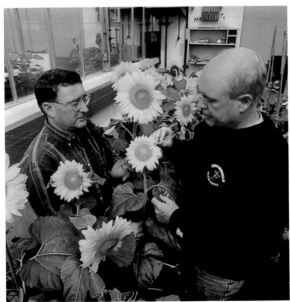

Agricultural Research Service, USDA

23-14 Scientists have found the gene that reduces fatty acids in sunflower oil, a popular vegetable oil used for frying.

Scientists foresee the day when people can receive immunity by eating a certain food instead of getting a shot. The edible vaccine would be grown in a plant or animal to replace the laboratory-prepared vaccine. This involves transferring genes to the food source to initiate the growth of the vaccine material.

In one example, goats are being developed to give milk that fights *malaria.* Malaria is a disease carried by mosquitoes. It affects a half-billion people and kills three million yearly. In another example, a new potato plant is carrying an edible vaccine for *E. coli,* a leading cause of foodborne illness in the United States.

Scientists are working on edible vaccines for many types of diseases and illnesses. Cancer and the common flu are just some of the illnesses that may be controlled by edible vaccines.

Is Bioengineering Safe?

The safety of foods produced through bioengineering concerns some consumers. Bioengineering that is well regulated poses little threat to people or the environment. Experts point out that bioengineered foods are just as safe as traditional foods. Developers must consult with the FDA before they can introduce a new bioengineered product. This process takes several years. It ensures that these products pass FDA's food safety assessment.

Many of the discoveries and advances in bioengineering begin in USDA research centers. See 23-15. The USDA also oversees field trials and large-scale production of bioengineered plants and animals. The Environmental Protection Agency (EPA) regulates the pest-resistant properties of bioengineered crops. These many checkpoints assure consumers and product developers of the safety of bioengineering.

Are Bioengineered Foods Labeled?

Most bioengineered foods will be so much like traditional foods that special labels

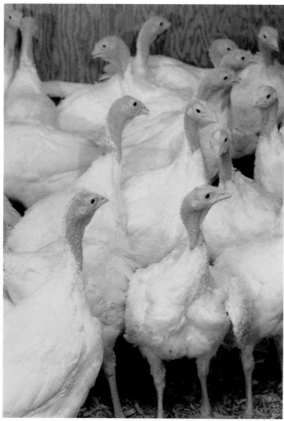

Agricultural Research Service, USDA

23-15 Nearly all U.S.-produced turkeys today come from the Beltsville Small White, named after USDA's Beltsville, Maryland, research center, where it was developed. It is prized for its wide breast and low weight (under 25 pounds).

will not be needed. However, labels will be required for the following:

- food that causes an allergic reaction in some people
- food whose nutrient content is changed (for example, a bioengineered carrot with more vitamin A)
- food that is new to the diet

New foods introduced to the public always require labeling. It does not matter whether the food is the result of bioengineering or traditional crossbreeding methods. *Broccoflower* is an example of a new food that required labeling. This green cauliflower was developed through traditional cross-breeding of broccoli and cauliflower.

● Functional Foods as Disease Fighters

The line between medicine and food is fast disappearing with a new category of foods called *functional foods*. A **functional food** is a food or food ingredient that provides health benefits beyond basic nutrition. This means the food is more than a source of nutrients. It also has the potential for preventing disease or promoting health.

An example of a functional food is broccoli. It is an excellent source of several vitamins and minerals plus fiber. However, certain phytochemicals in broccoli seem to stimulate cancer-fighting substances. (Phytochemicals were discussed in Chapter 8.) Other phytochemicals in broccoli seem to lower cholesterol levels and strengthen the immune system. If research confirms that broccoli provides all these benefits, its value goes far beyond the nutrients it provides. See 23-16.

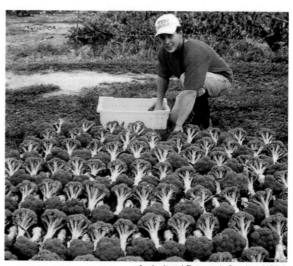

Agricultural Research Service, USDA

23-16 Broccoli sales are up because of discoveries linked to its phytochemicals. As a result, USDA scientists are finding ways to produce larger, more uniform stalks.

Broccoli is just one example of a traditional food that is considered a functional food. In fact, many fruits, vegetables, and grains seem to provide various health benefits. This is due to the beneficial phytochemicals they contain.

In addition to traditional foods, new products are being developed to perform one or more health functions. The development of functional foods is the biggest trend in new food products today. Meatlike dishes based on cereal or soy products were some of the first functional foods. Breakfast cereals, breads, baked goods, pasta, and frozen entrées are nearly ready for market.

Several factors are fueling the search for health-promoting substances in food. Rapid advances in science and technology are quickly revealing new facts about food and health. See 23-17. The growing desire throughout the general public to maintain a healthful diet is another factor. However, rising health care costs and the aging population are the main factors. Many older people would rather use food than drugs to preserve good health throughout life.

Phytochemicals are the largest, but not the only, active food components in functional foods. Dietary fiber and some fatty acids also seem to work as active components. Experts

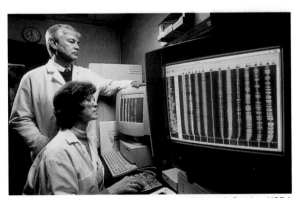

Agricultural Research Service, USDA

23-17 More powerful and sophisticated equipment is one of the reasons why scientific knowledge is expanding rapidly. These scientists are studying the DNA of a poultry virus.

agree more research is needed before the full effects of these food components are known. Some of the benefits reported to date include the following:

- reduced risk of diseases of the heart, eyes, intestinal tract, and reproductive system
- reduced risk of degenerative diseases
- lower blood cholesterol levels
- improved mental functions

You will hear functional foods sometimes called *nutraceuticals.* This is a term created by combining the words *nutrition* with *pharmaceuticals*, which are drugs. The new term indicates the druglike qualities that functional foods seem to have.

Food Safety Advances

A safe food supply is vitally important to the nutrition and fitness of a nation's citizens. The United States boasts one of the safest food supplies in the world, primarily because safety measures are constantly strengthened. This involves using safe practices at every step of growing, harvesting, processing, packaging, transporting, and selling food. (Then the consumer is responsible for food safety in the home.)

New technologies are used as tools to complement routine sanitation practices. Some of the new food safety technologies include competitive bacteria and DNA "fingerprinting." Technologies that make packaged foods safer include active packaging and irradiation.

Competitive Bacteria

Competitive bacteria prevent the growth of harmful organisms. They accomplish this by feeding on nutrients that would otherwise support harmful bacteria. This method of bacteria control was first used on pear orchards in 1995. See 23-18. Spraying the beneficial bacteria on the trees prevented *fire blight.* This disease causes plants to dry, turn brown, and stop producing fruit.

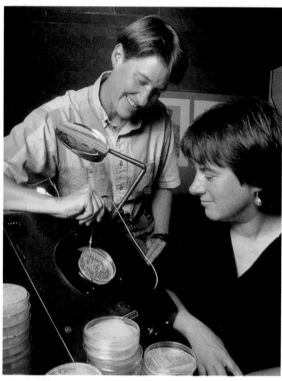

Agricultural Research Service, USDA

23-18 These plant scientists used bioengineering to develop the competitive bacteria used to combat disease in pear orchards.

Research is underway to find more uses of competitive bacteria. One example is the use of harmless bacteria to reduce *Salmonella* and *E. coli* in poultry. A mist of harmless bacteria is sprayed on newly hatched chicks. It introduces 29 bacteria naturally present in healthy adult chickens. As the birds fluff their feathers with their beaks, they ingest the spray. The "good" bacteria block sites in the chicks' intestines where harmful bacteria would take hold. Without food, harmful bacteria inside the poultry then die.

DNA Fingerprinting

DNA fingerprinting is a tracing process that identifies the microorganisms and food sources that cause contamination. It uses the same DNA procedure that links a criminal to a crime. DNA fingerprinting is a tool that provides quicker and highly accurate results to tests of possible poisoned food.

Acquiring facts through DNA fingerprinting helps officials make faster decisions about public health matters. These decisions may include investigations or *product recalls*. A **product recall** is the return to the manufacturer of defective or contaminated products.

Active Packaging

Active packaging is a type of food packaging process. The package interacts with the food or the gases inside. One version uses an agent that releases a specific gas, usually carbon dioxide, to retard the growth of microbes. This method is used to delay the spoilage of packaged produce and coffee.

Other types of active packaging absorb oxygen to delay the growth of spoilage bacteria. Organisms need oxygen to grow, so with less of it, their growth is slowed. The "active" part of the package is a separate component placed inside the package itself.

In addition to fighting microorganisms, active packaging can provide information. A special indicator strip on the outside of the package can sense time and temperature. If the package has not been kept at safe temperatures, the strip changes color. This color signal informs food handlers and consumers that food is not safe to eat.

Irradiation

Irradiation is the exposure of food to ionizing energy. Ionizing energy creates positive and negative charges. Irradiation kills food spoilage organisms and extends the freshness of perishable foods. It also stops the sprouting of vegetables and delays the ripening of produce. Irradiation does not change the food itself in any way. It is impossible, therefore, to detect food that has been exposed to irradiation.

The first food approved for irradiation by the FDA was for U.S. space program astronauts. If you have eaten any spices, you probably already sampled irradiated food. Spices are the most commonly irradiated food in the world. The other foods approved by the FDA for irradiation include fruits, vegetables, wheat, potatoes, pork, poultry, and red meat. The FDA requires a special symbol on the labels of irradiated food. See 23-19.

During irradiation, foods go through some chemical and nutritional changes. Electromagnetic waves strike molecules in the food product. The force breaks molecular bonds, and new compounds are produced, such as carbon dioxide, formic acid, and glucose. These substances are commonly found in all types of foods. No substances produced have been found to be harmful. Keeping food temperatures and oxygen levels in check during irradiation limits damage to nutrients.

Irradiation causes little change in flavor, texture, or color of most foods. However, this process cannot be used to kill salmonella in eggs because the egg whites are altered. On the other hand, irradiation can kill salmonella in poultry with no damage to the poultry.

Irradiation is a safe, effective, and thoroughly tested method for preserving food. However, many consumers do not understand this process. Their fears have slowed the use of this technology in the marketplace.

Fitness Trends

Physical activity once was a natural part of everyday life in the United States. Now most people must plan to incorporate it into their lives. As a result, many products and services are being offered to answer today's fitness needs.

Today's Inactive Lifestyle

When the United States was largely agricultural, most people lived on farms. They built their homes, raised their food, and made their clothing. Every day was a workday. Work started before sunrise and continued long after sunset. The daily tasks involved much physical activity, so hearty meals were the general rule.

During the 1800s, farm work was traded for factory work. Then, too, long workdays were common. Like farm work, many factory jobs were physically demanding.

Today, factory jobs are fewer and highly automated. See 23-20. Machines now perform most of the exhausting or complex motions that people formerly handled.

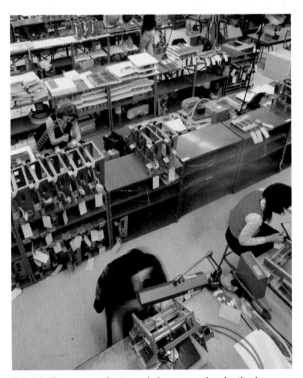

23-20 For many factory jobs, people do their work from a seated position.

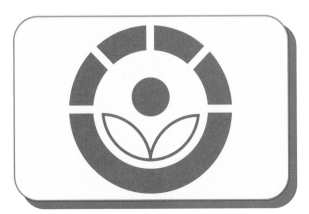

23-19 This international symbol, named a radura, is used to identify irradiated food.

More positions are opening in the rapidly growing service sector of the economy. The *service sector* employs people who provide assistance. Examples include dry cleaning, teaching, bus driving, and computer programming.

Besides changes in the workplace, much has changed in homes over the last few centuries. Most people no longer need to chop wood, start a fire to boil water, scrub dirty clothes on a washboard, and iron them. Dirty laundry is cleaned by simply tossing it into an automatic washing machine. Most clothes have finishes that make ironing unnecessary. All aspects of household upkeep require much less physical effort today.

Other developments of modern society also contribute to a decrease in physical activity. For example, few people walk or ride bikes to work or school. Elevators and escalators move you between the floors of a building or shopping mall. Instead of mowing lawns or painting, many people hire others to do the work.

You can see how the average lifestyle in the United States has shifted over the years. A society that was once physically active has become highly sedentary. This widespread lack of physical activity is one of the reasons for the obesity problem in the United States. The following American Dietetic Association statistics indicate the extent of the problem:

- Each year more than half of the population tries to either lower weight or maintain a recent weight loss. Most do not successfully keep off excess pounds. See 23-21.
- The number of overweight adults is continually rising. In the United States, over half the population is currently overweight, and a third is obese.

While excess weight can result from many factors, the number one cause is ingesting too many calories. (This fact was explained in Chapter 12, "The Energy Balancing Act.") With many people needing weight loss help, a new fitness industry has developed.

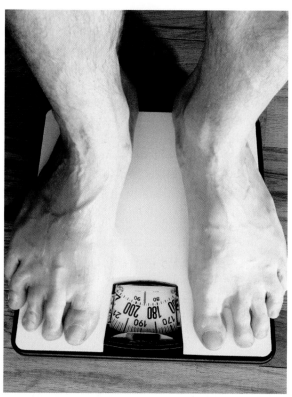

23-21 The bathroom scale prompts many people to try to lose weight.

● The Fitness Industry

Eating foods low in fats as a regular diet habit is one way people are trying to manage their weight. (The preference for lowfat foods was discussed earlier in this chapter.) In addition, more people are looking for ways to increase physical activity. As a result, the fitness industry has developed to supply their needs. A number of trends are shaping the products and services offered by this industry.

- **Fitness aids are numerous.** There are exercise machines and video tapes galore. Ads for these products appear on TV and in your favorite magazines. Computer software programs are available to link to home exercise equipment and monitor fitness progress. In addition, many books and TV programs feature exercise routines for young adults, women, and other population segments.

- **Sports apparel is increasing.** Not only do people want more exercise, but they also want special clothes for it. The all-purpose gym shoe is practically a thing of the past. See 23-22. Now there are special shoes for nearly every sport as well as for walking and running. To complement the shoes, there are complete lines of exercise and sports apparel. Many shopping malls have stores that sell only sports apparel or shoes.

- **Many corporations are encouraging employees to stay fit.** These companies help their employees use exercise as a way to reduce stress and stay healthy. They know that healthy employees work more productively. When space and funding permit, exercise facilities are built on site. In other cases, employees may receive discounts for using nearby health clubs. See 23-23.

- **Health care institutions are sponsoring fitness programs.** Traditionally, hospitals focused on making sick people well. Now many are interested in keeping healthy people fit so that illness is prevented or its effects are lessened. Hospitals and other health care providers are sponsoring programs with nearby health clubs and exercise facilities. These programs are often open to the general public. However, hospital patrons and members of health insurance programs are the primary targets.

- **Career opportunities in the fitness field are rapidly expanding.** A physical education teacher is just one of the many fitness-related professionals in your community. There is increasing demand for fitness experts and their professional advice. You

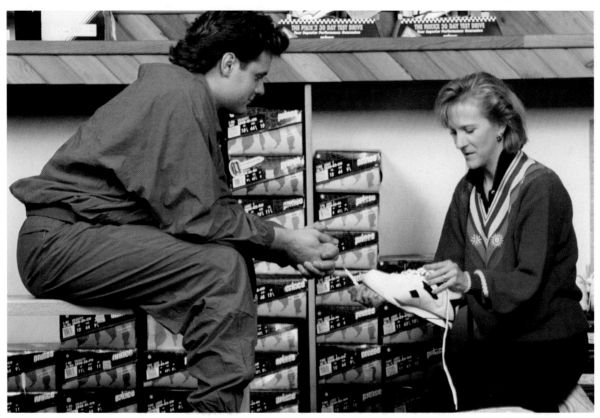

23-22 Numerous sportswear choices are available to satisfy everyone's comfort needs and style preferences.

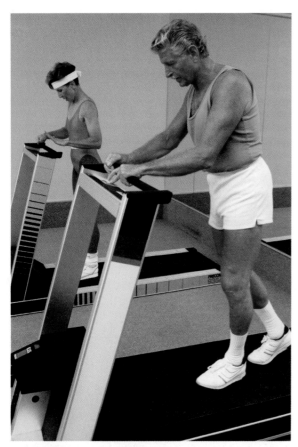

23-23 Many health clubs are open from sunrise to near midnight to allow customers the opportunity to fit exercise into their schedules.

see them in health clubs, but they are employed in a wide variety of careers. For example, they teach exercise science, test the equipment, and design fitness programs. See 23-24. Colleges are creating new degree programs and departments to address this expanding career area. You will learn more about it in Chapter 25, "A Career for You in Nutrition and Fitness."

Many products and services are being introduced to promote nutrition and fitness. It may become easier to incorporate a fitness routine into all stages of the life cycle. Staying fit does take time and effort, but the benefits to your health are great.

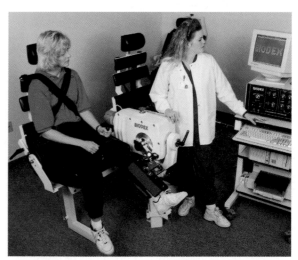

23-24 A physical therapy clinician is trained to exercise healing muscles and test their strength.

Summary

Food trends provide a glimpse of the future for food and nutrition. International cuisines will continue to shape U.S. food tastes. Public demand will stay strong for food that is fresh and convenient. Lowfat and fat free versions are likely to remain popular. Use of nonnutrient supplements is also growing, even though their safety and effectiveness are unproven.

Biotechnology offers enormous potential for many food improvements. It can increase food quality and quantity. It can add or increase nutrients in food. It can remove unwanted food components. It may even make some foods react like medicines and fight disease.

To keep food safe, new technologies will assist common sanitation practices. For example, special harmless bacteria can prevent the harmful types from growing. A highly accurate tracking method can trace the causes of food poisoning and impurity. Special packaging materials can slow the growth of spoilage organisms, and irradiation can kill them.

In the fitness area, many products and services will be available to help people stay in shape. A wide variety of self-help aids will help people stay fit. The sports apparel industry will continue to expand. Employers and health providers will encourage people to use fitness facilities. As the fitness field expands, so will career opportunities.

Check Your Knowledge

1. True or false. Foods with mild flavors are becoming more popular.

2. Describe what has been done to some supermarket produce to provide ready-to-eat convenience.

3. True or false. Fat affects a food's flavor, texture, mouth feel, and nutrient content.

4. Name a calorie-free fat replacer.

5. State briefly the positions of advocates and opponents of nonnutrient supplements.

6. What lets a person know that a nonnutrient supplement's claims have *not* been scientifically proven?

7. What part of an organism's cell does bioengineering change?

8. Bioengineering has the ability to ____.
   A. increase food quantity and quality
   B. enhance the nutrient content of food
   C. prevent disease
   D. All of the above.

9. True or false. The first bioengineered whole product was an insect-resistant apple.

10. What bioengineered food may be helpful in the fight against malaria?

11. When is a food label necessary on a bioengineered product?

12. How was broccoflower created?

13. Name two active components in food that seem to have disease-fighting or health-promoting qualities.

14. Why are functional foods sometimes called nutraceuticals?

15. True or false. Competitive bacteria can rapidly trace the causes of food poisoning or impurity.

16. Identify two benefits of active packaging.

17. Which of the following is *not* true about irradiation?
    A. It is safe, effective, and thoroughly tested.
    B. It is easy to detect in food.
    C. It is a food preservation method.
    D. It is commonly used to preserve spices.

18. Briefly contrast activity levels of the U.S. population today to 100 years ago.

19. Identify four signs that indicate the fitness industry is increasing.

20. Name two ways corporations are helping employees stay fit.

Put Learning into Action

1. Survey family members that are your parent's age or older. Ask them what foods or flavors they enjoy now that weren't available 10 years ago. Summarize your findings in a one-page report.

2. Visit an area supermarket. Find five foods that are available in lowfat versions. For each, compare the costs per serving of regular and lowfat versions. (Be sure to compare packages of nearly equal size and food of relatively similar type and ingredients. For example, some unfair comparisons include: a family size package versus a single serving, frozen juice versus canned juice, or a creamy salad dressing versus oil and vinegar.)

3. Interview the human resources director of a local company. Learn what programs or facilities the company provides to promote employee fitness. If the company has a brochure or policy statement on the subject of employee fitness, obtain a copy. Report your findings to the class.

Explore Further

1. Analyze a nonnutrient supplement to learn more about its claims. Look for products in local drugstores or supermarkets, or focus on a sample your teacher may bring to class. Study the product's label and ad. (The product's ad may be found in magazines or in the store where it is sold. If no ad is available, request a copy by writing to the manufacturer.) Are the product's claims safe? What helps you determine this? Write a brief research report on the product. Include a copy of the label, ad, and any other related items.

2. Research information about Gregor Mendel and his contribution to the science of plant breeding. What exactly did he do and learn? Use visual aids to explain his fundamental discoveries to the class.

3. Investigate a food, nutrition, or fitness theory that is currently being studied. Check the local Cooperative Extension Service office and other sources for information. Summarize the research done and the conclusions made to date. What are the potential benefits of the research? Who will benefit most from it? Write a two-page report summarizing your findings.

Chapter 24

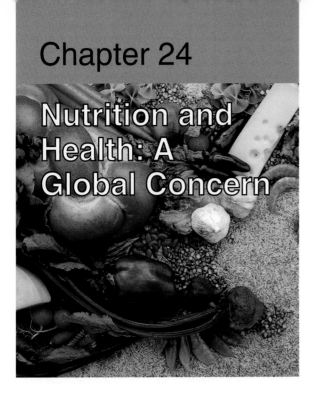

Nutrition and Health: A Global Concern

Learn the Language

developing nation
hunger
undernutrition
malnutrition
starvation
famine
food security
United Nations (U.N.)
underweight
stunted
wasted
hemorrhage

mortality rate
compassion
overpopulation
cash crop
congregate meal
commodity food
hunger myth
food policy
infrastructure
environmental
  sustainability
advocate

Objectives

After studying this chapter, you will be able to

- define terms related to global hunger.
- explain the major causes of hunger.
- refute common misconceptions about global hunger.
- describe how a nation's hunger problem can be solved through the following factors: economic progress, science and technology advances, effective infrastructure, slower population growth, and education.
- identify the primary organizations working to combat hunger in the United States and throughout the world.
- propose several ways individuals can help fight hunger.

The world's population, now around six billion people, is expected to jump beyond eight billion by 2025. The numbers are easier to understand when you consider the population increase on a daily basis. There are about 140,000 deaths per day and 365,000 births. As a result, the world's population increases daily by about 225,000 people. This is more than six million people per month.

Consider, too, that over 840 million people in the world's poorest countries are hungry. This figure does not account for the number of hungry people living in the United States and other wealthy countries. Will there be enough food to feed the people of the world? This chapter focuses on the issues related to meeting the world's food needs now and in the future. See 24-1.

The Hunger Problem

When food is scarce, hunger problems develop quickly. Some nations cannot raise enough food for their citizens and are too poor to buy it. The United Nations has identified 83 such countries, which are often called developing nations. A ***developing nation*** has a low economic level of living standards and industrial production.

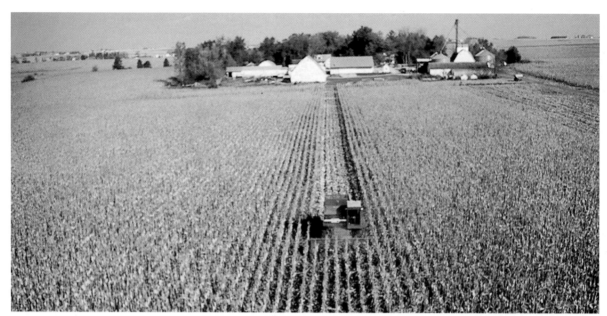

U.S. Department of Agriculture

24-1 Some countries share their abundance with starving nations, but this is only a temporary solution to global hunger.

The greatest numbers of hungry people are found in South and East Asia and parts of Africa. The most extreme hunger conditions are also found there. The average annual income is less than $1,500 per person in developing countries. In nearly 50 of these countries, average income ranges between $100 and $500 per year. Many families use 80 to 90 percent of their income to buy food. Quality and quantity of food are limited, so people must accept whatever food is available.

Industrialized nations face hunger problems, too. In most of these countries, enough food is available. However, many people lack the money to buy it. This is evident in Eastern Europe, where the hunger rate grows as food prices rise. It is also seen in the United States, where emergency food requests jump during periods of high unemployment.

● The Meaning of Hunger

Everyone has felt some form of hunger. You may be hungry as you read this chapter. Hours after you eat, your stomach lets you know that it wants food. A craving for food is the type of hunger that probably is most familiar to you. The meaning of **hunger** in this chapter, however, is a weakened state caused by prolonged lack of sufficient food. Other terms closely related to hunger are *undernutrition* and *malnutrition.*

- *Undernutrition* is eating too little food to maintain healthy body weight and normal activity levels. In developing nations, it is caused by lack of food, which is due to poverty. An indicator of undernutrition is low calorie intake. About one-fifth of the world's people live with this condition.

- *Malnutrition* is poor nutrition, usually endured for a long period. It can result from a nutritionally poor diet or some condition that prevents the body from using nutrients. The focus of this chapter is malnutrition caused by undernutrition. There are varying degrees of malnutrition. They range from underweight to stunted growth to progressive destruction of body tissue. The most common indicator of malnutrition is low protein intake. However, various ratios of weight, height, body mass, and age are used to measure the degree of malnutrition.

In developed countries, the average protein intake per person is 106 grams per day. The average protein intake in Bangladesh, a developing country, is 40 grams per day. See 24-2. The adult RDAs for protein range from 46 to 63 grams daily. What might you conclude about the general health status of many people in Bangladesh?

The most severe nutritional inadequacy is starvation. **Starvation** is the condition that results from a lack of food needed to sustain life. It often results in death. Starvation is very

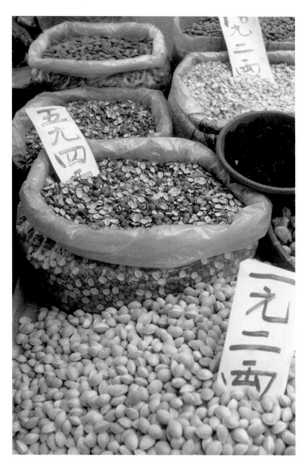

24-2 Approximately one cup of dry beans provides 40 grams of protein. This is below the recommended dietary allowance for everyone over 14 years old.

common when famines occur. A **famine** is an extreme scarcity of food for an extended period, perhaps years.

In the past, famines were often due to crop diseases or natural disasters. Modern science and swift emergency responses from other nations have helped eliminate these causes. Today famines mostly occur in war zones. They are caused by the intentional withholding of food from the "enemy" or the destruction of crops due to war.

The most common reason for global hunger is a lack of access to food due to poverty. The nations working to end hunger believe that, regardless of income level, all human beings deserve food security. **Food security** means always having access to the food needed for a healthy life. Many factors affect food security, especially the way governments run their countries.

Most countries are working to achieve food security for all people of the world. Some countries, however, are not willing to make the changes needed to create food security. The leaders of these nations view poverty and hunger as sad facts of life. They believe some citizens must endure food shortages so the leaders can keep comfortable lifestyles. Their beliefs have led to government policies that have allowed hunger to persist for years.

● Health Problems Related to Hunger

In a society where hunger is widespread, children and pregnant women always suffer first and most profoundly. When malnutrition occurs in the early years, its effect on a person is lifelong. People who are malnourished get sick more quickly and lack energy. They never grow as strong or as tall as they could. Mental ability and the drive to succeed decrease when hunger exists too long.

According to United Nations' figures, one-third to one-half of the children in developing nations die before age five. About 90 percent of childhood deaths are related to poor nutrition. Malnutrition often occurs when children are weaned from breast milk too early. Breast milk provides protein and other nutrients needed for normal growth. It also contains substances that fight infection. Available foods seldom match the nutritional quality of breast milk.

Malnourished women generally lack good health. Therefore, many have babies with low birthweights. These babies are more likely to become sick and die than heavier babies. Low-birthweight children may have underdeveloped organs or mental or physical disabilities. Poverty and malnutrition form a vicious cycle, as illustrated in 24-3. The cycle is repeated from one generation to the next.

People become more likely to get diseases and infections as their bodies age. This susceptibility increases for elderly people who are malnourished. At any age, an inadequate diet may also cause appetite loss, sluggish mental responses, and slower healing of wounds. These factors may reduce an elderly person's drive to try to obtain nutritious food.

Malnourished people often have a shorter life span than healthy, well-nourished individuals. In fact, 75 percent of the people born in the least developed countries die before age 50. Compare that to the global life expectancy today of 66 years.

Assessing the nutritional status of hungry people all over the world is a high priority of

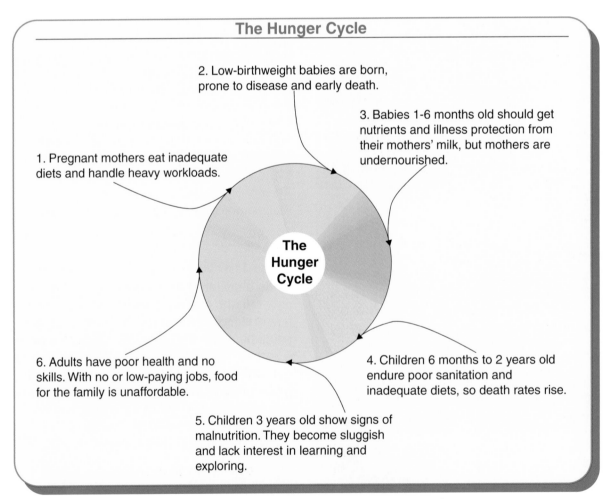

The Hunger Cycle

2. Low-birthweight babies are born, prone to disease and early death.

3. Babies 1-6 months old should get nutrients and illness protection from their mothers' milk, but mothers are undernourished.

1. Pregnant mothers eat inadequate diets and handle heavy workloads.

The Hunger Cycle

6. Adults have poor health and no skills. With no or low-paying jobs, food for the family is unaffordable.

4. Children 6 months to 2 years old endure poor sanitation and inadequate diets, so death rates rise.

5. Children 3 years old show signs of malnutrition. They become sluggish and lack interest in learning and exploring.

24-3 Once the hunger cycle begins, those in it are often powerless to stop it.

the **United Nations (U.N.)**. This is the organization formed by the nations of the world to promote international peace and security. The U.N. reports the following facts about the nutritional status of people in developing countries:

- Undernutrition—Twenty percent of the world's people do not get enough calories each day. This points to a general lack of carbohydrates.

- Malnutrition—Focusing just on children, over 190 million are *underweight*, 230 million are *stunted*, and 50 million are *wasted*. **Underweight** children have a weight below the healthy range. **Stunted** means having below-average height and never catching up. **Wasted** means having severe weight loss due to progressive destruction of body tissue. These statistics reflect widespread protein deficiency and risk of death. Malnutrition also occurs in adolescents and adults, but to a lesser degree.

- Vitamin A deficiency—Over 40 million children in at least 60 developing countries suffer from lack of vitamin A. This vitamin helps eyes function and affects all stages of body development. About 250,000 children go blind each year because they get too little vitamin A.

- Iodine deficiency—About 1.6 billion people in the world do not get enough iodine in their diets. The problem is not limited to developing countries. It exists in the United States and European countries as well. Iodine deficiency is the chief cause of preventable brain damage and mental retardation in newborn infants.

- Iron deficiency—About two billion people have a diet severely low in iron. This problem mainly affects women and preschool children. See 24-4. In some areas, more than half the women and children are anemic. Too little iron slows growth, makes the body prone to infections, and causes fatigue. It also increases a mother's risk of **hemorrhage** (uncontrollable bleeding) and

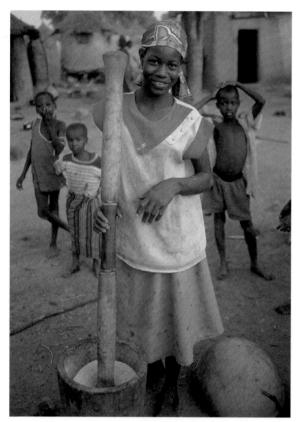

24-4 Many children in developing countries rarely eat meat, eggs, and other excellent sources of iron. Instead they rely on leafy greens and dry beans to avoid iron deficiency.

infections before, during, and after childbirth. About 20 percent of maternal deaths are linked to anemia.

- Zinc deficiency—The importance of zinc has often been overlooked. This is because no reliable method exists for examining the zinc stored in the body. Evidence is growing, however, that zinc deficiency is widespread. A lack of the nutrient causes poor growth, poor resistance to infections, and other health problems.

● Why Care About Hunger in the World?

Food scarcity problems affect all nations and all people, rich and poor alike. Everyone has a duty to help stop world hunger. There are at least four major reasons for ending hunger. These involve political, economic, humanitarian, and compassionate reasons.

● Political Reasons

A situation in one country can affect other countries. Why is this so? As trade between nations expands, nations become increasingly interdependent. For example, high food prices and hunger can lead to political unrest and armed conflict. A developing nation might lack the resources to address such a hunger problem and calm the unrest. Therefore, it might ask for help from developed nations. The developed nations have political reasons for providing requested help. They want to protect their trade relationship with the developing country.

Solving the food problems of poorer countries tends to reduce their political instability. Thus, world peace is directly affected by hunger issues. All the nations of the world benefit when they work together to solve global hunger problems.

● Economic Reasons

Starving people do not have the luxury of choosing from an array of foods. They must eat whatever food is available. Once basic needs for food are met, however, people gain interest in food variety. This fact gives developed countries with surplus crops an economic reason for wanting to end world hunger. A desire for food variety creates new markets for agricultural products.

Before a country's economic structure can be developed, families within that country must have the chance to earn a living. With enough income, families can break the poverty cycle. They are able to buy enough food to maintain physical health and strength. This enables them to contribute to their country's economic status. With improved economic well-being, the country will increase trade with other nations. With higher incomes, families can afford foods imported from other countries. See 24-5.

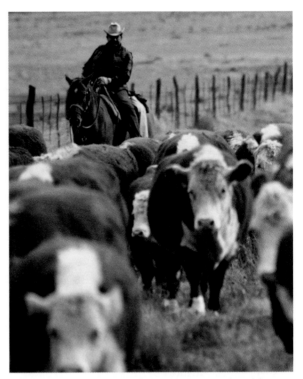

24-5 World demand for meat, such as beef from Argentina, is growing. However, family incomes must rise dramatically before imported meat is affordable.

● Humanitarian Reasons

Making sure people have food because it is one of their rights as human beings shows *humanitarian* concern. Most nations agree that people cannot feel a sense of self-respect until their basic human needs have been met. Along with adequate clothing and shelter, people need food to survive. When they have these necessities, people can believe they are worthwhile and their lives have value.

To what extent are human needs being met in various parts of the world? The United Nations collects data to profile the living conditions of people in different countries. Some indications of a nation's quality of life include the following:

- infant and child ***mortality rate***, or death rate

- life expectancy, or the average life span

- percent of the population with access to safe water
- percent of the population with adequate sanitation, such as food refrigeration and prompt waste removal
- primary school enrollment rate
- *per capita gross domestic product (GDP),* or the average value of goods and services produced yearly by each resident of the country

These are just some of the many statistics that help reveal a nation's living conditions and quality of life. Refer to 24-6 to see how these factors compare for the United States and five other countries. As you study the chart, keep in mind that a statistic is a midpoint between the highest and lowest numbers. Therefore, living conditions may be poor in one part of a country and comfortable in another at the same time.

Compassionate Reasons

A sense of obligation is the motivating force behind humanitarian concerns about hunger. *Compassion* goes one step further. **Compassion** is a deep sense of sadness for human suffering coupled with a strong desire to stop it.

When you feel compassion, you genuinely care about another person's feelings. You are emotionally moved by the pain and despair you see in a hungry person's eyes. You want to do more than stop hunger; you want to help repair that person's life and offer hope. Compassion is a deeply personal feeling that motivates you to go beyond a sense of obligation. A compassionate person willingly extends a helping hand to others.

Primary Causes of Hunger

There are many reasons for hunger in the world. The cause of hunger in one country may differ from that in another. Causes of hunger within a country can also change from one year to the next. As you might guess, poverty, overpopulation, and natural disasters are main causes of hunger. Other factors that affect hunger include

Indicators of Health and Living Conditions

Nation	Infant and Child Mortality (death rate per 1,000 for ages 1-4)	Life Expectancy at Birth (years of age)	Population with Safe Water (%)	Population with Adequate Sanitation (%)	Primary School Enrollment Rate (% of children covered by attendance requirements)	Per Capita GDP (U.S. $)
Afghanistan	257	45	39	8	48	250
Angola	292	47	32	16	88	410
Bolivia	102	61	63	58	95	800
Cambodia	170	53	36	14	118*	270
Haiti	134	54	37	25	56	250
United States	8	76	x	x	107*	26,980

x = not studied
* = Figures exceeding 100% indicate voluntary preschool enrollment.

Source: The State of the World's Children 1998, The World Bank

24-6 A dramatic difference in health and living conditions exists between the United States and developing countries.

government policies and environmental factors. Cultural practices and a lack of education play roles, too. Natural disasters cause short-term hunger problems. Other causes create ongoing hunger problems that require long-term solutions.

● **Poverty**

The main cause of hunger is lack of access to food because of poverty. Poor people do not have enough money to buy food. With no income, they cannot even buy the seeds, fertilizer, and tools needed to start a home garden.

Poverty often occurs in rural settings, but it also is an urban problem. The biggest difference between rural and urban poverty is the sanitation level. In crowded urban areas, unsanitary conditions abound. They threaten the health of the residents. See 24-7.

● **Overpopulation**

A large population may not be the cause of hunger, but it does strain food resources. When there are more people than the land can support, overpopulation results. *Overpopulation* is a population growth so rapid that it deteriorates the environment or the quality of life.

Usually, the fastest rates of population growth occur in the poorest nations. Couples there have large families for several reasons. They may not be able to obtain or afford birth control methods. They may feel intense social pressure to have large families. They also know that children contribute to household income. Therefore, having large families will allow them to earn more money.

● **Natural Disasters**

Earthquakes, hurricanes, and other natural disasters can wipe out food supplies. One U.S. representative who visited Bangladesh after a life-threatening flood said, "I saw tens of thousands of people who were homeless, barely existing. All their assets were wiped away with the flood. Their water is very contaminated. They need antibiotics. Their bridges and railways need repair."

Most natural disasters are likely to cause short-term, rather than long-term, hunger problems. The poorer the country, however,

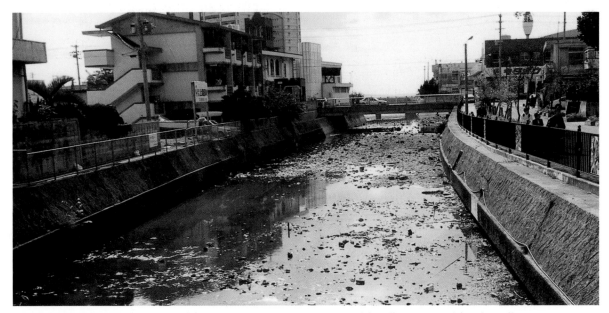

24-7 Unsanitary city streets and canals are a breeding ground for disease and food spoilage organisms. Over half the people in Asia and Africa will live in cities by the year 2025.

the harder it is to handle even short-term disasters. Stored food reserves can be used, but not every country has them. Food aid and hunger relief efforts provided by developed nations are often needed when disasters occur.

● **Government Policies**

A government's policies play a major role in removing or increasing hunger among its people. Policy decisions made by governments affect food production, market prices, and sales practices. Governments often make decisions about the types and quantities of crops to grow. These decisions affect how a nation's land, water, and other natural resources are used. Ultimately, all these decisions affect the poor.

Some policies promote urban or military development instead of rural development. Such policies make life tough for people in rural areas that lack suitable systems to produce, transport, and store food. Without these systems, large amounts of food become unusable. For example, almost half of all harvests in Latin America and Africa are lost to insect damage and unsanitary conditions. In West Africa, over one million gallons of milk must be thrown away each year. The milk spoils because it cannot be taken to cooling centers within three hours.

Sometimes governments decide to use their land for raising *cash crops* instead of staple crops. A ***cash crop*** is one that can be sold to an exporter. It is not consumed within the country and often is not a good source of nutrients. It is, however, a more profitable crop. Examples of crops grown for cash are coffee, nuts, and cacao beans. See 24-8. If rice, corn, wheat, or other staple crops were grown instead, local people could use them for food. Then the population would have a greater chance of obtaining a nutritionally adequate diet.

A government's policies during times of war often worsen a country's hunger problems. Money sent to a nation for food purchases is sometimes used for military

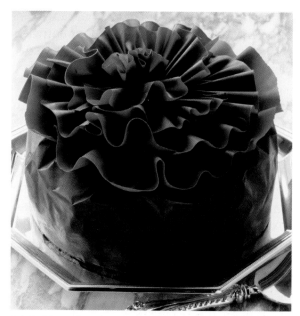

24-8 Chocolate is made from cacao beans, which are often grown as a cash crop in developing countries.

purchases instead. Food sent to feed the hungry may be diverted to the military, too.

● **Environmental Factors**

Deserts, mountains, and other harsh environments make growing food difficult. Often this results in too little food produced where people need it most. Overfished waters or polluted rivers compound a nation's food scarcity. Without proper care, the soil deteriorates and cannot support crops. When food cannot be grown locally, it must be imported from other countries. Imported food is usually much more expensive than locally grown food.

● **Culture**

Each ethnic culture has food traditions and beliefs that cause people to favor some foods and avoid others. Avoiding certain foods may not be a problem in a society where people eat a wide variety of foods. The situation is quite different when a forbidden food is the primary source of a required nutrient. For instance, animal foods and brewer's yeast are rich sources of vitamin B_{12}. However, most

Hindus in southern parts of India are vegetarians. They do not include these foods in their diets. Therefore, they are likely to be lacking in vitamin B$_{12}$. See 24-9.

Inadequate Education

People who lack education do not know what to do to improve their lives. They simply repeat what they have always done. For example, farmers in developing countries tend to grow the same crops in the same way year after year. The farmers are unaware that this repetition strips the soil of nutrients needed for crop growth. As a result, crop yields dwindle and the farmers sink ever deeper into poverty and hunger.

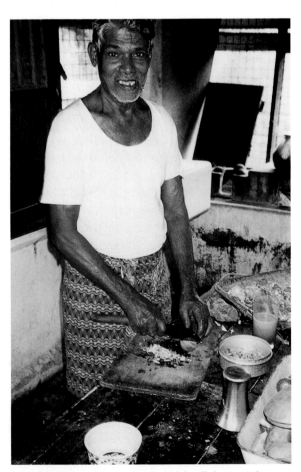

24-9 Highly seasoned vegetable dishes replace meat dishes in many parts of India.

Working Toward National Solutions

How can there be hunger in the United States when it produces more food than it needs? Even in this land of plenty, over 10 percent of the population falls below the poverty line. Many families in this population group do not earn enough income to buy adequate amounts of food. Many low-income families go hungry for several days each month.

Hunger in the United States

Who are the hungry in this country? They are the families using food stamps who run out of food before the end of the month. They are the people who experience difficult times, such as the loss of a job, 24-10.

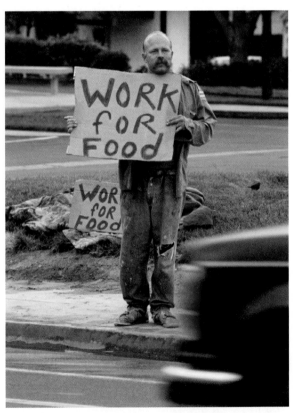

24-10 Hungry people live unnoticed in many communities until their situations become desperate.

Health emergencies and other misfortunes also cause people to rely on food donations and government programs.

About 30 to 70 million U.S. citizens lack nourishing food; safe, clean housing; and access to health care. With a poor start in life, children are given little opportunity to enter society's mainstream and develop productive adult lives.

The United States has made some gains in reducing hunger and malnutrition. However, the total number of people in poverty will probably increase in the near future. The main weapon against hunger remains, in large part, federal food and nutrition programs. However, private donations at the local level provide considerable food relief to area citizens.

National Programs

People need to know what resources exist to help them when they have food needs. The following five programs are available through the United States Department of Agriculture (USDA).

Food Stamp Program

The Food Stamp Program is designed to improve the diets of low-income families. Families who qualify receive food stamps based on their income levels. Fewer food stamps are provided as family income rises. Recipients use food stamps like cash to buy eligible foods at approved grocery stores. This assistance is not enough to purchase a nutritionally adequate diet. Families must add money to their food stamp allotment to meet their nutritional needs.

National School Feeding Programs

The School Breakfast Program provides a free breakfast, usually to all children in schools that offer it. The National School Lunch Program provides lunches free or at reduced prices. Also, the Special Milk Program is offered at selected schools and child care centers. It provides up to one free pint of milk daily for each child.

Many school children benefit from these government programs because selected schools charge the same prices to all students. Therefore, children from low-income families and their classmates pay less than true costs for food offered by the school. See 24-11. For example, a small carton of milk may cost 25¢ from the cafeteria. In a delicatessen, the same carton might cost 65¢.

WIC Program

The Supplemental Food Program for Women, Infants, and Children (WIC) is intended to help children get a healthy start in life. It focuses on pregnant and lactating (breast feeding) women and children up to

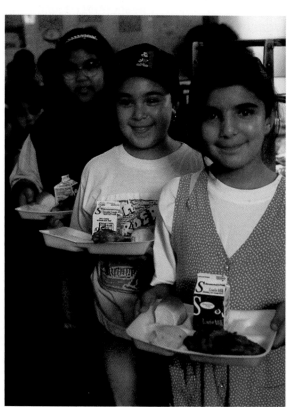

U.S. Department of Agriculture

24-11 Milk is the most common food offered through government programs to U.S. school children.

age five. The program is designed to help low-income mothers and children who are at nutritional risk. Local and state agencies provide vouchers for foods high in protein, iron, vitamin A, and vitamin C. Some of the foods provided are infant formula, cereal, juice, milk, cheese, and eggs.

● Congregate Meals Program

The Congregate Meals Program is designed to meet both the social and nutritional needs of people age 50 and older. A *congregate meal* is a group meal. Group meals are provided at local places of worship, community centers, or other facilities one or more days a week.

● Commodity Distribution Program

The Commodity Distribution Program gives surplus food to low-income people and organizations. A *commodity food* is a common, mass-produced item. Instant dry milk, flour, sugar, and cornmeal are often given out through this program. Perishable foods, such as butter, cheese, fruits, and vegetables, may also be issued. See 24-12.

Resources through this program may shrink as farm policies change and food costs continue to rise.

● Private Food Donations

Requests for donations of money and food to feed the hungry are made throughout the year. Food-raising efforts tend to cluster around fall harvest, cold weather, and major holidays. Religious groups and nonprofit organizations initiate many of the food drives, but they are not alone. Companies, local governments, and schools also make a special effort. Banks, shopping centers, and newspapers have become strong supporters of local food drives. Usually they urge customers to make donations, then they match those contributions.

Besides periodic food drives, many religious and community groups work to maintain a steady supply of food donations. They regularly supply food to hungry families in the area. They also try to keep reserves for emergency cases. These operations are called food banks, or *food pantries.*

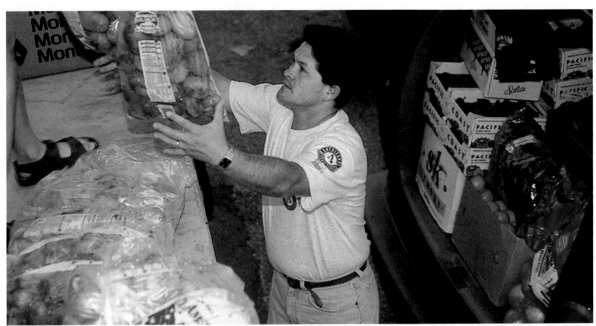

U.S. Department of Agriculture

24-12 Commodity foods include excess supplies of vegetables and fruits.

Some food banks are organized to work on a large scale. They take mass quantities of products donated by businesses, such as restaurants and food manufacturers. Then they distribute the food wherever the need is greatest.

Food items distributed by food banks are safe and wholesome but unsellable for various reasons. For instance, food cannot be sold if packages are lighter than the labeled weight or missing a component. Boxed dinners of macaroni and cheese with too little macaroni or no packet of sauce mix are two examples. They result from production plant errors that affect the packaging, not the food itself. Rather than destroy good food, companies donate it to food banks. The companies gain a tax benefit, and hungry people receive food that would otherwise go to waste.

● Working Toward Global Solutions

The United States, with 6 percent of the world's population, uses 30 to 40 percent of the world's resources. A person born in a developed nation will consume 30 times as much food as a person born in a developing nation. Unequal distribution of the world's resources means a few people live where there is plenty. However, most people live where there is very little. Consequently, where people are born determines what is available to them.

Solutions to problems as complex as global hunger are never easy. All the factors causing hunger must be understood before they can be addressed.

● Recognize the Hunger Myths

Hunger myths may be a big reason for the unsolved hunger problem. A *hunger myth* is a popular misconception about the cause of hunger. Recognizing that myths contain errors in thinking helps people focus on the real problems. Only then can workable solutions be found. Which of the following myths sound familiar to you?

● **Food Scarcity**
Myth: People go hungry because there is not enough food.
Fact: Currently there is enough grain available to provide every person with adequate calories every day. Often, however, where hunger exists, a few people in power have tight control over how food is produced and used. The food does not reach all the people who need it, 24-13.

● **Overpopulation**
Myth: Hunger exists where there are too many people to feed.
Fact: Population density by itself is not the cause of hunger. For example, Bolivia is a country in South America with many cultivated acres per person. Bolivia also has proportionately many more hungry people than Japan or the Netherlands does. Yet these countries have far less cultivated land per person than Bolivia.

High birthrates tend to occur in the same countries that have high infant death rates. High birthrates are related to low income and education levels.

● **Technology**
Myth: The solution to hunger is using improved technology to produce more food.
Fact: The food supply has more than doubled in the past 40 years, far outpacing the population growth. In spite of this, the number of hungry people has risen in some areas. Technology generally helps landowners who have political influence and access to bank credit. They, not the hungry, benefit from using the tools of high technology.

While wealthy farmers profit, poor farmers are sometimes replaced by more efficient equipment. See 24-14. Sometimes the poor are forced to sell their land to the wealthy. Poor farmers do not have the economic resources to take advantage of new

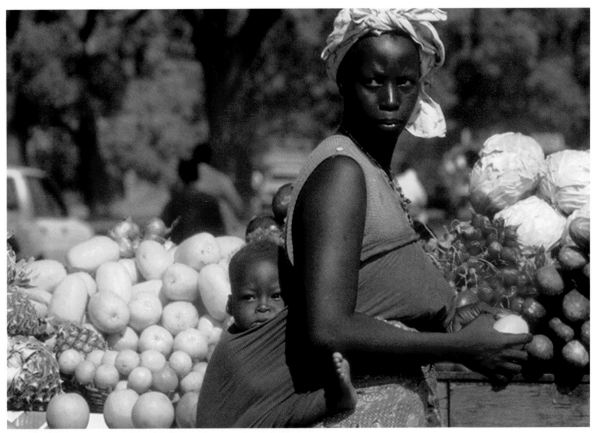

24-13 Food may be plentiful in markets near crop fields, but scarce in the rest of a country.

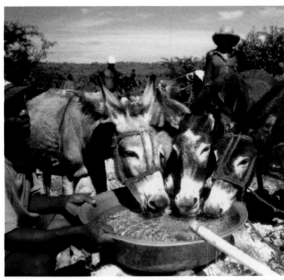

United Methodist Committee on Relief

24-14 One tractor replaces dozens of mules and the farmers who guide them.

technologies. Their quality of life continues on a downhill slide.

● **Location**

Myth: Feed the hungry people in poor countries and global hunger will be eliminated.

Fact: Hunger exists in wealthy as well as poor countries. Sometimes an effort used in an undeveloped country also works in a developed one. Countries working together can pool their knowledge in the fight to end hunger.

● **Foreign Aid**

Myth: Foreign aid is the most effective way to help end hunger.

Fact: Most food from foreign aid programs is not given, but sold, to the developing nations. Their governments often sell food to those who can afford to pay. If food is given away, it often goes to the military or those in power. As a result, purchased food may never reach the countryside where hunger is likely to exist.

● Goodwill

Myth: Everyone wants hunger to end.

Fact: Many people financially benefit from the hunger problem. People who are hungry are willing to work for very low wages. Wages may be as low as a dollar per day to produce export crops, such as coffee and bananas. See 24-15.

Corporations and governments stand to gain financially by paying low wages. In some countries, governments pay poor farmers a small fraction of the real market value of the crop. Often the wages are so low that farmers cannot afford to buy the crops they grow. Sometimes, too, food prices in the cities are set to benefit the government.

● Ignorance

Myth: Hungry people are too ignorant to change.

Fact: What appears to be ignorance is really passive behavior caused by hopelessness. The poor are very aware of the forces that keep them poor. Hope is renewed, however, when people start working together to initiate change.

If people are hungry because of an unjust system, then part of the solution is to change the system. Carefully examining causes of hunger can pinpoint the real factors at work.

● Focus on Hunger Solutions

In 1974, the countries working through the United Nations set an important goal. The goal was to make sure no child went to bed hungry by 1985. That goal was not reached in spite of massive relief efforts and dramatic agricultural advances.

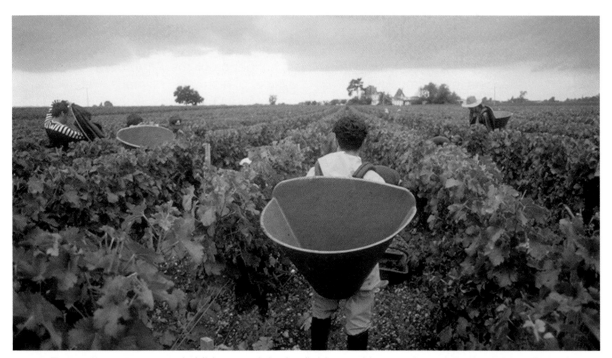

24-15 Even when parents and children work in the fields, total income is usually too low to lift the family from poverty.

In 1996, the nations of the world again set a goal to reduce world hunger. The goal is to reduce the number of undernourished people in the world at least 50 percent by the year 2015. Will the worldwide community of nations meet the goal this time?

Many factors are involved in combating world hunger, making simple solutions impossible. Giving food to needy people is one solution, but only a short-term answer. A food donation to a country does not ensure the country's future ability to buy or grow food for itself. It does not solve the hunger-causing problems. Consequently, it does not address the larger issues that remain after the relief effort ends. The hunger problem must be attacked on several fronts if hunger is to be eliminated.

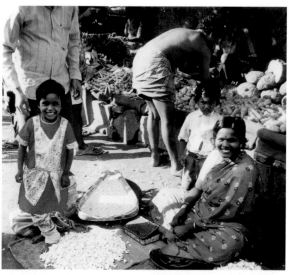

24-16 This family in India makes a comfortable living selling homegrown garlic, squash, carrots, and potatoes.

Economic Progress

Ending hunger requires finding ways to reduce poverty. One answer rests in a country's ability to use food policies to make economic progress. A *food policy* is a rule or regulation that affects food production, prices, and trade.

When governments support agricultural development, more food is produced. Countries that urge farmers to sell crops in the marketplace have growing markets. Farmers benefit, too, with increased wages. See 24-16. As their incomes rise, they become more able to buy foods they cannot grow at home.

Often poor countries must borrow money to start building an agricultural base. This means that developed countries must be willing to lend money. Developing countries may need to rely on support from financially stronger countries for many years. Cooperation among nations requires trust and goodwill.

Making national leaders aware of the hidden economic drawbacks of hunger is a high priority of the United Nations. Currently some leaders make little effort to end hunger. They fail to grasp that hunger is blocking their country's economic growth. Leaders are more willing to take steps to end hunger when they see how this will boost their country's economy.

Effective Infrastructure

The quality of a country's infrastructure directly affects how well that nation can solve its hunger problems. An *infrastructure* is a system of highways, railroads, waterways, and other public works. When this system is sound, seeds, fertilizer, and other supplies are easily moved to where they are needed. Food can be stored under safe and sanitary conditions. See 24-17.

Research and Technology Advances

Scientists have worked for decades to find ways to reduce the hunger problem. They made dramatic advances in seed quality, crop yields, and irrigation practices in the 1970s and 1980s. That worldwide effort, known as the *green revolution*, turned many brown fields green and productive.

The green revolution greatly increased grain yields worldwide. According to the National Research Council, improved wheat and rice seeds alone added 50 million tons of

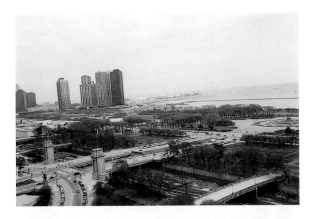

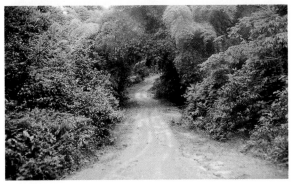

24-17 A nation's ability to move goods across roads, railways, and waterways affects the quality of life of its citizens.

grain annually. Other improved crops include maize (corn), beans, cassava (a starchy root vegetable), potatoes, and sorghum (a grain). Boosting crop yields is a goal that never ends.

Scientists are also searching for new varieties of food to expand food options. About 80,000 species of plants are considered edible, but the vast majority go unused. Finding ways to use other plants for food may provide some answers to the hunger problem. Scientists are especially interested in food sources that grow in less-than-ideal conditions, such as drought or unfertilized soil.

Besides these areas of research, scientists are exploring how to increase food yields by watering plants more efficiently. They are improving the protein content of plants to make existing foods more nourishing. They are also developing crops that are

more resistant to disease, insects, and the destructive effects of drought.

Making the land more productive presents yet more challenges. Any land can become desert when overplowed or overgrazed. Mountain regions, when cultivated, are prone to soil erosion. Cultivating grassland can destroy the natural resources needed for different species of animals. Clearing forests leaves soil too shallow and acidic for long-term crop use.

When good farmland is not available, other alternatives are explored. Some alternatives present creative ways to raise food, 24-18, but others are destructive. Removing forests, for example, will change the water flow and the ecology of the environment. By solving one problem today, will a new one appear tomorrow? Is it possible to foresee all the consequences of technology?

Technology must proceed carefully. The continued use of chemical pesticides and herbicides can contaminate the air, land, and water. Plants and animals that grow in the environment may be affected. People who rely on these plants and animals as food sources may also be affected. All antibiotics and hormones used to promote animal health and growth must be administered with care. Meat from these animals needs to be safe for people to eat.

Success in stamping out hunger calls for ***environmental sustainability***. This is the wise use of natural resources to preserve them for later use, 24-19. Fertile soil and pure water must last for future generations to use in producing food.

● Slower Population Growth

The rapidly expanding population puts great pressure on the world's limited food supplies. Population growth will cause 90 percent of the rate of increase in global food demand through the year 2010.

For decades, world leaders believed the earth could provide enough food to feed everyone. However, that assumption is being

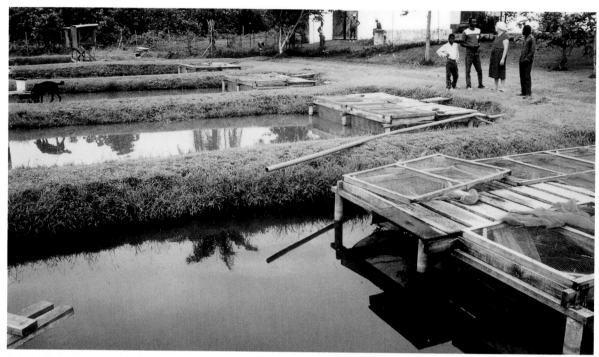

24-18 Fish farming makes excellent use of land and provides high-quality protein.

questioned. The United Nations now warns that global food availability cannot be taken for granted forever.

There are two main reasons for this reversal of thought. First, finding new land for growing crops is becoming harder. Second, crop yields are no longer keeping pace with the population growth. In other words, although the food supply increases, sometimes dramatically, the world population grows even faster.

Improving people's health status is one way to slow population growth. When infants live to adulthood, parents tend to limit the number of births. In countries where almost half the children die before age five, most families make no effort to limit births. Having many children is a way for the family to replace the children who will eventually die.

Improving the education in developing countries is also a key to slowing population growth. Women need to get more information on reproductive health. Only through education will they learn the benefits of spacing the births of their children. This will help them resist the social pressure to have a large family. Women need to learn how to meet the special nutritional needs pregnancy puts on their bodies, too.

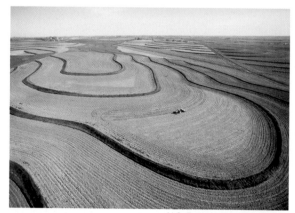

U.S. Department of Agriculture

24-19 One method of environmental sustainability is contour plowing. Crops are planted around the curves of the land instead of in straight rows. This prevents heavy rains from washing soil away.

Education

Education on many fronts is sorely needed to end global hunger. Teaching children and adults to read must be a main goal. With reading skills, people can learn to apply nutrition and sanitation principles. They will also learn how to recognize poor health and take steps to stay healthy.

Through education, adults learn job skills to earn a decent living, 24-20. They learn methods for successfully growing home gardens to raise most or part of the family's food. Farmers learn how to maintain the quality of the soil and boost crop yields.

Informed people can become a strong voice for change. Education empowers people to try to improve the conditions that negatively affect their families and communities. Raising the economic level of poor families through education is a major step toward ending hunger.

International Organizations and Programs

Many private and government agencies work to end global hunger. Some specialize in short-term crisis relief. Others work on long-term solutions, such as improving farming methods. Many provide materials for students to use in their studies. The roles of some key organizations are described here.

Food and Agricultural Organization (FAO). Increasing crop yields in developing nations is the focus of this organization. It is also concerned with the fair distribution of food to rural people. FAO works under the United Nations.

United Nations International Children's Emergency Fund (UNICEF). This group focuses on the needs of children. It sponsors the distribution of protein-rich foods to infants and children. UNICEF helps

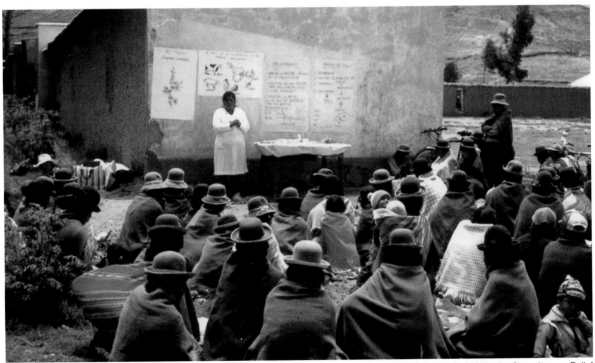

United Methodist Committee on Relief

24-20 Farmers in Bolivia learn about fish farming through this training program, sponsored by a religious organization.

in areas of the world where food and clean water are scarce and health services are inadequate. October is international UNICEF month. Special activities are held to help raise awareness and funds for the world's neediest children.

World Food Day (WFD). The U.S. National Committee for World Food Day sets aside October 16 as the annual day of caring. Information is shared about a wide range of issues related to world hunger. Food safety and land and water use are among the topics addressed.

World Health Organization (WHO). This United Nations organization is mainly concerned with health issues. They work to fight disease and promote and protect wellness of people all over the world. WHO also works with other agencies to improve the nutrient intakes of infants and mothers.

Many local groups also conduct hunger-relief programs abroad, 24-21. The American Red Cross, the Peace Corps, and Church World Service are among the organizations that help. Most invite the public to join their efforts. The number of organizations grows as people recognize that everyone has a role to play in ending world hunger.

● What Can One Person Do?

"Never doubt that a small group of people can change the world; indeed, it is the only thing that ever has." These are the words of Margaret Mead, a famous anthropologist. She believed that thoughtful, interested citizens can bring about change.

Becoming involved is the first step to creating change. Joining forces with others helps swell the ranks of organizations devoted to ending hunger. With more members, these organizations attract more notice from

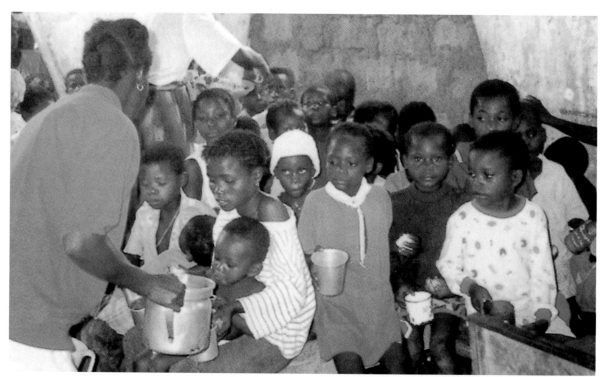

United Methodist Committee on Relief

24-21 Donations from church members make it possible for these children in war-stricken areas of Africa to receive food.

Hunger-Relief Organizations

America's Second Harvest
35 E. Wacker Drive, #2000
Chicago, IL 60601
800-771-2303
www.secondharvest.org

Bread for the World
50 F Street, NW, Suite 500
Washington, DC 20001
800-82-BREAD
www.bread.org

Freedom from Hunger
1644 DaVinci Court
Davis, CA 95616
800-708-2555
www.freedomfromhunger.org

Heifer Project International
P.O. Box 8058
Little Rock, AR 72203
800-422-0474
www.heifer.org

Mercy Corps
Dept. W
PO Box 2669
Portland, OR 97208-2669
800-292-3355
www.mercycorps.org

Oxfam America
26 West Street
Boston, MA 02111-1206
800-776-9326
www.oxfamamerica.org

Seeds of Hope Publishers
602 James
Waco, TX 76706
254-755-7745
www.seedspublishers.org

UNICEF House
3 United Nations Plaza
New York, NY 10017-4414
212-326-7000
www.unicef.org

U.S. National Committee for World Food Day
2175 K Street NW
Washington, DC 20437
202-653-2404
www.worldfooddayusa.org

Worldwatch Institute
1776 Massachusetts Ave., NW
Washington, D.C. 20036-1904
202-452-1999
www.worldwatch.org

24-22 These groups provide accurate information on hunger issues. Some suggest ways for concerned individuals to help.

decision makers. This, ultimately, helps the organizations' causes.

A person who speaks out on behalf of an issue or a problem is an *advocate*. Being an advocate for the poor and hungry means being willing to voice an opinion and take action. Advocates become involved by addressing problems with workable solutions. Here are some specific actions you might take to be an advocate for ending hunger.

- Volunteer your time at a local food pantry. You may be needed to help receive incoming food. You might assemble or distribute food packages. Perhaps you will handle housekeeping or record keeping duties.

- Become involved in fund-raising projects that support food programs for the hungry.

- Donate money or needed items to victims of natural disasters and other emergencies.

- Phone or write for information to learn more about the groups that fight hunger. See 24-22.

- Become familiar with problems of hunger and poverty in your community. Support programs that look at the whole issue and address underlying causes.

- Write to decision makers about hunger-related policies. The policies may involve food distribution, food production, nutrition education, or other subjects. Positive letters praising good decisions are as important as letters seeking change.

- Educate others about hunger in the world and in your community. Become an advocate for undernourished and malnourished people. Support policies that offer hungry people a chance to improve their diets and health.

- Find creative ways to help families who lack food. Providing garden space for growing vegetables is one way, 24-23. Donating excess food from home or volunteering to prepare meals for a needy family are other possibilities.

Finally, examine your lifestyle in relation to the use of the world's resources. How much food someone eats or the type of car he or she drives is not the critical issue. The lifestyle of excess and abundance enjoyed by many people in developed countries is the issue. Question whether possessing so many material goods prevents others from achieving a decent standard of living.

According to a common expression, "If you are not part of the solution, you are part of the problem." Each person can find a way to help end hunger. Think about what you can do, then do it. Solving global hunger requires the efforts of every healthy person.

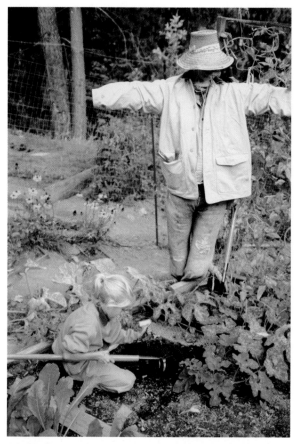

24-23 Gardening not only provides food, it can also give people hope for a brighter future.

Summary

Hunger is both a global and local problem. It occurs throughout the United States. It affects millions of people all over the world. The effects of hunger and malnutrition are most serious for children, pregnant women, and the elderly. A population with below-average weight and/or height often is a sign of widespread hunger.

Both rich and poor countries should care about hunger. Political and economic decisions in one country can affect all countries. On a humanitarian level, many people believe hunger should be ended because human beings deserve enough to eat. Compassionate people want to do more than simply provide food.

Some government leaders do little to end hunger in their countries. Poverty, disasters, or environmental factors can make it hard for people to get food. Culture, lack of education, and overpopulation can also add to hunger problems.

Federal food and nutrition programs help hungry people in the United States. They provide food and other resources to those in need. Private donations of food, money, and time also help reduce hunger problems locally.

Taking positive steps to end global hunger requires knowing the real causes. Scientific progress can expand food variety and improve ways to grow and harvest food. Slower population growth allows the existing food supply to reach more hungry people. Through education, people learn how to take better care of their health and resources. Many organizations are involved in the fight against global hunger. Some focus on short-term crisis relief. Others attack the long-term problems.

Individuals can help fight hunger, too. They can volunteer time to hunger-relief organizations. They can donate resources and help raise funds. Concerned people can also study the hunger facts, teach others, and support effective policies.

Check Your Knowledge

1. What is an indicator of undernutrition?
2. What is an indicator of malnutrition?
3. List the three degrees of malnutrition, from least to most severe.
4. Identify five nutrients cited by the United Nations as deficient in the diets of developing countries.
5. Name five indicators that describe the living conditions within a country.
6. What is the main cause of global hunger and starvation?
7. Besides poverty, identify five root causes of hunger.
8. List five programs run by the Department of Agriculture that address the food and nutrition needs of people in the United States.
9. True or false. High rates of infant births occur in the same countries that have high rates of infant deaths.
10. Explain why improved technology is not an answer to ending the hunger of poor farmers.
11. Explain the facts behind this myth: everyone wants hunger to end.
12. Why is giving food to needy people only a short-term solution to hunger?
13. How can an effective infrastructure reduce hunger?
14. True or false. Experts agree that the world will be capable of producing enough food in the future to feed everyone.
15. Name four ways education can help eliminate hunger.
16. What international organization focuses exclusively on helping hungry children?

17. List five ways an individual can help fight hunger.

Put Learning into Action

1. It is estimated that over six million people are added to the world population each month. Consider the number *six million* in terms of seconds of time. How much time does this represent?

2. Locate a soup kitchen or food pantry that serves your community. Volunteer after school or on weekends to assist with the program. Report your experience to the class.

3. Organize a food drive in your community to coincide with a holiday period. Invite the entire school to participate.

4. Prepare an argument, pro or con, to debate this statement: "Food assistance promotes dependence."

5. Interpret this statement made by Herbert Hoover: "Hunger is more destructive than armies, not only in human life, but in morale."

Explore Further

1. Analyze a typical diet of people from a developing nation. Use library references to learn about dietary patterns. In a written report, evaluate the nutrient content of the diet in relation to the RDAs.

2. Contact a hunger relief organization to learn about its accomplishments in fighting hunger. Find out how and where it operates. What are its proudest achievements and its future plans? How does it raise funds to operate? Make a brief report of your findings to the class.

3. Use the Internet to research the general living conditions of a country that may have serious hunger problems. Use the name of the country as your search word. Investigate infant mortality rate, life expectancy at birth, percent of the population with safe water and adequate sanitation, and per capita GDP. Include information about four additional factors that present a clearer picture of the country's hunger condition. Share your findings with the class.

Chapter 25

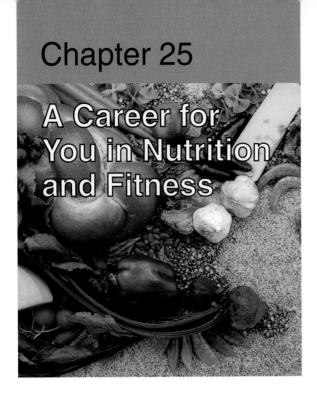

A Career for You in Nutrition and Fitness

Learn the Language

bachelor's degree
dietitian
dietetics
registered dietitian
  (RD)
master's degree
doctoral degree
dietetic technician
associate degree
preventive health
  care
certification
license
aptitude

ability
goal
employability skill
problem solving
entry-level job
portfolio
networking
resume
reference
job interview
mentor
ethics
entrepreneur

Objectives

After studying this chapter, you will be able to
- list common job titles, responsibilities, and qualifications for people in the nutrition and fitness career areas.
- cite reasons for certification and license requirements for many jobs in the nutrition and fitness field.
- explain how interests, aptitudes, values, and goals can affect career decisions.
- describe steps to take during the teen years to help prepare for a career.
- use effective techniques to find, keep, and leave a job.
- explore opportunities for entrepreneurs.

The future looks bright for nutrition and fitness professionals. Job opportunities are growing faster for these careers than for most other professions. A number of reasons account for this positive forecast.

Interest in the ways food and fitness can add to overall good health continues to grow. Senior citizens, who tend to be quite open to food and fitness information, are increasing in number. Employer-sponsored fitness programs are becoming more common. Health care providers are focusing efforts on preventive health care. These factors bring the services of nutrition and fitness experts to people who might not seek them otherwise. These factors also support career growth in both new and traditional job areas.

Nutrition and Fitness Professionals

Interest in nutrition and fitness can lead to more than a healthy life. It can become your career. Do you see yourself in any of these roles?
- teaching health and fitness at a community center
- working with a health care team to set nutrition guidelines for hospital patients

- helping a restaurant chain improve the nutrient quality of its meals
- working as a fitness instructor at a health club or sports center
- developing a snack food for active teens
- writing nutrition updates for newspaper and TV reports

Nutrition and fitness experts work in hospitals, schools, and exercise centers. They also work in restaurants, private offices, and many other settings. Most work directly with people. Others research, write, or develop new programs or products. See 25-1.

This broad area offers a range of career options that appeal to many interests. Nutrition and exercise sciences are very specialized areas. Therefore, many jobs require at least a four-year college degree, or **bachelor's degree**. Nutrition and fitness professionals include dietitians, dietetic technicians, and health and fitness specialists.

Dietitians

Many of the people working in the nutrition and fitness field are dietitians. A **dietitian**

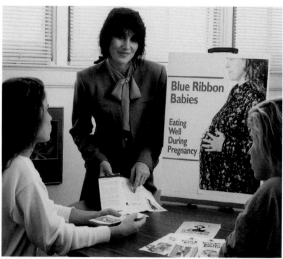

American Dietetic Association

25-1 Teaching students about life cycle nutrition is just one of many career roles a nutrition and fitness professional might fill.

is a person trained to apply nutrition principles to diet planning. This professional works with individuals and groups. He or she promotes good health through sound eating habits. The program of study that prepares a person to become a dietitian is called **dietetics**.

Dietitians can specialize in a number of areas. The widest range of options is open to dietitians who become registered. (Dietitians become registered through certification. You will read about this later in this chapter.) A **registered dietitian (RD)** is qualified to analyze a person's diet and perform diet treatment. Dietitians who are not registered are not qualified to plan diets for people. They often focus on teaching, writing, and research.

Business Dietitians

Dietitians in the business sector often work for food and drug companies and supermarket chains. They may also work for health and fitness centers, magazines, and newspapers. Their job duties may focus on product development or nutrition labeling. They may be involved with marketing, advertising, public relations, and communications. More jobs are opening up for registered dietitians in business settings.

Clinical Dietitians

A clinical dietitian is a member of a health care team. He or she works with doctors, nurses, pharmacists, and other medical professionals. Together, team members assess a patient's recovery goals and diet plans. Often, the clinical dietitian specializes in specific areas of health care. For instance, he or she may work mainly with diabetic and obese patients. Clinical dietitians work in hospitals, doctors' offices, clinics, and research labs. They are also employed in *hospices*. These are facilities to care for patients whose illnesses cannot be cured.

A clinical dietitian studies each patient's diet and food habits. He or she also tries to understand the family's influence on the patient's diet. Other job duties include teaching classes and helping patients change eating behaviors. Clinical dietitians must be registered dietitians.

Community Dietitians

Community dietitians work with people one-on-one and in groups. Their goal is to help people improve their quality of life. These professionals work in health agencies, child care centers, health and fitness clubs, and private homes. They often work with government programs that feed families, older adults, pregnant women, and children.

Community dietitians plan events to help people learn about the value of a healthful diet. They also speak to groups about current nutrition issues. People working in this field must be registered dietitians.

Consultant Dietitians

Consultant dietitians work under contract with food providers. These might include health care facilities, athletic centers, and nursing homes. Dietitians working in this role give dietetic advice to foodservice managers, 25-2.

Some consultant dietitians work in private practice. They perform diet assessments for clients. They may counsel patients referred by doctors. They may advise clients about topics such as how to lose weight or reduce cholesterol intake. They might also address other diet-related concerns, such as eating disorders and food allergies.

People who want to pursue careers in this area must be registered dietitians. They must have several years of experience, too.

Educator Dietitians

Educator dietitians work in colleges and universities. They may also work in community or technical schools. They teach the science of nutrition and fitness. Future doctors, nurses, and dietitians are among their students.

An advanced degree is required for this career area. Master's and doctoral degrees are advanced degrees. A *master's degree*

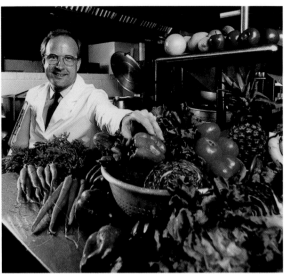

American Dietetic Association

25-2 In foodservice operations, consultant dietitians plan wholesome menus and sometimes help prepare the food.

involves about two years of school beyond a bachelor's degree. A *doctoral degree* requires about three to five more years of school beyond a master's degree.

Management Dietitians

Management dietitians supervise people who plan, prepare, and serve meals in schools and hospitals. They may also perform this role in restaurants, company dining rooms, and prisons. See 25-3. Their duties may include staff training, budgeting, and food purchasing. A person must be a registered dietitian to work as a management dietitian. He or she may need an advanced degree.

Research Dietitians

Research dietitians work in government and medical labs. They may also work for food and drug companies or universities. They do experiments or conduct studies to find answers to nutrition questions. They may study alternative foods or look into the ways foods and drugs interact. A career in this area almost always requires an advanced degree.

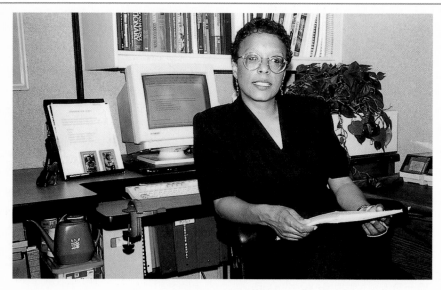

Meet a Dietitian

Norma Killough, RD, is a dietitian with the Michigan Department of Corrections. She and 11 other dietitians manage menu planning for 40,000 persons in the state's correctional system.

"Some individuals are here for a short while, but others are here for their entire lives," says Norma. "While people are under our control, we're responsible for their health."

According to Norma, there is another important reason for maintaining inmates' health. It costs less in the long run to house healthy people than those with medical needs caused by poor eating habits. Because the corrections system is supported by taxpayers, controlling costs is always important.

"Unfortunately the number of people entering the corrections system is growing, so our job gets bigger each year," says Norma. "This growth, however, provides opportunities for more dietitians to develop professional skills that can be used in many other areas of the food and nutrition industry."

She routinely works with administrators, attorneys, legislative staff, the general public, and the prisoners and their families. She believes that an ability to work with people from a variety of backgrounds is an important requirement for this job.

Her job requires her to stay organized, work independently, and take responsibility for decisions. She devotes considerable time to keeping up with the rapid changes in the foodservice industry. She takes pride in the fact that her staff's expertise is respected and sought by professionals from other disciplines.

Try to place yourself in Norma's shoes. Would this work interest you?

25-3 Planning and organizing is a big part of a management dietitian's work.

● Dietetic Technicians

A fairly new title in the nutrition and fitness field is *dietetic technician*. A **dietetic technician** is a member of a health care team. He or she works under the guidance of a registered dietitian. A dietetic technician may ask clients or patients about their eating habits. The technician can then help people make food choices that fit into their diet plans. The technician can also teach people about good nutrition and healthful ways to prepare foods.

A dietetic technician must take courses in an approved two-year college program. He or she will receive an *associate degree* after completing such a program.

Other Food Science Professionals

Interest is growing in the areas of nutrition, good health, and food safety. This has led to a variety of new careers in fields other than dietetics. These careers all require a strong science background and at least a bachelor's degree.

Some nutrition professionals become experts in human nutrition but do not pursue training in dietetics. They focus on understanding food components and their effects on the body. Many of these professionals conduct research, 25-4. They are looking for new ways that food affects health. Other nutrition professionals teach at the college level. Some develop healthful new products for food companies.

Some nutrition experts receive training in the health sciences. Those with bachelor's degrees may work in entry-level jobs in the health industry. However, many use their nutrition training to prepare for a career in medicine. Some wish to work in the fields of dentistry, nursing, or physical therapy.

Another career area for food science professionals blends health and food safety knowledge. Specialists with this background may work for food companies. They also work for water companies, drug manufacturers, and food packagers. These experts might help set up and enforce sanitation procedures for each stage of production.

Many health and food safety experts work for local, state, and national health departments. In these government jobs, some perform research. However, most conduct health inspections. They routinely check the sanitation of establishments that handle food, such as processing plants, restaurants, and schools.

Health and Fitness Specialists

The need for fitness professionals with nutrition knowledge is growing. People want experts who can tell them how to exercise correctly and eat healthfully to stay fit. Schools, community centers, and health clubs often hire health and fitness specialists. Many other jobs are also opening for people who are well versed in both of these areas.

This field is changing quickly. New job titles are being created to define new sets of work tasks. Many of the jobs described here require a bachelor's degree. In addition, many also require certification. (Certification is discussed later in this chapter.)

Corporate Fitness Specialists

Corporate fitness specialists work for companies. They design fitness programs to improve employees' state of wellness. They may focus on such issues as safety, stress, motivation, teamwork, and leadership. Some corporate fitness specialists work with community programs. They promote healthy lifestyles to people of all ages. They teach health and wellness in local health organizations. These experts are also called *health, exercise,* and *wellness specialists.*

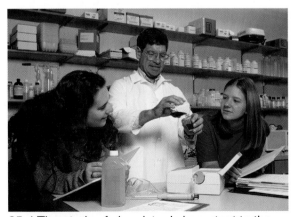

25-4 The study of chemistry is important to the training of a food researcher.

Exercise Leaders

Exercise leaders work with people in public and private settings. They show people how to do safe, effective exercises. These leaders may teach aerobics, aquatics, dance exercise, and other types of fitness classes. They design fitness programs that stress preventive health care. **Preventive health care** focuses on preserving health now to prevent poor health later. See 25-5.

Exercise Science Specialists

Exercise science specialists apply science and math principles to the structure of the body. They study human motion in work and rehabilitation tasks. This helps the specialists devise better ways to test and measure physical performance. These professionals are also known as *ergonomics specialists* or *human engineering specialists*.

These professionals may specialize in many areas. Some focus on studying the effects of exercise on the body's systems. They are called *exercise physiologists*. Others design the tools and equipment used to test performance and fitness levels. They are called *exercise test technologists*.

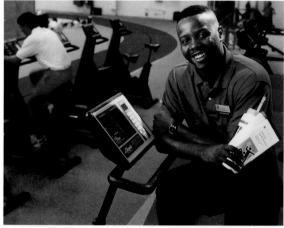

American Dietetic Association

25-5 An exercise leader may teach fitness classes and show people how to safely use exercise equipment.

Exercise Specialists

Exercise specialists work with patients in health care settings. They combine their background in fitness science with training in an allied health field. Allied fields include physical therapy and sports medicine. Exercise specialists help people with weakened conditions regain flexibility, strength, and coordination. They prescribe activities to meet each patient's needs and measure the results. They also treat sports injuries. Exercise specialists are trained to detect unhealthy eating habits and clarify nutrition misconceptions. They are also called *exercise therapists* or *physical therapists*.

Fitness Instructors

Fitness instructors often work one-on-one with people. They may serve as personal trainers or strength conditioners. They are hired by sports teams, health clubs, and individuals. Fitness instructors use counseling skills to urge their clients to adopt more healthful lifestyles. They assess clients' physical conditions. Then they suggest exercise and diet plans to enhance fitness. *Athletic trainer* and *weight training instructor* are other names for these fitness specialists.

Health and Fitness Directors

Health and fitness directors are the business managers of fitness facilities. See 25-6. They are in charge of choosing equipment, hiring and training staff, and scheduling programs. They may also handle the finances and contracts. Most of their customers are people who are hoping to take up healthier lifestyles. Sometimes these professionals are called *health club managers*.

Health Enhancement Instructors

Many schools teach physical education separately from health education. However, a growing number of schools combine the two into a program called *health enhancement*. The instructors of these programs teach

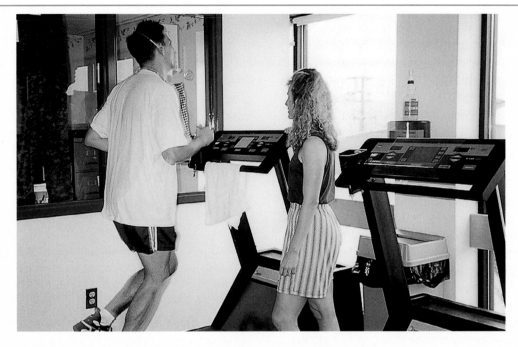

Meet a Fitness Director

Nadine Moody is a conditioning center director for a family-centered, community-based YMCA. She is in charge of the staff, equipment, and activities offered by the Y's conditioning center and weight room.

"I try to be a role model for a healthful lifestyle," says Nadine. "You have to love being energetic to be effective in this job." Besides managing the center, she conducts personal fitness training sessions and leads exercise classes for groups ranging in age from teens to seniors. Her classes focus on aerobics, muscle building, and strength renewal.

As a certified fitness trainer and aerobics instructor, Nadine is well qualified for her job. She is also CPR-certified. This means she is qualified to handle heart attacks, breathing problems, and other exercise-related emergencies.

Nadine's personality is well-suited for this work. She is friendly, upbeat, and eager to balance many responsibilities. "This job can sometimes be stressful, even for me," says Nadine. "You have to be willing to work hours that are convenient to your clients. This means weekends and hours that may not be convenient to you and your family."

Often she is invited to speak to community groups and work on joint projects. She also hires and trains new employees. In addition, she prepares materials to promote the Y's programs and manages extension sites for classes. Recently she began selling sports apparel on-site to help raise funds for equipment purchases.

Nadine enjoys working for the YMCA because she shares its values regarding fitness. The Y exists to promote healthful lifestyles for people of all ages, income levels, and ethnic backgrounds. According to Nadine, it also is a good place to pursue a career in the health and fitness field. Professionals with different specializations and experience levels are needed, and relocation is possible to many other sites.

Can you picture yourself doing Nadine's job? If so, the fitness field may be for you.

25-6 Fitness directors do not have nine-to-five jobs. They must be available whenever the business or its customers need them.

students in kindergarten through grade 12. Students begin to view good health as a lifetime goal that exercise helps them achieve. Students also learn various sports, exercises, dances, and games. They learn about good health and eating habits. The program goal is to have students value all forms of movement as ways to protect, maintain, and improve health.

Recreation Workers

Recreation workers put together a wide range of programs for groups of all ages. These programs stress fitness, fairness, and self-improvement. Recreation workers work in playgrounds, parks, and other public facilities. Sometimes they bring physical activities to groups who are less mobile. For instance, they make take programs to older adults in nursing homes. Recreation workers may be untrained volunteers as well as trained recreation aides. *Facility directors* and *recreation supervisors* might also be recreation workers.

Sports Instructors

Sports instructors teach individual or group sports in a wide range of settings. They might work at private clubs and resorts, summer camps, bowling alleys, and swimming pools. The instructors provide lessons for all skill levels from beginning to advanced. Sports instructors are also called *physical instructors*. In competitive events that require teamwork and game strategy, the instructor is called a *coach*.

Certification and License Requirements

People who work in jobs that deal with people's lives, health, or safety must often be certified and/or licensed. Doctors, dentists, and teachers are some examples. Many professionals in the nutrition and fitness field have these requirements, too. See 25-7.

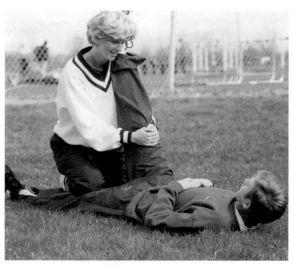

25-7 This athletic trainer must be certified to instruct athletes about how to prepare their bodies for competitive events.

Meeting certification and license requirements means a person has a clear grasp of the science involved. It also means the person has shown an ability to apply scientific principles correctly with each client. This keeps unqualified people from holding these important jobs. It also prevents the physical harm that may result from bad advice.

Certification is a special standing within a profession. This standing comes as a result of meeting certain requirements. A *license* is a work requirement set by a government agency. Often the license requirements are similar or identical to the certification requirements. The one main difference is license requirements carry the force of law. Performance standards of licensed professionals are controlled by the government.

Certification and license requirements usually address the following items:

- acceptable programs of study to complete
- minimum level of education or degree(s) required
- internship and/or on-the-job experience required

- minimum grade or score required on a national exam

Those who meet the requirements receive a certificate or license. Many professionals choose to display these documents at their workplaces. This allows clients to know they are dealing with qualified professionals.

Certificates and licenses usually have dates showing when they expire. Renewal is granted if the person has taken suggested courses and/or attended a required number of approved meetings. Requiring renewal on a regular basis makes sure professionals keep their knowledge and skills up-to-date.

All certification requirements and professional standards for careers in dietetics are set by the American Dietetic Association (ADA). For fitness careers, various groups are involved. One leading organization is the American College of Sports Medicine (ACSM). Another is the National Athletic Trainers Association (NATA).

New fitness organizations seem to appear all the time. They claim to represent certain areas of the fitness field. They may offer short workshops or home-study programs that promise to lead to jobs in nutrition and fitness. Unfortunately, graduates of these programs do not meet the minimum standards of the profession. When comparing graduates of different fitness programs, check the certification requirements set by the profession. People who meet and surpass them are well trained for health and fitness careers.

Initials after a person's name can be a sign of certification or licensing. For example, a certified health education specialist uses the initials *CHES*. A certified fitness director uses the initials *ACSM*. This is because the American College of Sports Medicine provides the certification. A certified dietitian is called a *registered dietitian*. He or she uses the initials *RD*. See 25-8. In states that require dietitians to be licensed, the initials *LD* are used.

When a license is a job requirement, the government controls the use of related titles and initials. For example, a person who uses

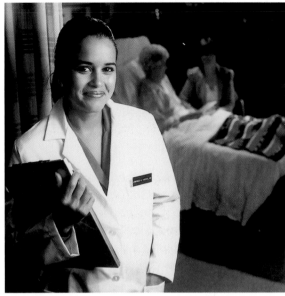

American Dietetic Association

25-8 The initials on the nameplate identify this professional as a registered dietitian. These professionals often work in hospitals, planning diets that help restore patients' health.

the initials *LD* or the title *Licensed Dietitian* must be qualified to do so. If not, fines or penalties may result.

Many states have license requirements for dietitians. Some have them for anyone using the term *nutritionist*. The licensing process for nutrition and fitness professionals in general is expanding. This is due to a growing number of complaints from consumers. Consumers are concerned about deceitful people who give harmful nutrition or exercise advice. Such *frauds* lack proper training. They are interested only in selling a product or service.

Professional associations, too, are expanding their certification efforts. They are trying to cover more job categories. Jobs that direct, counsel, or treat people are their main focus. Their goal is to keep unqualified people from spreading wrong information.

A quick, easy route is not enough to prepare you for a nutrition and fitness career. Recognized programs take years of study and preparation. They are developed with certification and license requirements in mind. They provide the training and experiences needed to meet these requirements on the first try. Your school counselor can tell you which schools offer reputable programs.

● Making a Positive Career Choice

Can you picture yourself working in the nutrition and fitness field? What type of jobs interest you most? One way to narrow the long list of career possibilities is to examine your interests, aptitudes, values, and goals, 25-9. Then you can focus on the career options that best suit you.

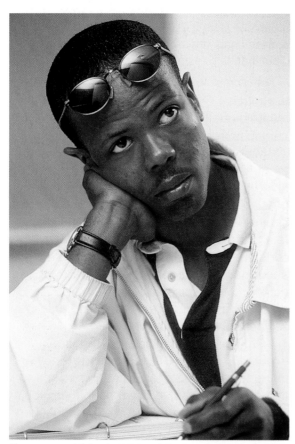

Photo courtesy of University Relations, MSU, Bruce A. Fox, photographer

25-9 Carefully thinking about your interests, aptitudes, values, and goals can help you choose a career that is right for you.

● Knowing Your Interests

Everyone has a unique set of interests, and no one knows yours better than you. One person's interests are not better than another's. Interests simply help define an individual. Knowing your interests is important in choosing a career because a job that includes your interests will be fun and exciting.

Career interests can be classified into three broad categories: people, information, and material items. Which do you most enjoy? Consider these categories and the types of jobs that most relate to each.

● Interest in People

Do you prefer to be with a group or on your own? Do you like projects that involve teamwork or those you accomplish yourself? Do you prefer to socialize or work alone on a hobby?

If you enjoy being around others, you are probably suited for a career that focuses on interacting with people. Counseling hospital patients and working with youth groups at a neighborhood center are examples of careers whose main interest is people. Those who focus on helping others truly care about the lives of people.

● Interest in Information

Do you like to keep track of facts and details? Do you regularly check information sources, such as magazines, newspapers, TV, or the Internet? Do you enjoy making discoveries?

If you like to gather facts and share what you know, you are probably suited for a career that focuses on information. Researching nutrition mysteries, reporting discoveries, and teaching are some of the careers that appeal to people whose primary interest is information.

● Interest in Material Items

Do you like to work with your hands? Do you enjoy assembling objects or taking items apart to find out how they operate? Do you like to spend time with hobbies or crafts?

If you enjoy developing items, whether beautiful or functional, a career that focuses on tools and material items could be ideal for you. Nutrition and fitness jobs that relate to this interest include developing new sports equipment, exercise programs, or healthful restaurant dishes.

● **Overlapping Interests**

Some jobs address two or more interest areas with almost equal emphasis. One example is writing, which focuses on information and material items. Another example is teaching, which focuses on people and gathering up-to-date information, 25-10. It is possible to find a career that addresses more than one area.

● Knowing Your Aptitudes and Abilities

When choosing a career, it is very important to consider your *aptitudes* and *abilities*. An **aptitude** is a natural talent. Most people have several aptitudes. These are the areas in which you excel and generally find the greatest satisfaction. They also tend to be the areas in which you develop your greatest skills. For example, people with an aptitude

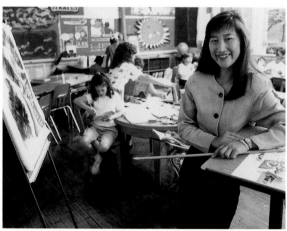

American Dietetic Association

25-10 Helping students make healthful food choices requires a love of teaching and an interest in nutrition facts.

for singing do it well even without practice. Because they enjoy singing, they also enjoy practicing. With more practice, their singing improves.

A person without an aptitude for singing may still be able to develop singing ability. An **ability** is a skill learned through practice. A person who practices frequently may be able to achieve some success in singing. However, that person is unlikely to achieve as much success as someone with natural singing aptitude.

The same is true in the world of employment. People who perform a job using a natural talent often do it better and quicker than others. For example, a person with little talent for math can develop a math ability through practice. However, if that person takes a job requiring math ability, the job is likely to be a struggle. A person with a natural math aptitude, on the other hand, will find the job easy and fun.

When you match yourself against your peers, in which areas do you excel? What can you do better than most of your friends? The activities you most enjoy are probably those you do best. Aptitude tests given by your school counselors can help you recognize your natural talents. This information can help you identify possible career paths that match your interests.

● Knowing Your Values

Your family, friends, and life experiences shape your *values,* which are beliefs or attitudes that are important to you. What you value will determine the way you live your life. For example, people who value peacefulness make their homes in the country or a quiet suburb. However, people who value nonstop excitement enjoy living in a big city.

Your values also affect your career choice. People who value independence, for example, want control over their work hours. They dislike nine-to-five jobs. People who value education want a job that pays for job-related degrees they earn while employed.

A person who values family life avoids jobs that requires constant travel. Carefully considering your values will point you to the job that best suits you. See 25-11.

Usually you can narrow the wide list of career options to a select few by considering your interests and aptitudes. Then your values help you determine which of those selections will make you happiest.

Identifying Your Career Goals

Most people can improve their lives by setting goals. *Goals* are the aims you strive to reach. Without goals, you will not know what direction to take when faced with choices. When you have goals, they become life plans that can help you identify the stepping-stones it takes to realize your dreams.

Short-term career goals are targets related to work you want to achieve within the next few months. Each short-term goal is a springboard to a long-term goal. Long-term career goals are the specific job destinations you plan to reach in a year or more. Many students have trouble focusing on their studies because they do not realize passing a class is a short-term career goal. It is one step in the path to a long-term career goal, such as getting a bachelor's degree in food-service management. Some long-term career goals, such as owning your own restaurant, take many years to reach. Working toward short-term goals now will help you reach long-term goals in the future.

Characteristics of Goals

Effective goals have certain characteristics. One such characteristic is a deadline. A short-term career goal may have a deadline of a few months. A long-term career goal, on the other hand, may have a deadline of a few years into the future. If you do not set deadlines, you may never reach your goals.

Effective goals are achievable. Trust yourself to know what is and is not reachable. Talk to your parents and listen to your friends. If the goal seems achievable to you, then go for it. You may be able to accomplish what others thought was impossible. See 25-12.

Effective goals are personal. Make the goal your goal, not someone else's. You must feel your dreams are right for you.

Effective goals are stated in a positive way. For instance, suppose you have a problem with tardiness. A negatively stated goal might be "I will not be late for class once this week." Stating this goal in a positive way, you might say "I will be on time every day this week." This will give you a more upbeat approach to making an improvement in your life.

Effective goals are specific. Saying "I will do better this semester" is too general. Saying "I will get at least a B in every class this semester" is more defined. A specific goal gives you more direction about what you need to do to reach your target.

Career Preparation

A professional career in the nutrition and fitness field will probably require a college degree. However, career preparation should not be postponed until then. Thinking about

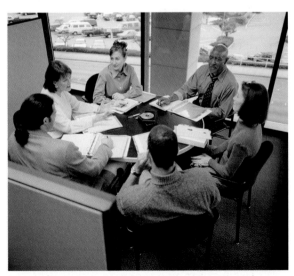

25-11 An informal office and dress code appeal to those who value casual clothing.

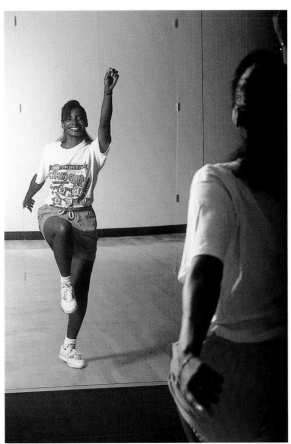

Photo courtesy of University Relations, MSU, Bruce A. Fox, photographer

25-12 Practicing a routine plays a key role in making a goal to perform well achievable.

your career goals now can prepare you for a smoother transition into the world of work.

There are several ways to begin preparing now for your future career. Take required classes and participate in career-related school activities. Develop the skills employers seek. Gain work experience by accepting a volunteer or paid position. Talk with people who can help you achieve your career goal. Assemble a portfolio to display your abilities to potential employers.

● Take Appropriate Courses

Classes in family and consumer sciences, life management, and health offer an introduction to nutrition and fitness concepts. Foods and nutrition courses in high school or vocational-technical schools may convince

an employer of a person's qualifications for a part-time job. These courses can help the college-bound student understand more difficult nutrition concepts later.

Nutrition and fitness college programs are heavily weighted in science. Many physical and biological sciences are required, such as chemistry, biology, and physiology. Several behavioral and social sciences are also required, such as psychology, sociology, and human behavior. Business, management, and communications are other courses that students of nutrition and fitness programs can expect to take. Taking introductory classes in these areas prepares students for future college courses.

While in high school, students heading for nutrition and fitness careers should also take computer classes. Today, practically every job involves computer use in some way. Computer skills acquired in high school will be an important part of professional skills, 25-13.

● Join Related Clubs and School Organizations

Leadership and team-building skills are practiced through participation in school organizations. This teamwork skill is viewed by employers as valuable preparation for job success. As a member of a team, you learn how to work with others to achieve group goals. Find out what school organizations are offered and take advantage of those that best suit your career plan.

Students interested in the management aspect of nutrition and fitness can join Future Business Leaders of America (FBLA). FBLA fosters an understanding of how the business system operates. It also promotes leadership, self-confidence, and other personal qualities important in a business career.

Another example of a school organization that offers leadership-building opportunities is Family, Career and Community Leaders of America (FCCLA). Students enrolled in family

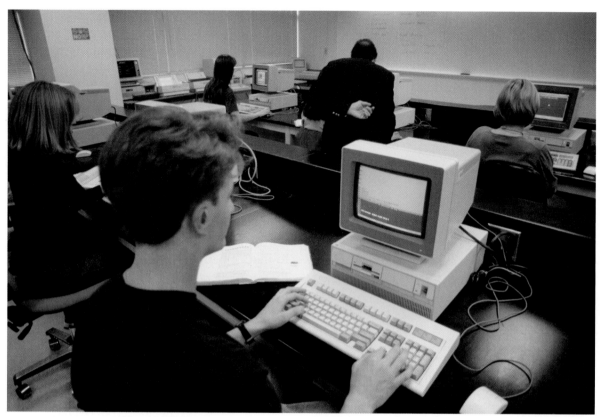

25-13 Learning computer skills prepares students for the workplace.

and consumer sciences, home economics, or life management classes can join FCCLA.

Also consider the sports and athletic options. Students destined for the fitness field will benefit from participation in various physical activities. They will also learn motivational techniques they can use later when helping others stay fit.

● Try Volunteering

Community service programs frequently depend on volunteer help. When you volunteer, you improve your community and learn about the world of work.

Food banks and community meal programs often need dependable volunteers to make their services possible. Volunteers to help serve meals and visit patients are also appreciated in hospitals and nursing homes. These and similar work experiences are ideal for anyone considering a career as a dietitian or a dietetic technician.

Opportunities to volunteer in the fitness field are numerous. Local park districts and neighborhood centers offer many options. Volunteers help recreation leaders and sports instructors with after-school, weekend, and summer programs. Recreation assistants also work in summer camps, swimming pools, and bowling alleys. Local tennis, golf, ski, and athletic clubs may offer other possibilities.

Besides preparing you for your future career, volunteering boosts your personal development. By helping others, you increase your self-esteem and self-worth. You gain valuable information about personal skills and abilities. These skills become useful in later jobs when you meet more complex problems and situations. See 25-14.

You can learn about volunteer opportunities by talking with your school counselor. Also check community bulletin boards. To find out about volunteering for a specific position, express your interest to its program

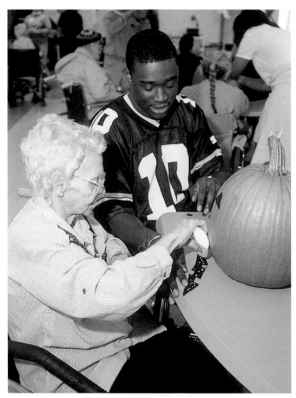

Photo courtesy of University Relations, MSU, Bruce A. Fox, photographer

25-14 Volunteering helps young people build communication skills and learn about what types of work they find most satisfying.

director. If that person cannot help you obtain the position you seek, he or she may know another employer who can. Later, when you are looking for a full-time job, these professionals may be invaluable sources to contact again.

● Acquire Employability Skills

School and volunteer experiences can help you develop employability skills. An *employability skill* is a competency that individuals need for successfully obtaining and keeping a job. Employers have identified several skills that are critical to job success in every career path.

You develop employability skills through many of your everyday activities at home and school. In your home, you learn how to work with others to meet family goals. In clubs and organizations, you make plans to complete group tasks. In classes, you participate in discussions, work on team projects, and acquire new knowledge. These experiences all help you acquire the following types of employability skills:

- Problem-solving skills—*Problem solving* is a process used to answer tough questions and resolve difficult situations. Often, problem solving involves adapting to a new way of doing things. Students who can problem solve effectively usually apply a five-step process. (1) Clearly identify the real problem. (2) List alternative courses of action. (3) Evaluate the consequences of each possible course of action. (4) Choose an alternative and take action. (5) Assess the outcome for reference when faced with future problems.

- Leadership skills—Employers want to know how you function as a leader in a group. If you have ever made a decision that helped others achieve a goal, you have used leadership skills. Leadership skills go hand in hand with problem-solving skills. Leaders often have to help individual group members resolve problems among themselves. Leaders also have to help the group as a whole overcome hurdles to reaching group goals. Leaders are eager to work with people to make change happen. Leaders need to be willing to take responsibility for their actions and the actions of the group. Leaders also need to be helpful, inspiring, open, flexible, and creative.

- Teamwork skills—A team can be defined as a small number of people with similar skills who share a common purpose. Effective team members focus on the aims of the group. All group members share leadership tasks, so everyone helps carry out group efforts. Like leaders, team members need problem-solving skills to help settle disputes and remove barriers to group goals. Team members also need communication skills so each person can express ideas fully and frankly. Being part of a team means striking a balance between group productivity and personal satisfaction.

- Communication skills—You will use oral, written, graphic, and electronic communications in most career areas. To be a good communicator, you need to be an attentive listener. You also need to be assertive enough to clearly express your point of view, 25-15.

- Creative thinking skills—Creativity is a capacity to question the ordinary. It is an ability to think in ways few other people have thought. Creative people can see problems from many angles. They look at a variety of solutions, some of which many be viewed as unusual. Problem-solving exercises help you build your creative thinking skills.

- Organizational skills—Organizational skills relate to your ability to make plans. Managing a schedule shows you know how to use time well. Keeping resources such as documents and supplies in order makes them easy to retrieve when needed. When you have organizational skills, your coworkers can count on you to meet deadlines as you complete your tasks.

- Technical skills—Most employers are willing to train an employee in the specific technical skills needed for a job. However, you must express a willingness to learn. You should also be able to show you have done well in your past learning opportunities.

When employers look for new employees, they try to hire people who already possess these employability skills. Therefore, begin practicing these skills now so you possess them when you begin the job-seeking process.

● Gain Work Experience

Part-time and summer jobs can help students become acquainted with various career fields. Most of the jobs available to students are *entry-level jobs*. An **entry-level job** requires few skills and pays minimal wages.

Most entry-level jobs in nutrition-related careers allow a person to observe how food is prepared and handled. Most entry-level jobs in fitness-related careers generally involve assisting at a camp, district park, or local playground, 25-16. Many of these jobs teach interpersonal skills in dealing with patients, clients, or customers.

The skills you acquire from an entry-level job can affect your entire life. Through your

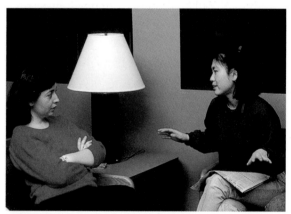

Photo courtesy of University Relations, MSU, Bruce A. Fox, photographer

25-15 Being able to clearly express ideas and opinions is an employability skill needed in any position that involves working with people.

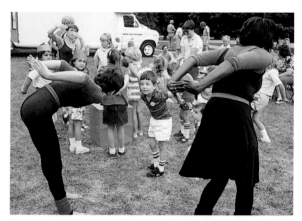

Photo courtesy of University Relations, MSU, Bruce A. Fox, photographer

25-16 Working with young children at a community playground or park would provide work experience related to a fitness career.

first jobs, you learn about yourself. You develop work habits and discover work nterests. You also learn which types of work you like best. On-the-job experiences give you an insider's view of work.

Your school may offer a supervised career-connections work experience. If so, take an active part in choosing a worksite for this experience that matches your needs and interests. This experience will give you a chance to explore the world of work, and it may help you begin a career. Your experiences will allow you to develop work-related skills. You will learn how to solve problems creatively within the work environment. In addition, the people you meet through this experience may become important connections to jobs in the future.

● Talk with Others

First talk with your school counselors about career choices that interest you. Guidance and career counselors are professionally trained to help you research suitable careers to match your strengths.

Have a counselor recommend someone in the community with experience in your area of interest who can discuss possible job options. Also visit with people who work in different job settings to gain a broader view of the diverse opportunities that exist. By talking with others, you can more fully understand all the career opportunities available.

● Develop a Portfolio

A student *portfolio* is an organized collection of papers, letters, pictures, and projects that shows what a person has accomplished. A portfolio provides a visible way to demonstrate your skills and achievements to others who might want to hire you. It becomes a personal advertisement about who you are and what skills you can offer.

Contents of the portfolio will vary. Change the materials in the portfolio to relate to the

requirements of the job you are seeking. If you use a three-ring binder, you can easily add or remove items. Carefully label and date all the items you include. See 25-17 for suggested items for your portfolio.

Display the items in your portfolio neatly and simply to showcase your skills. During job interviews, offer the employer an opportunity to review your portfolio. Be prepared to discuss any item you include in your portfolio, highlighting only the main points.

● Finding the Job You Want

Reaching your career goals takes years of planning and work. Your part-time work and volunteer experiences will help you decide what you enjoy most and least about work.

Your Personal Portfolio

What skills would each of the following examples illustrate to a potential employer?

- Transcript of completed courses
- National and state test results
- Recognitions and documented accomplishments
- Vocational-technical training records
- Evidence of involvement in extracurricular activities
- Samples of school papers and projects
- Letters of recommendations from teachers or former employers
- Photos, newspaper clippings, other documentation of completed projects
- List of committee positions held, with a brief description of what was learned and/or accomplished in each

25-17 Anything that clearly demonstrates a person's ability to do a job well can be included in a portfolio.

Well-prepared job candidates are more likely to be successful than those who leave career planning to the last minute. To get a job, you need to know how to locate job openings, write a resume, and prepare for job interviews.

Locating Jobs

Knowing how and where to find work is a valuable skill. When looking for a job, consider as many sources of information as possible. Your teachers, school counselors, parents, and adult friends may know some job openings for you to pursue.

Friends and relatives are often your most fruitful resources. Many jobs have been located through a friend of a friend. The process of connecting with the people you know is networking. **Networking** means alerting a wide circle of people about your interest in a job. By networking, you simply reach out for assistance. You will find that most people are happy to help you.

While you are networking, check other information sources about job openings. These include the following:

- Read the want ads in local newspapers and in state and national publications that serve the profession. Most advertised job openings appear in these classified ads. If you qualify for any, apply for the position by carefully following the directions provided.

- Check bulletin boards for job announcements, starting with those located in your school's career center. Community organizations may also post job announcements in public buildings. See 25-18.

- Search the Internet for job ads. Use the search word *careers.* Hundreds of data banks are available to you from companies, unions, trade associations, government agencies, and universities. Many employers use the Internet exclusively to post their computer- or technology-related positions.

- Attend job fairs and career days. At these events many employers have booths to promote available jobs. You can talk with

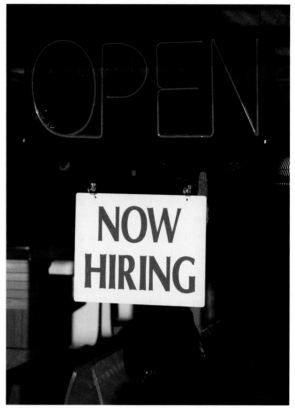

25-18 Local businesses often post signs announcing job openings.

employer representatives and learn more about the companies. Watch your local papers for career event announcements.

- Contact employment services. Public employment services exist solely to inform job-seekers of job openings in the state and beyond. Private employment agencies are business firms that receive job listings from employers who pay them a fee to fill the openings. Private agencies may specialize in specific types or levels of jobs. Public employment services are free, but private agencies may charge a fee for their service. Before using a private agency, make sure you first understand what your costs are, if any.

Getting the job you want will probably require a time-consuming search. Those who succeed say networking and hard work are the two key ingredients to a successful job search.

● **Recognizing a Safe Work Environment**

As you look for a job, you should be aware of the hazards that may be associated with the work environment. This will help you evaluate the environment to be sure safety standards are being met. For instance, work in a research laboratory may involve the use of dangerous chemicals. When you visit the laboratory, observe whether workers are wearing safety goggles and protective gloves. Check to see if chemicals are stored safely, too. This will help you determine whether guidelines for maintaining safe working conditions are being followed.

You will want to work for an employer who cares about the safety of the employees. The employer should also care about the safety of the people who use the goods or services you produce. Look for workplaces that meet the following conditions:

- Lighting is adequate to perform tasks without eyestrain.
- Traffic ways are clear of obstacles.
- Floors are dry.
- Ventilation is sufficient to maintain good air quality throughout the facility.
- Equipment is well maintained and safety guards and shields are in place.
- Hazardous materials are clearly labeled and properly stored.
- Employees wear necessary safety gear and protective clothing, 25-19.
- Sanitation standards are observed when working with food.

● **Writing a Resume**

A *resume* outlines on paper a person's job qualifications. It is a quick reference for the employer to determine if you seem qualified to handle a specific job. When you apply for a job, attach a copy of your resume to your letter of application. You may give an extra copy of your resume to the interviewer during a job interview.

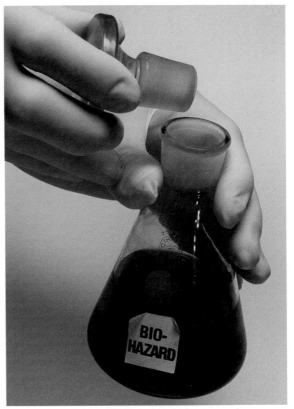

25-19 In a safe work environment, employees should wear gloves and other protective gear when handling hazardous materials.

You will want to carefully prepare your resume and type it on fine quality paper. Computer programs and high-quality printers create resumes that look professionally prepared. The appearance of a resume may be as important as the information in it. A well-prepared resume can make you stand out from the crowd of many applicants.

Examine the sample resume in 25-20. The information in your resume should show all the key facts about you and your accomplishments. A resume includes the following categories:

- name, address, and telephone number where you can be reached
- job objective in clear, simple language
- work experience, both volunteer and paid employment (including company names, addresses, service dates, and job titles)

Rochelle Smith
223 Elm Street
Hope, Michigan 48000
616-555-9999

Position Desired

Restaurant Hostess—To work on weekends and earn money for college.

Work Experience

Salvation Army Volunteer—Assists the supervision of children by preparing and serving snacks.

Salvation Army

Bob Benjamin, Director

1127 Hill Street

Hope, Michigan, 48000

616-555-1798

July, 2001–present

Family Cook

Prepares dinner twice a week for a five-member family.

June, 2000–present

Neighborhood Babysitter

Cooks and provides care for three children, ages 5-10, once a week during summers.

June, 2000–present

Education

Junior at South High School

122 Main Street

Hope, Michigan 48000

616-555-2912

College preparatory program with B+ grade average. Special classes in:

Computers

Speech and communications

Graduation date: June, 2004

Certified in CPR

Activities

President, FCCLA, 2001–02

Member of Students Against Destructive Decisions, 2000–02

Member of Student Council, 2000–01

Interests

Sports, cooking, and travel

References

References are available upon request.

25-20 A resume should be specific but brief. The job interview is the place for providing details.

- education information, including the school's name and address, the program of study, special courses completed relative to job success, grade average or grade point, and the graduation date
- activities and honors, including participation in school organizations
- interests and hobbies (optional)
- a final statement: "References will be provided upon request."

A **reference** is the name of a person who will speak highly of your skills and abilities. Usually a list with at least three references should be ready to give to employers. The list should include the names, titles, work addresses, phone numbers, fax numbers, and electronic mail addresses of your references. Get each person's permission before adding his or her name to your list.

For your references, select people who know you well and are respected in the community. Teachers, counselors, employers, and spiritual leaders are ideal choices. Never name family members or personal friends since their opinions may be viewed as biased.

Omit information about your race, ethnic background, religion, sex, marital status, or disabilities from your resume. This information is personal and has no bearing on whether you are qualified for the job. Also, equal opportunity laws prohibit employers from considering these facts in deciding whom to hire.

● The Job Interview

The **job interview** is a discussion between the job applicant and the person doing the hiring. The purpose of the job interview is to give you and the employer a chance to seek information and ask questions. The interviewer will want to know more about your work skills, likes and dislikes, and future goals. You will probably want to know more details about the position available.

For a successful job interview, you must first do your homework. This means preparing for the interview in much the same way as

you prepare for school assignments. Being ready for an interview requires the following:

- learning as much as possible about the employer and its business
- preparing a resume and a portfolio, highlighting the qualifications that relate to the job being considered
- listing questions to ask the employer about the job and opportunities for advancement
- practicing orally with a friend by answering questions the employer might ask

Practice mock interviews to gain confidence in your ability to answer questions well. Typical questions that interviewers might ask are listed in 25-21. If possible,

---

Common Interview Questions

The interviewer will probably begin by saying, "Tell me about yourself." Then expect the following questions:

- What types of work experience have you had?
- How do your past experiences relate to this position?
- What are your most (or least) favorite subjects in school? Why?
- How do you spend your spare time?
- What team projects have you worked on?
- How would you describe your ability to get along with people?
- How would you describe your strengths (or weaknesses)?
- Why should I hire you for this position?
- What type of job do you want in five years?
- What hours are you willing to work?
- What is your salary expectation?
- What would you do if . . . ? (This could involve any ethical dilemma or problem-solving situation related to the work environment.)

25-21 Practice answering these questions by speaking in front of a mirror or to a friend.

record the sessions on an audio or video cassette to replay your responses. Put yourself in an employer's shoes as you evaluate your interview. How did you appear during the session? Did you look composed and maintain eye contact? Repeated practice will help you look and feel more at ease.

Plan what you will wear to the interview and try to dress as much like the employees as possible. Looking neat, clean, and appropriately dressed reflects your potential for job success. Find out if the interview process includes a test and, if possible, prepare for it. Learn exactly where the interviewer's office is and plan to arrive at least ten minutes early. If you use public transportation, know the travel schedules.

After completing the job interview, send a follow-up letter right away. This letter should thank the interviewer for his or her time and express a continued interest in the job. This also is the opportunity to clarify any points about your qualifications that were raised during the interview. The letter should follow the form of a business letter.

If you do not get the job, try not to be discouraged. Often there are many applicants competing for the same job. Learn from this experience by evaluating what went well in the interview and what you would do differently. Then continue your job search. Try to be positive and think about all the other job opportunities that may be better than the job you did not get.

● Maintaining a Job

Once you have secured a job, you must be able to keep it and feel successful at what you do. You are responsible for performing work tasks according to accepted standards. Traits often cited as key to job success include a positive attitude and good communication skills. Employers also want to retain workers who are creative, flexible, and open to new ideas. Exhibiting these traits will help you keep your job.

Be patient during your first few weeks at a new job. Try not to be overly critical of yourself. Realize it takes time to learn who people are and how to get work done. Avoid comparing yourself to others who have more experience. Find someone at your job who can become your mentor. A **mentor** is a fellow worker who has years of experience and can help you with your questions and challenges. Following your mentor's example may help you maintain a job for years.

Part of becoming a professional is being willing to assess your strengths and limitations on the job. This is the first step toward improving areas in which you are weak. Take advantage of opportunities to stay up to date with the latest research and new resources that will help you do a better job. As your job skills develop, you will be able to do your work with greater ease and accuracy. This will help you and your employer feel satisfaction with your work and enable you to remain in your position. See 25-22.

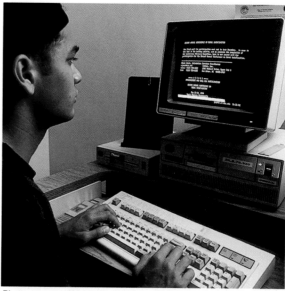

Photo courtesy of University Relations, MSU, Bruce A. Fox, photographer

25-22 Learning how to use new programs and equipment in the workplace will help employees keep their jobs.

Applying Professional Ethics

As a member of the workforce, you may face problems daily for which solutions are not always clear. The way you make decisions in these situations can affect your ability to maintain your job. You will need to apply professional ethics. *Ethics* are standards, guidelines, and codes that guide behaviors. Ethics should rule over every aspect of your job—every decision you make and every action you take. Without a code of ethics, you cannot be considered a professional.

What do you need to consider when applying ethics to a particular decision? Ask yourself the following questions:

- Are my actions aimed at improving the quality of life for others?
- Do my actions show I respect others regardless of their ethnic background, race, religion, sex, or age?
- Will my actions cause other people to have their freedoms denied?
- Do my actions show I respect the privacy and confidentiality of others?
- Do my actions reflect truthfulness and open communication?

Always allow ethics to guide your actions. Also, make a point of associating with other professionals who display high standards of ethics to the public.

Leaving a Job

People choose to leave their jobs for a number of reasons. Some people quit their jobs because they lose interest and want more challenging work experiences. Others choose to leave positions because the work is unpleasant or the work environment is unsafe. Some people feel their jobs are not giving them a chance to use their skills. Others feel stress because they do not feel they have all the skills needed to perform their jobs with ease.

Whatever the reasons for leaving a job, you can grow from analyzing the pros and cons of a work experience. A positive attitude and a willingness to learn from mistakes can make your next job more productive and satisfying. A new job can offer a chance to begin again and put your experience to work.

When you leave a job, it is important to behave professionally. Most employers request at least a two-week notice that you will be leaving. This gives your employer time to find someone else to take over your responsibilities. You should give this notice in writing. Briefly explain that you are leaving and give the date of your last day on the job. Some people also choose to state why they are resigning and mention where they will be working next. This type of information should be conveyed in a positive tone.

You do not want to anger an employer you may need to list as a reference someday. Therefore, avoid focusing on what you do not like about the job you are leaving. Instead, you might describe the challenges that attracted you to your new position. Remember that even unpleasant work experiences can provide chances to learn and grow as a professional. Be sure to thank your employer for the opportunities you have had in your present position.

Being an Entrepreneur

Would you like to start a business of your own someday? People who own and operate their own businesses are called *entrepreneurs.* Many opportunities for entrepreneurs exist in the area of nutrition and fitness. A dietitian may develop a program on drug-free muscle building to present to athletes at area schools. A fitness specialist may create an exercise program to help factory workers avoid repetitive-motion injuries. See 25-23.

Successful entrepreneurs have three key traits. First, entrepreneurs are innovative. They have the creativity to take an old idea and market it in a new way or to a new audience. Second, entrepreneurs are risk takers.

They are willing to invest their time and resources to put their business plan into action. The third trait of successful entrepreneurs is persistence. It takes persistence to repeatedly adapt your product or service until it fully meets the needs of your market. Most entrepreneurs are people who stick with their dreams. They know what needs to be done and they do it.

Entrepreneurs get their business ideas by doing market research. Entrepreneurs start by seeing consumer needs. Then they search for ways to meet those needs with new products or services. Suppose the owner of a local health club notices mothers leaving their young children with babysitters while they work out. This gives the owner an idea to offer a mother-child exercise class. The owner conducts market research by interviewing the mothers about the idea. The owner learns most mothers would prefer an aqua aerobics class that would allow them to swim with their children. Market research allowed this entrepreneur to find a way to expand her business to meet the needs of her clients.

Advances in technology also create new opportunities for entrepreneurs. Through technology, new research findings can be revealed and new products and services can be developed. For instance, technology might lead to the development of a testing device. This device could be used in a laboratory study to reveal new benefits of a certain phytochemical. This research could prompt an ambitious dietitian to develop and sell a line of drinks made from plants rich in this phytochemical. Technology comes into play again to invent the machine that will extract the plant juices used in the drinks.

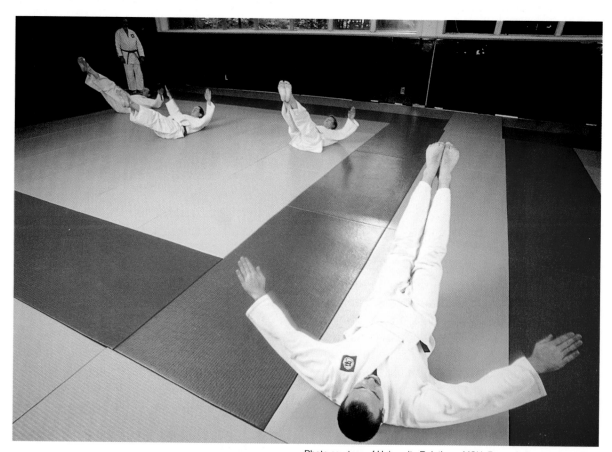

Photo courtesy of University Relations, MSU, Bruce A. Fox, photographer

25-23 An exercise specialist could turn an interest in Tai Chi into an entrepreneurial opportunity by offering classes.

Chapter 25 Review

Summary

Job opportunities in all areas of nutrition and fitness careers are expected to increase. Hospitals, school districts, and many other employers hire dietitians to plan diets. Dietetic technicians counsel patients and plan menus according to dietitians' directions. Other nutrition professionals teach, report, and research nutrition, sometimes as a prelude to entering other health professions. Fitness professionals promote exercise and more healthful lifestyles.

Entry-level positions are available in some nutrition and fitness areas. However, most professional careers in the field require a college degree. Many also require certification. Certification is earned by meeting special requirements set by the profession. Some government agencies may require a license. Proof of continued education is often needed for staying certified or licensed.

Students should examine their interests when considering career options. Recognizing personal aptitudes, abilities, values, and goals is also important. Together these factors help students identify the most suitable jobs and employers.

To prepare for a career, students can take several steps while they are in high school. They can choose the appropriate courses and participate in school organizations related to their goals. They can volunteer their help. These experiences will help students develop employability skills. Students can hold part-time or summer jobs to gain work experience. They can talk to professionals in the field and learn career information not available anywhere else. Once a career direction is known, students can develop portfolios to highlight their skills and accomplishments.

Whether pursuing part-time jobs now or dream jobs later, students need to know how to locate job openings. Job seekers should also practice writing resumes and interviewing for jobs. Students need to be willing to learn on the job and apply professional ethics in order to keep their jobs. They need to know the appropriate way to leave a job when the time comes. After gaining work experience, many employees choose to expand their careers by becoming entrepreneurs.

Check Your Knowledge

1. Give two reasons job opportunities for nutrition and fitness professionals are increasing.
2. What job function can only registered dietitians perform?
3. Name five areas of career specialization for dietitians.
4. What does a dietetic technician do?
5. True or false. Someone who studies nutrition and food safety is a dietetic technician.
6. Name and describe four career areas for fitness professionals.
7. Why do many nutrition and fitness careers require certification and/or a license?
8. What are the three main categories of job interests?
9. Explain the difference between aptitude and ability.
10. Why is it important to consider personal values when choosing a career?
11. Propose a long-term career goal and two short-term career goals that would help you reach it.
12. Name four ways students can begin preparing for their careers while still in school.
13. List five types of employability skills.
14. What should a portfolio contain?
15. List four ways to learn about job openings.
16. List five conditions that describe a safe work environment.
17. What is the purpose of a resume?
18. Cite four ways to prepare for a job interview.
19. What are two effective methods for maintaining a job and two points to remember when leaving a job?

20. How do market research and advances in technology help create business opportunities for entrepreneurs?

Put Learning into Action

1. Interview a nutrition or fitness professional about available careers in his or her field. Ask the professional what he or she did to meet any certification or license requirements.

2. Prepare a picture collage illustrating the various job opportunities related to nutrition or fitness. The collage should show people at work on their jobs.

3. Collect information from various colleges and universities offering nutrition and/or fitness programs. Create a display of the materials.

4. Make a list of the top 10 factors most important to you for job satisfaction. Compare responses with your classmates. Discuss why lists vary from person to person and how this influences career choices.

5. Imagine you have worked in a fast-food restaurant for the past nine months. Write a letter of resignation to your employer.

Explore Further

1. Research the job market outlook for nutrition or fitness careers. Use the Internet as a resource or refer to the *Occupational Outlook Handbook* from the U.S. Department of Labor. How do the starting salaries in nutrition and fitness careers compare with others?

2. Research a professional organization related to nutrition or fitness. Investigate the following: What is the organization's name and purpose? When did it begin? Who can become a member? Does it have a certification or continuing education program? What is the name of its professional journal? What does the journal report?

3. Identify the nutrition and/or fitness area that interests you most. Research the job requirements and employment opportunities. What courses and/or job experiences are needed to prepare you for this job?

4. Interview an employer in the nutrition and food science or fitness field. Ask the employer to identify the 10 top personal traits he or she looks for when hiring a new employee. After the interview, rate yourself for each trait the employer listed.

5. Research and analyze quality control standards for a safe working environment in the food industry. Share your findings in an oral report using visual aids.

6. Use the Internet to research a class or seminar being offered on a food and nutrition or fitness topic. Write a one-page proposal an employee might give an employer. In the proposal, describe the class and explain how it could help the employee stay current in his or her field.

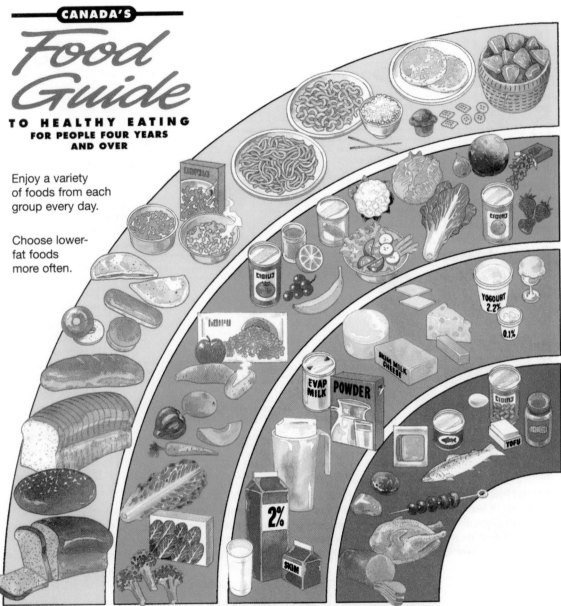

Health Canada Santé Canada

CANADA'S Food Guide TO HEALTHY EATING FOR PEOPLE FOUR YEARS AND OVER

Enjoy a variety of foods from each group every day.

Choose lower-fat foods more often.

Grain Products
Choose whole grain and enriched products more often.

Vegetables and Fruit
Choose dark green and orange vegetables and orange fruit more often.

Milk Products
Choose lower-fat milk products more often.

Meat and Alternatives
Choose leaner meats, poultry and fish, as well as dried peas, beans and lentils more often.

Canada

Health Canada

Recommended Nutrient Intakes

Dietary Reference Intakes: Vitamins

Life-Stage Group	Biotin (μg/d)	Folate (μg/d)[a]	Niacin (mg/d)[d]	Pantothenic Acid (mg/d)	Riboflavin (mg/d)	Thiamin (mg/d)	Vitamin A (μg/d)	Vitamin B$_6$ (mg/d)	Vitamin B$_{12}$ (μg/d)	Vitamin C (mg/d)	Vitamin D (μg/d)[f,g]	Vitamin E (mg/d)[h]	Vitamin K (μg/d)
Infants													
0–6 mo	5	65	2	1.7	0.3	0.2	400	0.1	0.4	40	5	4	2.0
7–12 mo	6	80	4	1.8	0.4	0.3	500	0.3	0.5	50	5	6	2.5
Children													
1–3 yr	8	150	6	2	0.5	0.5	300	0.5	0.9	15	5	6	30
4–8 yr	12	200	8	3	0.6	0.6	400	0.6	1.2	25	5	7	55
Males													
9–13 yr	20	300	12	4	0.9	0.9	600	1.0	1.8	45	5	11	60
14–18 yr	25	400	16	5	1.3	1.2	900	1.3	2.4	75	5	15	75
19–30 yr	30	400	16	5	1.3	1.2	900	1.3	2.4	90	5	15	120
31–50 yr	30	400	16	5	1.3	1.2	900	1.3	2.4	90	5	15	120
51–70 yr	30	400	16	5	1.3	1.2	900	1.7	2.4[e]	90	10	15	120
>70 yr	30	400	16	5	1.3	1.2	900	1.7	2.4[e]	90	15	15	120
Females													
9–13 yr	20	300	12	4	0.9	0.9	600	1.0	1.8	45	5	11	60
14–18 yr	25	400[b]	14	5	1.0	1.0	700	1.2	2.4	65	5	15	75
19–30 yr	30	400[b]	14	5	1.1	1.1	700	1.3	2.4	75	5	15	90
31–50 yr	30	400[b]	14	5	1.1	1.1	700	1.3	2.4	75	5	15	90
51–70 yr	30	400	14	5	1.1	1.1	700	1.5	2.4[e]	75	10	15	90
>70 yr	30	400	14	5	1.1	1.1	700	1.5	2.4[e]	75	15	15	90
Pregnancy													
≤18 yr	30	600[c]	18	6	1.4	1.4	750	1.9	2.6	80	5	15	75
19–30 yr	30	600[c]	18	6	1.4	1.4	770	1.9	2.6	85	5	15	90
31–50 yr	30	600[c]	18	6	1.4	1.4	770	1.9	2.6	85	5	15	90
Lactation													
≤18 yr	35	500	17	7	1.6	1.5	1,200	2.0	2.8	115	5	19	75
19–30 yr	35	500	17	7	1.6	1.5	1,300	2.0	2.8	120	5	19	90
31–50 yr	35	500	17	7	1.6	1.5	1,300	2.0	2.8	120	5	19	90

Food and Nutrition Board, Institute of Medicine, The National Academies

NOTE: This table represents Recommended Dietary Allowances (RDAs) in unshaded boxes and Adequate Intakes (AIs) in shaded boxes. RDAs and AIs may both be used as goals for individual intake. RDAs are set to meet the needs of almost all (97 to 98 percent) individuals in a group. For healthy human milk-fed infants, the AI is the mean intake. The AI for other life-stage and gender groups is believed to cover needs of all healthy individuals in the group, but lack of data or uncertainty in the data prevent being able to specify with confidence the percentage of individuals covered by this intake.

a As dietary folate equivalents (DFE). 1 DFE = 1 μg food folate = 0.6 μg of folic acid (from fortified food supplement) consumed with food = 0.5 μg of synthetic (supplemental) folic acid taken on an empty stomach.

b In view of evidence linking folate intake with neural tube defects in the fetus, it is recommended that all women capable of becoming pregnant consume 400 μg of synthetic folic acid from fortified foods and/or supplements in addition to intake of food folate from a varied diet.

c It is assumed that women will continue consuming 400 μg of folic acid until their pregnancy is confirmed and they enter prenatal care, which ordinarily occurs after the end of the periconceptional period—the critical time for formation of the neural tube.

d As niacin equivalents (NE). 1 mg of niacin = 60 mg of tryptophan; 0–6 months = preformed niacin (not NE).

e Because 10 to 30 percent of older people may malabsorb food-bound B$_{12}$, it is advisable for those older than 50 years to meet their RDA mainly by consuming foods fortified with B$_{12}$ or a supplement containing B$_{12}$.

f As cholecalciferol. 1 μg cholecalciferol = 40 IU vitamin D.

g In the absence of adequate exposure to sunlight.

h As α-tocopherol, which includes RRR-α-tocopherol, the only form of α-tocopherol that occurs naturally in foods, and the 2R-stereoisomeric forms of α-tocopherol (RRR-, RSR-, RRS-, and RSS-α-tocopherol) that occur in fortified foods and supplements. Does not include the 2S-stereoisomeric forms of α-tocopherol (SRR-, SSR-, SRS-, and SSS-α-tocopherol), also found in fortified foods and supplements.

Dietary Reference Intakes: Minerals

Life-Stage Group	Calcium (mg/d)	Fluoride (mg/d)	Iodine (µg/d)	Iron (mg/d)	Magnesium (mg/d)	Phosphorus (mg/d)	Selenium (mg/d)	Zinc (mg/d)
Infants								
0–6 mo	210	0.01	110	0.27	30	100	15	2
7–12 mo	270	0.5	130	11	75	275	20	3
Children								
1–3 yr	500	0.7	90	7	80	460	20	3
4–8 yr	800	1	90	10	130	500	30	5
Males								
9–13 yr	1,300	2	120	8	240	1,250	40	8
14–18 yr	1,300	3	150	11	410	1,250	55	11
19–30 yr	1,000	4	150	8	400	700	55	11
31–50 yr	1,000	4	150	8	420	700	55	11
51–70 yr	1,200	4	150	8	420	700	55	11
>70 yr	1,200	4	150	8	420	700	55	11
Females								
9–13 yr	1,300	2	120	8	240	1,250	40	8
14–18 yr	1,300	3	150	15	360	1,250	55	9
19–30 yr	1,000	3	150	18	310	700	55	8
31–50 yr	1,000	3	150	18	320	700	55	8
51–70 yr	1,200	3	150	8	320	700	55	8
>70 yr	1,200	3	150	8	320	700	55	8
Pregnancy								
≤18 yr	1,300	3	220	27	400	1,250	60	12
19–30 yr	1,000	3	220	27	350	700	60	11
31–50 yr	1,000	3	220	27	360	700	60	11
Lactation								
≤18 yr	1,300	3	290	10	360	1,250	70	13
19–30 yr	1,000	3	290	9	310	700	70	12
31–50 yr	1,000	3	290	9	320	700	70	12

Food and Nutrition Board, Institute of Medicine, The National Academies

NOTE: This table represents Recommended Dietary Allowances (RDAs) in unshaded boxes and Adequate Intakes (AIs) in shaded boxes. RDAs and AIs may both be used as goals for individual intake. RDAs are set to meet the needs of almost all (97 to 98 percent) individuals in a group. For healthy human milk-fed infants, the AI is the mean intake. The AI for other life-stage and gender groups is believed to cover needs of all healthy individuals in the group, but lack of data or uncertainty in the data prevent being able to specify with confidence the percentage of individuals covered by this intake.

DRI Values for Energy

Life-Stage Group	Energy (cal/d) Males	Energy (cal/d) Females
Infants		
0–6 mo	570	520
7–12 mo	743	676
Children		
1–2 yr	1,046	992
3–8 yr	1,742	1,642
Adolescents and Adults		
9–13 yr	2,279	2,071
14–18 yr	3,152	2,368
>18 yr	3,067[a]	2,403[b]
Pregnancy		
14–18 yr		
1st trimester		2,368
2nd trimester		2,708
3rd trimester		2,820
19–50 yr		
1st trimester		2,403[b]
2nd trimester		2,743[b]
3rd trimester		2,855[b]
Lactation		
14–18 yr		
1st 6 mo		2,698
2nd 6 mo		2,768
19–50 yr		
1st 6 mo		2,733[b]
2nd 6 mo		2,803[b]

Food and Nutrition Board, Institute of Medicine, The National Academies

a The intake that meets the average energy expenditure of healthy, moderately active individuals at the reference height, weight, and age. (See height and weight table.)

b Subtract 10 cal/day for males and 7 cal/day for females for each year of age above 19 years.

Dietary Reference Intakes: Macronutrients									
Life-Stage Group	Carbohy-drates (g/d)	Total Fiber (g/d)	Total Fat (g/d)	Protein[c] (g/d)	Life-Stage Group	Carbohy-drates (g/d)	Total Fiber (g/d)	Total Fat (g/d)	Protein[c] (g/d)
Infants					**Females**				
0-6 mo	60	ND[d]	31	9.1	9-13 yr	130	26	ND	34
7-12 mo	95	ND	30	13.5	14-18 yr	130	26	ND	46
Children					19-30 yr	130	25	ND	46
1-3 yr	130	19	ND	13	31-50 yr	130	25	ND	46
4-8 yr	130	25	ND	19	51-70 yr	130	21	ND	46
Males					>70 yr	130	21	ND	46
9-13 yr	130	31	ND	34	**Pregnancy**				
14-18 yr	130	38	ND	52	14-18 yr	175	28	ND	+25[e]
19-30 yr	130	38	ND	56	19-50 yr	175	28	ND	+25[e]
31-50 yr	130	38	ND	56	**Lactation**				
51-70 yr	130	30	ND	56	14-18 yr	210	29	ND	+25[f]
>70 yr	130	30	ND	56	19-50 yr	210	29	ND	+25[f]

Food and Nutrition Board, Institute of Medicine, The National Academies

NOTE: This table presents Recommended Dietary Allowances (RDAs) in unshaded boxes and Adequate Intakes (AIs) in shaded boxes. RDAs and AIs may both be used as goals for individual intake. RDAs are set to meet the needs of almost all (97 to 98 percent) individuals in a group. For healthy human milk-fed infants, the AI is the mean intake. The AI for other life-stage and gender groups is believed to cover needs of all healthy individuals in the group, but lack of data or uncertainty in the data prevent being able to specify with confidence the percentage of individuals covered by this intake.

[c] AI or RDA for reference individuals. (See height and weight table.) The RDA for men and women over age 19 is 0.36 g/lb (0.8 g/kg) body weight/day of protein.

[d] ND = not determined.

[e] The RDA for pregnancy is 25 g/day protein in addition to the RDA of the nonpregnant woman. This added amount is recommended only for the second half of pregnancy. For the first half of pregnancy, the protein requirements are the same as those of the nonpregnant woman.

[f] In addition to the RDA of the nonlactating adolescent or woman.

Upper Tolerable Intake Levels (UL[a])										
Nutrient	0-6 mo	7-12 mo	1-3 yr	4-8 yr	9-13 yr	14-18 yr	19-30 yr	31-50 yr	51-70 yr	>70 yr
Vitamins										
Biotin	ND[b]	ND	ND	ND	ND	ND	ND	ND	ND	ND
Folate	ND	ND	300 µg	400 µg	600 µg	800 µg	1,000 µg	1,000 µg	1,000 µg	1,000 µg
Niacin	ND	ND	10 mg	15 mg	20 mg	30 mg	35 mg	35 mg	35 mg	35 mg
Pantothenic acid	ND	ND	ND	ND	ND	ND	ND	ND	ND	ND
Riboflavin	ND	ND	ND	ND	ND	ND	ND	ND	ND	ND
Thiamin	ND	ND	ND	ND	ND	ND	ND	ND	ND	ND
Vitamin A	600 µg	600 µg	600 µg	900 µg	1,700 µg	2,800 µg	3,000 µg	3,000 µg	3,000 µg	3,000 µg
Vitamin B_6	ND	ND	30 mg	40 mg	60 mg	80 mg	100 mg	100 mg	100 mg	100 mg
Vitamin B_{12}	ND	ND	ND	ND	ND	ND	ND	ND	ND	ND
Vitamin C	ND	ND	400 mg	650 mg	1,200 mg	1,800 mg	2,000 mg	2,000 mg	2,000 mg	2,000 mg
Vitamin D	25 µg	25 µg	50 µg	50 µg	50 µg	50 µg	50 µg	50 µg	50 µg	50 µg
Vitamin E	ND	ND	200 mg	300 mg	600 mg	800 mg	1,000 mg	1,000 mg	1,000 mg	1,000 mg
Vitamin K	ND	ND	ND	ND	ND	ND	ND	ND	ND	ND
Minerals										
Calcium	ND	ND	2,500 mg	2,500 mg	2,500 mg	2,500 mg	2,500 mg	2,500 mg	2,500 mg	2,500 mg
Fluoride	0.7 mg	0.9 mg	1.3 mg	2.2 mg	10 mg	10 mg	10 mg	10 mg	10 mg	10 mg
Iodine	ND	ND	200 µg	300 µg	600 µg	900 µg	1,100 µg	1,100 µg	1,100 µg	1,100 µg
Iron	40 mg	40 mg	40 mg	40 mg	40 mg	45 mg	45 mg	45 mg	45 mg	45 mg
Magnesium	ND	ND	65 mg	110 mg	350 mg	350 mg	350 mg	350 mg	350 mg	350 mg
Phosphorus	ND	ND	3,000 mg	3,000 mg	4,000 mg	4,000 mg[c]	4,000 mg[c]	4,000 mg[c]	4,000 mg	3,000 mg
Selenium	45 µg	60 µg	90 µg	150 µg	280 µg	400 µg	400 µg	400 µg	400 µg	400 µg
Zinc	4 mg	5 mg	7 mg	12 mg	23 mg	34 mg	40 mg	40 mg	40 mg	40 mg

Food and Nutrition Board, Institute of Medicine, The National Academies

[a] The UL represents the maximum level of daily nutrient intake that is likely to pose no risk of adverse effects. Unless otherwise specified, the UL represents total intake from food, water, and supplements. Due to lack of suitable data, ULs could not be established for biotin, pantothenic acid, riboflavin, thiamin, vitamin B_{12}, or vitamin K. In the absence of ULs, extra caution may be warranted in consuming levels above recommended intakes. UL values are the same for males and females in all life-stage groups. UL values are also unaffected by pregnancy and lactation unless otherwise noted.

[b] Not determinable due to lack of data of adverse effects in this age group and concern with regard to lack of ability to handle excess amounts. Source of intake should be from food only to prevent high levels of intake.

[c] 3,500 mg during pregnancy.

SOURCES: These tables are adapted from the following DRI reports: *Dietary Reference Intakes for Calcium, Phosphorus, Magnesium, Vitamin D, and Fluoride* (1997); *Dietary Reference Intakes for Thiamin, Riboflavin, Niacin, Vitamin B_6, Folate, Vitamin B_{12}, Pantothenic Acid, Biotin, and Choline* (1998); *Dietary Reference Intakes for Vitamin C, Selenium, and Carotenoids* (2000); and *Dietary Reference Intakes for Vitamin A, Vitamin K, Arsenic, Boron, Chromium, Copper, Iodine, Iron, Manganese, Molybdenum, Nickel, Silicon, Vanadium, and Zinc* (2001). These reports may be accessed via www.nap.edu.

Nutritive Values of Foods

Appendix C

(Tr indicates nutrient present in trace amount.)

Item No. (A)	Foods, approximate measures, units, and weight (weight of edible portion only) (B)	(B)	Water (C) Percent	Food energy (D) Calories	Protein (E) Grams	Fat (F) Grams	Saturated fat (G) Grams	Cholesterol (H) Milligrams	Carbohydrate (I) Grams	Dietary fiber (J) Grams	Calcium (K) Milligrams	Iron (L) Milligrams	Potassium (M) Milligrams	Sodium (N) Milligrams	Vitamin A (O) Micrograms	Thiamin (P) Milligrams	Riboflavin (Q) Milligrams	Niacin (R) Milligrams	Vitamin C (S) Milligrams
		Grams																	
Beverages																			
Carbonated:[2]																			
Club soda	12 fl. oz.	355	100	0	0	0	0.0	0	0	0	18	Tr	0	78	0	0.00	0.00	0.0	0
Cola type:																			
Regular	12 fl. oz.	369	89	160	0	0	0.0	0	41	0	11	0.2	7	18	0	0.00	0.00	0.0	0
Diet, artificially sweetened	12 fl. oz.	355	100	Tr	0	0	0.0	0	Tr	0	14	0.2	7	32	0	0.00	0.00	0.0	0
Ginger ale	12 fl. oz.	366	91	125	0	0	0.0	0	32	0	11	0.1	4	29	0	0.00	0.00	0.0	0
Grape	12 fl. oz.	372	88	180	0	0	0.0	0	46	0	15	0.4	4	48	0	0.00	0.00	0.0	0
Lemon-lime	12 fl. oz	372	89	155	0	0	0.0	0	39	0	7	0.4	4	33	0	0.00	0.00	0.0	0
Orange	12 fl. oz.	372	88	180	0	0	0.0	0	46	0	15	0.3	7	52	0	0.00	0.00	0.0	0
Pepper type	12 fl. oz.	369	89	160	0	0	Tr	0	41	0	11	0.1	4	37	0	0.00	0.00	0.0	0
Root beer	12 fl. oz.	370	89	165	0	0	0.0	0	42	0	15	0.2	4	48	0	0.00	0.00	0.0	0
Cocoa and chocolate-flavored beverages. See Dairy Products																			
Coffee:																			
Brewed	6 fl. oz.	180	100	Tr	Tr	Tr	0.0	0	Tr	0	4	Tr	124	2	0	0.00	0.02	0.4	0
Instant, prepared (2 tsp. powder plus 6 fl. oz. water)	6 fl. oz.	182	99	Tr	Tr	Tr	0.0	0	1	0	2	0.1	71	Tr	0	0.00	0.03	0.6	0
Fruit drinks, noncarbonated:																			
Canned:																			
Fruit punch drink	6 fl. oz.	190	88	85	Tr	0	0.0	0	22	0	15	0.4	48	15	2	0.03	0.04	Tr	[4]61
Grape drink	6 fl. oz.	187	86	100	Tr	0	0.0	0	26	Tr	2	0.3	9	11	Tr	0.01	0.01	Tr	[4]64
Pineapple-grapefruit juice drink	6 fl. oz.	187	87	90	Tr	Tr	Tr	0	23	Tr	13	0.9	97	24	6	0.06	0.04	0.5	[4]110
Frozen:																			
Lemonade concentrate:																			
Undiluted	6-fl.-oz. can	219	49	425	Tr	Tr	Tr	0	112	1	9	0.4	153	4	4	0.04	0.07	0.7	66
Diluted with 4 1/3 parts water by volume	6 fl. oz.	185	89	80	Tr	Tr	Tr	0	21	Tr	2	0.1	30	1	1	0.01	0.02	0.2	13
Limeade concentrate:																			
Undiluted	6-fl.-oz. can	218	50	410	Tr	Tr	Tr	0	108	1	11	0.2	129	Tr	Tr	0.02	0.02	0.2	26
Diluted with 4-1/3 parts water by volume	6 fl. oz	185	89	75	Tr	Tr	0.0	0	20	Tr	2	Tr	24	Tr	Tr	Tr	Tr	Tr	4
Fruit juices. See type under Fruits and Fruit Juices.																			
Milk beverages. See Dairy Products.																			
Tea:																			
Brewed	8 fl. oz.	240	100	Tr	Tr	Tr	0.0	0	Tr	0	0	Tr	36	1	0	0.00	0.03	Tr	0
Instant, powder, prepared:																			
Unsweetened (1 tsp. powder plus 8 fl. oz. water)	8 fl. oz.	241	100	Tr	Tr	Tr	0.0	0	1	0	1	Tr	61	1	0	0.00	0.02	0.1	0
Sweetened (3 tsp. powder plus 8 fl. oz. water)	8 fl. oz.	262	91	85	Tr	Tr	Tr	0	22	0	1	Tr	49	Tr	0	0.00	0.04	0.1	0
Dairy Products																			
Butter. See Fats and Oils																			
Cheese:																			
Cheddar:																			
Cut pieces	1 oz.	28	37	115	7	9	0.6	30	Tr	0	204	0.2	28	176	86	0.01	0.11	Tr	0
	1 in.³	17	37	70	4	6	3.6	18	Tr	0	123	0.1	17	105	52	Tr	0.06	Tr	0
Shredded	1 cup	113	37	455	28	37	23.8	119	1	0	815	0.8	111	701	342	0.03	0.42	0.1	0
Cottage (curd not pressed down):																			
Creamed (cottage cheese, 4% fat):																			
Large curd	1 cup	225	79	235	28	10	6.4	34	6	0	135	0.3	190	911	108	0.05	0.37	0.3	Tr
Small curd	1 cup	210	79	215	26	9	6.0	31	6	0	126	0.3	177	850	101	0.04	0.34	0.3	Tr
Lowfat (2%)	1 cup	226	79	205	31	4	2.8	19	8	0	155	0.4	217	918	45	0.05	0.42	0.3	Tr

(A)	(B)	(C)	(D)	(E)	(F)	(G)	(H)	(I)	(J)	(K)	(L)	(M)	(N)	(O)	(P)	(Q)	(R)	(S)
Uncreamed (cottage cheese dry curd, less than 1/2% fat)	1 cup (145)	80	125	25	1	0.4	10	3	0	46	0.3	47	19	12	0.04	0.21	0.2	0
Cream	1 oz. (28)	54	100	2	10	6.2	31	1	0	23	0.3	34	84	124	Tr	0.06	Tr	0
Mozzarella, made with:																		
Whole milk	1 oz. (28)	54	80	6	6	3.7	22	1	0	147	0.1	19	106	68	Tr	0.07	Tr	0
Part skim milk (low moisture)	1 oz. (28)	49	80	8	5	3.1	15	1	0	207	0.1	27	150	54	0.01	0.10	Tr	0
Parmesan, grated:																		
Tablespoon	1 tbsp. (5)	18	25	2	2	1.0	4	Tr	0	69	Tr	5	93	9	Tr	0.02	Tr	0
Ounce	1 oz. (28)	18	130	12	9	5.4	22	1	0	390	0.3	30	528	49	0.01	0.11	0.1	0
Swiss	1 oz. (28)	37	105	8	8	5.0	26	1	0	272	Tr	31	74	72	0.01	0.10	Tr	0
Pasteurized process cheese:																		
American	1 oz. (28)	39	105	6	9	5.6	27	Tr	0	174	0.1	46	406	82	0.01	0.10	Tr	0
Swiss	1 oz. (28)	42	95	7	7	4.6	24	1	0	219	0.2	61	388	65	Tr	0.08	Tr	0
Pasteurized process cheese: food, American	1 oz. (28)	43	95	6	7	4.4	18	2	0	163	0.2	79	337	62	0.01	0.13	Tr	0
spread, American	1 oz. (28)	48	80	5	6	3.8	16	2	0	159	0.1	69	381	54	0.01	0.12	Tr	0
Cream, sweet:																		
Half-and-half (cream and milk)	1 cup (242)	81	315	7	28	17.3	89	10	0	254	0.2	314	98	259	0.08	0.36	0.2	2
	1 tbsp. (15)	81	20	Tr	2	1.1	6	1	0	16	Tr	19	6	16	0.01	0.02	Tr	Tr
Light, coffee, or table	1 cup (240)	74	470	6	46	28.8	159	9	0	231	0.1	292	95	437	0.08	0.36	0.1	2
	1 tbsp. (15)	74	30	Tr	3	1.8	10	1	0	14	Tr	18	6	27	Tr	0.02	Tr	Tr
Whipping, unwhipped (volume about double when whipped):																		
Light	1 cup (239)	64	700	5	74	46.1	265	7	0	166	0.1	231	82	705	0.06	0.30	0.1	1
	1 tbsp. (15)	64	45	Tr	5	2.9	17	Tr	0	10	Tr	15	5	44	Tr	0.02	Tr	Tr
Heavy	1 cup (238)	58	820	5	88	54.7	326	7	0	154	0.1	179	89	1,002	0.05	0.26	0.1	1
	1 tbsp. (15)	58	50	Tr	6	3.4	21	Tr	0	10	Tr	11	6	63	Tr	0.02	Tr	Tr
Whipped topping, (pressurized)	1 cup (60)	61	155	2	13	8.3	46	7	0	61	Tr	88	78	124	0.02	0.04	Tr	Tr
	1 tbsp. (3)	61	10	Tr	1	0.6	2	Tr	0	3	Tr	4	4	6	Tr	Tr	Tr	Tr
Cream, sour	1 cup (230)	71	495	7	48	29.9	102	10	0	268	0.1	331	123	448	0.08	0.34	0.2	2
	1 tbsp. (12)	71	25	Tr	3	1.8	5	1	0	14	Tr	17	6	23	Tr	0.02	Tr	Tr
Cream products, imitation (made with vegetable fat): Whipped topping:																		
Frozen	1 cup (75)	50	240	1	19	16.4	0	17	0	5	0.1	14	19	[5]65	0.00	0.00	0.0	0
	1 tbsp. (4)	50	15	Tr	1	1.1	0	1	0	Tr	Tr	1	1	[5]3	0.00	0.00	0.0	0
Pressurized	1 cup (70)	60	185	1	16	13.2	0	11	0	4	Tr	13	43	[5]33	0.00	0.00	0.0	0
	1 tbsp. (4)	60	10	Tr	1	0.8	0	1	0	Tr	Tr	1	2	[5]2	0.00	0.00	0.0	0
Ice cream. See Milk desserts, frozen.																		
Ice milk. See Milk desserts, frozen.																		
Milk: Fluid:																		
Whole (3.3% fat)	1 cup (244)	88	150	8	8	5.1	33	11	0	291	0.1	370	120	76	0.09	0.40	0.2	2
Lowfat (2%): No milk solids added	1 cup (244)	89	120	8	5	2.9	18	12	0	297	0.1	377	122	139	0.10	0.40	0.2	2
Milk solids added, label claim less than 10 g of protein per cup	1 cup (245)	89	125	9	5	2.9	18	12	0	313	0.1	397	128	140	0.10	0.42	0.2	2
Lowfat (1%): No milk solids added	1 cup (244)	90	100	8	3	1.6	10	12	0	300	0.1	381	123	144	0.10	0.41	0.2	2
Milk solids added, label claim less than 10 g of protein per cup	1 cup (245)	90	105	9	2	1.5	10	12	0	313	0.1	397	128	145	0.10	0.42	0.2	2
Fat free (skim): No milk solids added	1 cup (245)	91	85	8	Tr	0.3	4	12	0	302	0.1	406	126	149	0.09	0.34	0.2	2
Milk solids added, label claim less than 10 g of protein per cup	1 cup (245)	90	90	9	1	0.4	5	12	0	316	0.1	418	130	149	0.10	0.43	0.2	2
Buttermilk	1 cup (245)	90	100	8	2	1.3	9	12	0	285	0.1	371	257	20	0.08	0.38	0.1	2
Canned: Condensed, sweetened	1 cup (306)	27	980	24	27	16.8	104	166	0	868	0.6	1,136	389	248	0.28	1.27	0.6	8
Evaporated: Whole milk	1 cup (252)	74	340	17	19	11.6	74	25	0	657	0.5	764	267	136	0.12	0.80	0.5	5
Nonfat milk	1 cup (255)	79	200	19	1	0.3	9	29	0	738	0.7	845	293	298	0.11	0.79	0.4	3
Dried: Nonfat, instantized: Envelope, 3.2 oz., net wt.[6]	1 envelope (91)	4	325	32	1	0.4	17	47	0	1,120	0.3	1,552	499	[7]646	0.38	1.59	0.8	5

Nutritive Values of Foods – Continued
(Tr indicates nutrient present in trace amount.)

Item No. (A)	Foods, approximate measures, units, and weight (edible portion only) (B)		Water (C) Percent	Food energy (D) Calories	Protein (E) Grams	Fat (F) Grams	Saturated fat (G) Grams	Cholesterol (H) Milligrams	Carbohydrate (I) Grams	Dietary fiber (J) Grams	Calcium (K) Milligrams	Iron (L) Milligrams	Potassium (M) Milligrams	Sodium (N) Milligrams	Vitamin A (O) Micrograms	Thiamin (P) Milligrams	Riboflavin (Q) Milligrams	Niacin (R) Milligrams	Vitamin C (S) Milligrams
		Grams																	
	Milk beverages:																		
	Chocolate milk (commercial):																		
	Regular	1 cup	250	82	210	8	8	5.2	31	26	3	280	0.6	417	149	73	0.09	0.41	0.3	2
	Lowfat (2%)	1 cup	250	84	180	8	5	3.1	17	26	3	284	0.6	422	151	143	0.09	0.41	0.3	2
	Lowfat (1%)	1 cup	250	85	160	8	3	1.5	7	26	3	287	0.6	425	152	148	0.10	0.42	0.3	2
	Cocoa and chocolate-flavored beverages:																		
	Powder containing nonfat dry milk	1 oz.	28	1	100	3	1	0.7	1	22	Tr	90	0.3	223	139	Tr	0.03	0.17	0.2	Tr
	Powder without nonfat dry milk	3/4 oz.	21	1	75	1	1	0.4	0	19	1	7	0.7	136	56	Tr	Tr	0.03	0.1	Tr
	Eggnog (commercial)	1 cup	254	74	340	10	19	11.3	149	34	0	330	0.5	420	138	203	0.09	0.48	0.3	4
	Malted milk:																		
	Chocolate:																		
	Powder	3/4 oz.	21	2	85	1	1	0.5	1	18	Tr	13	0.4	130	49	5	0.04	0.04	0.4	0
	Shakes, thick:																		
	Chocolate	10-oz. container	283	72	335	9	8	6.5	30	60	Tr	374	0.9	634	314	59	0.13	0.63	0.4	0
	Vanilla	10-oz. container	283	74	315	11	9	5.3	33	50	Tr	413	0.3	517	270	79	0.08	0.55	0.4	0
	Milk desserts, frozen:																		
	Ice cream, vanilla:																		
	Regular (about 11% fat):																		
	Hardened	1/2 gal.	1,064	61	2,155	38	115	72.4	476	254	1	1,406	1.0	2,052	929	1,064	0.42	2.63	1.1	6
		1 cup	133	61	270	5	14	9.0	59	32	Tr	176	0.1	257	116	133	0.05	0.33	0.1	1
	Soft serve (frozen custard)	1 cup	173	60	375	7	23	12.9	153	38	Tr	236	0.4	338	153	199	0.08	0.45	0.2	1
	Ice milk, vanilla:																		
	Hardened (about 4% fat)	1/2 gal.	1,048	69	1,470	41	45	27.7	146	232	1	1,409	1.5	2,117	836	419	0.61	2.78	0.9	6
		1 cup	131	69	185	5	6	3.5	18	29	Tr	176	0.2	265	105	52	0.08	0.35	0.1	1
	Soft serve (about 3% fat)	1 cup	175	70	225	8	5	2.8	13	38	Tr	274	0.3	412	163	44	0.12	0.54	0.2	1
	Sherbet (about 2% fat)	1/2 gal.	1,542	66	2,160	17	31	17.9	113	469	0	827	2.5	1,585	706	308	0.26	0.71	1.0	31
		1 cup	193	66	270	2	4	2.2	14	59	0	103	0.3	198	88	39	0.03	0.09	0.1	4
	Yogurt:																		
	With added milk solids:																		
	Made with lowfat milk:																		
	Fruit-flavored[8]	8-oz. container	227	74	230	10	2	1.6	10	43	1	345	0.2	442	133	25	0.08	0.40	0.2	1
	Plain	8-oz. container	227	85	145	12	4	2.3	14	16	0	415	0.2	531	159	36	0.10	0.49	0.3	2
	Made with nonfat milk	8-oz. container	227	85	125	13	Tr	0.3	4	17	0	452	0.2	579	174	5	0.11	0.53	0.3	2
	Eggs																		
	Eggs, large (24 oz. per dozen):																		
	Raw:																		
	Whole, without shell	1 egg	50	75	80	6	6	1.6	274	1	0	28	1.0	65	69	78	0.04	0.15	Tr	0
	White	1 white	33	88	15	3	Tr	0.0	0	Tr	0	4	Tr	45	50	0	Tr	0.09	Tr	0
	Yolk	1 yolk	17	49	65	3	6	1.6	272	Tr	0	26	0.9	15	8	94	0.04	0.07	Tr	0
	Cooked:																		
	Fried in butter	1 egg	46	68	95	6	7	1.9	278	1	0	29	1.1	66	162	94	0.04	0.14	Tr	0
	Hard-cooked, shell removed	1 egg	50	75	80	6	6	1.6	274	1	0	28	1.0	65	69	78	0.04	0.14	Tr	0
	Poached	1 egg	50	74	80	6	6	1.6	273	1	0	28	1.0	65	146	78	0.03	0.13	Tr	0
	Scrambled (milk added) in butter. Also omelet	1 egg	64	73	110	7	8	2.2	282	2	0	54	1.0	97	176	102	0.04	0.18	Tr	Tr
	Fats and Oils																		
	Butter (4 sticks per lb.):																		
	Tablespoon (1/8 stick)	1 tbsp.	14	16	100	Tr	11	7.1	31	Tr	0	3	Tr	4	[9]116	[10]106	Tr	Tr	Tr	0
	Pat (1 in. square, 1/3 in. high; 90 per lb.)	1 pat	5	16	35	Tr	4	2.5	11	Tr	0	1	Tr	1	[9]41	[10]38	Tr	Tr	Tr	0
	Fats, cooking (vegetable shortenings)	1 cup	205	0	1,810	0	205	51.5	0	0	0	0	0.0	0	0	0	0.00	0.00	0.0	0
		1 tbsp.	13	0	115	0	13	3.3	0	0	0	0	0.0	0	0	0	0.00	0.00	0.0	0

(A)	(B)	g	(C)	(D)	(E)	(F)	(G)	(H)	(I)	(J)	(K)	(L)	(M)	(N)	(O)	(P)	(Q)	(R)	(S)
Margarine:																			
Imitation (about 40% fat), soft	8-oz container	227	58	785	1	88	14.5	0	1	0	40	0.0	[11]57	2,178	[12]2,254	0.01	0.05	Tr	Tr
	1 tbsp.	14	58	50	Tr	5	0.9	0	Tr	0	2	0.0	4	[11]134	[12]139	Tr	Tr	Tr	Tr
Regular (about 80% fat):																			
Hard (4 sticks per lb.):																			
Tablespoon (1/8 stick)	1 tbsp.	14	16	100	Tr	11	1.8	0	Tr	0	4	Tr	6	[11]132	[12]139	Tr	0.01	Tr	Tr
Pat (1 in. square, 1/3 in. high; 90 per lb.)	1 pat	5	16	35	Tr	4	0.8	0	Tr	0	1	Tr	2	47	[12]50	Tr	Tr	Tr	Tr
8-oz. container	8-oz. container	227	16	1,625	2	183	30.7	0	1	0	60	0.0	[11]86	2,449	[12]2,254	0.02	0.07	Tr	Tr
Soft	1 tbsp.	14	16	100	Tr	11	1.9	0	Tr	0	4	0.0	5	[11]151	[12]139	Tr	Tr	Tr	Tr
Spread (about 60% fat):																			
Hard (4 sticks per lb.):																			
Tablespoon (1/8 stick)	1 tbsp.	14	37	75	Tr	9	2.0	0	0	0	3	0.0	4	[11]139	[12]139	Tr	Tr	Tr	Tr
Pat (1 in. square, 1/3 in. high; 90 per lb.)	1 pat	5	37	25	Tr	3	0.7	0	0	0	1	0.0	1	50	[12]50	Tr	Tr	Tr	Tr
8-oz. container	8-oz. container	227	37	1,225	1	138	29.1	0	0	0	47	0.0	[11]68	2,256	[12]2,254	0.02	0.06	Tr	Tr
Soft	1 tbsp.	14	37	75	Tr	9	1.8	0	0	0	3	0.0	4	[11]139	[12]139	Tr	Tr	Tr	Tr
Oils, salad or cooking:																			
Corn	1 cup	218	0	1,925	0	218	29.4	0	0	0	0	0.0	0	0	0	0.00	0.00	0.0	0
	1 tbsp.	14	0	125	0	14	1.8	0	0	0	0	0.0	0	0	0	0.00	0.00	0.0	0
Safflower	1 cup	218	0	1,925	0	218	19.8	0	0	0	0	0.0	0	0	0	0.00	0.00	0.0	0
	1 tbsp.	14	0	125	0	14	1.3	0	0	0	0	0.0	0	0	0	0.00	0.00	0.0	0
Soybean oil, hydrogenated (partially hardened)	1 cup	218	0	1,925	0	218	31.4	0	0	0	0	0.0	0	0	0	0.00	0.00	0.0	0
	1 tbsp.	14	0	125	0	14	2.0	0	0	0	0	0.0	0	0	0	0.00	0.00	0.0	0
Sunflower	1 cup	218	0	1,925	0	218	25.0	0	0	0	0	0.0	0	0	0	0.00	0.00	0.0	0
	1 tbsp.	14	0	125	0	14	1.5	0	0	0	0	0.0	0	0	0	0.00	0.00	0.0	0
Salad dressings:																			
Commercial:																			
Blue cheese	1 tbsp.	15	32	75	1	8	1.5	3	1	Tr	12	Tr	6	164	10	Tr	0.02	Tr	Tr
French:																			
Regular	1 tbsp.	16	35	85	Tr	9	1.5	0	1	Tr	2	Tr	2	188	Tr	Tr	Tr	Tr	Tr
Low calorie	1 tbsp.	16	75	25	Tr	2	0.1	0	2	Tr	6	Tr	3	306	Tr	Tr	Tr	Tr	Tr
Italian:																			
Regular	1 tbsp.	15	34	80	Tr	9	1.0	0	1	Tr	1	Tr	5	162	3	Tr	Tr	Tr	Tr
Low calorie	1 tbsp.	15	86	5	Tr	Tr	0.2	0	2	Tr	1	Tr	4	136	Tr	Tr	Tr	Tr	Tr
Mayonnaise:																			
Regular	1 tbsp.	14	15	100	Tr	11	1.6	8	Tr	0	3	0.1	5	80	12	0.00	0.00	0.0	0
Imitation	1 tbsp.	15	63	35	Tr	3	0.5	4	2	0	Tr	0.0	2	75	9	0.00	0.00	0.0	0
Tartar sauce	1 tbsp.	14	34	75	Tr	8	1.5	4	1	Tr	3	0.1	11	182	9	Tr	Tr	0.0	Tr
Thousand island:																			
Regular	1 tbsp.	16	46	60	Tr	6	1.0	4	2	Tr	2	0.1	18	112	15	Tr	Tr	Tr	0
Low calorie	1 tbsp.	15	69	25	Tr	2	0.2	2	2	Tr	2	0.1	17	150	14	Tr	Tr	Tr	0
Prepared from home recipe:																			
Cooked type	1 tbsp.	16	69	25	1	2	0.5	9	2	Tr	13	0.1	19	117	20	0.01	0.02	Tr	Tr
Vinegar and oil	1 tbsp.	16	47	70	0	8	1.5	0	Tr	0	0	0.0	1	Tr	1	0.00	0.00	0.0	0
Fish and Shellfish																			
Clams:																			
Raw, meat only	3 oz	85	82	65	11	1	0.1	43	2	0	59	2.6	154	102	26	0.09	0.15	1.1	9
Crabmeat, canned	1 cup	135	77	135	23	3	0.3	135	1	0	61	1.1	149	1,350	14	0.11	0.11	2.6	0
Fish sticks, frozen, reheated, (stick, 4 by 1 by 1/2 in.)	1 fish stick	28	52	70	6	3	0.9	26	4	Tr	11	0.3	94	53	5	0.03	0.05	0.6	0
Haddock, breaded, fried[14]	3 oz	85	61	175	17	9	3.2	75	7	1	34	1.0	270	123	20	0.06	0.10	2.9	0
Halibut, broiled, with butter and lemon juice	3 oz	85	67	140	20	6	0.5	62	Tr	0	14	0.7	441	103	174	0.06	0.07	7.7	1
Salmon:																			
Canned (pink), solids and liquid	3 oz	85	71	120	17	5	1.7	34	0	0	[15]167	0.7	307	443	18	0.03	0.15	6.8	0
Sardines, Atlantic, canned in oil, drained solids	3 oz	85	62	175	20	9	1.7	85	0	0	[15]371	2.6	349	425	56	0.03	0.17	4.6	0
Scallops, breaded, frozen, reheated	6 scallops	90	59	195	15	10	2.5	70	10	Tr	39	2.0	369	298	21	0.11	0.11	1.6	1
Shrimp:																			
Canned, drained solids	3 oz	85	70	100	21	1	0.2	128	1	0	98	1.4	1	1,955	15	0.01	0.03	1.5	0
French fried (7 medium)[16]	3 oz	85	55	200	16	10	3.8	168	11	Tr	61	2.0	189	384	26	0.06	0.09	2.8	0
Tuna, canned, drained solids:																			
Oil pack, chunk light	3 oz	85	61	165	24	7	1.3	55	0	0	7	1.6	298	303	20	0.04	0.09	10.1	0
Water pack, solid white	3 oz	85	63	135	30	1	0.2	48	0	0	17	0.6	255	468	32	0.03	0.10	13.4	0

Nutritive Values of Foods – Continued
(Tr indicates nutrient present in trace amount.)

Item No. (A)	Foods, approximate measures, units, and weight (weight of edible portion only) (B)	(B) Grams	Water (C) Percent	Food energy (D) Calories	Protein (E) Grams	Fat (F) Grams	Saturated fat (G) Grams	Cholesterol (H) Milligrams	Carbohydrate (I) Grams	Dietary fiber (J) Grams	Calcium (K) Milligrams	Iron (L) Milligrams	Potassium (M) Milligrams	Sodium (N) Milligrams	Vitamin A (O) Micrograms	Thiamin (P) Milligrams	Riboflavin (Q) Milligrams	Niacin (R) Milligrams	Vitamin C (S) Milligrams
Fruits and Fruit Juices																			
	Apples:																		
	Raw:																		
	Unpeeled, without cores:																		
	2-3/4-in. diam. (about 3 per lb. with cores)	1 apple 138	84	80	Tr	Tr	0.1	0	21	3	10	0.2	159	Tr	7	0.02	0.02	0.1	8
	Peeled, sliced	1 cup 110	84	65	Tr	Tr	0.1	0	16	2	4	0.1	124	Tr	5	0.02	0.01	0.1	4
	Dried, sulfured	10 rings 64	32	155	1	Tr	Tr	0	42	6	9	0.9	288	1856	0	0.00	0.10	0.6	2
	Apple juice, bottled or canned[19]	1 cup 248	88	115	Tr	Tr	Tr	0	29	Tr	17	0.9	295	7	Tr	0.05	0.04	0.2	20[2]
	Applesauce, canned:																		
	Sweetened	1 cup 255	80	195	Tr	Tr	Tr	0	51	3	10	0.9	156	8	3	0.03	0.07	0.5	20[4]
	Unsweetened	1 cup 244	88	105	Tr	Tr	Tr	0	28	3	7	0.3	183	5	7	0.03	0.06	0.5	20[3]
	Apricots:																		
	Raw, without pits (about 12 per lb. with pits)	3 apricots 106	86	50	1	Tr	Tr	0	12	2	15	0.6	314	1	277	0.03	0.04	0.6	11
	Canned (fruit and liquid):																		
	Heavy syrup pack	1 cup 258	78	215	1	Tr	Tr	0	55	3	23	0.8	361	10	317	0.05	0.06	1.0	8
	Juice pack	1 cup 248	87	120	2	Tr	Tr	0	31	3	30	0.7	409	10	419	0.04	0.05	0.9	12
	Dried:																		
	Uncooked (28 large or 37 medium halves per cup)	1 cup 130	31	310	5	1	Tr	0	80	6	59	6.1	1,791	13	941	0.01	0.20	3.9	3
	Apricot nectar, canned	1 cup 251	85	140	1	Tr	Tr	0	36	2	18	1.0	286	8	330	0.02	0.04	0.7	20[2]
	Avocados, raw, whole, without skin and seed:																		
	California (about 2 per lb. with skin and seed)	1 avocado 173	73	305	4	30	4.5	0	12	6	19	2.0	1,097	21	106	0.19	0.21	3.3	14
	Bananas, raw, without peel:																		
	Whole (about 2-1/2 per lb. with peel)	1 banana 114	74	105	1	1	0.2	0	27	2	7	0.4	451	1	9	0.05	0.11	0.6	10
	Blackberries, raw	1 cup 144	86	75	1	1	0.3	0	18	6	46	0.8	282	Tr	24	0.04	0.06	0.6	30
	Blueberries:																		
	Raw	1 cup 145	85	80	1	1	Tr	0	20	4	9	0.2	129	9	15	0.07	0.07	0.5	19
	Frozen, sweetened	10-oz. container 284	77	230	1	Tr	0.1	0	62	6	17	1.1	170	3	12	0.06	0.15	0.7	3
	Cantaloupe. See Melons																		
	Cherries:																		
	Sour, red, pitted, canned, water pack	1 cup 244	90	90	2	Tr	0.1	0	22	2	27	3.3	239	17	184	0.04	0.10	0.4	5
	Sweet, raw, without pits and stems	10 cherries 68	81	50	1	1	0.1	0	11	Tr	10	0.3	152	Tr	15	0.03	0.04	0.3	5
	Cranberry juice cocktail, bottled, sweetened	1 cup 253	85	145	Tr	Tr	0.1	0	38	Tr	8	0.4	61	10	1	0.01	0.04	0.1	21[108]
	Cranberry sauce, sweetened, canned, strained	1 cup 277	61	420	1	Tr	Tr	0	108	3	11	0.6	72	80	6	0.04	0.06	0.3	6
	Dates:																		
	Whole, without pits	10 dates 83	23	230	2	Tr	0.2	0	61	6	27	1.0	541	2	4	0.07	0.08	1.8	0
	Fruit cocktail, canned, fruit and liquid:																		
	Heavy syrup pack	1 cup 255	80	185	1	Tr	Tr	0	48	3	15	0.7	224	15	52	0.05	0.05	1.0	5
	Juice pack	1 cup 248	87	115	1	Tr	Tr	0	29	3	20	0.5	236	10	76	0.03	0.04	1.0	7
	Grapefruit:																		
	Raw, without peel, membrane and seeds (3-3/4 in. diam., 1 lb. 1 oz., whole, with refuse)	1/2 grapefruit 120	91	40	1	Tr	Tr	0	10	1	14	0.1	167	Tr	22[1]	0.04	0.02	0.3	41
	Grapefruit juice:																		
	Canned:																		
	Unsweetened	1 cup 247	90	95	1	Tr	Tr	0	22	Tr	17	0.5	378	2	2	0.10	0.05	0.6	72
	Sweetened	1 cup 250	87	115	1	Tr	Tr	0	28	Tr	20	0.9	405	5	2	0.10	0.06	0.8	67
	Frozen concentrate, unsweetened																		
	Diluted with 3 parts water by volume	1 cup 247	89	100	1	Tr	0.1	0	24	Tr	20	0.3	336	2	2	0.10	0.05	0.5	83
	Grapes, European type (adherent skin), raw:																		
	Thompson seedless	10 grapes 50	81	35	Tr	Tr	0.1	0	9	Tr	6	0.1	93	1	4	0.05	0.03	0.2	5
	Grape juice:																		
	Canned or bottled	1 cup 253	84	155	1	Tr	0.1	0	38	2	23	0.6	334	8	2	0.07	0.09	0.7	20[Tr]
	Frozen concentrate, sweetened:																		
	Diluted with 3 parts water by volume	1 cup 250	87	125	Tr	Tr	0.1	0	32	Tr	10	0.3	53	5	2	0.04	0.07	0.3	21[60]
	Lemons, raw, without peel and seeds (about 4 per lb. with peel and seeds)	1 lemon 58	89	15	1	Tr	Tr	0	5	2	15	0.3	80	1	2	0.02	0.01	0.1	31

(A)	(B)	(C)	(D)	(E)	(F)	(G)	(H)	(I)	(J)	(K)	(L)	(M)	(N)	(O)	(P)	(Q)	(R)	(S)
Lemon juice: Canned or bottled, unsweetened	1 cup, 244	92	50	1	1	0.1	0	16	1	27	0.3	249	[2]351	4	0.10	0.02	0.5	61
Frozen, single-strength, unsweetened	6 fl. oz. can, 244	92	55	1	1	0.1	0	16	1	20	0.3	217	2	3	0.14	0.03	0.3	77
Lime juice: Canned, unsweetened	1 cup, 246	93	50	1	1	0.1	0	16	1	30	0.6	185	[2]339	4	0.08	0.01	0.4	16
Melons, raw, without rind and cavity contents: Cantaloupe, orange-fleshed (5 in. diam., 2-1/3 lb., whole, with rind and cavity contents)	1/2 melon, 267	90	95	2	1	0.1	0	22	2	29	0.6	825	24	861	0.10	0.06	1.5	113
Honeydew (6-1/2 in. diam., 5-1/4 lb., whole, with rind and cavity contents)	1/10 melon, 129	90	45	1	Tr	Tr	0	12	1	8	0.1	350	13	5	0.10	0.02	0.8	32
Nectarines, raw, without pits (about 3 per lb. with pits) 1 nectarine	1 nectarine, 136	86	65	1	Tr	0.1	0	16	2	7	0.2	288	Tr	100	0.02	0.06	1.3	7
Oranges, raw: Whole, without peel and seeds (2-5/8 in. diam., about 2-1/2 per lb., with peel and seeds)	1 orange, 131	87	60	1	Tr	Tr	0	15	3	52	0.1	237	Tr	27	0.11	0.05	0.4	70
Orange juice: Raw, all varieties	1 cup, 248	88	110	2	Tr	0.1	0	26	Tr	27	0.5	496	2	50	0.22	0.07	1.0	124
Canned, unsweetened	1 cup, 249	89	105	1	Tr	Tr	0	25	Tr	20	1.1	436	5	44	0.15	0.07	0.8	86
Frozen concentrate: Diluted with 3 parts water by volume	1 cup, 249	88	110	2	Tr	Tr	0	27	Tr	22	0.2	473	2	19	0.20	0.04	0.5	97
Orange and grapefruit juice, canned	1 cup, 247	89	105	1	Tr	Tr	0	25	Tr	20	1.1	390	7	29	0.14	0.07	0.8	72
Peaches: Raw: Whole, 2-1/2 in. diam., peeled, pitted (about 4 per lb. with peels and pits)	1 peach, 87	88	35	1	Tr	Tr	0	10	2	4	0.1	171	Tr	47	0.01	0.04	0.9	6
Canned, fruit and liquid: Heavy syrup pack	1 cup, 256	79	190	1	Tr	Tr	0	51	3	8	0.7	236	15	85	0.03	0.06	1.6	7
Juice pack	1 cup, 248	87	110	2	Tr	Tr	0	29	4	15	0.7	317	10	94	0.02	0.04	1.4	9
Dried: Uncooked	1 cup, 160	32	380	6	1	0.1	0	98	12	45	6.5	1,594	11	346	Tr	0.34	7.0	8
Frozen, sliced, sweetened 10 oz. container	10-oz container, 284	75	265	2	Tr	Tr	0	68	4	9	1.1	369	17	81	0.04	0.10	1.9	[21]268
	1 cup, 250	75	235	2	Tr	Tr	0	60	4	8	0.9	325	15	71	0.03	0.09	1.6	[21]236
Pears: Raw, with skin, cored: Bartlett, 2-1/2 in. diam. (about 2-1/2 per lb. with cores and stems)	1 pear, 166	84	100	1	1	Tr	0	25	4	18	0.4	208	Tr	3	0.03	0.07	0.2	7
Bosc, 2-1/2 in. diam. (about 3 per lb. with cores and stems)	1 pear, 141	84	85	1	1	Tr	0	21	3	16	0.4	176	Tr	3	0.03	0.06	0.1	6
Canned, fruit and liquid: Heavy syrup pack	1 cup, 255	80	190	1	Tr	Tr	0	49	5	13	0.6	166	13	1	0.03	0.06	0.6	3
Juice pack	1 cup, 248	86	125	1	Tr	Tr	0	32	5	22	0.7	238	10	1	0.03	0.03	0.5	4
Pineapple: Raw, diced	1 cup, 155	87	75	1	1	Tr	0	19	2	11	0.6	175	2	4	0.14	0.06	0.7	24
Canned, fruit and liquid: Heavy syrup pack: Crushed, chunks, tidbits	1 cup, 255	79	200	1	Tr	Tr	0	52	1	36	1.0	265	3	4	0.23	0.06	0.7	19
Juice pack: Chunks or tidbits	1 cup, 250	84	150	1	Tr	Tr	0	39	2	35	0.7	305	3	10	0.24	0.05	0.7	24
Pineapple juice, unsweetened, canned	1 cup, 250	86	140	1	Tr	Tr	0	34	Tr	43	0.7	335	3	1	0.14	0.06	0.6	27
Plums, without pits: Raw: 2-1/8 in. diam. (about 6-1/2 per lb. with pits)	1 plum, 66	85	35	1	Tr	Tr	0	9	1	3	0.1	114	Tr	21	0.03	0.06	0.3	6
Canned, purple, fruit and liquid: Heavy syrup pack	1 cup, 258	76	230	1	Tr	Tr	0	60	3	23	2.2	235	49	67	0.04	0.10	0.8	1
Juice pack	1 cup, 252	84	145	1	Tr	Tr	0	38	3	25	0.9	388	3	254	0.06	0.15	1.2	7
Prunes, dried: Uncooked	4 extra large or 5 large prunes, 49	32	115	1	Tr	Tr	0	31	4	25	1.2	365	2	97	0.04	0.08	1.0	2
Cooked, unsweetened, fruit and liquid	1 cup, 212	70	225	2	Tr	Tr	0	60	14	49	2.4	708	4	65	0.05	0.21	1.5	6
Prune juice, canned or bottled	1 cup, 256	81	180	2	Tr	Tr	0	45	3	31	3.0	707	10	1	0.04	0.18	2.0	10
Raisins, seedless: Cup, not pressed down	1 cup, 145	15	435	5	1	0.2	0	115	5	71	3.0	1,089	17	1	0.23	0.13	1.2	5

Nutritive Values of Foods – Continued
(Tr indicates nutrient present in trace amount.)

Nutrients in Indicated Quantity

Item No. (A)	Foods, approximate measures, units, and weight (weight of edible portion only) (B)		Water (C) Per-cent	Food energy (D) Cal-ories	Pro-tein (E) Grams	Fat (F) Grams	Satur-ated fat (G) Grams	Cho-lesterol (H) Milli-grams	Carbo-hydrate (I) Grams	Dietary fiber (J) Grams	Calcium (K) Milli-grams	Iron (L) Milli-grams	Potas-sium (M) Milli-grams	Sodium (N) Milli-grams	Vitamin A (O) Micro-grams	Thiamin (P) Milli-grams	Ribo-flavin (Q) Milli-grams	Niacin (R) Milli-grams	Vitamin C (S) Milli-grams
		Grams																	
Raspberries:																			
	Raw	1 cup	123	87	60	1	1	Tr	0	14	5	27	0.7	187	Tr	16	0.04	0.11	1.1	31
	Frozen, sweetened	10-oz. container	284	73	295	2	Tr	Tr	0	74	5	43	1.8	324	3	17	0.05	0.13	0.7	47
	Rhubarb, cooked, added sugar	1 cup	240	68	280	1	Tr	Tr	0	75	5	348	0.5	230	2	17	0.04	0.06	0.5	8
Strawberries:																			
	Raw, capped, whole	1 cup	149	92	45	1	1	Tr	0	10	2	21	0.6	247	1	4	0.03	0.10	0.3	84
Tangerines:																			
	Raw, without peel and seeds (2-3/8 in. diam., about 4 per lb., with peel and seeds)	1 tangerine	84	88	35	1	Tr	Tr	0	9	1	12	0.1	132	1	77	0.09	0.02	0.1	26
Watermelon, raw, without rind and seeds:																			
	Piece (4 by 8 in wedge with rind and seeds; 1/16 of 32-2/3 lb. melon, 10 by 16 in.)	1 piece	482	92	155	3	2	0.6	0	35	1	39	0.8	559	10	176	0.39	0.10	1.0	46
Grain Products																			
	Bagels, plain or water, enriched, 3-1/2 in. diam.[24]	1 bagel	68	29	200	7	2	0.1	0	38	2	29	1.8	50	245	0	0.26	0.20	2.4	0
	Biscuits, baking powder, 2 in. diam. (enriched flour, vegetable shortening):																			
	From home recipe	1 biscuit	28	28	100	2	5	1.2	Tr	13	Tr	47	0.7	32	195	3	0.08	0.08	0.8	Tr
	From mix	1 biscuit	28	29	95	2	3	0.8	Tr	14	1	58	0.7	56	262	4	0.12	0.11	0.8	Tr
	From refrigerated dough	1 biscuit	20	30	65	1	2	2.0	1	10	Tr	4	0.5	18	249	0	0.08	0.05	0.7	0
	Breads:																			
	Cracked-wheat bread (3/4 enriched wheat flour, 1/4 cracked wheat flour):[25]																			
	Slice (18 per loaf)	1 slice	25	35	65	2	1	0.2	0	12	2	16	0.7	34	106	Tr	0.10	0.09	0.8	Tr
	French or Vienna bread, enriched:[25]																			
	Slice:																			
	French, 5 by 2-1/2 by 1 in.	1 slice	35	34	100	3	1	0.2	0	18	1	39	1.1	32	203	Tr	0.16	0.12	1.4	Tr
	Vienna, 4-3/4 by 4 by 1/2 in.	1 slice	25	34	70	2	1	0.2	0	13	1	28	0.8	23	145	Tr	0.12	0.09	1.0	Tr
	Italian bread, enriched:																			
	Slice, 4-1/2 by 3-1/4 by 3/4 in.	1 slice	30	32	85	3	Tr	0.3	0	17	1	5	0.8	22	176	0	0.12	0.07	1.0	0
	Pita bread, enriched, white, 6-1/2 in. diam.	1 pita	60	31	165	6	1	0.1	0	33	1	49	1.4	71	339	0	0.27	0.12	2.2	0
	Pumpernickel (2/3 rye flour, 1/3 enriched wheat flour):[25]																			
	Slice, 5 by 4 by 3/8 in.	1 slice	32	37	80	3	1	0.1	0	16	1	23	0.9	141	177	0	0.11	0.17	1.1	0
	Raisin bread, enriched:[25]																			
	Slice (18 per loaf)	1 slice	25	33	65	2	1	0.3	0	13	1	25	0.8	59	92	Tr	0.08	0.15	1.0	Tr
	Rye bread, light (2/3 enriched wheat flour, 1/3 rye flour):[25]																			
	Slice, 4-3/4 by 3-3/4 by 7/16 in.	1 slice	25	37	65	2	1	0.2	0	12	2	20	0.7	51	175	0	0.10	0.08	0.8	0
	Wheat bread, enriched:[25]																			
	Slice (18 per loaf)	1 slice	25	37	65	2	1	0.2	0	12	1	32	0.9	35	138	Tr	0.12	0.08	1.2	Tr
	White bread, enriched:[25]																			
	Slice (18 per loaf)	1 slice	25	37	65	2	1	0.2	0	12	1	32	0.7	28	129	Tr	0.12	0.08	0.9	Tr
	Slice (22 per loaf)	1 slice	20	37	55	2	1	0.2	0	10	1	25	0.6	22	101	Tr	0.09	0.06	0.7	Tr
	Cubes	1 cup	30	37	80	2	1	0.2	0	15	1	38	0.9	34	154	Tr	0.14	0.09	1.1	Tr
	Crumbs, soft	1 cup	45	37	120	4	2	0.3	0	22	1	57	1.3	50	231	Tr	0.21	0.14	1.7	Tr
	Whole-wheat bread:[25]																			
	Slice (16 per loaf)	1 slice	28	38	70	3	1	0.3	0	13	2	20	1.0	50	180	Tr	0.10	0.06	1.1	Tr
	Bread stuffing (from enriched bread), prepared from mix:																			
	Dry type	1 cup	140	33	500	9	31	2.4	0	50	4	92	2.2	126	1,254	273	0.17	0.20	2.5	0

(A)	(B)	(C)	(D)	(E)	(F)	(G)	(H)	(I)	(J)	(K)	(L)	(M)	(N)	(O)	(P)	(Q)	(R)	(S)
Moist type	1 cup	203	420	9	26	3.0	67	40	4	81	2.0	118	1,023	256	0.10	0.18	1.6	0
Breakfast cereals:																		
Hot type, cooked:																		
Corn (hominy) grits:																		
Regular and quick, enriched	1 cup	242	145	3	Tr	0.1	0	31	5	0	[27]1.5	53	280	[29]0	[27]0.24	[27]0.15	[27]2.0	0
Instant, plain	1 pkt.	137	80	2	Tr	Tr	0	18	Tr	7	[27]1.0	29	343	0	[27]0.18	[27]0.08	[27]1.3	0
Cream of Wheat®:																		
Regular, quick, instant	1 cup	244	140	4	Tr	0.1	0	29	1	[30]54	[30]10.9	46	31,325	0	[30]0.24	[30]0.07	[30]1.5	0
Mix'n Eat, plain	1 pkt.	142	100	3	Tr	Tr	0	21	Tr	[30]20	[30]8.1	38	241	[30]376	[30]0.43	[30]0.28	[30]5.0	[30]15
Malt-O-Meal®	1 cup	240	120	4	Tr	Tr	0	26	1	5	[30]9.6	31	332	0	[30]0.48	[30]0.24	[30]5.8	[30]15
Oatmeal or rolled oats:																		
Regular, quick, instant, nonfortified	1 cup	234	145	6	2	0.4	0	25	4	19	1.6	131	342	4	0.26	0.05	0.3	0
Instant, fortified:																		
Plain	1 pkt.	177	105	4	2	0.3	0	18	3	[27]163	[27]6.3	99	[27]285	[27]453	[27]0.53	[27]0.28	[27]5.5	0
Ready-to-eat:																		
All-Bran® (about 1/3 cup)	1 oz.	28	70	4	1	0.1	0	21	10	23	[30]4.5	350	320	[30]375	[30]0.37	[30]0.43	[30]5.0	[30]15
Cap'n Crunch® (about 3/4 cup)	1 oz.	28	120	1	3	2.2	0	23	1	5	[27]7.5	37	213	4	[27]0.50	[27]0.55	[27]6.6	[30]15
Cheerios® (about 1-1/4 cup)	1 oz.	28	110	4	2	0.3	0	20	2	48	[30]4.5	101	307	[30]375	[30]0.37	[30]0.43	[30]5.0	[30]15
Corn Flakes (about 1-1/4 cup):																		
Toasties®	1 oz.	28	110	2	Tr	Tr	0	24	1	1	[30]0.7	33	297	[30]375	[30]0.37	[30]0.43	[30]5.0	0
40% Bran Flakes:																		
Kellogg's® (about 3/4 cup)	1 oz.	28	90	4	1	0.1	0	22	6	14	[30]8.1	180	264	[30]375	[30]0.37	[30]0.43	[30]5.0	[30]15
Froot Loops® (about 1 cup)	1 oz.	28	110	2	1	0.2	0	25	1	3	[30]4.5	26	145	[30]375	[30]0.37	[30]0.43	[30]5.0	[30]15
Golden Grahams® (about 3/4 cup)	1 oz.	28	110	2	1	2.9	Tr	24	1	17	[30]4.5	63	346	[30]375	[30]0.37	[30]0.43	[30]5.0	[30]15
Grape-Nuts® (about 1/4 cup)	1 oz.	28	100	3	Tr	Tr	0	23	3	11	1.2	95	197	[30]375	[30]0.37	[30]0.43	[30]5.0	[30]15
Honey Nut Cheerios® (about 3/4 cup)	1 oz.	28	105	3	1	0.1	0	23	1	20	[30]4.5	99	257	[30]375	[30]0.37	[30]0.43	[30]5.0	[30]15
Nature Valley® Granola (about 1/3 cup)	1 oz.	28	125	3	5	5.0	0	19	2	18	0.9	98	58	2	0.10	0.05	0.2	0
Product 19® (about 3/4 cup)	1 oz.	28	110	3	Tr	Tr	0	24	1	3	[30]18.0	44	325	[30]1,501	[30]1.50	[30]1.70	[30]20.0	[30]60
Raisin Bran:																		
Kellogg's® (about 3/4 cup)	1 oz.	28	90	3	1	0.2	0	21	5	10	[30]3.5	147	207	[30]288	[30]0.28	[30]0.34	[30]3.9	0
Rice Krispies® (about 1 cup)	1 oz.	28	110	2	Tr	Tr	0	25	Tr	4	[30]1.8	29	340	[30]375	[30]0.37	[30]0.43	[30]5.0	[30]15
Shredded Wheat (about 2/3 cup)	1 oz.	28	100	3	1	0.2	0	23	4	11	1.2	102	3	0	0.07	0.08	1.5	0
Special K® (about 1-1/3 cup)	1 oz.	28	110	6	Tr	Tr	Tr	21	Tr	8	[30]4.5	49	265	[30]375	[30]0.37	[30]0.43	[30]5.0	[30]15
Frosted Flakes,																		
Kellogg's® (about 3/4 cup)	1 oz.	28	110	1	Tr	Tr	0	26	1	1	[30]1.8	18	230	[30]375	[30]0.37	[30]0.43	[30]5.0	[30]15
Golden Crisps® (about 3/4 cup)	1 oz.	28	105	1	Tr	Tr	0	25	1	3	[30]1.8	42	75	[30]375	[30]0.37	[30]0.43	[30]5.0	[30]15
Total® (about 1 cup)	1 oz.	28	100	3	1	0.1	0	22	4	48	[30]18.0	106	352	[30]1,501	[30]1.50	[30]1.70	[30]20.0	[30]60
Wheaties® (about 1 cup)	1 oz.	28	100	3	Tr	0.1	0	23	3	43	[30]4.5	106	354	[30]375	[30]0.37	[30]0.43	[30]5.0	[30]15
Buckwheat flour, light, sifted	1 cup	98	340	12	1	0.2	0	78	6	11	1.0	314	2	0	0.08	0.04	0.4	0
Cakes prepared from cake mixes with enriched flour:[35]																		
Angel food:																		
Piece, 1/12 of cake	1 piece	53	125	3	Tr	0.1	0	29	1	44	0.2	71	269	0	0.03	0.11	0.1	0
Coffeecake, crumb:																		
Piece, 1/6 of cake	1 piece	72	230	5	7	1.3	47	38	1	44	1.2	78	310	32	0.14	0.15	1.3	Tr
Devil's food with chocolate frosting:																		
Piece, 1/16 of cake	1 piece	69	235	3	8	3.2	37	40	2	41	1.4	90	181	31	0.07	0.10	0.6	Tr
Cupcake, 2-1/2 in. diam.	1 cupcake	35	120	2	4	1.9	19	20	1	21	0.7	46	92	16	0.04	0.05	0.3	Tr
Gingerbread:																		
Piece, 1/9 of cake	1 piece	63	175	2	4	1.6	1	32	2	57	1.2	173	192	0	0.09	0.11	0.8	Tr
Yellow with chocolate frosting:																		
Piece, 1/16 of cake	1 piece	69	235	3	8	3.3	36	40	1	63	1.0	75	157	29	0.08	0.10	0.7	Tr
Cakes prepared from home recipes using enriched flour:																		
Carrot, with cream cheese frosting:[36]																		
Piece, 1/16 of cake	1 piece	96	385	4	21	5.5	74	48	1	44	1.3	108	279	15	0.11	0.12	0.9	1
Fruitcake, dark:[36]																		
Piece, 1/32 of cake, 2/3 in. arc	1 piece	43	165	2	7	0.5	20	25	2	41	1.2	194	67	13	0.08	0.08	0.5	16
Plain sheet cake:[37]																		
Without frosting:																		
Piece, 1/9 of cake	1 piece	86	315	4	12	3.3	61	48	Tr	55	1.3	68	258	41	0.14	0.15	1.1	Tr
With uncooked white frosting:																		
Piece, 1/9 of cake	1 piece	121	445	4	14	2.9	70	77	1	61	1.2	74	275	71	0.13	0.16	1.1	Tr

Nutritive Values of Foods – Continued
(Tr indicates nutrient present in trace amount.)

Nutrients in Indicated Quantity

Item No. / Foods, approximate measures, units, and weight (weight of edible portion only) (A)(B)		Grams	Water (C) Percent	Food energy (D) Calories	Protein (E) Grams	Fat (F) Grams	Saturated fat (G) Grams	Cholesterol (H) Milligrams	Carbohydrate (I) Grams	Dietary fiber (J) Grams	Calcium (K) Milligrams	Iron (L) Milligrams	Potassium (M) Milligrams	Sodium (N) Milligrams	Vitamin A (O) Micrograms	Thiamin (P) Milligrams	Riboflavin (Q) Milligrams	Niacin (R) Milligrams	Vitamin C (S) Milligrams
Pound:[38]																			
Slice, 1/17 of loaf	1 slice	30	22	120	2	5	0.3	32	15	Tr	20	0.5	28	96	60	0.05	0.06	0.5	Tr
Cakes, commercial, made with enriched flour:																			
Pound:																			
Slice, 1/17 of loaf	1 slice	29	24	110	2	5	3.2	64	15	Tr	8	0.5	26	108	41	0.06	0.06	0.5	0
Snack cakes:																			
Devil's food with creme filling (2 small cakes per pkg.)	1 small cake	28	20	105	1	4	0.9	15	17	Tr	21	1.0	34	105	4	0.06	0.09	0.7	0
Sponge with creme filling (2 small cakes per pkg.)	1 small cake	42	19	155	1	5	0.5	7	27	Tr	14	0.6	37	155	9	0.07	0.06	0.6	0
White with white frosting:																			
Piece, 1/16 of cake	1 piece	71	24	260	3	9	2.8	3	42	1	33	1.0	52	176	12	0.20	0.13	1.7	0
Yellow with chocolate frosting:																			
Piece, 1/16 of cake	1 piece	69	23	245	2	11	3.3	38	39	1	23	1.2	123	192	30	0.05	0.14	0.6	0
Cheesecake:																			
Piece, 1/12 of cake	1 piece	92	46	280	5	18	10.6	170	26	2	52	0.4	90	204	69	0.03	0.12	0.4	5
Cookies made with enriched flour:																			
Brownies with nuts:																			
Commercial, with frosting, 1-1/2 by 1-3/4 by 7/8 in.	1 brownie	25	13	100	1	4	1.1	14	16	1	13	0.6	50	59	18	0.08	0.07	0.3	Tr
Chocolate chip:																			
Commercial, 2-1/4 in. diam., 3/8 in. thick	4 cookies	42	4	180	2	9	3.1	5	28	1	13	0.8	68	140	15	0.10	0.23	1.0	Tr
From refrigerated dough, 2-1/4 in. diam., 3/8 in. thick	4 cookies	48	5	225	2	11	3.2	22	32	1	13	1.0	62	173	8	0.06	0.10	0.9	0
Oatmeal with raisins, 2-5/8 in. diam., 1/4 in. thick	4 cookies	52	4	245	3	10	1.7	2	36	2	18	1.1	90	148	12	0.09	0.08	1.0	0
Peanut butter cookie, from home recipe, 2-5/8 in. diam.[25]	4 cookies	48	3	245	4	14	2.1	0	28	1	21	1.1	110	142	5	0.07	0.07	1.9	0
Sandwich type (chocolate or vanilla), 1-3/4 in. diam., 3/8 in. thick	4 cookies	40	2	195	2	8	1.7	0	29	1	12	1.4	66	189	0	0.09	0.07	0.8	0
Sugar cookie, from refrigerated dough, 2-1/2 in. diam., 1/4 in. thick	4 cookies	48	4	235	2	12	2.8	29	31	Tr	50	0.9	33	261	11	0.09	0.06	1.1	0
Vanilla wafers, 1-3/4 in. diam., 1/4 in. thick	10 cookies	40	4	185	2	7	1.4	25	29	Tr	16	0.8	50	150	14	0.07	0.10	1.0	0
Corn chips	1 oz. package	28	1	155	2	9	1.3	0	16	1	35	0.5	52	233	11	0.04	0.05	0.4	1
Cornmeal:																			
Degermed, enriched:																			
Dry form	1 cup	138	12	500	11	2	0.3	0	108	10	8	5.9	166	1	61	0.61	0.36	4.8	0
Cooked	1 cup	240	88	120	3	Tr	0.1	0	26	4	2	1.4	38	0	14	0.14	0.10	1.2	0
Crackers:[39]																			
Cheese:																			
Plain, 1 in. square	10 crackers	10	4	50	1	3	0.9	6	6	Tr	11	0.3	17	112	5	0.05	0.04	0.4	0
Sandwich type (peanut butter)	1 sandwich	8	3	40	1	2	0.4	1	5	Tr	7	0.3	17	90	Tr	0.04	0.03	0.6	0
Graham, plain, 2-1/2 in. square	2 crackers	14	5	60	1	1	0.4	0	11	Tr	6	0.4	36	86	0	0.02	0.03	0.6	0
Saltines[40]	4 crackers	12	4	50	1	1	0.3	4	9	Tr	3	0.5	17	165	0	0.06	0.05	0.6	0
Snack-type, standard	1 round cracker	3	3	15	Tr	1	0.1	0	2	Tr	3	0.1	4	30	Tr	0.01	0.01	0.1	0
Wheat, thin	4 crackers	8	3	35	1	1	0.7	0	5	1	3	0.3	17	69	Tr	0.04	0.03	0.4	0
Croissants, made with enriched flour, 4-1/2 by 4 by 1-3/4 in.	1 croissant	57	22	235	5	12	6.7	13	27	1	20	2.1	68	452	13	0.17	0.13	1.3	0
Danish pastry, made with enriched flour:																			
Plain without fruit or nuts:																			
Round piece, about 4-1/4 in. diam., 1 in. high	1 pastry	57	27	220	4	12	2.3	49	26	Tr	60	1.1	53	218	17	0.16	0.17	1.4	Tr
Fruit, round piece	1 pastry	65	30	235	4	13	2.3	56	28	0	17	1.3	57	233	11	0.16	0.14	1.4	Tr
Doughnuts, made with enriched flour:																			
Cake type, plain, 3-1/4 in. diam., 1 in. high	1 doughnut	50	21	210	3	12	1.9	20	24	1	22	1.0	58	192	5	0.12	0.12	1.1	Tr
Yeast-leavened, glazed, 3-3/4 in. diam., 1-1/4 in. high	1 doughnut	60	27	235	4	13	3.5	21	26	1	17	1.4	64	222	Tr	0.28	0.12	1.8	0

(A)	(B)	(C)	(D)	(E)	(F)	(G)	(H)	(I)	(J)	(K)	(L)	(M)	(N)	(O)	(P)	(Q)	(R)	(S)
English muffins, plain, enriched	1 muffin	57	140	5	1	0.1	0	27	2	96	1.7	331	378	0	0.26	0.19	2.2	0
French toast, from home recipe	1 slice	65	155	6	7	2.0	112	17	Tr	72	1.3	86	257	32	0.12	0.16	1.0	Tr
Macaroni, enriched, cooked (cut lengths, elbows, shells):																		
Firm stage (hot)	1 cup	130	190	7	1	0.1	0	39	2	14	2.1	103	1	0	0.23	0.13	1.8	0
Muffins made with enriched flour, 2-1/2 in. diam., 1-1/2 in. high:																		
From home recipe:																		
Blueberry[25]	1 muffin	45	135	3	5	1.1	19	20	7	54	0.9	47	198	9	0.10	0.11	0.9	1
Bran[36]	1 muffin	45	125	3	6	1.2	24	19	3	60	1.4	99	189	30	0.11	0.13	1.3	3
From commercial mix (egg and water added):																		
Blueberry	1 muffin	45	140	3	5	0.7	45	22	1	15	0.9	54	225	11	0.10	0.17	1.1	Tr
Bran	1 muffin	45	140	3	4	1.1	28	24	4	27	1.7	50	385	14	0.08	0.12	1.9	0
Corn	1 muffin	45	145	3	6	1.3	42	22	2	30	1.3	31	291	16	0.09	0.09	0.8	Tr
Noodles (egg noodles), enriched, cooked	1 cup	160	200	7	2	0.5	50	37	2	16	2.6	70	3	34	0.22	0.13	1.9	0
Noodles, chow mein, canned	1 cup	45	220	6	11	2.0	5	26	2	14	0.4	33	450	0	0.05	0.03	0.6	0
Pancakes, 4 in. diam.:																		
Buckwheat, from mix (with buckwheat and enriched flours), egg and milk added	1 pancake	27	55	2	2	0.5	20	6	1	59	0.4	66	125	17	0.04	0.05	0.2	Tr
Plain:																		
From mix (with enriched flour), egg, milk, and oil added	1 pancake	27	60	2	2	0.1	16	8	Tr	36	0.7	43	160	7	0.09	0.12	0.8	Tr
Piecrust, made with enriched flour and vegetable shortening, baked:																		
From home recipe, 9 in. diam.	1 pie shell	180	900	11	60	15.5	0	79	3	25	4.5	90	1,100	0	0.54	0.40	5.0	0
From mix, 9 in. diam.	Piecrust for 2-crust pie	320	1,485	20	93	27.6	0	141	6	131	9.3	179	2,602	0	1.06	0.80	9.9	0
Pies, piecrust made with enriched flour, vegetable shortening, 9 in. diam.:																		
Apple:																		
Piece, 1/6 of pie	1 piece	158	405	3	18	3.3	0	60	3	13	1.6	126	476	5	0.17	0.13	1.6	2
Blueberry:																		
Piece, 1/6 of pie	1 piece	158	380	4	17	4.6	0	55	2	17	2.1	158	423	14	0.17	0.14	1.7	6
Cherry:																		
Piece, 1/6 of pie	1 piece	158	410	4	18	4.7	0	61	2	22	1.6	166	480	70	0.19	0.14	1.6	0
Creme:																		
Piece, 1/6 of pie	1 piece	152	455	3	23	7.4	8	59	0	46	1.1	133	369	65	0.06	0.15	1.1	0
Custard:																		
Piece, 1/6 of pie	1 piece	152	330	9	17	4.2	169	36	2	146	1.5	208	436	96	0.14	0.32	0.9	0
Lemon meringue:																		
Piece, 1/6 of pie	1 piece	140	355	5	14	2.2	143	53	2	20	1.4	70	395	66	0.10	0.14	0.8	4
Peach:																		
Piece, 1/6 of pie	1 piece	158	405	4	17	4.4	0	60	2	16	1.9	235	423	115	0.17	0.16	2.4	5
Pecan:																		
Piece, 1/6 of pie	1 piece	138	575	7	32	5.2	95	71	5	65	4.6	170	305	54	0.30	0.17	1.1	0
Pumpkin:																		
Piece, 1/6 of pie	1 piece	152	320	6	17	4.2	109	37	6	78	1.4	243	325	416	0.14	0.21	1.2	0
Pies, fried:																		
Apple	1 pie	85	255	2	14	6.5	14	31	2	12	0.9	42	326	3	0.09	0.06	1.0	1
Cherry	1 pie	85	250	2	14	2.0	13	32	2	11	0.7	61	371	19	0.06	0.06	0.6	1
Popcorn, popped:																		
Air-popped, unsalted	1 cup	8	30	1	Tr	Tr	0	6	1	1	0.2	20	Tr	3	0.03	0.01	0.2	0
Popped in vegetable oil, salted	1 cup	11	55	1	3	0.5	0	6	1	3	0.3	19	86	2	0.01	0.02	0.1	0
Sugar syrup coated	1 cup	35	135	2	1	1.3	0	30	2	2	0.5	90	Tr	3	0.13	0.02	0.4	0
Pretzels, made with enriched flour:																		
Twisted, dutch, 2-3/4 by 2-5/8 in.	1 pretzel	16	65	2	1	0.1	0	13	Tr	4	0.3	16	258	0	0.05	0.04	0.7	0
Twisted, thin, 3-1/4 by 2-1/4 by 1/4 in.	10 pretzels	60	240	6	2	0.4	0	48	2	16	1.2	61	966	0	0.19	0.15	2.6	0
Rice:																		
Brown, cooked, served hot	1 cup	195	230	5	1	0.4	0	50	4	23	1.0	137	0	0	0.18	0.04	2.7	0
White, enriched:																		
Commercial varieties, all types:																		
Cooked, served hot	1 cup	205	225	4	Tr	0.2	0	50	1	21	1.8	57	0	0	0.23	0.02	2.1	0
Instant, ready-to-serve, hot	1 cup	165	180	4	0	0.1	0	40	1	5	1.3	0	0	0	0.21	0.02	1.7	0

Nutritive Values of Foods – Continued
(Tr indicates nutrient present in trace amount.)

Nutrients in Indicated Quantity

Item No. (A)	Foods, approximate measures, units, and weight (weight of edible portion only) (B)	Weight (Grams)	Water (C) Percent	Food energy (D) Calories	Protein (E) Grams	Fat (F) Grams	Saturated fat (G) Grams	Cholesterol (H) Milligrams	Carbohydrate (I) Grams	Dietary fiber (J) Grams	Calcium (K) Milligrams	Iron (L) Milligrams	Potassium (M) Milligrams	Sodium (N) Milligrams	Vitamin A (O) Micrograms	Thiamin (P) Milligrams	Riboflavin (Q) Milligrams	Niacin (R) Milligrams	Vitamin C (S) Milligrams
Rolls, enriched:																			
Commercial:																			
Dinner, 2-1/2 in. diam., 2 in. high	1 roll	28	32	85	2	2	0.5	Tr	14	1	33	0.8	36	155	Tr	0.14	0.09	1.1	Tr
Frankfurter and hamburger (8 per 11-1/2 oz. pkg.)	1 roll	40	34	115	3	2	0.5	Tr	20	1	54	1.2	56	241	Tr	0.20	0.13	1.6	Tr
Hard, 3-3/4 in. diam., 2 in. high	1 roll	50	25	155	5	2	0.3	Tr	30	1	24	1.4	49	313	0	0.20	0.12	1.7	0
Hoagie or submarine, 11-1/2 by 3 by 2-1/2 in.	1 roll	135	31	400	11	8	1.2	Tr	72	4	100	3.8	128	683	0	0.54	0.33	4.5	0
Spaghetti, enriched, cooked:																			
Firm stage, "al dente," served hot	1 cup	130	64	190	7	1	0.1	0	39	2	14	2.0	103	1	0	0.23	0.13	1.8	0
Toaster pastries	1 pastry	54	13	210	2	6	0.8	0	38	1	104	2.2	91	248	52	0.17	0.18	2.3	4
Tortillas, corn	1 tortilla	30	45	65	2	1	0.1	0	13	2	42	0.6	43	1	8	0.05	0.03	0.4	0
Waffles, made with enriched flour, 7 in. diam.:																			
From mix, egg and milk added	1 waffle	75	42	205	7	8	1.7	59	27	1	179	1.2	146	515	49	0.14	0.23	0.9	Tr
Wheat flours:																			
All-purpose or family flour, enriched:																			
Sifted, spooned	1 cup	115	12	420	12	1	0.2	0	88	3	18	5.1	109	2	0	0.73	0.46	6.1	0
Cake or pastry flour, enriched, sifted, spooned	1 cup	96	12	350	7	1	0.1	0	76	2	16	4.2	91	2	0	0.58	0.38	5.1	0
Self-rising, enriched, unsifted, spooned	1 cup	125	12	440	12	1	0.2	0	93	3	331	5.5	113	1,349	0	0.80	0.50	6.6	0
Whole-wheat, from hard wheats, stirred	1 cup	120	12	400	16	2	0.4	0	85	15	49	5.2	444	4	0	0.66	0.14	5.2	0
Legumes, Nuts, and Seeds																			
Almonds, shelled:																			
Slivered, packed	1 cup	135	4	795	27	70	6.7	0	28	13	359	4.9	988	15	0	0.28	1.05	4.5	1
Beans, dry:																			
Cooked, drained:																			
Lima	1 cup	190	64	260	16	1	0.2	0	49	14	55	5.9	1,163	4	0	0.25	0.11	1.3	0
Canned, solids and liquid:																			
White with:																			
Pork and tomato sauce	1 cup	255	71	310	16	7	1	10	48	12	138	4.6	536	1,181	33	0.20	0.08	1.5	5
Red kidney	1 cup	255	76	230	15	1	Tr	0	42	5	74	4.6	673	968	1	0.13	0.10	1.5	0
Black-eyed peas, dry, cooked (with residual cooking liquid)	1 cup	250	80	190	13	1	0.2	0	35	12	43	3.3	573	20	3	0.40	0.10	1.0	0
Brazil nuts, shelled	1 oz.	28	3	185	4	19	4.6	0	4	2	50	1.0	170	1	Tr	0.28	0.03	0.5	Tr
Carob flour	1 cup	140	3	255	6	Tr	0.1	0	126	41	390	5.7	1,275	24	Tr	0.07	0.07	2.2	Tr
Cashew nuts, salted:																			
Dry roasted	1 cup	137	2	785	21	63	12.5	0	45	4	62	8.2	774	[41]877	0	0.27	0.27	1.9	0
Roasted in oil	1 cup	130	4	750	21	63	12.4	0	37	4	53	5.3	689	[42]814	0	0.55	0.23	2.3	0
Chestnuts, European (Italian), roasted, shelled	1 cup	143	40	350	5	3	0.6	0	76	9	41	1.3	847	3	3	0.35	0.25	1.9	37
Chick-peas, cooked, drained	1 cup	163	60	270	15	4	0.4	0	45	8	80	4.9	475	11	Tr	0.18	0.09	0.9	0
Coconut:																			
Dried, sweetened, shredded	1 cup	93	13	470	3	33	29.3	0	44	13	14	1.8	313	244	0	0.03	0.02	0.4	1
Filberts (hazelnuts), chopped	1 cup	115	5	725	15	72	5.3	0	18	9	216	3.8	512	1	8	0.58	0.13	1.3	1
	1 oz.	28	5	180	4	18	1.3	0	4	2	53	0.9	126	Tr	2	0.14	0.03	0.3	Tr
Lentils, dry, cooked	1 cup	200	72	215	16	1	0.1	0	38	5	50	4.2	498	26	4	0.14	0.12	1.2	Tr
Macadamia nuts, roasted in oil, salted	1 cup	134	2	960	10	103	15.3	0	17	12	60	2.4	441	[43]348	1	0.29	0.15	2.7	0
Mixed nuts, with peanuts, salted:																			
Dry roasted	1 oz.	28	2	170	5	15	2.0	0	7	3	20	1.0	169	[44]190	Tr	0.06	0.06	1.3	0
Roasted in oil	1 oz.	28	2	175	5	16	2.5	0	6	3	31	0.9	165	[44]185	1	0.14	0.06	1.4	Tr
Peanuts, roasted in oil, salted	1 cup	145	2	840	39	71	9.9	0	27	10	125	2.8	1,019	[45]626	0	0.42	0.15	21.5	0
Peanut butter	1 tbsp.	16	1	95	5	8	1.5	0	3	1	5	0.3	110	75	0	0.02	0.02	2.2	0
Peas, split, dry, cooked	1 cup	200	70	230	16	1	0.1	0	42	6	22	3.4	592	26	14	0.30	0.18	1.8	2
Pecans, halves	1 cup	108	5	720	8	73	5.8	0	20	5	39	2.3	423	1	14	0.92	0.14	1.0	1
	1 oz.	28	5	190	2	19	1.5	0	5	1	10	0.6	111	Tr	4	0.24	0.04	0.3	Tr
Pistachio nuts, dried, shelled	1 oz.	28	4	165	6	14	1.7	0	7	3	38	1.9	310	2	7	0.23	0.05	0.3	Tr

(A)	(B)	(C)	(D)	(E)	(F)	(G)	(H)	(I)	(J)	(K)	(L)	(M)	(N)	(O)	(P)	(Q)	(R)	(S)
Refried beans, canned	1 cup	290	295	18	3	1.0	0	51	14	141	5.1	1,141	1,228	0	0.14	0.16	1.4	17
Sesame seeds, dry, hulled	1 tbsp.	8	45	2	4	2.9	0	1	3	11	0.6	33	3	1	0.06	0.01	0.4	0
Soy products:																		
Tofu, piece 2-1/2 by 2-3/4 by 1 in.	1 piece	120	85	9	5	0.9	0	3	1	108	2.3	50	8	0	0.07	0.04	0.1	0
Sunflower seeds, dry, hulled	1 oz.	28	160	6	14	1.9	0	5	2	33	1.9	195	1	1	0.65	0.07	1.3	Tr
Walnuts:																		
Black, chopped	1 cup	125	760	30	71	4.5	0	15	6	73	3.8	655	1	37	0.27	0.14	0.9	Tr
English or Persian, pieces or chips	1 cup	120	770	17	74	6.7	0	22	5	113	2.9	602	12	15	0.46	0.18	1.3	4
Meat and Meat Products																		
Beef, cooked:[46]																		
Cuts braised, simmered, or pot roasted:																		
Relatively fat such as chuck blade:																		
Lean and fat, piece, 2-1/2 by 2-1/2 by 3/4 in.	3 oz.	85	325	22	26	11.6	87	0	0	11	2.5	163	53	Tr	0.06	0.19	2.0	0
Relatively lean, such as bottom round:																		
Lean and fat, piece, 4-1/8 by 2-1/4 by 1/2 in.	3 oz.	85	220	25	13	3.6	81	0	0	5	2.8	248	43	Tr	0.06	0.21	3.3	0
Ground beef, broiled, patty, 3 by 5/8 in.:																		
Lean	3 oz.	85	230	21	16	7.0	74	0	0	9	1.8	256	65	Tr	0.04	0.18	4.4	0
Regular	3 oz.	85	245	20	18	7.9	76	0	0	9	2.1	248	70	Tr	0.03	0.16	4.9	0
Liver, fried, slice, 6-1/2 by 2-3/8 by 3/8 in.[47]	3 oz.	85	185	23	7	3.0	410	7	0	9	5.3	309	90	48,9,120	0.18	3.52	12.3	23
Roast, oven cooked, no liquid added:																		
Relatively fat, such as rib:																		
Lean and fat, 2 pieces, 4-1/8 by 2-1/4 by 1/4 in.	3 oz.	85	315	19	26	14.3	72	0	0	8	2.0	246	54	Tr	0.06	0.16	3.1	0
Relatively lean, such as eye of round:																		
Lean and fat, 2 pieces, 2-1/2 by 2-1/2 by 3/8 in.	3 oz.	85	205	23	12	6.2	62	0	0	5	1.6	308	50	Tr	0.07	0.14	3.0	0
Steak:																		
Sirloin, broiled:																		
Lean and fat, piece, 2-1/2 by 2-1/2 by 3/4 in.	3 oz.	85	240	23	15	8.7	77	0	0	9	2.6	306	53	Tr	0.10	0.23	3.3	0
Beef, canned, corned	3 oz.	85	185	22	10	7.0	80	0	0	17	3.7	51	802	Tr	0.02	0.20	2.9	0
Beef, dried, chipped	2.5 oz.	72	145	24	4	0.5	46	0	0	14	2.3	142	3,053	Tr	0.05	0.23	2.7	0
Lamb, cooked:																		
Chops, (3 per lb. with bone):																		
Lean and fat	2.2 oz.	63	220	20	15	3.5	77	0	0	16	1.5	195	46	Tr	0.04	0.16	4.4	0
Leg, roasted:																		
Lean and fat, 2 pieces, 4-1/8 by 2-1/4 by 1/4 in.	3 oz.	85	205	22	13	7.8	78	0	0	8	1.7	273	57	Tr	0.09	0.24	5.5	0
Rib, roasted:																		
Lean and fat, 3 pieces, 2-1/2 by 2-1/2 by 1/4 in.	3 oz.	85	315	18	26	14.5	77	0	0	19	1.4	224	60	Tr	0.08	0.18	5.5	0
Pork, cured, cooked:																		
Bacon:																		
Regular	3 medium slices	19	110	6	9	3.3	16	Tr	0	2	0.3	92	303	0	0.13	0.05	1.4	6
Canadian-style	2 slices	46	85	11	4	1.3	27	1	0	5	0.4	179	711	0	0.38	0.09	3.2	10
Ham, light cure, roasted:																		
Lean and fat, 2 pieces, 4-1/8 by 2-1/4 by 1/4 in.	3 oz.	85	205	18	14	6.8	53	0	0	6	0.7	243	1,009	0	0.51	0.19	3.8	0
Ham, canned, roasted, 2 pieces, 4-1/8 by 2-1/4 by 1/4 in.	3 oz.	85	140	18	7	3.2	35	Tr	0	6	0.9	298	908	0	0.82	0.21	4.3	49,19
Luncheon meat:																		
Canned, spiced or unspiced, slice, 3 by 2 by 1/2 in.	2 slices	42	140	5	13	4.6	26	1	0	3	0.3	90	541	0	0.15	0.08	1.3	Tr
Cooked ham (8 slices per 8 oz. pkg.):																		
Regular	2 slices	57	105	10	6	1.9	32	2	0	4	0.6	189	751	0	0.49	0.14	3.0	49,16
Extra lean	2 slices	57	75	11	3	0.9	27	1	0	4	0.4	200	815	0	0.53	0.13	2.8	49,15
Pork, fresh, cooked:																		
Chop, loin (cut 3 per lb. with bone):																		
Broiled:																		
Lean and fat	3.1 oz.	87	275	24	19	4.6	84	0	0	3	0.7	312	61	3	0.87	0.24	4.3	Tr
Ham (leg), roasted:																		
Lean and fat, piece, 2-1/2 by 2-1/2 by 3/4 in.	3 oz	85	250	21	18	0.7	79	0	0	5	0.9	280	50	2	0.54	0.27	3.9	Tr
Rib, roasted:																		
Lean and fat, piece, 2-1/2 by 2-1/2 by 3/4 in.	3 oz.	85	270	21	20	6.7	69	0	0	9	0.8	313	37	3	0.50	0.24	4.2	Tr
Shoulder cut, braised:																		
Lean and fat, 3 pieces, 2-1/2 by 2-1/2 by 1/4 in.	3 oz.	85	295	23	22	9.6	93	0	0	6	1.4	286	75	3	0.46	0.26	4.4	Tr
Sausages:																		
Bologna, slice (8 per 8 oz. pkg.)	2 slices	57	180	7	16	3.2	31	2	0	7	0.9	103	581	0	0.10	0.08	1.5	49,12
Braunschweiger, slice (6 per 6 oz. pkg.)	2 slices	57	205	8	18	3.1	89	2	0	5	5.3	113	652	2,405	0.14	0.87	4.8	496

Nutritive Values of Foods – Continued
(Tr indicates nutrient present in trace amount.)

Nutrients in Indicated Quantity

Foods, approximate measures, units, and weight (weight of edible portion only) (A, B)	Grams	Water % (C)	Food energy Cal. (D)	Protein g (E)	Fat g (F)	Saturated fat g (G)	Cholesterol mg (H)	Carbohydrate g (I)	Dietary fiber g (J)	Calcium mg (K)	Iron mg (L)	Potassium mg (M)	Sodium mg (N)	Vitamin A µg (O)	Thiamin mg (P)	Riboflavin mg (Q)	Niacin mg (R)	Vitamin C mg (S)
Brown and serve (10-11 per 8 oz. pkg.), browned — 1 link	13	45	50	2	5	1.7	9	Tr	0	1	0.1	25	105	0	0.05	0.02	0.4	0
Frankfurter (10 per 1 lb. pkg.), cooked (reheated) — 1 frankfurter	45	54	145	5	13	4.9	23	1	0	5	0.5	75	504	0	0.09	0.05	1.2	12[49]
Salami:																		
Dry type, slice (12 per 4 oz. pkg.) — 2 slices	20	35	85	5	7	2.5	16	1	0	2	0.3	76	372	0	0.12	0.06	1.0	5[49]
Sandwich spread (pork, beef) — 1 tbsp.	15	60	35	1	3	0.9	6	2	Tr	2	0.1	17	152	1	0.03	0.02	0.3	0
Veal, medium fat, cooked, bone removed:																		
Cutlet, 4-1/8 by 2-1/4 by 1/2 in., braised or broiled — 3 oz.	85	60	185	23	9	7.6	109	0	0	9	0.8	258	56	Tr	0.06	0.21	4.6	0
Rib, 2 pieces, 4-1/8 by 2-1/4 by 1/4 in., roasted — 3 oz.	85	55	230	23	14	6.1	109	0	0	10	0.7	259	57	Tr	0.11	0.26	6.6	0
Mixed Dishes and Fast Foods																		
Mixed dishes:																		
Beef and vegetable stew, from home recipe — 1 cup	245	82	220	16	11	4.9	71	15	2	29	2.9	613	292	568	0.15	0.17	4.7	17
Beef potpie, from home recipe, baked, piece, 1/3 of 9 in. diam. pie[51] — 1 piece	210	55	515	21	30	8.4	42	39	3	29	3.8	334	596	517	0.29	0.29	4.8	6
Chicken a la king, cooked, from home recipe — 1 cup	245	68	470	27	34	12.7	221	12	1	127	2.5	404	760	272	0.10	0.42	5.4	12
Chicken chow mein:																		
Canned — 1 cup	250	89	95	7	Tr	0.0	8	18	2	45	1.3	418	725	28	0.05	0.10	1.0	13
Chili con carne with beans, canned — 1 cup	255	72	340	19	16	3.4	28	31	4	82	4.3	594	1,354	15	0.08	0.18	3.3	8
Chop suey with beef and pork, from home recipe — 1 cup	250	75	300	26	17	5.7	68	13	4	60	4.8	425	1,053	60	0.28	0.38	5.0	33
Macaroni (enriched) and cheese:																		
Canned[52] — 1 cup	240	80	230	9	10	4.2	24	26	1	199	1.0	139	730	72	0.12	0.24	1.0	Tr
From home recipe[38] — 1 cup	200	58	430	17	22	8.9	44	40	1	362	1.8	240	1,086	232	0.20	0.40	1.8	1
Spaghetti (enriched) in tomato sauce with cheese:																		
Canned — 1 cup	250	80	190	6	2	0.0	3	39	2	40	2.8	303	955	120	0.35	0.28	4.5	10
From home recipe — 1 cup	250	77	260	9	9	2.0	8	37	2	80	2.3	408	955	140	0.25	0.18	2.3	13
Spaghetti (enriched) with meatballs and tomato sauce:																		
Canned — 1 cup	250	78	260	12	10	2.1	23	29	6	53	3.3	245	1,220	100	0.15	0.18	2.3	5
From home recipe — 1 cup	248	70	330	19	12	3.3	89	39	8	124	3.7	665	1,009	159	0.25	0.30	4.0	22
Fast food entrees:																		
Cheeseburger:																		
Regular — 1 sandwich	112	46	300	15	15	6.7	44	28	0	135	2.3	219	672	65	0.26	0.24	3.7	1
4 oz. patty — 1 sandwich	194	46	525	30	31	10.2	104	40	0	236	4.5	407	1,224	128	0.33	0.48	7.4	3
Chicken, fried. See Poultry and Poultry Products.																		
Enchilada — 1 enchilada	230	72	235	20	16	15.0	19	24	0	322	11.0	2,180	4,451	352	0.18	0.26	Tr	Tr
English muffin, egg, cheese, and bacon — 1 sandwich	138	49	360	18	18	8.6	213	31	1	197	3.1	201	832	160	0.46	0.50	3.7	1
Fish sandwich:																		
Regular, with cheese — 1 sandwich	140	43	420	16	23	6.2	56	39	Tr	132	1.8	274	667	25	0.32	0.26	3.3	2
Large, without cheese — 1 sandwich	170	48	470	18	27	5.6	91	41	Tr	61	2.2	375	621	15	0.35	0.23	3.5	1
Hamburger:																		
Regular — 1 sandwich	98	46	245	12	11	3.2	32	28	0	56	2.2	202	463	14	0.23	0.24	3.8	1
4 oz. patty — 1 sandwich	174	50	445	25	21	9.7	71	38	0	75	4.8	404	763	28	0.38	0.38	7.8	1
Pizza, cheese, 1/8 of 15 in. diam. pizza[51] — 1 slice	120	46	290	15	9	2.9	56	39	2	220	1.6	230	699	106	0.34	0.29	4.2	2
Taco — 1 taco	81	55	195	9	11	4.6	21	15	1	109	1.2	263	456	57	0.09	0.07	1.4	1
Poultry and Poultry Products																		
Chicken:																		
Fried, flesh, with skin:[53]																		
Batter dipped:																		
Breast, 1/2 breast (5.6 oz. with bones) — 4.9 oz.	140	52	365	35	18	4.9	119	13	Tr	28	1.8	281	385	28	0.16	0.20	14.7	0

(A)	(B)	(C)	(D)	(E)	(F)	(G)	(H)	(I)	(J)	(K)	(L)	(M)	(N)	(O)	(P)	(Q)	(R)	(S)
Drumstick (3.4 oz. with bones)	2.5 oz.	72	53	195	16	11	3.0	62	6	Tr	12	1.0	134	194	19	0.08	0.15	3.7	0
Roasted, flesh only:																		
Breast, 1/2 breast (4.2 oz. with bones and skin)	3.0 oz.	86	65	140	27	3	0.9	73	0	0	13	0.9	220	64	5	0.06	0.10	11.8	0
Drumstick, (2.9 oz. with bones and skin)	1.6 oz.	44	67	75	12	2	1.4	41	0	0	5	0.6	108	42	8	0.03	0.10	2.7	0
Chicken liver, cooked	1 liver	20	68	30	5	1	1.6	126	Tr	0	3	1.7	28	10	983	0.03	0.35	0.9	3
Duck, roasted, flesh only	1/2 duck	221	64	445	52	25	9.2	197	0	0	27	6.0	557	144	51	0.57	1.04	11.3	0
Turkey, roasted, flesh only:																		
Dark meat, piece, 2-1/2 by 1-5/8 by 1/4 in.	4 pieces	85	63	160	24	6	4.0	72	0	0	27	2.0	246	67	0	0.05	0.21	3.1	0
Light meat, piece, 4 by 2 by 1/4 in.	2 pieces	85	66	135	25	3	2.7	59	0	0	16	1.1	259	54	0	0.05	0.11	5.8	0
Poultry food products:																		
Chicken:																		
Canned, boneless	5 oz.	142	69	235	31	11	3.1	88	0	0	20	2.2	196	714	48	0.02	0.18	9.0	3
Frankfurter (10 per 1-lb. pkg.)	1 frankfurter	45	58	115	6	9	2.5	45	3	0	43	0.9	38	616	17	0.03	0.05	1.4	0
Roll, light (6 slices per 6 oz. pkg.)	2 slices	57	69	90	11	4	1.1	28	1	0	24	0.6	129	331	14	0.04	0.07	3.0	0
Turkey:																		
Gravy and turkey, frozen	5 oz. package	142	85	95	8	4	1.0	26	7	Tr	20	1.3	87	787	18	0.03	0.18	2.6	3
Loaf, breast meat (8 slices per 6 oz. pkg.)	2 slices	42	72	45	10	1	0.5	17	0	0	3	0.2	118	608	0	0.02	0.05	3.5	0
Patties, breaded, battered, fried (2.25 oz.)	1 patty	64	50	180	9	12	2.7	40	10	Tr	9	1.4	176	512	7	0.06	0.12	1.5	540
Roast, boneless, frozen, seasoned, light and dark meat, cooked	3 oz.	85	68	130	18	5	2.2	45	3	0	4	1.4	253	578	0	0.04	0.14	5.3	0

Soups, Sauces, and Gravies

(A)	(B)	(C)	(D)	(E)	(F)	(G)	(H)	(I)	(J)	(K)	(L)	(M)	(N)	(O)	(P)	(Q)	(R)	(S)
Soups:																		
Canned, condensed:																		
Prepared with equal volume of milk:																		
Clam chowder, New England	1 cup	248	85	165	9	7	2.9	22	17	1	186	1.5	300	992	40	0.07	0.24	1.0	3
Cream of chicken	1 cup	248	85	190	7	11	4.6	27	15	Tr	181	0.7	273	1,047	94	0.07	0.26	0.9	1
Cream of mushroom	1 cup	248	85	205	6	14	5.1	20	15	1	179	0.6	270	1,076	37	0.08	0.28	0.9	2
Tomato	1 cup	248	85	160	6	6	2.9	17	22	1	159	1.8	449	932	109	0.13	0.25	1.5	68
Prepared with equal volume of water:																		
Bean with bacon	1 cup	253	84	170	8	6	1.5	3	23	9	81	2.0	402	951	89	0.09	0.03	0.6	2
Beef broth, bouillon, consommé	1 cup	240	98	15	3	1	0.3	Tr	Tr	0	14	0.4	130	782	0	Tr	0.05	1.9	0
Beef noodle	1 cup	244	92	85	5	3	1.1	5	9	1	15	1.1	100	952	63	0.07	0.06	1.1	Tr
Chicken noodle	1 cup	241	92	75	4	2	0.7	7	9	1	17	0.8	55	1,106	71	0.05	0.06	1.4	Tr
Chicken rice	1 cup	241	94	60	4	2	0.5	7	7	1	17	0.7	101	815	66	0.02	0.02	1.1	Tr
Clam chowder, Manhattan	1 cup	244	90	80	4	2	0.4	2	12	1	34	1.9	261	1,808	92	0.06	0.05	1.3	3
Pea, green	1 cup	250	83	165	9	3	1.8	0	27	5	28	2.0	190	988	20	0.11	0.07	1.2	2
Vegetable beef	1 cup	244	92	80	6	2	0.9	5	10	Tr	17	1.1	173	956	189	0.04	0.05	1.0	2
Vegetarian	1 cup	241	92	70	2	2	0.3	0	12	Tr	22	1.1	210	822	301	0.05	0.05	0.9	1
Dehydrated:																		
Prepared with water:																		
Chicken noodle	1 pkt. (6 fl. oz.)	188	94	40	2	1	0.3	2	6	Tr	24	0.4	23	957	5	0.05	0.04	0.7	Tr
Tomato vegetable	1 pkt. (6 fl. oz.)	189	94	40	1	1	0.4	0	8	1	6	0.5	78	856	14	0.04	0.03	0.6	5
Sauces:																		
From dry mix:																		
Cheese, prepared with milk	1 cup	279	77	305	16	17	9.3	53	23	1	569	0.3	552	1,565	117	0.15	0.56	0.3	2
From home recipe:																		
White sauce, medium[55]	1 cup	250	73	395	10	30	6.4	32	24	Tr	292	0.9	381	888	340	0.15	0.43	0.8	2
Ready to serve:																		
Barbecue	1 tbsp.	16	81	10	Tr	Tr	Tr	0	2	Tr	3	0.1	28	130	14	Tr	Tr	0.1	1
Soy	1 tbsp.	18	68	10	2	0	Tr	0	2	0	3	0.5	64	1,029	0	0.01	0.02	0.6	0
Gravies:																		
Canned:																		
Beef	1 cup	233	87	125	9	5	2.7	7	11	1	14	1.6	189	117	0	0.07	0.08	1.5	0
Chicken	1 cup	238	85	190	5	14	3.4	5	13	Tr	48	1.1	259	1,373	264	0.04	0.10	1.1	0
Mushroom	1 cup	238	89	120	3	6	0.8	0	13	Tr	17	1.6	252	1,357	0	0.08	0.15	1.6	0
From dry mix:																		
Brown	1 cup	261	91	80	3	2	0.8	2	14	Tr	66	0.2	61	1,147	0	0.04	0.09	0.9	0
Chicken	1 cup	260	91	85	3	2	0.5	3	14	Tr	39	0.3	62	1,134	0	0.05	0.15	0.8	3

Sugars and Sweets

(A)	(B)	(C)	(D)	(E)	(F)	(G)	(H)	(I)	(J)	(K)	(L)	(M)	(N)	(O)	(P)	(Q)	(R)	(S)
Candy:																		
Caramels, plain or chocolate	1 oz.	28	8	115	1	3	1.9	1	22	Tr	42	0.4	54	64	Tr	0.01	0.05	0.1	Tr

Nutritive Values of Foods – Continued
(Tr indicates nutrient present in trace amount.)

Nutrients in Indicated Quantity

Item No. Foods, approximate measures, units, and weight (weight of edible portion only) (A)	Measure (B)	Grams (B)	Water Percent (C)	Food energy Calories (D)	Protein Grams (E)	Fat Grams (F)	Saturated fat Grams (G)	Cholesterol Milligrams (H)	Carbohydrate Grams (I)	Dietary fiber Grams (J)	Calcium Milligrams (K)	Iron Milligrams (L)	Potassium Milligrams (M)	Sodium Milligrams (N)	Vitamin A Micrograms (O)	Thiamin Milligrams (P)	Riboflavin Milligrams (Q)	Niacin Milligrams (R)	Vitamin C Milligrams (S)
Chocolate:																			
Milk, plain	1 oz.	28	1	145	2	9	5.2	6	16	1	50	0.4	96	23	10	0.02	0.10	0.1	Tr
Milk, with almonds	1 oz.	28	2	150	3	10	4.8	5	15	2	65	0.5	125	23	8	0.02	0.12	0.2	Tr
Milk, with peanuts	1 oz.	28	1	155	4	11	3.4	5	13	2	49	0.4	138	19	8	0.07	0.07	1.4	Tr
Milk, with rice cereal	1 oz.	28	2	140	2	7	4.5	6	18	1	48	0.2	100	46	8	0.01	0.08	0.1	Tr
Semisweet, small pieces (60 per oz.)	1 cup or 6 oz.	170	1	860	7	61	29.8	0	97	10	51	5.8	593	24	3	0.10	0.14	0.9	Tr
Sweet (dark)	1 oz.	28	1	150	1	10	5.9	0	16	2	7	0.6	86	5	1	0.01	0.04	0.1	Tr
Fudge, chocolate, plain	1 oz.	28	8	115	1	3	1.5	1	21	Tr	22	0.3	42	54	Tr	0.01	0.03	0.1	Tr
Gum drops	1 oz.	28	12	100	Tr	Tr	0.0	0	25	0	2	0.1	1	10	0	0.00	Tr	Tr	0
Hard	1 oz.	28	1	110	0	Tr	0.0	0	28	0	Tr	0.1	1	7	0	0.00	0.00	0.0	0
Jelly beans	1 oz.	28	6	105	Tr	Tr	0.0	0	26	0	1	0.3	11	7	0	0.00	Tr	Tr	0
Marshmallows	1 oz.	28	17	90	1	0	0.0	0	23	Tr	1	0.5	2	25	0	0.00	Tr	Tr	0
Custard, baked	1 cup	265	77	305	14	15	6.2	278	29	0	297	1.1	387	209	146	0.11	0.50	0.3	1
Gelatin dessert prepared with gelatin dessert powder and water	1/2 cup	120	84	70	2	0	0.0	0	17	0	2	Tr	Tr	55	0	0.00	0.00	0.0	0
Honey, strained or extracted	1 cup	339	17	1,030	1	0	0.0	0	279	Tr	17	1.7	173	17	0	0.02	0.14	1.0	3
Jams and preserves	1 tbsp.	20	29	55	Tr	Tr	0.0	0	14	Tr	4	0.2	18	2	Tr	Tr	0.01	Tr	Tr
Jellies	1 tbsp.	18	28	50	Tr	Tr	Tr	0	13	Tr	2	0.1	16	5	Tr	Tr	0.01	Tr	1
Popsicle, 3 fl. oz. size	1 popsicle	95	80	70	0	0	0.0	0	18	0	0	Tr	4	11	0	0.00	0.00	0.0	0
Puddings:																			
Canned: Chocolate	5 oz. can	142	68	205	3	11	9.5	1	30	1	74	1.2	254	285	31	0.04	0.17	0.6	Tr
Canned: Vanilla	5 oz. can	142	69	220	2	10	9.5	1	33	Tr	79	0.2	155	305	Tr	0.03	0.12	0.6	Tr
Dry mix, prepared with whole milk: Chocolate: Instant	1/2 cup	130	71	155	4	4	2.4	14	27	2	130	0.3	176	440	33	0.04	0.18	0.1	1
Rice	1/2 cup	132	73	155	4	4	2.3	15	27	1	133	0.5	165	140	33	0.10	0.18	0.6	1
Vanilla: Instant	1/2 cup	130	73	150	4	4	2.3	15	27	Tr	129	0.1	164	375	33	0.04	0.17	0.1	1
Sugars:																			
Brown, pressed down	1 cup	220	2	820	0	0	0.0	0	212	0	187	4.8	757	97	0	0.02	0.07	0.2	0
White: Granulated	1 cup	200	1	770	0	0	0.0	0	199	0	3	0.1	7	5	0	0.00	0.00	0.0	0
White: Granulated	1 tbsp.	12	1	45	0	0	0.0	0	12	0	Tr	Tr	Tr	Tr	0	0.00	0.00	0.0	0
Powdered, sifted, spooned into cup	1 cup	100	1	385	0	0	0.0	0	99	0	1	0.1	4	2	0	0.00	0.00	0.0	0
Syrups:																			
Chocolate-flavored syrup or topping: Thin type	2 tbsp.	38	37	85	1	Tr	0.2	0	21	1	6	0.8	85	36	13	0.02	0.08	0.1	0
Fudge type	2 tbsp.	38	25	125	2	5	2.2	0	22	Tr	38	0.5	82	42	0	0.04	0.08	0.8	0
Molasses, cane, blackstrap	2 tbsp.	40	25	85	0	0	0.0	0	22	0	274	10.1	1,171	38	0	0.02	0.08	0.8	0
Table syrup (corn and maple)	2 tbsp.	42	25	122	0	0	0.0	0	32	0	187	4.8	757	97	0	0.02	0.07	0.2	0
Vegetables and Vegetable Products																			
Alfalfa seeds, sprouted, raw	1 cup	33	91	10	1	Tr	Tr	0	1	1	11	0.3	26	2	5	0.03	0.04	0.2	3
Asparagus, green: Cooked, drained: From raw: Cuts and tips	1 cup	180	92	45	5	1	0.2	0	8	4	43	1.2	558	7	149	0.18	0.22	1.9	49
From frozen: Cuts and tips	1 cup	180	91	50	5	1	0.2	0	9	4	41	1.2	392	7	147	0.12	0.19	1.9	44
Bamboo shoots, canned, drained	1 cup	131	94	25	2	1	0.1	0	4	3	10	0.4	105	9	1	0.03	0.03	0.2	1

(A)	(B)	(C)	(D)	(E)	(F)	(G)	(H)	(I)	(J)	(K)	(L)	(M)	(N)	(O)	(P)	(Q)	(R)	(S)
Beans:																		
Lima, immature seeds, frozen, cooked, drained:																		
Thick-seeded types (Ford-hooks)	1 cup	170	74	170	10	1	0.2	0	32	12	37	2.3	694	90	32	0.13	0.10	1.8	22
Snap:																		
Cooked, drained:																		
From raw (cut and French style)	1 cup	125	89	45	2	Tr	Tr	0	10	4	58	1.6	374	4	5783	0.09	0.12	0.8	12
From frozen (cut)	1 cup	135	92	35	2	Tr	Tr	0	8	4	61	1.1	151	18	5871	0.06	0.10	0.6	11
Canned, drained solids (cut)	1 cup	135	93	25	2	Tr	Tr	0	6	2	35	1.2	147	59339	6047	0.02	0.08	0.3	6
Beets:																		
Canned, drained solids, diced or sliced	1 cup	170	91	55	2	Tr	Tr	0	12	4	26	3.1	252	61466	2	0.02	0.07	0.3	7
Beet greens, leaves and stems, cooked, drained	1 cup	144	89	40	4	Tr	Tr	0	8	4	164	2.7	1,309	347	734	0.17	0.42	0.7	36
Broccoli:																		
Cooked, drained:																		
From raw:																		
Spears, cut into 1/2 in. pieces	1 cup	155	90	45	5	Tr	Tr	0	9	2	177	1.8	253	17	218	0.13	0.32	1.2	97
From frozen:																		
Chopped	1 cup	185	91	50	6	Tr	Tr	0	10	5	94	1.1	333	44	350	0.10	0.15	0.8	74
Brussels sprouts, cooked, drained:																		
From frozen	1 cup	155	87	65	6	1	0.2	0	13	6	37	1.1	504	36	91	0.16	0.18	0.8	71
Cabbage, common varieties:																		
Raw, coarsely shredded or sliced	1 cup	70	93	15	1	Tr	Tr	0	4	1	33	0.4	172	13	9	0.04	0.02	0.2	33
Cooked, drained	1 cup	150	94	30	1	Tr	0.1	0	7	4	50	0.6	308	29	13	0.09	0.08	0.3	36
Cabbage, red, raw, coarsely shredded or sliced	1 cup	70	92	20	1	Tr	Tr	0	4	2	36	0.3	144	8	3	0.04	0.02	0.2	40
Carrots:																		
Raw, without crowns and tips, scraped:																		
Whole, 7-1/2 by 1-1/8 in., or strips, 2-1/2 to 3 in. long	1 carrot or 18 strips	72	88	30	1	Tr	Tr	0	7	2	19	0.4	233	25	2,025	0.07	0.04	0.7	7
Cooked, sliced, drained:																		
From frozen	1 cup	146	90	55	2	Tr	Tr	0	12	6	41	0.7	231	86	2,585	0.04	0.05	0.6	4
Cauliflower:																		
Raw, (flowerets)	1 cup	100	92	25	2	Tr	Tr	0	5	2	29	0.6	355	15	2	0.08	0.06	0.6	72
Cooked, drained:																		
From frozen (flowerets)	1 cup	180	94	35	3	Tr	Tr	0	7	4	31	0.7	250	32	4	0.07	0.10	0.6	56
Celery, pascal type, raw:																		
Stalk, large outer, 8 by 1-1/2 in. (at root end)	1 stalk	40	95	5	Tr	Tr	Tr	0	1	1	14	0.2	114	35	5	0.01	0.01	0.1	3
Collards, cooked, drained:																		
From frozen (chopped)	1 cup	170	88	60	5	1	0.2	0	12	6	357	1.9	427	85	1,017	0.08	0.20	1.1	45
Corn, sweet:																		
Cooked, drained:																		
From raw, ear 5 by 1-3/4 in.	1 ear	77	70	85	3	1	0.2	0	19	2	2	0.5	192	13	6317	0.17	0.06	1.2	5
From frozen:																		
Ear, trimmed to about 3-1/2 in. long	1 ear	63	73	60	2	Tr	0.1	0	14	2	2	0.4	158	3	6313	0.11	0.04	1.0	3
Kernels	1 cup	165	76	135	5	1	Tr	0	34	4	3	0.5	229	8	6341	0.11	0.12	2.1	4
Canned:																		
Cream style	1 cup	256	79	185	4	1	0.2	0	46	4	8	1.0	343	64730	6325	0.06	0.14	2.5	12
Whole kernel, vacuum pack	1 cup	210	77	165	5	1	0.2	0	41	4	11	0.9	391	65571	6351	0.09	0.15	2.5	17
Cucumber, with peel, slices, 1/8 in. thick (large, 2-1/8 in. diam.; small, 1-3/4 in. diam.)	6 large or 8 small slices	28	96	5	Tr	Tr	Tr	0	1	Tr	4	0.1	42	1	1	0.01	0.01	0.1	1
Eggplant, cooked, steamed	1 cup	96	92	25	1	Tr	0.1	0	6	4	6	0.3	238	3	6	0.07	0.02	0.6	1
Kale, cooked, drained:																		
From frozen, chopped	1 cup	130	91	40	4	1	Tr	0	7	2	179	1.2	417	20	826	0.06	0.15	0.9	33
Lettuce, raw:																		
Butterhead, as Boston types:																		
Head, 5 in. diam.	1 head	163	96	20	2	Tr	Tr	0	4	4	52	0.5	419	8	158	0.10	0.10	0.5	13
Crisphead, as iceberg:																		
Head, 6 in. diam.	1 head	539	96	70	5	1	0.2	0	11	4	102	2.7	852	49	178	0.25	0.16	1.0	21
Wedge, 1/4 of head	1 wedge	135	96	20	1	Tr	Tr	0	3	1	26	0.7	213	12	45	0.06	0.04	0.3	5
Pieces, chopped or shredded	1 cup	55	96	5	1	Tr	Tr	0	1	1	10	0.3	87	5	18	0.03	0.02	0.1	2
Mushrooms:																		
Raw, sliced or chopped	1 cup	70	92	20	1	Tr	Tr	0	3	Tr	4	0.9	259	3	0	0.07	0.31	2.9	2
Canned, drained solids	1 cup	156	91	35	3	Tr	Tr	0	8	4	17	1.2	201	663	0	0.13	0.03	2.5	0

Nutritive Values of Foods – Continued
(Tr indicates nutrient present in trace amount.)

Nutrients in Indicated Quantity

Item No. (A)	Foods, approximate measures, units, and weight (weight of edible portion only) (B)	Grams	Water (C) Percent	Food energy (D) Calories	Protein (E) Grams	Fat (F) Grams	Saturated fat (G) Grams	Cholesterol (H) Milligrams	Carbohydrate (I) Grams	Dietary fiber (J) Grams	Calcium (K) Milligrams	Iron (L) Milligrams	Potassium (M) Milligrams	Sodium (N) Milligrams	Vitamin A (O) Micrograms	Thiamin (P) Milligrams	Riboflavin (Q) Milligrams	Niacin (R) Milligrams	Vitamin C (S) Milligrams
	Onions:																		
	Raw:																		
	Chopped — 1 cup	160	91	55	2	Tr	Tr	0	12	3	40	0.6	248	3	0	0.10	0.02	0.2	13
	Cooked (whole or sliced), drained — 1 cup	210	92	60	2	Tr	Tr	0	13	2	57	0.4	319	17	0	0.09	0.02	0.2	12
	Onion rings, breaded, par-fried, frozen, prepared — 2 rings	20	29	80	1	5	1.7	0	8	Tr	6	0.3	26	75	5	0.06	0.03	0.7	Tr
	Parsley:																		
	Freeze-dried — 1 tbsp.	0.4	2	Tr	Tr	Tr	Tr	0	Tr	1	1	0.2	25	2	25	Tr	0.01	Tr	1
	Peas, edible pod, cooked, drained — 1 cup	160	89	65	5	Tr	0.1	0	11	4	67	3.2	384	6	21	0.20	0.12	0.09	77
	Peas, green:																		
	Canned, drained solids — 1 cup	170	82	115	8	1	0.2	0	21	6	34	1.6	294	[66]372	131	0.21	0.13	1.2	16
	Frozen, cooked, drained — 1 cup	160	80	125	8	Tr	Tr	0	23	8	38	2.5	269	139	107	0.45	0.16	2.4	16
	Peppers:																		
	Hot chili, raw — 1 pepper	45	88	20	1	Tr	Tr	0	4	1	8	0.5	153	3	[67]484	0.04	0.04	0.4	109
	Sweet (about 5 per lb., whole), stem and seeds removed:																		
	Raw — 1 pepper	74	93	20	1	Tr	Tr	0	4	1	4	0.9	144	2	[68]39	0.06	0.04	0.4	[69]95
	Potatoes, cooked:																		
	Baked (about 2 per lb., raw):																		
	With skin — 1 potato	202	71	220	5	Tr	0.1	0	51	5	20	2.7	844	16	0	0.22	0.07	3.3	26
	Flesh only — 1 potato	156	75	145	3	Tr	Tr	0	34	2	8	0.5	610	8	0	0.16	0.03	2.2	20
	Boiled (about 3 per lb., raw):																		
	Peeled after boiling — 1 potato	136	77	120	3	Tr	Tr	0	27	2	7	0.4	515	5	0	0.14	0.03	2.0	18
	French fried, strip, 2 to 3-1/2 in. long, frozen:																		
	Oven heated — 10 strips	50	53	110	2	4	3.8	0	17	1	5	0.7	229	16	0	0.06	0.02	1.2	5
	Fried in vegetable oil — 10 strips	50	38	160	2	8	2.5	0	20	2	10	0.4	366	108	0	0.09	0.01	1.6	5
	Potato products, prepared:																		
	Au gratin:																		
	From dry mix — 1 cup	245	79	230	6	10	6.4	12	31	4	203	0.8	537	1,076	76	0.05	0.20	2.3	8
	Hashed brown, from frozen — 1 cup	156	56	340	5	18	7.0	0	44	3	23	2.4	680	53	0	0.17	0.03	3.8	10
	Mashed:																		
	From home recipe: Milk and margarine added — 1 cup	210	76	225	4	9	2.2	4	35	4	55	0.5	607	620	42	0.18	0.08	2.3	13
	Potato chips — 10 chips	20	3	105	1	7	3.1	0	10	1	5	0.2	260	94	0	0.03	Tr	0.8	8
	Pumpkin:																		
	Canned — 1 cup	245	90	85	3	1	0.4	0	20	6	64	3.4	505	12	5,404	0.06	0.13	0.9	10
	Radishes, raw, stem ends, rootlets cut off — 4 radishes	18	95	5	Tr	Tr	Tr	0	1	Tr	4	0.1	42	4	0	Tr	0.01	0.1	4
	Spinach:																		
	Raw, chopped — 1 cup	55	92	10	2	Tr	Tr	0	2	2	54	1.5	307	43	369	0.04	0.10	0.4	15
	Cooked, drained:																		
	From frozen (leaf) — 1 cup	190	90	55	6	Tr	Tr	0	10	4	277	2.9	566	163	1,479	0.11	0.32	0.8	23
	Canned, drained solids — 1 cup	214	92	50	6	1	0.2	0	7	6	272	4.9	740	[72]683	1,878	0.03	0.30	0.8	31
	Squash, cooked:																		
	Summer (all varieties), sliced, drained — 1 cup	180	94	35	2	1	0.2	0	8	2	49	0.6	346	2	52	0.08	0.07	0.9	10
	Winter (all varieties), baked, cubes — 1 cup	205	89	80	2	1	0.3	0	18	6	29	0.7	896	2	729	0.17	0.05	1.4	20
	Sweet potatoes:																		
	Cooked (raw, 5 by 2 in.; about 2-1/2 per lb.):																		
	Baked in skin, peeled — 1 potato	114	73	115	2	Tr	Tr	0	28	4	32	0.5	397	11	2,488	0.08	0.14	0.7	28
	Candied, 2-1/2 by 2 in. piece — 1 piece	105	67	145	1	3	1.4	8	29	2	27	1.2	198	74	440	0.02	0.04	0.4	7
	Canned:																		
	Vacuum pack, piece 2-3/4 by 1 in. — 1 piece	40	76	35	1	Tr	Tr	0	8	1	9	0.4	125	21	319	0.01	0.02	0.3	11
	Tomatoes:																		
	Raw, 2-3/5 in. diam. (3 per 12 oz. pkg.) — 1 tomato	123	94	25	1	Tr	0.1	0	5	1	9	0.6	255	10	139	0.07	0.06	0.7	22
	Canned, solids and liquid — 1 cup	240	94	50	2	1	0.1	0	10	2	62	1.5	530	[73]391	145	0.11	0.07	1.8	36

(A)	(B)	(C)	(D)	(E)	(F)	(G)	(H)	(I)	(J)	(K)	(L)	(M)	(N)	(O)	(P)	(Q)	(R)	(S)
Tomato juice, canned	1 cup	244	40	2	Tr	Tr	0	10	1	22	1.4	537	[74]881	136	0.11	0.08	1.6	45
Tomato products, canned:																		
Paste	1 cup	262	220	10	2	0.3	0	49	11	92	7.8	2,442	[75]170	647	0.41	0.50	8.4	111
Puree	1 cup	250	105	4	Tr	Tr	0	25	6	38	2.3	1,050	750	340	0.18	0.14	4.3	88
Sauce	1 cup	245	75	3	Tr	Tr	0	18	3	34	1.9	909	[77]1,482	240	0.16	0.14	2.8	32
Turnip greens, cooked, drained:																		
From frozen (chopped)	1 cup	164	50	5	1	0.2	0	8	7	249	3.2	367	25	1,308	0.09	0.12	0.8	36
Vegetable juice cocktail, canned	1 cup	242	45	2	Tr	Tr	0	11	1	27	1.0	467	883	283	0.10	0.07	1.8	67
Vegetables, mixed:																		
Canned, drained solids	1 cup	163	75	4	Tr	Tr	0	15	3	44	1.7	474	243	1,899	0.08	0.08	0.9	8
Frozen, cooked, drained	1 cup	182	105	5	Tr	Tr	0	24	5	46	1.5	308	64	778	0.13	0.22	1.5	6
Water chestnuts, canned	1 cup	140	70	1	Tr	Tr	0	17	1	6	1.2	165	11	1	0.02	0.03	0.5	2

1 Value not determined.
2 Mineral content varies depending on water source.
3 Blend of aspartame and saccharin; if only sodium saccharin is used, sodium is 75 mg; if only aspartame is used, sodium is 23 mg.
4 With added ascorbic acid.
5 Vitamin A value is largely from beta-carotene used for coloring.
6 Yields 1 qt. of fluid milk when reconstituted according to package directions.
7 With added vitamin A.
8 Carbohydrate content varies widely because of amount of sugar added and amount and solids content of added flavoring. Consult the label if more precise values for carbohydrate and calories are needed.
9 For salted butter; unsalted butter contains 12 mg sodium per stick, 2 mg per tbsp., or 1 mg per pat.
10 Values for vitamin A are year-round average.
11 For salted margarine.
12 Based on average vitamin A content of fortified margarine. Federal specifications for fortified margarine require a minimum of 15,000 IU per pound.
14 Dipped in egg, milk, and breadcrumbs; fried in vegetable shortening.
15 If bones are discarded, value for calcium will be greatly reduced.
16 Dipped in egg, breadcrumbs, and flour; fried in vegetable shortening.
18 Sodium bisulfite used to preserve color; unsulfited product would contain less sodium.
19 Also applies to pasteurized apple cider.
20 Without added ascorbic acid. For value with added ascorbic acid, refer to label.
21 With added ascorbic acid.
22 For white grapefruit; pink grapefruit have about 310 IU or 31 RE.
23 Sodium benzoate and sodium bisulfite added as preservatives.
24 Egg bagels have 44 mg cholesterol and 22 IU or 7 RE vitamin A per bagel.
25 Made with vegetable shortening.
27 Nutrient added.
28 Cooked without salt. If salt is added according to label recommendations, sodium content is 540 mg.
29 For white corn grits. Cooked yellow grits contain 145 IU or 14 RE.
30 Value based on label declaration for added nutrients.
31 For regular and instant cereal. For quick cereal, phosphorus is 102 mg and sodium is 142 mg.
32 Cooked without salt. If salt is added according to label recommendations, sodium content is 390 mg.
33 Cooked without salt. If salt is added according to label recommendations, sodium content is 324 mg.
34 Cooked without salt. If salt is added according to label recommendations, sodium content is 374 mg.
35 Excepting angel food cake, cakes were made from mixes containing vegetable shortening and frostings were made with margarine.
36 Made with vegetable oil.

37 Cake made with vegetable shortening; frosting with margarine.
38 Made with margarine.
39 Crackers made with enriched flour except for rye wafers and whole-wheat wafers.
40 Made with lard.
41 Cashews without salt contain 21 mg sodium per cup or 4 mg per oz.
42 Cashews without salt contain 22 mg sodium per cup or 5 mg per oz.
43 Macadamia nuts without salt contain 9 mg sodium per cup or 2 mg per oz.
44 Mixed nuts without salt contain 3 mg sodium per oz.
45 Peanuts without salt contain 22 mg sodium per cup or 4 mg per oz.
46 Outer layer of fat was removed to within approximately 1/2 inch of the lean. Deposits of fat within the cut were removed.
47 Fried in vegetable shortening.
48 Value varies widely.
49 Contains added sodium ascorbate. If sodium ascorbate is not added, ascorbic acid content is negligible.
51 Crust made with vegetable shortening and enriched flour.
52 Made with corn oil.
53 Fried in vegetable shortening.
54 If sodium ascorbate is added, product contains 11 mg ascorbic acid.
55 Made with enriched flour, margarine, and whole milk.
57 For green varieties; yellow varieties contain 101 IU or 10 RE.
59 For regular pack; special dietary pack contains 3 mg sodium.
60 For green varieties; yellow varieties contain 142 IU or 14 RE.
61 For regular pack; special dietary pack contains 78 mg sodium.
63 For yellow varieties; white varieties contain only a trace of vitamin A.
64 For regular pack; special dietary pack contains 8 mg sodium.
65 For regular pack; special dietary pack contains 6 mg sodium.
66 For regular pack; special dietary pack contains 3 mg sodium.
67 For green peppers; red peppers contain 350 IU or 35 RE.
68 For green peppers; red peppers contain 4,220 IU or 422 RE.
69 For green peppers; red peppers contain 141 mg ascorbic acid.
72 With added salt; if none is added, sodium content is 58 mg.
73 For regular pack; special dietary pack contains 31 mg sodium.
74 With added salt; if none is added, sodium content is 24 mg.
75 With no added salt; if salt is added, sodium content is 2,070 mg.
76 With no added salt; if salt is added, sodium content is 998 mg.
77 With salt added.

Glossary

A

ability. A skill learned through practice. (25)

absorption. The passage of nutrients from the digestive tract into the circulatory system. (3)

acid. A compound that has a pH lower than 7. (9)

acid-base balance. The maintenance of the correct level of acidity of a body fluid. (7)

active packaging. A type of food package that interacts with the food or the atmosphere inside the package. (23)

addiction. A psychological or physical dependence on a drug. (19)

Adequate Intake (AI). A value set for nutrients for which research is too inconclusive to determine an RDA. (4)

adipose tissue. Tissue in which the body stores lipids. (6)

adolescence. The period of life between childhood and adulthood. (11)

advocate. A person who speaks out on behalf of an issue or problem. (24)

aerobic activity. An activity that uses large muscles and is done at a moderate, steady pace for fairly long periods. The heart and lungs are able to meet the muscles' oxygen needs throughout an aerobic activity. (15)

agility. The ability to change body position with speed and control. (15)

alcoholism. An addiction to alcohol. (19)

amenorrhea. An abnormal cessation of menstrual periods. (9)

amino acid. One of the building blocks of protein molecules. (7)

amphetamine. A stimulant drug. (19)

anabolic steroid. An artificial hormone used to build a more muscular body. (19)

anaerobic activity. An activity in which the muscles are using oxygen faster than the heart and lungs can deliver it. (15)

anorexia nervosa. An eating disorder typified by an intense fear of weight gain that leads to self-starvation. (14)

antibody. A protein made by the immune system to defend the body against infection and disease. (7)

antidepressant. A drug that alters the nervous system and relieves depression. (14)

antioxidant. A substance that reacts with free radicals (unstable single oxygen molecules) to protect other substances from harmful effects of the free radicals. (8)

aptitude. A natural talent. (25)

aseptic packaging. A food packaging process that involves packing sterile food in sterile containers within a sterile atmosphere. (2)

assertiveness. A person's boldness to express what he or she thinks and feels in a way that does not offend others. (17)

associate degree. A degree received after graduating from a two-year college program. (25)

atherosclerosis. Hardened and narrowed arteries caused by plaque deposits. (6)

ATP (adenosine triphosphate). The storage form of energy in the body. (3)

B

bachelor's degree. A four-year college degree. (25)

bacteria. Single-celled microorganisms that live in soil, water, and the bodies of plants and animals. (20)

balance. The ability to keep the body in an upright position while standing still or moving. (15) A sense of proportional distribution given to life's roles and responsibilities. (17)

basal metabolic rate (BMR). The rate at which the body uses energy for basal metabolism. (12)

basal metabolism. The amount of energy required to support the operation of all internal body systems except digestion. (12)

base. A compound that has a pH greater than 7. (9)

beriberi. The thiamin deficiency disease, which is characterized by weakness, loss of appetite, irritability, poor arm and leg coordination, and a tingling throughout the body. (8)

bile. A digestive juice produced by the liver to aid fat digestion. (3)

binge eating disorder. An eating disorder that involves repeatedly eating very large amounts of food without a follow-up behavior to prevent weight gain. (14)

bingeing. Uncontrollable eating of huge amounts of food. (14)

bioelectrical impedance. A process that measures body fat by measuring the body's resistance to a low-energy electrical current. (12)

bioengineering. The science of changing the genetic makeup of an organism. (23)

biofeedback. A technique of focusing on involuntary bodily processes, such as breathing and pulse rate, in order to control them. (18)

blood lipid profile. A medical test that measures the amounts of cholesterol, triglycerides, HDL, and LDL in the blood. (6)

body composition. The percentage of different types of tissues in the body, such as fat, muscle, and bone. (12)

body mass index (BMI). A calculation of body weight and height used to define underweight, healthy weight, overweight, and obesity. (12)

botanical. A plant material or part of a plant. (23)

budget. A spending plan that outlines how to use sources of income to meet various fixed and flexible expenses. (21)

buffer. A compound that can counteract an excess of acid or base in a fluid. (7)

bulimia nervosa. An eating disorder that involves uncontrollable eating of huge amounts of food followed by an inappropriate behavior to prevent weight gain. (14)

burnout. A lack of energy and motivation to work toward goals. (17)

C

calorie density. The concentration of energy in a food. (12)

cancer. A disease in which abnormal cells grow out of control. (6)

carbohydrate loading. A technique used by endurance athletes to trick the muscles into storing more glycogen for extra energy. (16)

carbohydrates. One of the six classes of nutrients that includes sugars, starches, and fibers. Carbohydrates are the body's main source of energy. (5)

cardiorespiratory fitness. The body's ability to take in adequate amounts of oxygen and carry it efficiently through the blood to body cells. (15)

cash crop. A crop that can be sold to an exporter. (24)

certification. Special standing within a profession as a result of accomplishing certain requirements. (25)

cholesterol. A white, waxy lipid made by the body that is part of every cell. Cholesterol is also found in foods of animal origin. (6)

chylomicron. A ball of triglycerides thinly coated with cholesterol, phospholipids, and proteins formed to carry absorbed dietary fat to body cells. (6)

chyme. A mixture of gastric juices and food formed in the stomach during digestion. (3)

cirrhosis. A liver disease in which liver cells die, causing the liver to lose its ability to work. (19)

coagulation. The blood clotting process that stops bleeding. (8)

coenzyme. A nonprotein compound (usually a vitamin) that combines with an enzyme to form an active enzyme system. (8)

cofactor. A substance that acts with enzymes to increase enzyme activity. (9)

collagen. A protein substance in the connective tissue that holds cells together. (8)

commodity food. A common, mass-produced item, such as instant dry milk, flour, sugar, or cornmeal. (24)

communication. The sending of a message from one source to another. (17)

comparison shopping. Assessing prices and quality of similar products to choose those that best meet a consumer's needs and price range. (22)

compassion. A deep sense of sadness for human suffering coupled with a strong desire to stop it. (24)

competitive bacteria. Bacteria that prevent the growth of pathogens. (23)

complementary proteins. Two or more incomplete protein sources that can be combined to provide all the essential amino acids. (7)

complete protein. A protein that contains all the essential amino acids. (7)

complex carbohydrate. A polysaccharide. Starch and fiber are complex carbohydrates. (5)

compromise. A solution to a problem that blends ideas from two differing parties. (17)

conflict. Disagreement. (17)

congenital disability. A condition existing from birth that limits a person's ability to use his or her body or mind. (11)

congregate meal. A group meal. (24)

constipation. A condition that occurs when the feces become massed and hard in the large intestine, making expulsion infrequent. (3)

consumer. Someone who buys and uses products and services. (22)

contaminant. An undesirable substance that unintentionally gets into food. (20)

convenience food. A food item that is purchased partially or completely prepared. (21)

coordination. The ability to integrate the use of two or more parts of the body. (15)

coronary heart disease (CHD). Disease of the heart and blood vessels. Atherosclerosis and hypertension are the two most common forms of CHD. (6)

crash diet. A weight-loss plan that provides fewer than 1,200 calories per day. (13)

cretinism. Severe mental retardation and dwarfed physical features of an infant caused by the mother's iodine deficiency during pregnancy. (9)

cross-contamination. The transfer of harmful bacteria from one food to another food. (20)

culture. The beliefs and social customs of a group of people. (2)

D

daily hassles. Minor stressors that produce tension. (18)

Dietary Reference Intakes (DRIs). A set of nutrient reference values that can be used to plan and assess diets for healthy people. (4)

Daily Values. Recommended nutrient intakes, which are based on daily calorie needs, used as references on food labels. (4)

deficiency disease. A sickness caused by a lack of a nutrient. (7)

dehydration. A state in which the body contains a lower than normal amount of body fluids. (10)

denaturation. A change in shape that happens to protein molecules when they are exposed to heat, acids, bases, salts of heavy metals, or alcohol. (7)

dental caries. Tooth decay. (5)

depressant. A drug that decreases the activity of the central nervous system. (19)

designer drug. A lab-created imitation of an illegal drug. (19)

developing nation. A country with a very low economic level of living standards and industrial production. (24)

diabetes mellitus. A lack of or an inability to use the hormone insulin, which results in a buildup of glucose in the bloodstream. (5)

diagnosis. The identification of a disease. (1)

diarrhea. Frequent expulsion of watery feces. (3)

diet. All the foods and beverages a person consumes. (1)

Dietary Guidelines for Americans. A set of seven recommendations developed by the United States Departments of Agriculture and Health and Human Services to help healthy people over age two know what to eat to stay healthy. (4)

dietetic technician. A member of a health care team who works under the guidance of a registered dietitian. (25)

dietetics. The program of study that prepares a person to become a dietitian. (25)

dietitian. A person trained to apply nutrition principles to diet planning for achieving good health. (25)

digestion. The process by which the body breaks down food, and the nutrients in food, into simpler parts for use in growth, repair, and maintenance. (3)

disaccharide. A carbohydrate made up of two sugar units. Sucrose, lactose, and maltose are the disaccharides. (5)

distress. Harmful stress. (18)

diuretic. A substance that increases urine production. (10)

diverticulosis. A disorder in which many abnormal pouches form in the intestinal wall. (3)

DNA fingerprinting. A process that traces the cause of a food poisoning or impurity. (23)

doctoral degree. An advanced degree that requires about three to five years of school beyond a master's degree. (25)

drug. Any substance other than food or water that changes the way the body or mind operates. (19)

drug abuse. The use of a drug for other than medical reasons. (19)

drug misuse. Using a medicine in a way it was not intended to be used. (19)

E

eating disorder. An abnormal eating pattern that endangers physical and mental health. (14)

electronic shopping. A method of buying items over the Internet using a home computer. (22)

employability skill. A competency that individuals need for successfully obtaining and keeping a job. (25)

emulsifier. A substance, such as a phospholipid, that can mix with water and fat. (6)

endurance athlete. An athlete involved in a sport, such as marathon bicycling or distance swimming, that requires sustained muscle efforts for several hours at a time. (16)

energy. The ability to do work. (12)

enriched food. A food that has had vitamins and minerals added back that were lost in the refining process. (8)

entrepreneur. Someone who owns and operates his or her own business (25)

entry-level job. A job that requires few skills and pays minimal salary. (25)

environmental contaminant. A substance released into the air or water by industrial plants. (20)

environmental cue. An event or situation around a person that triggers him or her to eat. (13)

environmental quality. The state of the physical world, including the condition of water, air, and food. (1)

environmental sustainability. The wise use of natural resources to preserve them for later use. (24)

enzyme. A complex protein produced by cells to speed a specific chemical reaction in the body. (3)

epithelial cells. The surface cells that line the outside of the body, cover the eyes, and line the passages of the lungs, intestines, and reproductive tract. (8)

erythrocyte hemolysis. A vitamin E deficiency condition that is sometimes seen in premature babies and is characterized by broken red blood cells, resulting in weakness and listlessness. (8)

essential amino acid. An amino acid that cannot be made by the body and must, therefore, be supplied by the diet. (7)

essential fatty acid. A fatty acid needed by the body for normal growth and development that cannot be made by the body and, therefore, must be supplied by the diet. (6)

Estimated Average Requirement (EAR). A nutrient recommendation estimated to meet the needs of half the healthy people in a group. (4)

ethics. Standards, guidelines, and codes that guide behavior. (25)

ethnic food. A food that is typical of a given racial, national, or religious culture. (2)

extracellular water. The water outside the cells. (10)

F

fad diet.   An eating plan that is popular for a short time because it promises rapid weight loss. (13)

famine.   An extreme scarcity of food for an extended period, perhaps years. (24)

fasting.   Refraining from consuming most or all sources of calories. (13)

fat replacer.   An ingredient used in food products to replace some or all of the fat typically found in those products. (6)

fat-soluble vitamin.   A vitamin, specifically vitamin A, D, E, or K, that dissolves in fats. (8)

fatty acid.   An organic compound made up of a chain of carbon atoms to which hydrogen atoms are attached and having an acid group at one end. (6)

feces.   Solid wastes that result from digestion. (3)

female athlete triad.   A set of three related medical problems—disordered eating, amenorrhea, and osteoporosis—common among female athletes. (14)

fetal alcohol syndrome (FAS).   A set of symptoms that can occur in a newborn whose mother drinks alcohol while pregnant. (11)

fetus.   A developing human from eight weeks after conception until birth. (11)

fiber.   Indigestible polysaccharides that make up the tough, fibrous cell walls of plants. (5)

fight or flight response.   Physical reactions to stress that happen as the body gathers its resources to conquer danger or escape to safety. (18)

flexibility.   The ability to move body joints through a full range of motion. (15)

fluorosis.   A spotty discoloration of teeth caused by high fluoride intake. (9)

food additive.   A substance added to food products to cause desired changes in the products. (22)

food allergy.   A reaction of the immune system to certain proteins found in food. (3)

foodborne illness.   A disease transmitted by food. (20)

food diary.   A record of the kinds and amounts of all foods and beverages consumed for a given time. (4)

food-drug interaction.   A physical or chemical effect a drug has on a food or a food has on a drug. (19)

Food Guide Pyramid.   A research-based visual tool used to help people plan healthful diets. (4)

food norm.   Typical standard or pattern related to food and eating behaviors. (2)

food policy.   A rule or regulation that affects food production, prices, or trade. (24)

food processing.   Any procedure performed on food to prepare it for consumers. (22)

food security.   Always having access to the food needed for a healthy life. (24)

food taboo.   A social custom that prohibits the use of certain edible resources as food. (2)

fortified food.   A food that has one or more nutrients added during processing. (8)

free radical.   A highly reactive, unstable single oxygen molecule, which can generate a harmful chain reaction that can damage tissue. (8)

functional food.   A food or food ingredient that provides health benefits beyond basic nutrition. (23)

G

gallstones.   Small crystals that form from bile in the gallbladder. (3)

gastric juices.   A mixture of hydrochloric acid, digestive enzymes, and mucus produced by the stomach that helps digest food. (3)

gastrointestinal (GI) tract.   A muscular tube leading from the mouth to the anus through which food passes as it is digested. (3)

generic drug.   A drug available under its generic name. (19)

generic product.   An unbranded product, which can be identified by plain, simple packaging. (22)

glucose.   A monosaccharide that circulates in the bloodstream and serves as the body's source of energy. (5)

glycogen.   The body's storage form of glucose (also known as *animal starch*). (5)

goal.   An aim a person strives to reach. (25)

goiter.   An enlargement of the thyroid gland. (9)

GRAS (generally recognized as safe) list. A list prepared by the U.S. Food and Drug Administration of about 700 substances that have proved to be safe to use in food processing. (22)

growth spurt. A period of rapid physical growth. (11)

H

habit. A routine behavior that is often difficult to break. (13)

hallucinogen. A drug that causes the mind to create images that do not really exist. (19)

healthy weight. Describes an adult with a body mass index of 18.5 to 24.9. (12)

heart attack. The death of heart tissue caused by blockage of an artery carrying nutrients and oxygen to that tissue. (6)

heart rate. The number of times the heart beats per minute. (15)

heartburn. A burning pain in the middle of the chest caused by stomach acid flowing back into the esophagus. (3)

hemoglobin. An iron-containing protein that helps red blood cells carry oxygen from the lungs to cells throughout the body and carbon dioxide from body tissues back to the lungs for excretion. (9)

hemorrhage. Uncontrollable bleeding. (24)

herbicide. A plant killer, used primarily to control weeds. (23)

high-density lipoprotein (HDL). A lipoprotein that picks up cholesterol from around the body and transfers it to other lipoproteins for transport back to the liver for removal from the body. (6)

holistic medicine. An approach to health care that focuses on all aspects of patient care—physical, mental, and social. (1)

hormone. A chemical produced in the body and released into the bloodstream to regulate specific body processes. (5)

hunger. A weakened state caused by prolonged lack of food. (24)

hunger myth. A popular misconception about the cause of hunger. (24)

hydrogenation. The process of breaking the double carbon bonds in unsaturated fatty acids and adding hydrogen to make the fatty acid more saturated. (6)

hygiene. Practices that promote good health. (20)

hypertension. Abnormally high blood pressure; an excess force on the walls of the arteries as blood is pumped from the heart. (6)

hypoglycemia. A low blood glucose level. (5)

hypothesis. A suggested answer to a scientific question, which can be tested and verified. (1)

I

illegal drug. A drug that is unlawful to buy or use. (19)

immunity. High resistance to a disease. (23)

impulse buying. Making unplanned purchases. (22)

incomplete protein. A protein that is missing or short in one or more of the essential amino acids. (7)

indigestion. A difficulty in digesting food. (3)

infant. A child in the first year of life. (11)

infrastructure. A system of highways, railroads, waterways, and other public works. (24)

inhalant. A substance that is inhaled for its mind-numbing effects. (19)

insoluble fiber. An indigestible carbohydrate from plants that does not dissolve in water. (5)

insulin. A hormone secreted by the pancreas to regulate blood glucose level. (5)

intracellular water. The water inside body cells. (10)

iron-deficiency anemia. A condition in which the number of red blood cells declines, causing the blood to have a decreased ability to carry oxygen to body tissues. (9)

irradiation. The exposure of food to ionizing energy. (23)

J

job interview. A discussion between a job applicant and a person who is hiring employees. (25)

K

ketone bodies. Compounds formed from fatty acids the nervous system can use for energy when carbohydrates are not available. (12)

ketosis. An abnormal buildup of ketone bodies in the bloodstream. (12)

kilocalorie. The unit used to measure the energy value of food. (3)

kosher food. Foods prepared according to Jewish dietary laws. (2)

kwashiorkor. A protein deficiency disease. (7)

L

lactation. The production of breast milk by a mother's body following the birth of a baby. (11)

lactic acid. A product formed in the muscles as the result of the incomplete breakdown of glucose during anaerobic activity. (16)

lactose intolerance. An inability to digest lactose, the main carbohydrate in milk, due to a lack of the digestive enzyme lactase. (5)

lecithin. A phospholipid made by the liver and found in many foods. (6)

legume. A plant that has a special ability to capture nitrogen from the air and transfer it to protein-rich seeds. (7)

license. A work requirement set by the government. (25)

life-change events. Major stressors, such as death, divorce, and legal problems, that can greatly alter a person's lifestyle. (18)

life cycle. A series of stages through which people pass between birth and death. (11)

life expectancy. The average length of life of people living in the same environment. (1)

lipid. A group of compounds that includes triglycerides (fats and oils), phospholipids (lecithin), and sterols (cholesterol). (6)

lipoprotein. Fat droplets coated by proteins so they can be transported in the bloodstream. (6)

low-birthweight baby. A baby that weighs less than 5½ pounds (2,500 g) at birth. (11)

low-density lipoprotein (LDL). A lipoprotein that carries cholesterol made by the liver through the bloodstream to body cells. (6)

lubricant. A substance that reduces friction between surfaces. (10)

M

macromineral. Mineral required in the diet in an amount of 100 or more milligrams per day. (9)

malnutrition. Poor nutrition usually endured for a long period. (24)

marasmus. A wasting disease caused by a lack of calories and protein. (7)

master's degree. An advance degree that requires about two years of school beyond a bachelor's degree. (25)

mastication. Chewing. (3)

maximum heart rate. The highest speed at which the heart muscle is able to contract. (15)

meal management. Using resources to meet goals related to preparing and serving food. (21)

medicine. A drug used to treat an ailment or improve a disabling condition. (19)

megadose. A concentrated level of a substance many times higher than its natural occurrence in the diet. (23)

menopause. The time in a woman's life when menstruation ends due to a decrease in production of the hormone estrogen. (9)

mental health. The way a person feels about himself or herself, life, and the world. (1)

mentor. A coworker who has years of experience and can help a newer worker with questions and challenges in the workplace. (25)

metabolism. All the chemical changes that occur as cells produce energy and materials needed to sustain life. (3)

micromineral. Mineral required in the diet in an amount of less than 100 milligrams per day. (9)

microorganism. A living being so small it can be seen only under a microscope. (20)

minerals. An inorganic element needed in small amounts as a nutrient to perform various functions in the body. (9)

monosaccharide. A carbohydrate made up of single sugar units. Glucose, fructose, and galactose are the monosaccharides. (5)

monounsaturated fatty acid. A fatty acid that has only one double bond between carbon atoms in a carbon atom chain. (6)

mortality rate. A death rate. (24)

mouth feel. The textural sensation of a food as perceived by the tongue. (23)

muscular endurance. The ability to use a group of muscles over and over without getting tired. (15)

myoglobin. An iron-containing protein that carries oxygen and carbon dioxide in muscle tissue. (9)

N

narcotic. A drug that brings on sleep, relieves pain, or dulls the senses. (19)

national brand. A brand that is distributed and advertised throughout the country by a major company. (22)

negative stress. Stress that can reduce a person's effectiveness by causing him or her to be fearful and perform poorly. (18)

networking. Alerting a wide circle of people about an interest in a job. (25)

night blindness. A condition in which the cells in the eyes adjust slowly to dim light, causing night vision to become poor. (8)

nitrogen balance. A comparison of the nitrogen a person consumes with the nitrogen he or she excretes. (7)

nonessential amino acid. An amino acid that can be synthesized by the body from other amino acids. (7)

nonnutrient supplement. A pill, power, or liquid that claims to promote health but has not been proven to do so. (23)

nonverbal communication. The sending of a message from one source to another without the use of words. (17)

nutrient. A basic component of food that nourishes the body. (1)

nutrient density. A comparison of the nutrients provided by a food with the calories provided by the food. (4)

nutrition. The sum of the processes by which a person takes in and uses food substances. (1)

O

obese. Describes an adult with a body mass index of 30 or more. (12)

olestra. The first calorie-free fat replacer. (23)

omega-3 fatty acids. A certain type of polyunsaturated fatty acids found in fish oils and shown to have a positive effect on heart health. (6)

opiate. A narcotic drug, such as codeine, morphine, opium, or heroin, made from the opium poppy. (19)

optimum health. A state of wellness characterized by peak physical, mental, and social well-being. (1)

organic food. A food produced without the use of synthetic fertilizers, pesticides, or growth hormones. (22)

osmosis. The movement of water across a semipermeable membrane to equalize the concentrations of solution on each side of the membrane. (9)

osteomalacia. A vitamin D deficiency disease in adults that causes the bones to become misshapen. (8)

osteoporosis. A condition in which bones become porous and fragile due to a loss of minerals. (9)

outpatient treatment. Medical care that does not require a hospital stay. (14)

overdose. Taking an unsafe quantity of a drug. (19)

overpopulation. A population growth so rapid that it deteriorates the environment or the quality of life. (24)

over-the-counter (OTC) drug. A legal drug that can be bought without a prescription written by a physician. (19)

overweight. Describes an adult with a body mass index of 25 to 29.9. (12)

P

parasite. An organism that lives off another organism, which is called a host. (20)

peer pressure. The influence people in a person's age and social group have on his or her behavior. (1)

pellagra. The niacin deficiency disease, which is characterized by diarrhea and dermatitis and can lead to dementia and death. (8)

peristalsis. A series of squeezing actions by the muscles in the gastrointestinal tract that helps move food through the tract. (3)

pernicious anemia. A deficiency disease caused by an inability to absorb vitamin B_{12}, which is characterized by fatigue; weakness; a red, painful tongue; and a tingling or burning in the skin. (8)

personality. All the characteristics that make each person unique. (17)

pesticide residue. Chemical pesticide particles left in food after it is prepared for consumption. (20)

pH. A term used to express a substance's acidity or alkalinity as measured on a scale from 0 (extreme acid) to 14 (extreme base). (9)

phospholipids. A class of lipids that have a phosphorus-containing compound in their chemical structures, which allows them to combine with both fat and water to form emulsions. (6)

physical fitness. A state in which all body systems function together efficiently. (15)

physical health. The fitness of the body. (1)

phytochemicals. Health-enhancing nonnutrient compounds in plant foods that are active in the body at the cellular level. (8)

placenta. An organ that forms inside the uterus during pregnancy in which blood vessels from the mother and the fetus are entwined, enabling the transfer of materials carried in the blood. (11)

plaque. A buildup of fatty compounds made up largely of cholesterol that form on the inside walls of arteries. (6)

polysaccharide. A carbohydrate made up of many sugar units that are linked in straight or branched chains. (5)

polyunsaturated fatty acid. A fatty acid that has two or more double bonds between carbon atoms in a carbon atom chain. (6)

portfolio. An organized collection of papers, letters, pictures, and projects that shows what a person has accomplished. (25)

positive stress. Stress that motivates a person to accomplish challenging goals. (18)

posture. The position of the body when standing or sitting. (15)

power. The ability to do maximum work in a short time. (15)

premature baby. A baby born before the 35th week of pregnancy. (11)

premature death. Death that occurs due to lifestyle behaviors that lead to a fatal accident or the formation of an avoidable disease. (1)

prescription drug. A medicine that can only be obtained from a pharmacy with a written order from a doctor. (19)

preventive health care. Preserving health now to prevent poor health later. (25)

problem solving. A process used to answer tough questions and resolve difficult situations. (25)

product recall. The return to the manufacturer of defective or contaminated products. (23)

progressive muscle relaxation. A relaxation technique that involves slowly tensing and then relaxing different groups of muscles. (18)

protein. An energy-yielding nutrient composed of carbon, hydrogen, oxygen, and nitrogen. (7)

protein-energy malnutrition (PEM). A condition caused by a lack of calories and proteins in the diet. (7)

protozoa. Single-celled animals. (20)

provitamin. A compound the body can convert to the active form of a vitamin. (8)

psychoactive drug. A drug that affects the central nervous system. (19)

puberty. The time during which a person develops sexual maturity. (11)

purging. Clearing food from the digestive system. (14)

Q

quality of life. A person's satisfaction with his or her looks, lifestyle, and responses to daily events. (1)

R

rancid. Describes a fat in which the fatty acid molecules have combined with oxygen, causing them to break down, which makes the fat spoil and gives it an unpleasant smell and taste. (6)

reactant. A substance that enters into a chemical reaction and is changed by it. (10)

reaction time. The amount of time it takes to respond to a signal once the signal is received. (15)

Recommended Dietary Allowances (RDAs). Suggested levels of nutrient intake to meet the needs of most healthy people. (4)

reference. The name of a person who will speak highly of an individual's skills and abilities. (25)

refined sugar. A carbohydrate sweetener that is separated from its natural source for use as a food additive. (5)

registered dietitian (RD). The only professional who is qualified to analyze a person's diet and perform diet treatment. (25)

relationship. A connection a person forms with another person. (17)

resting heart rate. The speed at which a person's heart muscle contracts when he or she is sitting quietly. (15)

resume. An outline of a person's job qualifications. (25)

rickets. A deficiency disease in children caused by a lack of vitamin D and characterized by soft, misshapen bones. (8)

risk factor. A characteristic or behavior that influences a person's chance of being injured or getting a disease. (1)

S

sanitation. Maintaining clean conditions to help prevent disease. (20)

satiety. The feeling of fullness a person has after eating food. (5)

saturated fatty acid. A fatty acid that has no double bonds in its chemical structure and, therefore, carries a full load of hydrogen atoms. (6)

scientific method. The process researchers use to find answers to their questions. (1)

scurvy. The vitamin C deficiency disease, characterized by tiredness, weakness, shortness of breath, aching bones and muscles, swollen and bleeding gums, lack of appetite, slow healing of wounds, and tiny bruises on the skin. (8)

secondhand smoking. The inhaling of smoke released into the air when someone else is smoking. (19)

sedentary activity. An activity that requires a lot of sitting. (12)

self-actualization. A person's belief that he or she is doing his or her best to reach full human potential. (17)

self-concept. The idea a person has about himself or herself. (17)

self-esteem. The worth or value a person assigns himself or herself. (17)

self-talk. A person's internal conversations about himself or herself and the situations he or she faces. (18)

service sector. The part of the economy that employs people who provide assistance. (23)

serving size. The amount of a food item customarily eaten at one time. (4)

side effect. A reaction caused by a drug along with its intended reaction. (19)

simple carbohydrate. A monosaccharide or disaccharide. (5)

skinfold test. A test in which a caliper is used to measure the thickness of a fold of skin to estimate how much of the thickness is due to subcutaneous fat. (12)

smokeless tobacco. Tobacco products that are not intended to be smoked, such as chewing tobacco or snuff. (19)

social development. Learning how to get along with others. (17)

social health. The way a person gets along with other people. (1)

soluble fiber. An indigestible carbohydrate from plants that dissolves in water. (5)

solvent. A liquid in which substances can be dissolved. (10)

soul food. Traditional food of the African American ethnic group. (2)

speed. The quickness with which a person is able to complete a motion. (15)

staple food. A mainstay food in the diet. (2)

starch. A polysaccharide that is the storage form of energy in plants. (5)

starvation. The condition that results from a lack of food and water needed to sustain life. (24)

status food. A food that has a social impact on others. (2)

sterols. A class of lipids, including some hormones, vitamin D, and cholesterol, that have complex molecules made up of rings of carbon atoms with attached chains of carbon, hydrogen, and oxygen. (6)

stimulant. A kind of psychoactive drug that speeds up the nervous system. (19)

store brand. A brand that is sold in only specific chains of food stores. (22)

strength. The ability of the muscles to move objects. (15)

stress. The inner agitation a person feels when he or she is exposed to change. (18)

stressor. A source of stress. (18)

stroke. The death of brain tissue caused by blockage of an artery carrying nutrients and oxygen to that tissue. (6)

stunted. Having below-average height. (24)

subcutaneous fat. Fat that lies underneath the skin. (12)

sugars. A collective term used to refer to all the monosaccharides and disaccharides. (5)

supplement. A concentrated source of a nutrient, usually in pill, liquid, or powder form. (5)

support system. A group of people who can provide a person with physical help and emotional comfort. (18)

T

target heart rate zone. The range of heartbeats per minute at which the heart muscle receives the best workout; 60 to 90 percent of maximum heart rate. (15)

teamwork. Effort of two or more people toward a common goal. (17)

technology. The application of a certain body of knowledge. (2)

theory. A principle that tries to explain something that happens in nature. (1)

thermic effect of food. The energy required to complete the processes of digestion, absorption, and metabolism. (12)

thyroxine. A hormone produced by the thyroid gland that helps control metabolism. (9)

toddler. A child between one and three years of age. (11)

tolerance. The ability of the body and mind to become less responsive to a drug. (19)

toxicity. A poisonous condition. (8)

toxin. Poison. (20)

trans-fatty acid. A fatty acid with an odd molecular shape that forms when oils are partially hydrogenated. (6)

trend. A general pattern or direction. (23)

triglycerides. The major type of fat found in foods and in the body. Triglycerides consist of three fatty acids attached to glycerol. (6)

trimester. A span of about 13 to 14 weeks that represents one-third of the pregnancy period in humans. (11)

U

ulcer. An open sore in the lining of the stomach or small intestine. (3)

undernutrition. Eating too little food to maintain healthy body weight and normal activity levels. (24)

underweight. Describes an adult with a body mass index below 18.5. (12)

unit price. A product's cost per standard unit of weight or volume. (22)

United Nations. The organization formed by the nations of the world to promote international peace and security. (24)

unsaturated fatty acid. A fatty acid that has at least one double bond between two carbon atoms in a carbon atom chain and, therefore, is missing at least two hydrogen atoms. (6)

Upper Tolerable Intake Level (UL). The maximum level at which a nutrient is unlikely to cause harm to most people. (4)

V

vaccine. A weakened strain of a disease-causing organism. (23)

value. A belief or attitude that is important to someone. (2)

vegetarianism. The practice of eating a diet consisting entirely or largely of plant foods. (7)

verbal communication. The sending of a message from one source to another through the use of words. (17)

very low-density lipoprotein (VLDL). A lipoprotein that carries triglycerides and cholesterol made by the liver through the bloodstream to body cells. (6)

villi. Tiny, fingerlike projections that cover the wall of the small intestine. (3)

virus. A disease-causing agent that is the smallest type of life-form. (20)

vitamin. An organic compound needed in tiny amounts as a nutrient to regulate body processes. (8)

W

wasted. Having severe weight loss due to progressive destruction of body tissue. (24)

water intoxication. A rare condition caused by drinking too much water and consuming too few electrolytes. (10)

water-soluble vitamin. A vitamin, specifically vitamin C or one of the B-complex vitamins, that dissolves in water. (8)

weight cycling. A lifelong pattern of weight gain and loss. (13)

weight management. Attaining healthy weight and keeping it throughout life. (13)

wellness. The state of being in good health. (1)

withdrawal. Symptoms experienced by a person who stops taking a drug to which he or she is addicted. (19)

Index